THE SPIRIT IN AROMATHERAPY

of related interest

Essential Oils
A Handbook for Aromatherapy Practice
2nd edition
Jennifer Peace Rhind
ISBN 978 1 84819 089 4
eISBN 978 0 85701 072 8

Fragrance and Wellbeing
Plant Aromatics and Their Influence
on the Psyche
Jennifer Peace Rhind
ISBN 978 1 84819 090 0
eISBN 978 0 85701 073 5

Listening to Scent
An Olfactory Journey with
Aromatic Plants and their Extracts
Jennifer Peace Rhind
ISBN 978 1 84819 125 9
eISBN 978 0 85701 171 8

A Sensory Journey
Meditations on Scent for Wellbeing
Jennifer Peace Rhind
Card Set
ISBN 978 1 84819 153 2
eISBN 978 0 85701 175 6

Mudras of India
A Comprehensive Guide to the Hand
Gestures of Yoga and Indian Dance
Cain Carroll and Revital Carroll
Foreword by Dr David Frawley
ISBN 978 1 84819 109 9
eISBN 978 0 85701 067 4

THE SPIRIT IN AROMATHERAPY

Working with Intuition

GILL FARRER-HALLS

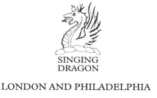

SINGING
DRAGON

LONDON AND PHILADELPHIA

First published in 2014
by Singing Dragon
an imprint of Jessica Kingsley Publishers
73 Collier Street
London N1 9BE, UK
and
400 Market Street, Suite 400
Philadelphia, PA 19106, USA

www.singingdragon.com

Front cover image source: John F. B. Miles (www.tibetanart.com)

Library of Congress Cataloging in Publication Data
Farrer-Halls, Gill, author.
  The spirit in aromatherapy : working with intuition / Gill Farrer-Halls.
    pages cm
  Includes bibliographical references and index.
  ISBN 978-1-84819-209-6 (alk. paper)
  1. Aromatherapy. I. Title.
  RM666.A68F37 2014
  615.3'219--dc23
                                        2014004228

British Library Cataloguing in Publication Data
A CIP catalogue record for this book is available from the British Library

ISBN 978 1 84819 209 6
eISBN 978 0 85701 159 6

Printed and bound in Great Britain

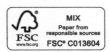

CONTENTS

ACKNOWLEDGEMENTS

I offer my heartfelt thanks to the many people who have enriched my understanding and practice of aromatherapy. Along the way I learned something of value from you all: at the beginning of the journey from my fellow students and teachers, then friends, colleagues and clients and my own students. I continue to read and study books, both old and new, which helps remind me that there is always more to learn about the art of aromatherapy. I also respectfully thank my spiritual teachers, whose kindness and wisdom is immeasurable.

Particular thanks are due to my dear friend and fellow aromatherapist, Ueli Morgenthaler, for his original suggestions about fragrant language, which inspired me to develop my own ideas into a coherent thesis for this book. And finally I offer my deep gratitude to Robert Beer for supplying the cover image from the collection of John F. B. Miles's work, and for his unwavering support and love during the writing of this book.

Introduction

A great deal has already been written about aromatherapy, and between all of the many books, the basic principles of our subject are comprehensively covered. In addition, the professional practitioner has already studied, trained and qualified and, through working with clients, has subsequently gained a great deal of invaluable 'hands-on' experience of all aspects of aromatherapy. The question arises of whether, as professional aromatherapist or keen amateur, we really need another book on aromatherapy at all. The publication in 2013 (by Singing Dragon, also the publisher of this title) of the recently updated version of Jennifer Peace Rhind's *Essential Oils: A Handbook for Aromatherapy Practice* is a triumph. This excellent book is comprehensive, thorough and reflects years, even decades, of research; it will be hard to surpass.

However, what follows is not another formal textbook outlining some of the different aspects of aromatherapy.

Instead I have tried to write something more personal and unusual, maybe from some perspectives even a little quirky. This book explores the intuitive approach to aromatherapy. Although intuition and meditation are not unfamiliar concepts to many aromatherapists, and have been written about to some extent in other aromatherapy titles, this book provides an in-depth discussion of how we can develop and then use intuition to benefit our clients and ourselves. It will, it is hoped, prove useful to the experienced professional because it seeks to go far beyond the basic skills taught on training courses and what has already been written about in many of the aromatherapy books available. And I suggest there is always more we can learn about the art of aromatherapy.

We all have individual strengths and specialist areas within our subject; my own lie in learning through play, experimentation and, above all, meditation and intuition. I consider myself fortunate that my teacher was Patricia Davis at the London School of Aromatherapy, and my class was the last one that she taught. Her approach resonated with me as we shared an interest in Buddhism and meditation, which influenced the teaching style and content of the course. Such a spiritual approach emphasised the principles of holism and synergy and particularly encouraged deep inner reflection and developing intuition around both the essential oils and each client's individual needs. As someone who has maintained a daily practice for nearly thirty years and done many retreats, meditation is integral to my whole life. Thus my understanding, philosophy and practice of aromatherapy are deeply informed by my experience of meditation and Buddhism.

Inevitably the qualities of calm, focus and intuitive insight brought about by meditating regularly over a long period of time have influenced my personal practice of aromatherapy. This inner awareness – or as a wonderful Tibetan Buddhist teacher called Lama Yeshe described it, inner wisdom – strengthens and reinforces intuition. Intuition in aromatherapy may be regarded as lacking credibility from some perspectives and is perhaps sometimes dismissed as superficial, uneducated or even simply wacky. However, when intuition arises in someone who has trained and thoroughly learned the 'outer' theory of aromatherapy, then I would argue that this 'inner' sense complements such knowledge. Or, as Lama Yeshe used to frequently say, 'Trust your inner wisdom dear.'

Thus I believe there is a place on the professional aromatherapist's bookshelf for a new title that offers an approach to aromatherapy based on intuitive awareness and meditative insight. *The Spirit in Aromatherapy: Working with Intuition* has been written with professional aromatherapists in mind, especially those who wish to develop further their intuitive skills to enhance their practice of aromatherapy. I think the book will also appeal to anyone who would like to explore a spiritual and intuitive approach to using essential oils.

Practising professional aromatherapists believe – and rightly so – that they know enough about aromatherapy already to work effectively with their clients. So this book aims to build upon, develop and extend existing skills, rather than reiterating what the competent aromatherapist already knows. In this way I believe the purpose of the book is for people to perhaps be able to learn to see things in a different way. As Hamlet reminded his friend: 'There are more things in heaven and earth, Horatio, Than are dreamt of in your philosophy' (*Hamlet*, Act 1, Sc. 5, l. 166–167). In other words, it is always useful to keep an open mind to alternative ways of working. I hope the reader may learn some new skills and techniques and a different approach to aromatherapy through developing their intuition and applying meditative calm and inner wisdom in their work.

The culture and philosophy of contemporary aromatherapy

Since I qualified as an aromatherapist about twenty-five years ago, there have been, of course, several significant changes within the culture of aromatherapy. As a practitioner, a teacher and examiner, and researching the subject as an author, I have witnessed changes not only in the theory and practice of aromatherapy, but also in the general perception of aromatherapy from clients and the general public. In the early days of my aromatherapy career when meeting new people and being asked the usual question, 'What do you do?' the reply to my answer was often, 'Aroma-what?' Nowadays it appears almost everyone is familiar with the terms 'aromatherapy' and 'aromatherapist' and has some idea of what aromatherapy involves.

One of the delights of aromatherapy is that there is a diversity of different approaches. Such diversity encourages discussion and debate, and we can learn a lot from those whose knowledge, opinions and understanding of aromatherapy differs from our own philosophy. The idea that one qualified, experienced aromatherapist's views are better than another's, or that one of us is right and the other wrong, is not only arrogant but also limiting. Although, quite understandably, we each believe that our own individual approach to aromatherapy is best, by remaining open to hearing others' views we may discover limitations, or the lack of something, in our own philosophy. There is always more we can learn about aromatherapy as the theory and practice, and we as aromatherapists, evolve and progress continuously.

So it was with interest that I observed the development of the scientific approach to aromatherapy over the last couple of decades, even though this differs from my own philosophy. Deepening the understanding of the chemistry underpinning essential oils, together with embracing the scientific methodology of rigorous clinical trials and studies, has been necessary not only to enrich our understanding of aromatherapy and therefore to be better practitioners, but also to counter criticism from the scientific and medical worlds that our healing practice lacked empirically verifiable evidence of efficacy. The rise of the scientific approach in aromatherapy has, directly and indirectly, facilitated aromatherapists to be able to work in the National Health Service (NHS), in hospitals and in palliative care and to be accorded respect as professionals in their work. A sound scientific basis may also help the aromatherapy world deal better with the potential introduction of regulation, or restriction of use, of essential oils from national and international legislative organisations.

For aromatherapy to be truly holistic, all approaches need to be considered and evaluated and then included when felt to be appropriate. New ways of understanding and practising aromatherapy have also developed alongside the scientific and intuitive, and it is heartening to see aromatherapists integrating into their practice aspects of Ayurveda, Chinese Five Elements, chakras and meridians, along with different styles and advanced techniques of massage and bodywork. Today aromatherapists may also work with crystals, flower remedies, colour healing or astrology. New essential oils are discovered and introduced into aromatherapy, and an ever-developing range of base oils are increasingly available, as well as the incorporation of hydrosols into aromatherapy practice.

Alongside all these new developments, aromatherapy has also spread around the world. As aromatherapy is introduced into new countries and cultures, it is informed by the traditions and indigenous healing plants it encounters. I had the great pleasure of working as a teacher and examiner in Japan for a decade, visiting twice a year for two to three weeks each time. While there I learned, among other customs, that while it is common practice for the British aromatherapist to use 3 per cent essential oils in base oil for full-body massage and perhaps 2 per cent for facial massage, in Japan often they find these dilutions too strong and prefer respectively 2 per cent and 1 per cent. In Tokyo I first encountered yuzu (*citrus medicus junos*, *citrus ichangensis × citrus reticulata var. austera*), an indigenous healing plant of Japan; this delightful citrus essential oil is now available and used in British aromatherapy. This is just two of many such examples of how aromatherapy has developed over time and around the world. No doubt, in the years to come aromatherapy will continue to evolve and innovate in exciting and currently unimaginable ways.

In this book I offer a personal, intuitive and meditative approach to deepening our insight into, and understanding and appreciation of, essential oils, their selection and blending, and bodywork. This is not a way of working that I consciously chose, but simply an extension of how I already exist in the world into the realm of aromatherapy. It's been an amazing journey and I'm delighted to have the opportunity here to share with others the best of what I have learned along the way.

CHAPTER 1

A Fragrant Language

In this chapter we will explore how developing a personalised fragrant language around individual essential oils and blends can help us to know them in more depth. We often take for granted the descriptions we are taught and have read of how an essential oil or a blend smells. For instance, when we read or hear about lavender being described as having a sweet, floral, herbaceous, fresh top note with a balsamic woody undertone we don't tend to question whether this is actually our experience of smelling lavender or not. However, personally when I smell lavender, for example, I don't find the fragrance especially sweet. I find that words such as 'soft' and 'gentle', 'clean' and 'calm' have much more personal resonance for me.

By investigating how we each individually respond to the essential oils and blends we use, we can begin to develop our own personal fragrant language. Creating a personalised vocabulary in this way can help us deepen our appreciation and understanding of essential oils, how they may affect our clients and how we can create blends in a different, perhaps more personally authentic, way. When we create our own fragrant vocabulary it can be said that we have named our feelings about and experience of the fragrance of essential oils and thereby own the language. These descriptions then have much more resonance for us.

Language has considerable power and influence over how we interpret and function in our lives and in the wider world. For instance, the familiar Biblical phrase 'In the beginning was the Word' gives us an idea of the essential primacy for humans of language. Another, this time fragrant, example is the name of the commercial perfume Samsara. All Buddhists and Hindus, and many others, know that this is not a particularly desirable name for a perfume as the word means 'trapped in the cycle of birth, death and rebirth'. But the word sounds exotic to the person, perhaps living in the West, who does not know its meaning. No doubt this is the reason why the perfume company's marketing department decided to use it, although they should perhaps have checked the etymology of the word more carefully before selecting it. The name will have only a limited appeal; anyone who knows the meaning of the word 'samsara' will find the perfume name amusing or ridiculous and therefore unenticing. Thus we can see that there is a lot in a name, and also in the whole vocabulary and use of language to describe the perfume of essential oils.

Language is the instrument of theory. Addressing the question I raised earlier in the introduction of whether yet another book on aromatherapy may be desirable, one of the concerns I did not discuss there was the issue of how to make the theory of aromatherapy more directly relevant to the practice. Although we definitely need to study theoretical information about our subject and learn and understand it in order to be as well informed as we possibly can, aromatherapy is a practical discipline so inevitably any book is limited. We also learn experientially – 'on the job' – in our aromatherapy practice and crucially by playing and experimenting with individual oils and blends well beyond our student years until this playful trying out of essential oils becomes an integral part of our lives. In this spirit I believe the ongoing process of developing our own fragrant vocabulary will facilitate creating a bridge between the language of aromatherapy theory and its practice.

How to develop a personal fragrant language
Take an essential oil you know well, like I did with lavender above. Smell and appreciate the perfume, while you read all the descriptions of it in the various books on your aromatherapy bookshelf. Then smell the fragrance of the essential oil again, this time with pen and paper to hand. Begin to scribble down words and phrases as they arise in your mind, focusing on those with personal meaning and resonance for you, and that you

feel describe the fragrance for you, even if tangentially or bizarrely. Your own words may be some of the same words on the pages in front of you, but also observe new words as they surface in your mind that you feel describe the fragrance. When your mind goes blank, smell the oil again and remind yourself of its perfume. Then repeat the experiment several times over the days and weeks after your first attempt. Create a written record with space to add new words and phrases as they arise, and then choose another oil to begin working with.

After you have worked with ten or perhaps twenty different oils, try returning to your first one. This time see if you can develop your fragrant language further and deeper. As language becomes more complex it becomes more evocative, so, for example, the figurative language of similes and metaphors that work with comparison may describe something in more depth and breadth than individual words do. For instance, to my personal list of words that I use to describe lavender I may add, 'laundry hanging on the washing line on a windy spring morning', 'walking through a meadow after rain', 'resting on the bottom of the ocean', 'hazy purple dreamtime' and 'perfumed like a summer evening'.

Try to avoid clichés unless they have personal meaning for you. For instance, in aromatherapy literature we are often told that lavender may be associated with our grannies, as that generation of women often used lavender water as a simple eau de toilette and lavender sachets in the wardrobe to keep clothes fresh. However, if you don't have a personal memory of your granny using lavender, then you will be trying to use someone else's memories, words and associations to describe the perfume of lavender and so this will have much less effect than an original, personal memory or evocation.

Once you have created an index of personal descriptions of the perfumes of essential oils you may notice how your memory and recall of individual oils has changed. When you bring to mind a particular essential oil, what will likely surface first in your mind are the words and phrases you have created for yourself, rather than the usual descriptions. In this way your personal fragrant language may add another dimension to how you choose to use and blend oils, both for your own use and for clients. The list of words below offers some suggestions to help you begin to develop your own fragrant vocabulary.

Words commonly used to describe fragrance

A: alluring, amber, animalistic, anise-like, aromatic

B: balancing, balsamic, bitter, bittersweet, bright

C: calming, camphoraceous, chypre, citrus, clarifying, clean, clear, clove-like, comforting, confident, cosseting

D: delicate, dry

E: earthy, energetic, enlightening, enlivening, erotic, euphoric, evocative, exhilarating, exotic

F: feminine, fiery, floral, fortifying, fresh, fruity

G: gentle, grassy, green

H: harmonious, hay-like, heady, heavy, herbaceous, herbal, honeyed, hypnotic

I: incense-like, intense, invigorating, inviting

L: leafy, lemon, light, lingering, liquorice-like, lively, loud, luxurious

M: masculine, medicinal, mellow, minty, mossy, musky, mysterious

N: narcotic, nutty

O: opulent, oriental

P: passionate, peaceful, penetrating, peppery, persistent, pervasive, powerful, profound, provocative, pungent

R: radiant, resinous, responsive, rich, rosy

S: sedative, seductive, sensual, sensuous, sharp, smoky, soft, soothing, sour, spicy, spiritual, sporty, stimulating, strengthening, strident, sultry, sweet

T: tangy, tar-like, tea-like, tenacious, terpenic, turpentine-like

U: uplifting

V: vanilla, vibrant, violet-like, vivacious, volatile, voluptuous

W: warm, woody

Y: young

Observe that these words come from different realms of perception, association and classification. Unsurprisingly, many come from nature, such as 'earthy', 'woody', 'rosy', 'minty' and 'leafy'. From cooking, with its associated tastes and smells, we have 'peppery', 'lemon', 'herbal', 'bitter', 'sweet', 'honeyed', 'nutty', etc. The feel on our skin and senses brings 'soft', 'hot', 'gentle', 'vibrant', 'sensuous', etc. The world of perfumery gives us 'chypre', 'classic', 'floral', 'oriental', etc. There are, of course, more words that you can add to this list and also other categories. For instance, some people find a strong association with colours when they smell essential oils, and if this works for you it can be useful too. Lavender and purple or mauve, and lemon or bergamot and yellow, are obvious examples, but you may find other, perhaps deeply personal, examples, too. Try to come up with some other words and distinguish other realms for yourself, as certain words may fit into several categorisations; what's important is that the words are meaningful to you personally.

Characterology

Another approach that draws on the use of fragrant language is the work of Philippe Mailhebiau in his book *Portraits in Oils: The Personality of Aromatherapy Oils and Their Link with Human Temperaments* (1995).

Mailhebiau used the term 'characterology' to describe essential oils in terms of personality, with character traits similar to humans. Like Marguerite Maury, the well-known pioneer in aromatherapy, he believed that an individualistic therapeutic method facilitated a deeply personal way to select essential oils to treat a client. He wrote of how this broadened the scope of aromatherapy beyond the physiochemical action of essential oils alone by also using the psychosensory effect of the oils on individuals for whom the chosen oils shared a similar temperament. He believed working with essential oils in this creative and expansive way would stimulate personal growth, something I have found to be true in my own journey of exploring essential oils.

In the monographs of his interesting (and to the modern aromatherapist, sometimes unpredictable and surprising) selection of essential oils he trawls myth and legend, and poetry and literature to uncover archetypal traits and the personality or character of individual oils. His book contains many riches and treasures, and I have browsed through it for inspiration whenever I have felt stuck in my understanding of an essential oil or felt myself to be lacking intuition around creating a blend. In particular, Mailhebiau's inclusion of snippets of poetry, legends and literature can help expand considerably our fragrant language and facilitate finding our own unique way of describing the perfume of essential oils.

Chemistry and smell

To begin with a word and then delve into the areas of your mind, such as the limbic system, for a smell to match the word is unusual in daily life. The normal way we operate is to smell something first, assess it and then act according to the information. For instance, we may smell a food item, notice that it smells bad, realise it has gone off or turned rancid, know that it would be a mistake to eat the food as it would likely make us ill and decide to throw it away.

Yet when we study aromatherapy theory we often read descriptions of how an essential oil is supposed to smell before we have actually opened a bottle and sniffed the contents. Operating this way round makes it harder to memorise and retain the information; our brain struggles to fully integrate the information given. We also don't fully appreciate the descriptions of how an essential oil smells until we have actually used that oil in massage blends, in the bath, in a burner and so forth.

However, when we learn by playing and experimenting with individual oils, trying out blends and different proportions in our mixtures we have 'learned by smelling'. We tend to remember with much greater ease the individual fragrances of oils and how they combine in blends, as well as what works and what doesn't. In this way we learn to trust our experiential work and also learn from our own and our clients' responses to individual oils and blends.

In contrast, we may strive to remember all the constituents and properties of essential oils when we read about and study them, unless we can link the theory to the actual physical manifestations of the oils. One of the difficulties we may have with remembering the different chemical constituents of essential oils – unless we are trained in chemistry – is the unfamiliarity of the names. However, it is worth noting that it is the constituents that usually give essential oils their individual aromas. This means that with practice and over time we can learn to recognise each group of constituents by noticing a similarity in their fragrance.

Even if a chemical constituent is only present in small quantities it may still sometimes dominate the smell of an essential oil. All the different constituents blend into the overall fragrance of an oil, but by comparing the aromas of two essential oils from the same family of constituent – for example, esters – we can learn to distinguish what an ester smells like. Esters tend to have a sweet, fruity aroma that most people find pleasant, so they are a good place to begin. By selecting two – or more – essential oils that have a high ester content and comparing their fragrances, you may be able to learn to recognise the typical ester smell. Exercises such as this may help you remember better the names of the constituents of essential oils.

Once we have learned how to pick out the different components of an essential oil from its fragrance, if we smell an oil we are unfamiliar with we can take a guess at what the major components of it may be and then we can also guess what that oil may be useful for. It has been suggested that this skill may form part of our intuitive understanding of essential oils. This idea offers an exciting link between chemistry and intuition, and may contribute to how we formulate a blend holistically.

Beyond words

Developing a fragrant language is about more than just discovering words and vocabulary to describe the fragrance of essential oils for us personally. Drawing from Mailhebiau's idea of essential oils having a character and traits, we can try working out some characterologies of oils for ourselves that are personally meaningful. Another excellent book to help us discover character traits of essential oils is Robert Tisserand's *The Art of Aromatherapy* (1997). In his studies of individual oils he offers suggestions on whether a particular oil is yin/feminine or yang/masculine, and thus whether it is hot or cool, dry or moist, dark or light, active or passive and also its planetary ruler (and thus we can also perhaps deduce some information from the relevant astrological signs).

Although we use language in creating a character study of essential oils, such an anthropomorphic exercise also takes us into the realms of creative imagination and feeling, thereby adding yet another dimension to our understanding of essential oils and their fragrances. Remember it's important to smell the oil you are trying to describe as you write your character description; you need to combine your sense of smell and the feelings the fragrance evokes within you with your creative imagination, archetypal images and fantasy.

To continue with the example of lavender I have used throughout this chapter, here is a brief character study that evokes this ubiquitous and wonderful essential oil for me.

> Lavender is a woman on the cusp of becoming old, but with an ageless demeanour. She is soft and quiet, and serene and patient; when I am troubled or behave like an agitated child her soothing maternal qualities are calming, helping to ameliorate stress and grief. She embodies tranquillity, like the cool freshness of a mountain stream and offers protection from anger, pain and hostility. Moving in an elegant and gracious way, the gift of healing radiates from her hands and heart; she promotes restful sleep and inner peace. She bestows a gaze of love and compassion upon all whom she encounters. The essence of her being is sacred and spiritual; she is Tara and Demeter, and embodies the spirit of the mother goddess.

This character study may evoke lavender for you and be a good starting point for you to devise your own version. However, if it doesn't work for you then try to find your own way to describe the archetypal qualities of lavender in a characterisation that does evoke the fragrance and quality of the essential oil for you.

What is the purpose of fragrant language and characterology?

No doubt the approach described in this chapter to deepening our understanding of essential oils may seem a little bizarre to some readers, but I hope all of you find something of value in the ideas discussed and the suggested exercises. I believe this playful but practical approach helps us find ways to choose and blend essential oils using our intuition. This can be described as doing 'inner work' to learn about essential oils alongside the 'outer work' of reading and studying. The next chapter will further discuss how we work with intuition and essential oils in this way.

CHAPTER 2

Intuition

For a blend of essential oils to be truly holistic we need the outer knowledge of chemistry and theory of essential oils to work together with the inner wisdom of intuition and experience gained from practice in the creation of a mixture. The individual essential oils also need to come together to create a synergy – to have both therapeutic and aesthetic value in each treatment and to harmonise the physical, mental, emotional, psychological and spiritual aspects of the client. In this way we seek to create a perfect harmony with our blends.

We spend years learning about aromatherapy, reinforcing our knowledge of essential oils through further study and experience of blending for clients. All this learned and experiential knowledge and intuitive knowing then has to come together in the therapy room during a brief consultation with a client, followed by an even briefer few minutes to create a blend. It is often difficult to unite this mass of information into a coherent whole that makes sense of the individual client and what she is presenting with at that time. In this scenario, to go deeper than an initial assessment of the client's requirements and move beyond a reliance on oils and blends we know work well can represent quite a challenge.

Client versus symptoms

So, how can we develop further and deepen our blending skills? In trying to do the best for our client it is easy to slip into a pattern in which we give primacy to the symptoms the client presents with rather than the actual human being sitting in front of us – even if we investigate the causes of their symptoms. I have noticed too that sometimes in continuing professional development (CPD) workshops that include a massage component, students who are experienced aromatherapists may sometimes show a little lack of empathy with the person they are massaging. It's easy to unconsciously slip into the mind-set – and indeed, the hands-on experience – of 'Oh, it's just another body,' although of course this would never be a conscious thought. But the repetition of seeing clients, day after day, year after year can lead to losing a little of that 'in the moment' caring approach to each individual we are so conscious of and try so hard to maintain when we first start working professionally.

Such a mind-set equally affects how we create blends. It's all too easy to assess a client's symptoms during the consultation, recall that we have had success with certain oils and blends for these issues and simply repeat the same old formulas. Developing our intuitive skills can help redress slipping into these overfamiliar patterns of massage and blending and reinforce a client-based attitude.

What is intuition?

The word 'intuition' comes from the Latin verb *intueri*, which translates as 'to look inside' or 'to contemplate'. Thus intuition is often considered to be a kind of inner perception or understanding – the ability to acquire knowledge by responding to unconscious cues without inference or the use of conscious reason. There are many other definitions, such as that intuition is a sensing beyond conscious understanding, or a gut feeling located somatically in the body rather than the mind. Intuition is the perception of the unconscious stimulated by a heightened observation that goes far beyond surface reality. Intuition is an implicit understanding attained without conscious reasoning, but that draws upon previous learning. Intuition is a deep intelligence rooted below the level of consciousness; it arrives in a flash of inspiration often referred to as the Aha! moment. Intuition is a comprehensive inner knowing, which draws from previous practical experience and theoretical knowledge.

However we choose to define it, intuition offers us views, opinions, understanding, information, judgements and beliefs that we cannot empirically verify, nor can we explain rationally how we acquired such insights. Throughout the ages intuition has intrigued thinkers from various disciplines, especially in the religious, esoteric and spiritual domains, where it is often considered a mystical experience, and in the more scientific subjects of psychology and neuropsychology. Along with artistic and creative ability, intuition is commonly believed to be a right-brain activity, while factual, logical analysis and reasoning are considered left-brain activities.

However, as some scientists have suggested that intuition is associated with innovation in scientific discovery, it seems that intuition may offer a bridge between how the two different sides of the brain function. This is demonstrated by the classic tale of the scientist Kekulé, who said that he had discovered the ring shape of the benzene molecule after having a reverie or daydream of a snake seizing its own tail. This ancient archetypal symbol, known as the ouroborus, came to him intuitively in a vision – but only after many years of studying the nature of carbon–carbon bonds. Thus it seems that the theory of science and years of 'outer learning' may well work together harmoniously with intuition to prompt the unconscious to bring forth a universal symbol (or other such intuitive insight), which then enriches our understanding of phenomena and helps make new discoveries.

Intuition and psychology

In Jungian psychology, Carl Jung defined intuition as 'perception via the unconscious', to mean using our underlying sense perception as a starting point or catalyst to bring forth ideas, images, possibilities and even ways out of blocked situations, by an unconscious process. Jung said that a person in whom intuition was dominant, a so-called intuitive type, acted not on the basis of rational judgement but relied on the sheer intensity of their perception. In everyday life this would likely manifest as a preponderance to react to situations intuitively, but to have some recourse to rational thought as well. Very few people are actually clear-cut 'black and white' as the theory may suggest.

Psychology also posits the phrase 'empathic accuracy' as an alternative way of describing intuition. This refers to how accurately one person, the perceiver, can infer the thoughts and feelings of another person, the target. Similar to the phrase 'accurate empathy' coined by the psychologist Carl Rogers, empathic accuracy is an important aspect of what the psychologist William Ickes has called 'everyday mind reading'. There is an obvious link here with aromatherapy. In an aromatherapy treatment – both in the consultation and the actual massage – we deliberately evoke within ourselves empathy with our client to better understand, even 'feel with' the client, their symptoms and their issues. In this way we could be said to have 'read' the client and gained useful information to help enhance their treatment.

The reliability of intuition depends somewhat upon past knowledge and experience. Thus an aromatherapist who has extensive experience of dealing with clients will usually tend to have better instincts and intuition in treating clients than a relative beginner. However, experience does not always guarantee accurate intuition. Although the chances of it being more reliable are greater, a recently qualified practitioner with highly developed intuitive skills can be just as, if not more, effective.

Children tend to be closely in touch with their intuition, and it is natural for them to behave intuitively in all aspects of daily life. It is only when we reach an age at which we become conditioned or socialised into behaviour acceptable to a society that tends not to value, or even much use, intuition that some people lose their intuitive skills. Interestingly, it is claimed that anyone has the potential to develop intuition if that outcome is desired strongly enough, regardless of how powerful or weak a person's innate intuitive abilities may be. In light of the above comments, I suggest that this potential is a 'refinding' of intuition rather than a case of developing intuitive skills for the first time.

Once we have developed, or refound, our innate intuition we can then make appropriate decisions quickly, but still can rarely identify a conscious rationale. For instance, during an aromatherapy consultation we can read nonverbal facial cues and body language and acquire information in this way, before the client tells us what we have already discovered or deduced for ourselves. This understanding of nonverbal communication is central to how intuition operates, and so we can observe clients and immediately 'know' some of what they require from their treatment. Even if we are unable to articulate why or how we know this information, or what prompted the knowledge to surface in consciousness, we can still act upon it. When this occurs we can intimate that intuition is working as a preconscious or unconscious process. Thus as an 'inner knowing' rooted in experience, intuition is invaluable when assessing clients and what they want and need from an aromatherapy treatment. This intuitive understanding of the client and their needs leads naturally to intuitive selection and blending of essential oils.

Intuition in the spiritual domain

As mentioned earlier, intuition may be considered to be an integral part of the spiritual experience within many different religious and esoteric philosophies. In some traditions intuition is associated with the concepts of transcendence and spirit – a going beyond oneself to a higher realm. In other traditions, as well as within the ideas of Jung, intuition is regarded to be transformative and is considered alongside individuation – the striving to find 'wholeness' within oneself or to be united with God or another spiritual source. Intuition tends to arise as a flash of illumination – the Aha! moment – that can be seen as an intervention, or a gift, from divine providence, perhaps to stimulate the evolution of consciousness and spiritual insight. Such illumination offers a link between earthly knowledge or insight derived from religious practice and the higher spiritual planes.

There is a common assumption and acceptance that intuition cannot be judged or interpreted by logical reasoning, nor by empirically verifiable scientific criteria, but this in no way detracts from the validity of the spiritual intuitive experience. In fact, in some spiritual and esoteric traditions psychic and psycho-spiritual phenomena such as intuition, visions, out-of-body experiences, speaking in tongues and so forth are actively encouraged, and are celebrated when they occur.

All the different religions offer spiritual practices that facilitate the development of intuition, although this is often considered as a by-product rather than the main aim of religious practice. Nonetheless, it is from the spiritual practices of prayer, contemplation, devotional acts, ritual and meditation that we as aromatherapists can learn to enrich and extend our innate intuitive abilities. You do not have to become 'religious' or adopt all the tenets of a particular religion (unless you want to) to benefit from prayer, meditation, etc., although it is helpful to appreciate the values that underpin the religion. These values have a particular and individual expression in each religion, but are essentially universal; love, compassion, humility and the desire to be of benefit to and serve others are values everyone can espouse without necessarily having 'belief' in God or another divine being.

Developing intuition

Most aromatherapists will already have cultivated and developed their innate intuitive abilities to a greater or lesser extent, as the intimate nature of aromatherapy massage lends itself to such an approach. For many of us intuition is part and parcel of how we work; it is not something we need to think about consciously, nor strive for. We simply intuit information about our clients, their needs and desires and the essential oil blends with which to treat them, as well as massaging intuitively according to what we 'feel' and 'read' from the client.

However, as someone who meditates daily, and has done for many years, I suggest the regular practice of meditation can help strengthen intuition and reinforce 'being present' with the client. For the experienced aromatherapist it can be easy to slip off into reverie and extraneous thoughts while working with a client, as I know only too well myself. But by not being fully present with the client for the duration of their treatment, we may miss the subtle cues and signs the person unconsciously manifests that we may otherwise intuit information from and then act upon.

Unless I can be fully present with the person I am working with for the duration of their session, then I feel I am short-changing them in some way, even if the aromatherapy treatment is deemed successful and the client is happy with the outcome. Significantly, I have found meditation to be a wonderful and effective practice to help me remain fully present in each and every moment – and thus to be able to use my intuition to the fullest advantage. In the next chapter we will explore meditation and techniques that can benefit the aromatherapist, not only to help stay fully present with the client as much as possible, but also to use meditation to stimulate and develop our innate intuition. And having full recourse to our intuition, alongside our theoretical knowledge and understanding, and experience, helps us to be truly holistic aromatherapists.

CHAPTER 3

Meditation and Aromatherapy

Traditionally, meditation is practised as part of the path to awakening or enlightenment, but along the way we may experience many other benefits before we reach full realisation. Meditation is not an end in itself; it's a method usually practised to find peace and calm, awareness and inner wisdom and to be fully present in each and every moment. In this way the regular practice of meditation can transform giving aromatherapy massage into a profound, even spiritual, experience for both aromatherapist and client. Essentially, meditation consists of concentration and enquiry: concentration helps you to develop stillness, single pointed attention and tranquillity; enquiry helps you cultivate clarity of mind. Above all, meditation is a journey of self-discovery.

As aromatherapists we can meditate to become more self-aware and consequently more aware of our clients, their individual needs and requirements from their aromatherapy treatment. Practising meditation helps bring about the realisation of the interconnectedness of all things – an understanding that mind/body and self/other are essentially non-dual, or not different from each other. This realisation of non-duality gives rise to a corresponding sense or feeling of being at one with the universe – a state of being that facilitates healing on many levels for both ourselves and our clients.

Meditation involves withdrawing from the distractions of the external world to examine the inner world of the mind, bodily sensations and feelings. Exploring our inner world also helps us discover our innate intuitive faculties. Once we have developed awareness of our intuition we become more receptive to hearing and acting upon its messages. The Tibetan word for meditation is *sgom*, which translates as 'to become familiar with'. This means that meditation requires continual, regular effort; the occasional sporadic attempt will not produce the desired result of calm, focused awareness and intuitive insight.

When we practise meditation we become familiar with the mind. This may seem a strange idea because we use our minds all the time, so you may think you are already familiar with your mind. However, in reality we spend most of our time following random thoughts, fantasies about the future and nostalgic dreams of the past. These are simply the contents of the mind, which we tend to follow blindly and unquestioningly. Meditation trains the mind to be aware of this process and to discover what lies beneath this apparently ceaseless mental chatter.

The correct practice of meditation is not an attempt to suppress the thoughts and feelings that naturally occur. What we try to do is observe this ongoing process of thoughts and sensations as they arise and pass, and recognise them for what they are – fleeting, transient and insubstantial. Then we can recognise that our thoughts and feelings are not the actual mind itself, merely objects of the mind. In meditation we train the mind to maintain awareness of thoughts as they arise and then follow through with the decision not to indulge in thinking them. Of course, this is extremely difficult to accomplish, as our minds have wandered freely ever since we were conscious. But gradually, over time and with a lot of practice, we begin to glimpse the nature of mind that lies beneath our superficial thoughts.

We can describe the mind as being like a deep ocean with hidden depths. Usually we are just conscious and aware of the waves on the top, rising and breaking, like the thoughts that arise and pass on the surface of the mind. In the same way waves are swallowed up into the vastness of the ocean, so thoughts are effortlessly absorbed back into our minds. When we meditate we try to catch glimpses of the ocean's hidden depths – what lies between the end of one thought and the beginning of another. This is the pure nature of the mind.

Meditation allows us to rest in being present in the here and now; there is nothing to do when we sit in meditation except to be aware of thoughts, sensations and feelings as they arise and slip away. Yet meditation is not passive. On the contrary, meditation is about really being alive and conscious of each precious moment of life. Once the mental baggage of superficial thoughts has been cleared away we can see that the mind is bright and vibrant, and then we are able to respond with clarity and creative imagination to whatever situation we encounter. This spaciousness of mind facilitates being kind and compassionate to others and ourselves, while focused attention brings insight and wisdom to deal in a skilful way with whatever arises.

We can all meditate because meditation does not require adherence to a particular religion, nor any special talent or great cleverness, just an open mind and the willingness to keep practising day after day. The Thai Buddhist teacher Venerable Dhammasami describes meditation as simply applying mindfulness without thinking nor speculating, not forming opinions nor judgements. In this way, we cultivate a mindful, spacious awareness that awakens us to our potential to live life fully in every moment. T.S. Eliot (1986 [1943]) described this in 'Burnt Norton' in *Four Quartets* as being '[a]t the still point of the turning world'. He captures the sense of needing to find that deep inner still silence in order to radiate out and function skilfully in a world that is in ceaseless motion. So, in our work as aromatherapists, when we can access this still point in ourselves through meditation, we become better practitioners, more able intuitively to tune in to and become aware of the needs of our clients.

Forms of meditation

There are many different forms of meditation. Most are practised sitting still, but there are movement meditations as well such as walking meditation, yoga and t'ai chi. Any of the movement meditations can help our bodies to stay supple, and to move with fluidity and grace as we perform aromatherapy massage. However, the most useful meditations offer more profound benefits to practitioners of aromatherapy; they are the simple, basic forms, which underpin all meditation practices. These are watching the breath or *samatha*, insight meditation or vipassana, and just sitting, known as zazen or *shikantaza*.

Watching the breath, or mindfulness of breathing, is the best meditation to start with and also to return to at any time. This fundamental practice, common to many traditions, calms and focuses the mind. We simply sit still and quiet and observe each inhalation and each exhalation, although of course the mind wanders a great deal and we must remind ourselves to return our attention to the breath each time we notice that we have become distracted by a thought, feeling or sensation. Mindfulness of breathing is almost always used to begin any meditation session as well as being a complete meditation practice in itself.

Insight meditation alternates between mindfulness of breathing and enquiry. The emphasis is on awareness

– of the breath coming and going, of thoughts, feelings and sensations arising and passing, of sounds beginning and ending. Whichever object of meditation you choose to focus your awareness on, you become aware of its impermanence or unreliability. Normally we think that if something exists it will continue to be like that, but with insight meditation, when we enquire into the nature of phenomena we notice that it is the case that things change – they fluctuate and are unstable.

We notice our breath moves from shallow to deep, the sound of a car passing becomes louder and then softer, a feeling of sadness may change into a moment of self-pity, the sensation of an itch comes and goes. Our mind will wander and follow random thoughts during this meditation too, or we may become agitated or mentally dull; when this occurs it's time to return to simple mindfulness of breathing. Once your awareness is focused again, try to observe thoughts, sensations and feelings that come and go without grasping or rejecting them but enquiring into how they exist.

Just sitting, or zazen, comes from the Japanese *shikantaza*, and is also referred to as silent illumination. Just sitting forms part of Soto Zen Buddhism, which originated in China, although it is now practised mainly in Japan and Korea. Silent illumination means not having a specific object of meditation, such as a mantra or watching the breath, and also refers to the clarity of mind without thoughts.

As the name suggests, in this meditation you just sit still without thinking or doing anything else at all. In just sitting meditation you pay attention to keeping the physical posture of your body sitting absolutely still and your concentration is focused on the moment. You remain open to whatever manifests in the moment, but without the mind commenting or judging; thoughts, feelings, sounds, smells and sensations arise and pass. Normally we grasp, reject or judge these things, or create stories about or desire them, or our thoughts wander off elsewhere, but in this practice we try to have a still, clear mind as well as a still, quiet body. As always the mind will wander, but when you notice you have been thinking or daydreaming then you bring your attention back to sitting still in the moment.

How to meditate: Mindfulness of breathing

The easiest posture for the beginner in meditation is to sit upright on a hard chair, with both feet flat on the floor, hands folded loosely together in the lap. However, if you prefer you can sit cross-legged or in half-lotus posture on a floor cushion with another cushion folded under your bottom so you lean forward slightly to stabilise your posture. If you like you can experiment with both positions to see which is more comfortable for you.

You need to be able to sit comfortably without adjusting your posture for however long you wish to meditate for; at the beginning this will be only ten to fifteen minutes. It's important to sit with a straight back, not rigid and tense but relaxed and upright. Try to avoid moving or fidgeting for the duration of the session. Eyes can be half-open, focused on the floor in front of you, or closed altogether.

- Take a few moments to settle and resolve to sit still for the entire meditation session. Make the commitment to meditate as well as you can and to let go of your thoughts, fantasies and memories for the duration of the meditation.

- Set an alarm clock for ten or fifteen minutes and then forget about the time. If this seems very short afterwards, then try twenty minutes next time. If it seems very long, persevere with ten-minute sessions.

- Take a few deep breaths, and imagine any stress or tension leaving your body along with the air you exhale; you can visualise this negativity as black smoke if you find it helpful. Then let your breath flow naturally. Bring your attention to your breathing by focusing either on the light sensation of breath entering and leaving at the tip of your nostrils, or the sensation of the rising and falling of your abdomen. Try both methods, and then stick with the one that suits you best. Do not keep alternating between them; this is just a distraction.

- Be mindful that you are here, now, in the present moment, and all you are doing is watching the breath come and go. Notice the rhythm of your breathing; be aware of whether it is shallow or deep, fast or slow, but do not judge how you breathe or try to change it in any way – there is no 'good' or 'bad' way of breathing in meditation. Be aware that your body breathes of its own accord; breathing is not a conscious activity you have to initiate or do.

• Check your posture is still balanced and upright and that you have not slouched or become tense. Be aware of the sensations of your body touching the chair or cushion, of your feet on the floor and the feeling of clothing touching your skin. You may be able to feel the air circulating around you if the window is open.

• When a thought arises, be aware of it as just a thought. Let it go. You do not have to follow it, however attractive it may seem. You have made the decision to meditate for a set time and you can think all your thoughts afterwards.

• Be aware that your mind will wander a lot when you begin meditating. It often seems as if there are many more thoughts than normal, but this is not the case; you are just noticing them. Don't be annoyed or judge yourself harshly, but do keep on trying. Each time you become aware you are following a thought or feeling, bring your attention gently back to the breath, and try to keep it there.

- Be one with your breathing, and feel how the in-breath and the out-breath connect you to your environment. Rest in awareness, alert but relaxed.

- When the alarm sounds, slowly bring your attention to your surroundings. Do not rush off immediately; take some time to evaluate the experience. Resolve to meditate again soon and move thoughtfully into your daily life.

Benefits of meditating

You may be wondering by now how, or if, meditation can in some way make you a better aromatherapist or perhaps a better person. Although meditation can and does wreak several positive changes in how we live in the world and the manner in which we approach our work, some of these changes are subtle and may take quite some time to manifest. However, even after only a few meditation sessions you will feel more connected to the 'still point' inside. As your intuition dances in this quiet inner space, serenity and calm evolve, and insights begin to manifest that will deepen and strengthen your aromatherapy practice.

One benefit of meditating is realised by becoming more accepting of ourselves and how we behave by understanding more of how the world and we ourselves actually exist. Everyone wants to find happiness and avoid suffering, but often we go about this business of life from an incorrect perspective. We tend to seek happiness in phenomena outside of ourselves. Perhaps we think that owning beautiful objects, eating delicious food, achieving fame and success and having an ideal relationship will bring us happiness. These things certainly bring pleasure for a while, but they cannot bring lasting happiness, because all these things are impermanent and will therefore change.

For instance, recall an object you felt you really must have – a beautiful dress, a stunning piece of jewellery or a dream home. If you were lucky enough to be able to acquire this precious object, no doubt for a while it gave enormous pleasure. But after a while the pleasure faded, you began to take the object for granted, it broke or you became bored with it or realised you no longer liked it much. You began to crave something else instead that suddenly appeared highly desirable.

Meditation helps us realise that none of these things are intrinsically desirable, and that these objects, or our feelings about them, will change. When we meditate we watch as our feelings shift and change, arise and pass. We can recall the beautiful dress purchased last year no longer fits, or has torn or faded, or we no longer like it; either it or we, or both, have changed. We can also notice that the feeling of desire has a pattern and is habitual. This craving for something arises often, but the feeling is never satisfied for long; it always wants something new.

Craving does not bring us happiness. Realising this by examining the feeling in meditation actually helps lessen craving a little, and so when it does appear we can recognise it for what it is: simply a desire that will arise and pass whether or not it is fulfilled. The contemporary Buddhist teacher Stephen Batchelor says that meditation does not add anything to life, but it recovers what has been lost. In other words, by enquiring into the nature and meaning of life itself, by exploring its mystery, we can learn to live with more equanimity and thereby accept better and more realistically both happiness and dissatisfaction.

How to meditate: Insight meditation

Insight meditation is the most useful practice in which to consider the points made above by enquiring into the nature of phenomena, our feelings and patterns such as craving. Begin as you would for mindfulness of breathing, and spend five to ten minutes allowing the mind to calm and settle by watching the breath.

- Gradually your mind will slow down and you can begin to observe thoughts arising and passing. Start to enquire into your thoughts and feelings, analyse them and try to see where they come from, what their cause is and what effect they may have.

- If your mind begins to wander and drift into fantasies, return to watching the breath. Once your concentration strengthens, return to enquiry and analysis.

- Try hard to penetrate a thought or feeling with your intellect, and question what you habitually think you know about it. Allow your intuitive feelings to interact with your analysis, be creative and spacious and open to new insights.

- Check what mood you are in, or what the predominant emotional feeling is, and then see whether there is any physical sensation accompanying the mood. How do you feel? Enquire into these emotions, sensations and feelings.

- You can think of insight meditation as an internal debate that questions all of your assumptions and enquires into all possible interpretations and angles. You are not looking for definitive answers, so keep the questioning flexible and open.

- Insight meditation can be difficult, but just keep going and be aware that all things come to pass. Doubts, questions and old, painful memories and feelings will probably arise from time to time, but stay with the process. Remember, whenever you get distracted return to watching the breath for a while.

- As you watch thoughts and feeling arise and pass look out for the tendencies you have that take you away from your concentration. Do you have a tendency to daydream, to speculate, or to judge, or to obsessively revisit the past? Note your tendencies and see what you can learn from them.

- When issues, difficult feelings and doubts arise, look at them carefully and analyse them too. You can learn from anything and everything that arises during meditation.

• When the alarm sounds to remind you that your meditation has finished, spend a few minutes quietly watching the breath, before you resume your daily activities.

Informal meditation in daily life

Meditation is not an activity confined only to formal meditation sessions. To fully experience its benefits we need to bring the quality of meditation into our daily life, including our work as aromatherapists. In this way mindfulness can help transform our lives. For instance, instead of mindlessly reacting in habitual ways, like getting angry and frustrated in a traffic jam, we can remind ourselves that there is nothing inherently irritating about being stuck in traffic; it is only our reaction that causes the problem. If you simply accept the situation – that you are going to arrive later than you intended, and there is absolutely nothing you can do to alter this fact – then you don't have to sit there feeling impatient and angry. You can relax and maybe even do some mindfulness of breathing. Informal meditation helps us regard such situations as opportunities to be mindful and to watch the breath instead of wasting time being angry.

The prime tool of meditation is our own mind, and as we are never apart from our minds we have plenty of opportunities for informal meditation. For instance, we can use informal meditation for pleasure. Watching the breath mindfully can enhance our enjoyment of looking at a beautiful view in nature by putting us in close touch with our bodily sensations and feelings, so we are present to the whole experience. In this way we really feel part of the beautiful vista and our experience becomes non-dual; we feel at one with nature. This is a natural inclination for many people anyway, but doing it consciously transforms the experience into something special as we become more aware of the mystery of life. Informal meditation helps us live life fully in the here and now, appreciating every precious moment, not idling life away in daydreams.

We can also regard giving aromatherapy massage as a form of informal meditation. The calmness and single pointed focus we have learned from meditating helps us remain fully present with clients while treating them. We observe and read the client's behaviour, facial expressions and body language as easily as we interpret their words during the consultation, thereby using fully all our faculties including our intuition. We feel a real empathy for the client's issues and needs. Certain essential oils and blends may come to mind, and we 'know' they will be helpful for this client on this particular occasion.

When we come to do the massage, we feel grounded and centred in our own body, in touch with our breathing. We feel open and caring towards the person lying on the massage couch and pleased we have the opportunity to offer the healing touch of aromatherapy massage. When we place our hands on the client we feel aware this is another human being, just like us, someone who wishes to find happiness and avoid suffering. We connect with the rhythm of their breathing and feel their life force pulsing through their body.

We stay fully present to the experience of giving this person a massage, and avoid slipping off into daydreams, fantasies and distracting thoughts, such as what we may eat for lunch. As the fragrance of the blend evolves we notice the subtle transformation, and we feel each tiny change as the client responds to the healing touch of our hands. We maintain a deep connection with the person, being fully with them right until the end of the treatment, while also maintaining awareness of the temperature, light and all other features of the room. We can call this way of working aromatherapy massage meditation.

How to meditate: Just sitting

Each of the three meditation techniques described in this chapter offers a slightly different method and emphasis to find calm, single pointed concentration and inner wisdom. But the importance of and focus on being in the moment in just sitting meditation is especially helpful to transform aromatherapy massage into a meditation, because it facilitates being completely with the client in every moment. However, because the object of this meditation technique – being in the moment – is less tangible than watching the breath or enquiring into thoughts and feelings, you may also find this meditation a little harder. Thus I suggest practising both the other two meditations for a while first, until you feel comfortable with the techniques and notice the benefits of meditating, before you try just sitting.

The Zen teacher Taisen Deshimaru describes just sitting as the process of becoming intimate with oneself, of finding our inner stillness. We try to uncover the non-abiding mind, the mind that rests nowhere, which is beyond all thought and relativity. Yet this is nothing other than our ordinary everyday mind that lies beneath the flow of superficial thoughts. It is said that continual introspection, or 'turning back' of the mind from thoughts and other distractions, arouses an inner potential (including intuition), which eventually breaks through into ordinary everyday consciousness. There is a strong tradition that once you have realisations from this meditation you should go out and live and work in the world so all may benefit. Thus it is most fitting to take the skills and benefits of this meditation into our aromatherapy work.

- Start as you would for mindfulness of breathing, but pay extra close attention to your posture. You may like to sit facing the wall, as this is the posture traditionally adopted in just sitting. Make sure your back is straight, that you are sitting upright – relaxed not tense, comfortable but not slouching. Spend five to ten minutes allowing the mind to calm and settle by watching the breath.

- In just sitting it is enough just to be, without intention, analysis, effort nor imagination. The human mind is essentially free, not clinging to anything; in just sitting we learn to uncover this mind, and then we can see who we really are.

- It is necessary to concentrate on your posture but you must also forget about the body and embrace this apparent contradiction. If you experience pain, try not to become distracted by it nor move. Pain and discomfort often dissipate of their own accord, so try allowing the pain to just be, without doing anything. Of course, if the pain becomes intense you will need to shift position, but try to move once only and not to fidget or give the pain any extra energy.

- The more completely the mind is at rest, the more deeply the body is at rest. Out of stillness our whole life arises, so to live life fully it's important to get in touch with stillness. Just let go of thoughts, opinions and everything else that the mind grasps at.

- Be aware of thoughts as they arise, but do not try to control or suppress them, yet be vigilant in not following them. Whenever you become distracted, return your attention to being in the moment, to just sitting.

- When you notice momentary gaps between thoughts, this is pure awareness, but the instant you think this you lose it. Try to be aware without thinking. Being fully present is not letting the mind rest anywhere; the moment it rests or alights upon something thoughts arise.

- The mind is like a mirror; it reflects thoughts but is not the thoughts themselves. It is said that enlightenment is already present, staring us right in the face, thereby doing away with the duality of practising meditation and realisation.

- Just sit in the moment, silent and still. When the bell rings to end the session, spend a few moments reflecting upon your meditation. Then try to take the quality of fully being in the moment with you as you move on with your daily life.

Practising any, or all, of these meditations regularly will help you cultivate your ability to be quiet and peaceful and to find clarity and insight. You will discover you gradually become a better listener and more able to empathise with and understand your clients. As this gift of creative intuitive awareness manifests, you will feel more in touch with life and its meaning, and can bring these qualities into your aromatherapy work.

Try meditating alongside doing the exercises for developing your own fragrant language and personal understanding of essential oils described in Chapter I, as these all complement and enrich one another. There is also another meditation – a visualisation ritual described in the following chapter – that you will likely experience more intensely the more you practise the meditations described here.

CHAPTER 4

Ancient and Modern Magic in Aromatherapy

Working intuitively with essential oils and absolutes is a deep, reflective process, which may almost be described as alchemical. Although individual essential oils are powerful healing substances in themselves, far from the 'base metals' of alchemy, when we combine oils together to make blends, we are trying to create something precious, like the 'precious metals' of gold and silver the alchemists were aiming for in their transformative processes. Many of the blends we create bear a similarity to the elusive elixir of life the alchemists were seeking; they go beyond a simple physical and emotional healing to the enhancement of life itself, even if not attaining the mythical Fountain of Youth or mystical Philosopher's Stone. But most of all, when we approach working with essential oils and creating blends using our intuition, then we bring in elements of spirituality, mythology and magic that are integral to the philosophy of alchemy.

The familiar idea of alchemists trying to transform base metal into gold is, however, a superficial perspective; from a deeper understanding the alchemical process is a metaphor for refining human life into its true – and spiritual – nature. The real alchemists were on a spiritual quest aiming for an inner transformation, a purification of the human psyche into what they called the quintessence or soul. Some alchemists included in their experiments 'chymical' oils bought from the apothecary along with other substances to be tested. They would have known that aromatics were so highly prized by ancient civilisations that they were burned as offerings to the divine. So as they observed the oils evaporate into ether through their various distillations and experiments, alchemists may have also realised that this created yet another metaphor for their philosophy of transformation: the purified human soul, its quintessence, yearns to become one with God.

We saw in Chapter 1 how drawing from myth, legend and archetypal imagery can help us formulate our own personal fragrant language, and how this can deepen our understanding and appreciation of individual essential oils and blends. In Chapter 3 the discussion of how meditation can deepen and enhance aromatherapy massage revealed how meditation is rooted in spiritual philosophy and esoteric practice. Both of these approaches can help develop our innate intuitive faculties, as described in Chapter 2. Now we will see what magic may have to offer the contemporary aromatherapist to further develop her intuition. However, the very word 'magic' can effect in some people a knee-jerk reaction of negativity and judgement, perhaps a condemning of this much-misunderstood and maligned tradition, so we will consider first which of the many elements of magic, past and present, may be able to enrich our aromatherapy work.

The term 'magic' is wide ranging and can mean different things to different people depending on the individual's belief system and values, their prejudice – both positive and negative – and which form of magic is being referred to. Generally speaking, magic is often misunderstood and interpreted according to narrow ideas, such as black magic, white magic, the casting of spells and so forth. Yet magic goes far beyond such superficial and narrow concepts. There are entire magical traditions such as Wicca, and traditions rooted in magic such as shamanism, paganism, Druidry and the ancient Anglo-Saxon tribal wisdom known as Wyrd.

There are also magical features in most religions. Sometimes these aspects become so familiar within a culture that they become unremarkable and it is easy to forget that they are magic. For instance, in Christian cultures the imbibing of the sacrament of bread and wine as symbols of Christ's body and blood is taken for granted. Yet what is this transubstantiation if not a form of magic? Thus we can surmise there is a great deal more to magic than is often supposed, and much to learn from it that may prove useful.

Magic can be described as using intention, ritual and belief or faith in supernatural phenomena to achieve particular ends that may not be realised by mundane everyday methods. Sometimes summed up as the power of mind over matter, this concept is demonstrated well by the placebo effect. This is how people recover from the symptoms of a particular illness because they have been told they have been given medicine to cure their malady, when in fact what they actually swallowed was a sugar pill. The cure is 'magical' in the sense that it cannot be rationally or scientifically verified, although it is apparent that the human mind/body organism has ways of healing itself when given appropriate suggestions, triggers or catalysts.

For the contemporary aromatherapist, it is magic as part of the natural healing tradition and essential oils coming from nature that are of particular interest. There are, however, also elements of magic present in the contemporary practice of aromatherapy itself. In the professional training at the London School of Aromatherapy we included practical exercises to stimulate and develop the flow of energy in the hands, and discussion about the aura and subtle energies, including meridians and pressure points, all of which have magical aspects. But it is the protective visualisation undertaken just before giving an aromatherapy massage that demonstrates most powerfully a form of magic. We taught our students how to visualise a shower of white light pouring over them, or to visualise drawing golden circles of light around themselves, to prevent taking on negative energies released from the client as part of their healing process. We also taught how to flick the fingers during massage to release these energies.

However, in each class there were always some who rolled their eyes in disbelief when we taught protective visualisations, and we knew that these students were unlikely to follow our instructions. A few months into their course some, if not all, of these students would seek out one of us tutors and tell her of problems with taking on negative energy after practising massage, although they tended to use somewhat different language to describe their experiences. When the tutor gently enquired if the student was doing the protective visualisations she or he would guiltily shake their head and reveal they had thought this was just superstitious nonsense. The tutor would then reiterate the importance of protective visualisations and remind the student of how to do them. Once these sceptical students opened their minds to the magic of protective visualisations and wholeheartedly embraced doing them, their problems with taking on negative energy were largely solved.

Traditional healers

It is valuable to consider what we have perhaps lost from the modern way of working in aromatherapy but can possibly recover from looking at how some of our predecessors practised their healing arts, rather than following the common tendency to just seek out the latest new development. We can regard this as a way forward that draws from the past, by taking a look at witches, early herbalists and the 'wise healing women', both actual and archetypal. What can we learn, or recover, from these traditional healers to contribute to an intuitive, magical way of working in contemporary aromatherapy?

From my early years I have always thought of myself as 'witchy'. As a young child I read about potpourri – long before it became fashionable and easily available – and tried to create my own version, attempting to dry rose petals and herbs from my mother's garden, and then adding spices from her kitchen. The results were disastrous, as I had no knowledge of the processes or correct ingredients or proportions, but I remember my experiments were exciting, fun and rewarding to do, although disappointing at the end. There were many further attempts to make all sorts of witchy potions, but with distinctly mixed success.

Also, at a young age I was reprimanded severely for making garlands of red berries, hanging them around my neck and then taking off all my clothes and dancing around a pretend fire in the woods at the bottom of our garden. My parents were horrified at such – to them – outrageous behaviour and also worried the berries might have been poisonous. But I was always drawn to such ritualistic activities in nature – a childish magic – because it felt normal and natural. So when to my delight in my twenties I discovered aromatherapy and embarked upon a professional training, my natural instincts led me to carry on experimenting with essential oils in a similar fashion to the witchy ways of my childhood.

I remember buying my first bottles of essential oils, and then lying on the rug in a patch of sun in the sitting room and playing with the bottles in the sunlight, peering into the mysterious depths of the liquids encased in the dark glass. Then investigating the oils inside the bottles – learning about colour and viscosity by playing with the oils as well as by frequently sniffing the entrancing smells. I constantly experimented with individual oils and blends in my meditation practice, baths, burners, room sprays, perfumes and anything else I could think of, such as adding oils to un-fragranced liquid soaps, fabric conditioners and moisturisers.

But the most fun and excitement came from experimenting with each new essential oil I bought – creating blends and then practising massage with fellow students and friends with the results. The outcomes were sometimes unexpected; many blends were delightful and only a very few unsuccessful, although these could be interesting too – and we learn as much from our mistakes, if not more, as we do from our triumphs. One blend containing the inadvertent slip-up of too many drops of violet leaf left both my friend and me distinctly woozy after doing a massage swap. But no harm was done; the sensation was pleasant enough, and this was a good lesson in respecting the power of essential oils. I found I learned as much from my intuitive experimenting with oils, blends and massage as I did from my studies, and the two ways of learning certainly complemented each other, leading to a genuinely holistic appreciation of essential oils and aromatherapy practice.

This intuitive, free and experimental way of working looks back to the days of antiquity, to the early healing women, witches and herbalists when knowledge was acquired through trial and error and from being passed on in an oral tradition. This healing tradition was mainly female, although there were wise men herbalists and witches too. Without modern science, and before the evolution beyond a select few of reading and writing or communication beyond one's immediate locality, it was essential for the individual healer to acquire information about plants and their healing or poisonous qualities through experimenting, being in close touch with nature and their intuition, and learning from a respected elder healer. These wise healing women, witches and herbalists were regarded almost as doctors among most village people, as only the rich could afford the professional doctors of the day with their leeches and bloodletting and eventually their chemicals.

Natural healers were held in high esteem, but also much feared because they held the power of this esoteric knowledge. They could of course harm as well as heal. Although harm was caused mostly unintentionally in flawed attempts to heal, unethical healers and witches could, and did, poison and place curses or spells to wreak illness and chaos, and so all natural healers were dreaded as well as respected. This mostly female anarchic power was deeply threatening to the patriarchal ordering of society, and led to terrible persecution of these healers, herbalists and witches, which eventually drove this way of working underground. In the process much of the ancient healing herbal lore was destroyed, ridiculed, lost or hidden.

I have always regarded these wise healing women, herbalists and witches of the long distant past as early, primitive practitioners of the natural healing tradition, of which the modern practice of aromatherapy is one of the latest manifestations. Of course, now we have the tremendous benefit of knowledge and science of aromatic plants and essential oils undreamed of in the early days, and this informs a great deal of our work today. But in our understandable enthusiasm for this scientific knowledge and way of understanding what essential oils are composed of and how they work on the human body, we can lose sight of the intuitive wisdom and insight of these ancient natural healers.

I suggest the truly holistic aromatherapist today needs to be aware of and needs to consider both approaches, to trust both scientific knowledge and her own intuitive inner wisdom. In fact, this book on intuitive aromatherapy can be regarded as a tribute to these early pioneers in our field of natural plant healing and an acknowledgement of the important role they played. By incorporating what is useful to modern aromatherapy today from their experimental and intuitive way of working, we also pay respect to and honour the terrible price they suffered for practising their healing arts.

A word of caution

There are risks associated with this intuitive experimental method of working with essential oils and massage, and it is important to be aware of the potential to cause harm and avoid doing so. Certainly in the old ways of healing there were grievous errors and mistakes, causing harm or even death, as well as healing successes. Intuition itself can also occasionally be mistaken, and it is always a good idea to check a new blend we have arrived at through using our intuition by further research. We have aromatherapy books and course notes and, now with the ubiquitous internet, the modern aromatherapist is indeed fortunate to have access to a wealth of information and scientific understanding about essential oils, anatomy and knowledge from all the disciplines that inform our work.

However, the risks of working intuitively are minimal for the professional aromatherapist who has studied all the necessary theory, undertaken extensive practice and then qualified. For instance, when we study anatomy we learn about muscles, bones, the attachments between them, the location of organs, the structure of the skin and so forth. So when we place our hands on a client and begin to massage we already know how to avoid doing harm because we know where the organs, bones and muscles are and how they work. Thus we can allow intuition – our inner wisdom – to inform deviations from the standard massage routine to tailor the massage to the client's individual needs. We literally feel and sense the best way to help the client, using both learned knowledge, previous experience and intuition.

It can be a little different with essential oils and blends. In most cases when we intuitively select several essential oils and then blend them according to what we 'feel' is right, our learned knowledge informs our intuition and we create an effective, holistic blend. However, on rare occasions this methodology doesn't always work perfectly. An interesting example is ginger, and both theoretical knowledge and intuition can be flawed when working with this oil. When we study spice oils we learn it is essential to use them carefully as they can be potential skin irritants because they have hot and stimulating properties. Thus, both intuitively and drawing from our theoretical knowledge we may create a blend including ginger to warm and stimulate and use a low dilution to avoid any chance of skin irritation.

Yet when we go back and check our notes and textbooks we realise this is only part of the picture. Some authorities, such as Franchomme and Penoel, regard ginger as an anti-inflammatory rather than a rubefacient, thus cooling rather than warming (cited in Rhind 2013). It is suggested that the herbal preparation and the distilled essential oil differ considerably; Battaglia quotes Holmes as saying the oil contains no pungent components, thus diverging significantly from the herbal extract (cited in Rhind 2013).

So although ginger 'feels' warming – and on a psychological/emotional level there is general agreement that this is true – how it works on the physical level and the skin is possibly not yet fully appreciated. Perhaps the qualities of ginger depend on how much is used; maybe in small amounts ginger is cooling but in stronger dilutions it is warming. Thus, by intuitively choosing ginger for a rubefacient effect and using only a small amount because it is a spice oil – to avoid potential skin irritation – we may inadvertently be causing an anti-inflammatory effect. This interesting and fascinating topic reminds us there is always more to explore and learn about essential oils, both scientifically and intuitively.

My own personal intuitive feelings around ginger are interestingly concerned neither with rubefacient nor anti-inflammatory qualities, although I appreciate its warming effect on the emotions and also tend to use this oil more in winter than summer. For me ginger is first and foremost a tonic – fortifying and strengthening, good in blends for exhaustion and convalescence, for stagnant circulation and digestion, indigestion and for those feeling weak, overwhelmed and finding it difficult to cope with everyday life. Words I associate with ginger include 'rich', 'exotic', 'opulent', 'expansive' and 'recuperative' and for me this language informs the qualities described above.

Traditional ways of working

There are several ways the contemporary aromatherapist can benefit from the traditional ways of working of the wise women healers of the past. We have already reflected on developing intuition, and then incorporating this inner wisdom into how we practise selecting and blending essential oils and doing aromatherapy massage. Now we can consider how this valuable and esoteric healing knowledge was passed on from one healer to another.

It is likely that many of the wise women healers attracted disciples: their daughters, or other local girls and young women who became interested in learning the ways of healing. These apprentices would have worked closely with their erudite elders, learning to find the places where healing plants grew, how to distinguish them from similar other plants, which part of the plant to use, how and when to collect the plant and how to prepare it into a healing potion, ointment and so forth. All this information was learned from watching and working with the respected elder, along with practising how things were done, and by listening to and remembering the knowledge imparted, often by regular recitation. There would have been other healing substances to learn about as well, mostly derived from animals, stones, clays and so forth. This way of learning, known as the oral tradition, was the main way to learn before reading, writing and books were widely available.

Although having books, the internet and being able to read and write are wonderful, valuable tools of education they do, however, encourage a more solitary way of learning. We study alone, read books and write essays without much contact with a teacher or classmates. Of course, on a professional aromatherapy training course we attend classes, listen to lectures, have discussions and watch massage demonstrations and practise with a partner, but nonetheless a lot of our work is still done alone. Then, after qualifying, we set out to build up a practice, take on clients and work mainly in isolation from our teachers and peers.

The requirement to do continuing professional development (CPD) hours each year is an important way to ensure an ongoing learning process. However, I believe we aromatherapists could do a lot more to be mutually supportive, to work and play together, and to share and learn with one another. Some years ago when I worked on the International Federation of Aromatherapists council for a couple of terms, I researched and wrote a paper about introducing supervision. The idea was to encourage newly qualified aromatherapists to spend time with a well-experienced teacher/practitioner to discuss issues with clients, ways of working and so forth and to be generally supported in their work. I had already run quite a few supervision CPD classes, and feedback indicated that this work was of much benefit to the participants. However, supervision was not taken up formally as it transpired there were too many difficulties in its implementation.

Nonetheless, I would encourage aromatherapists to consider supervision. The word can evoke some negative connotations, but I do not regard supervision as checking up on, interference, intrusion or critical intervention; rather I find it is supportive and can be of mutual benefit, more like the way the traditional healing women must have worked. Perhaps a more appropriate word than supervision is mentoring. I remember several students from my London School of Aromatherapy days who, even several years after qualifying, would from time to time phone me for advice, to discuss a particular client or just to chat about their aromatherapy practice because they felt unsupported and isolated. I wished then that we had retained this supportive aspect of the traditional old ways of working. But we cannot now return to the old days and this is probably for the best.

However, it is a good idea to find appropriate ways to support one another and maintain good communication, as it can be an isolating, lonely experience working as an aromatherapist in the modern world. There are aromatherapy conferences where we can meet one another and network, but although valuable they are infrequent and crowded occasions and can lack the space and time needed for intimate, informal communication. So as well as meeting at conferences, doing CPD classes and perhaps undertaking supervision – either in groups or individual sessions – we can also develop the system of doing massage swaps with one another. I feel this offers a way of keeping in touch with our fellow students or aromatherapy friends and – as well as massage – provides a forum for swapping ideas, information, concerns, successes and simply embracing being with a fellow aromatherapist on a human level, that is, an informal 'time out' and sharing that would have formed an integral part of how the wise women healers of the past worked, played and learned.

Experience has shown how important it is to receive massage as well as to give it. If we do not from time to time feel the sensations of receiving a whole body massage, and notice the effect of the overall treatment and particular strokes and techniques, then we can lose sensitivity when we massage others. Such sensitivity also informs intuition. Of course, many aromatherapists will already have a 'swap buddy' or perhaps several. A friend and I, from our old student days more than twenty-five years ago, still get together every once in a while and do swaps as we always did; the day together remains of great benefit to us both.

We can also do swaps with other complementary therapists, and this is a good way of learning and extending skills and techniques, as an adjunct to attending CPD classes. Over the years I have done swaps with practitioners of Reiki, Alexander Technique, Thai massage, deep tissue massage and Shiatsu, among others. The most blissful occasion I recall was with an osteopath friend when we treated each other on a beach in Goa; so swaps can open up delightful new ways of working too.

This informal sharing of time and knowledge, playing and experimenting with oils, blends and massage techniques together, and indulging in the familiar ritual of chatting over a cup of tea as well as giving each other a massage, is both timeless and invaluable. With a massage swap friend or supervisor we can express feelings, unconscious material, fears and uncertainties that we might never otherwise have the opportunity to talk about. Spending time together in this manner keeps us connected to our tradition of aromatherapy in a personal and human way. And this timeless human interaction that the early healers would have also shared, speaking freely and voicing unconscious thoughts and feelings is yet another way of developing our intuition.

CHAPTER 5

Aromatherapy Ritual

Spiritual and Sacred Use of Essential Oils

Meditation, ritual and other mystical practices share the aim of transforming the mundane experience of duality, in which mind, body and spirit or soul are regarded as being separate entities, into a state where they become unified in consciousness. Mental, physical and spiritual awareness thereby merge into a single identity that is not perceived as mind, body or spirit because it is all three simultaneously. In this state we become one with our mind/body/spirit continuum and also with the world around us, a recognition of our interdependence with all beings and phenomena. When we work as healers from this perspective we lose the sense of ego, that 'I' heal 'another', and intuit that rather we facilitate healing to happen, a more genuine, holistic and humble approach.

We have already discussed meditation and how, with regular practice, this can take our work as aromatherapists on to a deeper, more intuitive level, and also considered the magical aspects of aromatherapy. So in this chapter we look at what ritual is, and how it can contribute to an intuitive practice of aromatherapy. Meditation, magic and ritual share certain characteristics: they need to be performed regularly with focused intent in order to be optimally effective, there are conscious and unconscious expectations, and often they have some form of spiritual or religious significance and ceremonial features. For instance, when Christians go to church on Sundays they fulfil the conscious need to worship within their belief system. The ritual aspects of the service and prayer encourage participants to reflect on their faith and to consider the fundamental questions of existence, such as the meaning of life and death, and some, at least, of these musings will be unconscious.

Rituals, as well as many forms of meditation and prayer, require appropriate preparations; they can be powerful and transformative experiences, and rushing into them unprepared is foolish. All rituals begin with clearing and calming the mind through meditation and then bringing attention to your intentions: what you want to achieve by doing the ritual. Sometimes called psychic centring, this preparatory reflective time beforehand unites your intention, vision, will and belief and allows unconscious desires and intuitive insights to come into consciousness.

Once the mind is calm and clearly focused on the ritual then purification, often referred to in ritual terminology as banishing, can be performed. This is an outer act that reflects the inner process of 'banishing' the stream of mundane thoughts that distract from doing the ritual with calm clear attention. Many places of worship require you to leave your shoes at the door, symbolising the casting off of mundane, everyday concerns as well as usefully keeping the sacred space physically clean. Some traditions require the head or other body parts to be covered as a symbol of respect, and some also require the ritual washing of the mouth, feet or hands to symbolise inner purity. Before performing the ritual described below you can simply remove your shoes and wash your hands as symbols of outer purity, which reflects and reinforces the inner purity of the mind after meditation, while having clean hands is also appropriate for anointing yourself with oil.

The place in which you perform your ritual is important, and you need to create a simple, physical scared space. In a similar fashion to creating an inner sacred space by calming and clearing the mind and focusing on your intention, you also create an outer sacred space that is private, away from the noise and busyness of everyday life. Sometimes described as the place between the worlds where divine and earthly can meet, a sacred space is created by preparation rather than being intrinsically sacred. Thus, a quiet ordinary room cleared of mundane, secular objects, ritually and mindfully cleaned and with the door shut to delineate the boundaries between the sacred space and everything outside it is sufficient. Once you have purified the mind by meditating and created the sacred space by physical preparation, then you can begin the ritual. There are many other ritual preparations that can also be included once you have some experience of performing rituals, but it's best to begin with simplicity and not detract from the power of the ritual itself.

The ritual described here is a version of a guided visualisation meditation ritual, like a simple shamanic journeying, which I have adapted to use with essential oils. Rituals often include the burning of aromatics such as incense, or ritual anointing with scented oils, so this contemporary aromatherapy ritual is in keeping with traditional rituals. Vaporising and self-anointing with an essential oil, together with guided visualisation and imagination, facilitates a deeper, more intuitive appreciation of the essential oil you choose to work with. The ritual may even bring about a visionary or imaginary encounter with the plant spirit, although probably not in the way you may at first imagine.

For the sceptically minded, the very idea of this ritual may push the boundaries of credibility, but try to keep an open mind; you will never know what may happen unless you attempt it. But you do need to have the intention to perform the ritual correctly and with respect; a sneering, negative attitude will sabotage the potential of the ritual's effectiveness. Feel free to experiment and make changes to the ritual described to create a personally meaningful version, although be mindful to retain the spirit of the original. When you find, or develop, a ritual that 'works' for you, there is an Aha! moment of recognition, as archetypal images and glimpses of universal truth slip from the unconscious into consciousness and reveal themselves to you as intuitive inner wisdom.

Ritual with essential oil

Begin by fulfilling all the preparations as described above so you have created a scared space and spent sufficient time in it calming the mind with meditation. Then bring your attention to the objective of the ritual, which is to deepen your knowledge and appreciation of your chosen essential oil, and learn to 'know' it in a different, more intuitive way. Spend ten to fifteen minutes focusing on your objectives for the ritual. Allow your intuition to help you choose which essential oil you want to work with in this ritual; it may be the first oil that springs to mind, the first bottle your hand selects or, after pondering the question for some minutes, the oil that comes through strongest.

Make up a roll-on bottle with your essential oil diluted in base oil; use a perfume strength dilution of 10 to 20 per cent, depending on power of fragrance and possible skin-irritant qualities or other safety issues of the oil. Prepare an essential oil burner with tea light and water, and then add ten to fifteen drops of your chosen essential oil and light the tea light. Use tepid to hot water to allow the oil to diffuse slowly, as the ritual will take half to three-quarters of an hour.

- Sit comfortably in your usual meditation posture, with the oil burner close by. You may like to request a higher spiritual source, god or goddess, or the plant spirit of the essential oil itself to help you fulfil the aim of your ritual. Then mindfully and with intention anoint yourself: apply the roll-on oil to wrists, behind the ears and arms, legs or ankles if uncovered. You could recite an invocation or prayer to reinforce your intention to increase your learning and knowledge of the oil through the ritual. Use your intuition to help you discover the appropriate words.

- Bring your attention to your breathing, and let the mind settle in meditation. As you become aware of the fragrance of the essential oil from both the burner and the roll-on observe the feelings and sensations the fragrance evokes. Let your awareness be suffused with the fragrance.

- With eyes closed and mind open, visualise yourself sitting in your sacred space, permeated by the fragrance of the oil. Allow feelings, images and associations evoked by the fragrance to arise; if anything strikes you as interesting or important explore the image, association or feeling.

- Now visualise the sacred space expanding far beyond the confines of the room; it can be helpful to see this as white mist clearing away and revealing space on the other side. Visualise yourself slowly walking into the mist. After a while the mist clears and you enter into a Garden of Eden: a primitive, natural timeless place of nature full of every kind of plant from around the world growing prolifically together. You may perhaps visualise this place as rainforest – humid and steamy with sunlight blocked by the canopy of giant trees high above. The place is beautiful but primal; you sense you are exploring the terrain as the first person; you feel excited but a little apprehensive as you enter the unknown. Spend some time exploring all the plants you encounter in your imagination.

- After a while you hear the sound of a waterfall and slowly walk towards it through the abundance of plants. You need to push through tangled hanging vines and creepers and watch your step so as not to trip over giant roots. Be aware of the scent of your essential oil and feel that it is guiding you safely along the path towards the sound of falling water.

- Now visualise yourself arriving in front of the waterfall: a huge cascade of water tumbling into a pool fringed by dense undergrowth. Carefully pick your way towards the waterfall until you are standing so close you can feel the spray on your skin. Take a deep breath and duck into the waterfall; feel the water pour over you as you fumble through the darkness to find your way out. The fragrance of the oil gives you courage and helps you break on through to the other side.

• Once through the waterfall, focus on the fragrance of the essential oil. Feel how it has permeated your senses through your skin and by you inhaling the vapour from the burner, and how the plant spirit has guided you to this place. Now bring to mind the plant of the essential oil and visualise it growing in its natural habitat; this is the place you have arrived at on the other side of the waterfall. Create a sensory picture in your imagination. What does the place feel like? What does the plant look like? Is the plant young or old? Is it winter or summer, dry or wet? Is it day or nightfall? Is it one plant or many? All the while let the fragrance wash over you and help bring your imagination to vivid life.

• For instance, if your chosen essential oil is lavender, you may find yourself sitting at the edge of a vast lavender field with bushes of lavender in long rows stretching as far as the eye can see. It is dusk after a long, hot, dry day, and the fragrance of lavender rises as the welcome fresh cool of evening descends. A wind stirs and the bushes softly rustle, wafting the scent on the breeze. Gradually the vibrant purple of lavender flowers becomes one with the dark night, but the smell remains with you, filling your senses.

- When you feel ready, let the visualisation fade and bring your attention back to your breathing. Let the mind calm and settle in meditation. As thoughts, feelings, sensations and images arise, enquire into them; see if something has come through from your visualisation ritual. When you feel ready to finish, pay respect and offer thanks to the fragrant spirit of the essential oil for guiding and supporting you through the ritual. Then gradually open your eyes and be present to the experience of sitting in your sacred space. Spend a little time reflecting on your ritual. Finally, get up, walk over to and open the door, and leave the room to formally close down the sacred space and end the ritual.

Take adequate time to reflect on the ritual soon afterwards and write down any insights into the plant or essential oil that came to you. If you enjoyed doing the ritual, make a conscious resolve to do it again a few more times, maybe working with a different essential oil on each occasion. Perhaps not much came through to consciousness, or maybe you actually felt or 'saw' in your imagination the plant spirit. But however little or much came into your consciousness during the ritual, seeds were sown in your unconscious that will manifest when the time is right. Thus it can be helpful to regard the plant spirit as insights and intuitive wisdom about the oil that manifest gradually, rather than as an actual physical presence or representation – although of course if your unconscious gifted you a vision of a plant spirit, then treasure it and work with it in further rituals.

Essential oils as amulets

One of my favourite aromatherapy books is *Marguerite Maury's Guide to Aromatherapy* (1989). I have always found Maury's ideas, personality and energy inspirational, and her brilliant concept of the Individual Prescription has informed my own work in several ways. She describes the Individual Prescription, or Mixture, as meeting the requirements of each person in their unique disposition and temperament shaped by their individual circumstances. By selecting essential oils that have an affinity with the person, which represent and reflect who that person is, we can work with them to strengthen their positive attributes and redress any negativities. In particular, the Individual Prescription is normalising and balancing, helping to bring harmony to the person on their journey through life.

I have worked with clients using their Individual Prescription as both a massage oil and in a roll-on perfume to use at home. The roll-on bottles fit neatly into a pocket or handbag, so in fact can be applied in almost any circumstances if required. As the client's issues resolved or changed subtly, so did the Individual Prescription modify to reflect the person's current physical, emotional, spiritual and psychological condition. Drawing from a broad sense of the Individual Prescription, I also began to work with mood perfumes, both for clients and with students, to explore the particular emotional, psychological and spiritual aspects of essential oils.

This way of working turned out to be most effective. Clients reported that whenever they used their roll-on perfume it evoked the experience of the massage, as the fragrance was the same and therefore reminded them of the occasion of their treatment. Thus clients found that their recollection of the relaxed calm state of the massage, evoked by the fragrance, helped them to find calm in their current situation. I also found that telling clients this would likely happen whenever they used their roll-on reinforced their experience of wearing the perfume. Used in this way, the roll-on perfume became a form of fragrant amulet that, whenever needed, the client could turn to and use for support beyond the confines of the treatment.

Also known as charms or talismans, amulets are objects of power traditionally used to bring good luck and repel evil spirits or avoid bad luck. Amulets are most often physical objects. If small enough, they can be worn around the neck. Alternatively, small amulets can be kept in a pocket to be held in the hand, unseen by others if required, when necessary. They are sacred objects, often imbued with religious significance such as the Christian cross, Native American totem or Hindu lingam.

However, a roll-on perfume created from a person's Individual Prescription can work equally well as an amulet. Used over time, amulets develop a psychic charge, and this works together with any intrinsic quality – in this case the healing qualities of the essential oils – but most of all with the person's belief in the efficacy of their amulet. Suggesting to the client that regularly applying the roll-on in a personal ritualised way will be of benefit to them creates in their mind faith and belief in the power of the amulet, so it will also work on unconscious levels together with the physical and emotional effects of the oils. This encourages the potential for transformation, personal and spiritual growth and healing on all levels to be realised, and empowers the client to be actively involved in their healing process.

CHAPTER 6

Essential Oils and Absolutes

Even the most experienced aromatherapist can fall into patterns or habits of choosing oils and blends that are limited in the context of the extensive repertoire of essential oils and absolutes at our disposal. We may find ourselves over-relying upon blends and individual oils we discovered to be effective in the early days of our professional work. As our career progresses we may find that essential oils we once used extensively fall from grace, or that we gradually come to neglect essential oils that are difficult to blend in favour of easier options. Maybe we no longer always explore new essential oils as they become available for aromatherapy, or we have lost touch with the passion of discovering unfamiliar oils and blends. Possibly we sometimes overlook the fact that if we, or a client, like the fragrance of an essential oil or blend and are attracted to it, then this is intuition – our inner wisdom – informing us that the oil or blend will be of benefit in some way.

The earlier chapters have discussed various methods and techniques to help avoid these limitations. Here we will discuss absolutes and the issues surrounding their use in aromatherapy, and also consider a relatively newly introduced essential oil to aromatherapy with a particular resonance with the intuitive, spiritual approach. Palo santo may be familiar to some aromatherapists, but is not yet widely used, except possibly in the United States. Sometimes described as tricky to work with, palo santo can be difficult to blend because of its strong and unusual fragrance, but such challenges are useful to stimulate creativity and help avoid the limiting habits of blending described above.

An essential oil to discover

Palo santo (Bursera graveolens)

Major constituents are Limonene, alpha-Terpineol, beta-Bisaolene and Carvone and trans-Carveol. This intriguing, mystical essential oil works in both physical and metaphysical realms. It belongs to the same family as frankincense, myrrh and elemi, which – along with its name in Spanish meaning holy wood – gives us a good idea of its character. There is limited information on safety to date, but palo santo is generally thought to be non-toxic and non-sensitising, but it can be a skin-irritant if used in high concentrations. It is best to avoid it during pregnancy.

The aroma is described as buttery with a fascinating mint top note with hints of citrus; it is a fresh smelling essential oil with a clean, rich, uplifting and spiritual scent with similarities to both frankincense and elemi. It is strong, with an intense, powerful and at first almost sickly sweet, woody base note, but, after a few moments, the sickliness passes and the fragrance becomes more harmonious. The fragrance from the wood smoke is less intense than the essential oil and easier to appreciate. Like frankincense, when you smell the oil you can feel the body responding by taking deep, long, slow breaths. Palo santo adds an intense and spiritual note to blends.

Therapeutic properties

There remains much to be learned about the constituents and properties of palo santo as this essential oil is quite newly introduced into aromatherapy. However, information so far indicates that palo santo is considered to be antiseptic, anti-inflammatory, nervine, expectorant and antibacterial. Useful in a chest oil blend to help bronchial coughs, colds and influenza, it has been reported anecdotally to also help with headaches, allergies and asthma. In full-body massage palo santo helps relieve tense, painful muscles, inflammation and stiff joints. In skin care it is reputed to help regenerate healthy new skin cells.

Psychotherapeutic, spiritual and emotional benefits

Palo santo helps alleviate stress, sadness, negativity, panic and anxiety. An intense spiritual essential oil, palo santo lends itself to all forms of spiritual practice, especially meditation, and ritual; this is one of its most valuable properties. In meditation palo santo is said to promote a deep connection to the spiritual source or God. The oil promotes and enhances deep relaxation and brings about inner calm and tranquillity, while also enhancing concentration, creativity and learning. Reputed to create a heavenly presence, the smoke of burning palo santo wood is used in Ayahuasca ceremonies to release negative energy and purify and cleanse the spirit.

Its qualities in spiritual practices overlap especially with frankincense, but also myrrh, juniper and sage. It has been said that palo santo brings good fortune to those who are open to its magic. The intense calming fragrance of palo santo helps you find peace and clarity in the moment, creating happy, positive feelings. A shaman told me that palo santo is also used in rituals to help harmonise the energies between men and women, or perhaps to help men integrate more fully their anima and women their animus.

Traditional healing use

The wood and smoke especially, and to a limited extent the essential oil, of palo santo have been used for their therapeutic benefits in the traditional ethnobotanical medicine of the Andes for thousands of years, especially in Peru and Ecuador by shamans and healers. You can still find shamans and healers known as curanderos, in the Andes using palo santo in their ceremonies and healing rituals, thereby keeping alive this traditional aspect of their culture. It is believed the magic of palo santo lies in the alchemical process that happens after the death of a wise, old branch or tree. In order for palo santo to gain its magical and medicinal properties it must die a natural death. After death the wood lies in its natural habitat for four to ten years to complete its metamorphosis. Only then it is believed that its sacred, medicinal and mystical properties come alive.

Palo santo is a powerful insect repellent. The natives in Ecuador use the smoke from burning wood, as well as the oil, to protect themselves from insects such as mosquitoes and also to fragrance their homes. In folk medicine it is used to treat flu, colds, coughs, asthma and allergies as well as psoriasis, acne, wounds and sprains, and to relieve stress, headaches, anxiety, depression and inflammation. In massage oil, palo santo helps arthritis, pain and muscle aches. It is believed to stimulate the immune system and calm the nervous system to speed recovery from illness, and palo santo bark is also simmered in hot water and drunk as a tea.

The bark and other aromatic parts of the tree are burned by shamans and medicine people in ceremonies to clear, cleanse, heal and purify negative energies in the home. Much used in ancestral rituals, shamans use palo santo to clear bad energy from their bodies. It is also used to alleviate emotional pain and offer psychic protection and in healing shamanic rituals.

SUSTAINABILITY AND PROVENANCE

Palo santo aromatic trees are mostly wild crafted and sustainably harvested by local communities in the dry tropical forests of Ecuador and along the South American coastline. Palo santo trees in Ecuador and Peru are protected by national government and can only be harvested under strict conditions. Palo santo oil is concentrated and deposited in the interior of the tree trunk, a process that takes about ten years. Only aged trees and branches that fall naturally to the ground are used, and the average life of the tree is eighty to ninety years.

The essential oil is steam distilled in small quantities using traditional methods employed for many generations to ensure a high-quality essential oil produced with love and respect for the environment. Distillation produces a thin yellow or light brown essential oil. I find palo santo blends well with frankincense, elemi and myrrh, also holy basil, marjoram, rosemary, clary sage, roman chamomile, bergamot and lemon. It is best to add it drop by drop as the powerful fragrance can easily overwhelm a blend.

As the use of this potent essential oil has spread beyond South America, palo santo has caught the attention of Western scientific researchers and is being studied for possible anti-cancer effects.

Absolutes

These lovely additions to the aromatherapist's repertoire are not universally popular. There was, and for some aromatherapists still is, unease about the use of absolutes in aromatherapy. Such concern arises mostly from the method of solvent extraction, which leaves minute traces of solvents in the resulting absolute. However, modern methods of solvent extraction use less toxic solvents and now incorporate an ethanol stage, which removes all but the tiniest traces of the primary solvent. And some absolutes – as well as some essential oils – derived by carbon dioxide (CO_2) extraction rather than solvents are also more easily obtainable these days. Another concern is that there are miniscule amounts of non-volatiles in absolutes, and it is largely unknown what role they may play. Many absolutes are also very expensive. If an absolute seems comparatively cheap it may be adulterated, so it's important to buy them only from reputable suppliers.

I have always been drawn to absolutes intuitively and have used some of them therapeutically and in perfumes throughout my aromatherapy career. When I did a perfumery course some years ago, I was pleased to discover that perfumers regard absolutes very highly, and in many cases they are more valued than essential oils. One of the reasons cited is that during steam distillation to produce essential oil many of the delicate water-soluble components are lost, but that through solvent or CO_2 extraction pretty much everything survives the process and is present – in however miniscule amounts – in the absolute. Therefore, absolutes are the truest aromatic representation of the plant material; they are complete and thus could be described as more holistic than essential oils.

It is easy to 'sniff test' this theory with lavender, as lavender absolute is now quite easy to obtain. Try comparing the fragrance of one or more of the lavender essential oils with lavender absolute and see for yourself whether you find the absolute has more breadth and depth and smells more like the plant. Although it is highly likely that the essential oil with its proven reputation will remain the preferred choice for aromatherapy therapeutic practice, the absolute may prove to be useful as well. Blending the essential oil together with the absolute produces an interesting complex lavender fragrance with therapeutic value.

As perfumers use many absolutes extensively in their perfumes, and have done so for many decades with little cause for concern regarding safety or toxicity, we can deduce that a carefully selected few are also safe to use in aromatherapy in small amounts. Perhaps the miniscule traces of unknown compounds may even have a beneficial effect in combination with the other identifiable components present in the whole absolute. There are, however, always exceptions, and we should use absolutes with due care. For instance, recently some in the perfume industry have been recommending against the use of oak moss because of concerns with dermal sensitisation, so oak moss should best be avoided in aromatherapy too.

However, for the experienced professional practitioner who wishes to explore using absolutes (beyond rose and jasmine) in therapeutic practice then a delightful fragrant journey awaits. There is a range of high-quality absolutes now available. I find the intense, delightful scents of absolutes facilitates the intuitive, spiritual approach to aromatherapy, helping the therapist work with inner calm and awareness, while the client may more easily enter a deeply relaxed state, which encourages the healing process. But it is a personal decision, up to each aromatherapist to decide for herself whether to use absolutes or not, and even pure CO_2 extracted absolutes are unlikely to appeal to every aromatherapist.

I worked for a couple of years in therapy rooms in Covent Garden, a busy central London location. Clients tended to arrive highly stressed from working and travelling around in such a high-pressure environment, and I observed how they benefited considerably from massage blends incorporating absolutes that soothe nervous tension. I realised that no matter how pure the oils used in the therapy room are, the minute that people stepped out of the door onto the street they encountered air full of traffic fumes and all the other toxic airborne waste of a major city. This experience led me to believe that the therapeutic potential of some absolutes outweighs concerns about their use. I remain convinced the therapeutic value of some absolutes is significant, although it is important to use only the best quality. However, it should be noted this is a personal hypothesis, without any scientific verification.

Many aromatherapists already use rose and jasmine absolutes routinely, and may be interested to include others that appear to offer therapeutic benefit. Although the physiological actions of most absolutes may not yet be much documented, it is clear they positively affect the emotions and psyche. Absolutes tend to be deeply relaxing and euphoric, reducing stress and nervous tension. They make us feel good – a reason underpinning the long history of wearing perfume.

Unsurprisingly, given their extensive use in high-class perfumery, absolutes add a wonderful fragrant note to blends, lifting the overall scent, and just this in itself has a beneficial effect. As the smell is so powerful and concentrated, 0.5 to 1 per cent of an absolute is sufficient in a typical massage blend to enrich the overall aroma and have a therapeutic effect. I have found that using 2 to 2.5 per cent for a massage blend containing absolutes rather than the more standard 3 per cent generally works best. Below are three absolutes (alongside rose and jasmine of course) that I have found to be especially effective in aromatherapy massage, although there are several others that also seem to offer benefits.

Violet leaf (Viola Odorata or occasionally Alba)

Both the leaves and flowers of violet have a long history of traditional use in herbal medicine, stretching as far back in time as the eleventh century, when the mystic Hildegard of Bingen used violets to treat breast tumours, apparently with some success. Although herbal preparations tend to have different properties to essential oils and absolutes, the long and continuous use of violets would indicate violet leaf absolute also has some healing properties. Marguerite Maury mentioned using violet, and modern aromatherapy practice does include violet leaf, with several textbooks including descriptions of its constituents and properties.

Violet leaf absolute has a deep, mysterious, leafy-green fragrance, reminiscent of fresh mown hay, herbaceous hints and an elusive, delicate floral top note. It is much used in perfumery for its green note and as a fixative. The scent of violets has been described as being able to 'comfort and strengthen the heart'. It blends very well with rose, and also with lavender, basil, clary sage, roman chamomile, geranium, neroli, frankincense, cumin, yuzu and bergamot.

Feminine, deep, dark and mysterious, violet leaf has powerful yin energy and can help with female conditions of menstrual pains and irregularities. Its cooling yin quality helps soothe cystitis and also dry, red, itchy and sensitive skin, and violet leaf helps with thread veins and problem skin generally. Especially suited to mature skin, it may have anti-ageing regenerative properties. Violet leaf is reputed to be a liver decongestant and circulatory stimulant, and may help with bronchitis, rheumatism and sore throat and mouth infections.

However, perhaps its most useful effect is on the psyche, spirit and emotions. Professor Paolo Rovesti has used a range of essential oils and absolutes including violet leaf to help people with psychological disturbances. He comments that 'people feel transported into a different, more agreeable and acceptable world' after treatment (Rovesti cited in Tisserand 1997, pp.97–98). Violet leaf has a tonic effect on the nervous system and is good for nervousness, nervous exhaustion and tension;

it also helps with insomnia, dizziness, headaches and migraine.

Emotionally, violet leaf comforts grief and loss; it is soothing and encourages independence and acceptance of change and letting go. I found it particularly helpful in massage blends, often combined with rose, when I worked with people living with human immunodeficiency virus (HIV) and acquired immunodeficiency syndrome (AIDS). Especially helpful for those who are emotionally or psychologically disturbed or distressed, violet leaf's feminine character helps facilitate calm introspection, going deep into the psyche to uncover unresolved issues to bring about intuitive insight.

Linden blossom (Tilia Vulgaris)

This gorgeous scented absolute comes from the flowers of the lime or linden tree. The flowers have a long history of traditional use in herbal medicine, especially as a herbal infusion or tisane, which is used as a tea to calm the nerves and digestion and to promote restful sleep. Culpepper described linden flowers as a 'good cephalic and nervine, excellent for apoplexy, epilepsy, vertigo and palpitations of the heart' (cited in Lawless 1992, pp.122–123), and it would appear the absolute shares some of these qualities, as its powerful fragrance is so deeply calming.

Linden blossom is used in perfumery for its exquisite fragrance. It is also mentioned in a few aromatherapy textbooks; for instance in her excellent and comprehensive *The Encyclopaedia of Essential Oils* (1992), Julia Lawless lists linden blossom as helping cramps, indigestion, liver pains, headaches, insomnia, migraine, nervous tension and stress-related conditions. However, linden blossom does not yet much feature in aromatherapy therapeutic practice, although it may become more widely embraced as it becomes better known.

Linden blossom has an intense, sweet, floral, honeyed fragrance with herbaceous, hay-like and green notes. If you are fortunate to live near a lime tree, try standing underneath it when the flowers are in full bloom to appreciate its exquisite scent, which is so deliciously calming and relaxing it can be difficult to move on. I find linden blossom blends especially well with the citrus oils, which lighten the powerful heavy sweetness. It also blends with other florals, roman chamomile, clary sage, frankincense, elemi, black pepper, ginger and holy basil.

Deeply relaxing and soothing, linden blossom is excellent for nervous tension, anxiety, exhaustion, hysteria and all stress-related conditions. It seems to have a calming, sedative and tonic action and I have found linden blossom to work much like rose, jasmine, melissa and neroli. The powerful fragrance induces an almost hypnotic state in which clients can emotionally more easily let go of troubling issues and also physical tension in the body.

As with all absolutes, a little goes a long way, especially when linden blossom is used to ameliorate headaches and an overactive mind, as using too much can actually bring on a headache. But one, two or a maximum of three drops in a relaxing massage blend can really help bring about a deep, calm healing state, transporting the client to a sweetly scented meditative and transformative inner space.

*Narcissus (*Narcissus poeticus*)*

Narcissus has a long tradition of use, as far back in time as when the Arabs were beginning to distil essential oils for formulating into perfumes. The Romans also used narcissus in perfume. There are spiritual connotations as narcissus, mixed with other fragrant oils, is used in India as an anointing oil before entering into temples for prayer, puja and meditation. The name comes from the Greek *narkao*, meaning 'to be numb', and Narcissus also features in Greek legend.

The god Narcissus was a handsome young male god, but so vain that he fell in love with his own image reflected in a pool of water. Unfortunately for Narcissus, the pool belonged to the nymph Echo. She became incensed when Narcissus preferred to gaze adoringly at his own image, completely neglecting to look at her and appreciate her beauty. So enraged was Echo that she commanded the water nymphs who lived by the pool to seize his soul, whereupon he died. His fate was to spring up every year as a spring flower.

This legend gives an idea of the character of Narcissus as being introspective and uninterested in, or literally 'numb' to, others. Unhealthy narcissism is when people are unable to form intimate relationships; they have such an inflated self-love they are unable to detect their own flaws. However, healthy narcissism is a natural part of growing up, and forms the basis of adult self-esteem and healthy ego. Narcissus absolute is narcotic and sedative, and therefore may help create introspection – a looking inward that when directed can be healthy self-assessment rather than unproductive navel gazing.

The fragrance is heady, sweet, green herbaceous with a beguiling heavy floral note. Narcissus is used in top-end perfumes. It enhances most blends and works particularly well with other florals, clove bud, cardamom, sandalwood and patchouli. There is little documented use in aromatherapy, but I have found narcissus beneficial in blends when there is hysteria, a need to 'switch off' from work or obsession. Narcissus is valuable to include in blends for spiritual enquiry and self-growth, and to bring about a languid, hypnotic, soporific, relaxed state. Great care is needed with narcissus, as it is emetic and irritant when too much is used. However, one or two drops maximum in a massage blend can be effective and beneficial.

I once had a client – an actress – who was creative and powerful; she knew exactly what she wanted and intended to have it. Unable to find a more conventional blend that satisfied her, after several attempts I came up with lavender: 5 drops, basil: 3 drops and narcissus:

2 drops in 20ml of almond oil, thus just over 2 per cent total. She adored this blend and requested it at every treatment. It worked very well for her, allowing her to switch off from whatever role she was playing, facilitating a useful introspective mood and bringing about deep relaxation. I also appreciated this surprisingly lovely blend and have used it on other occasions with equal success.

ENDNOTE

My heartfelt hope is that this book on intuitive aromatherapy will enrich the practice of professionals and offer insights, new ways of working and inspiration to all of you who love, play and work with essential oils. What has been described here is, however, more than just tips on enhancing the work of aromatherapists. Developing intuition is not only about using it as a skill to facilitate and enhance our aromatherapy work, although that is of fundamental importance in this context. Cultivating intuitive ability is also a path of self-growth – part of a spiritual journey that can benefit all areas of our lives.

I hope you take sufficient time to embrace fully the information and different exercises, meditations and rituals offered in the book and then put them into practice with an open mind and heart. In this way you create a process of learning about and developing intuitive skills that will last a lifetime if you are willing to seriously engage with this inner growth work.

If we delve deep into our psyches we discover what lies beneath the surface of superficial thoughts and mundane behaviour. We uncover aspects of ourselves that, when brought into the light of consciousness and integrated, contribute to fulfilling the potential of what it means to be a human being. Then we live our lives more abundantly, and the wiser, more compassionate and more skilful we become, the better able we are to practise our healing arts for the benefit of all.

BIBLIOGRAPHY

Ashcroft-Nowicki, D. (1990) *First Steps in Ritual*. London: Thorsons.

Auel, J. M. (1980) *The Clan of the Cave Bear: Earth's Children*. London: Hodder and Stoughton.

Batchelor, M. (2001) *Meditation for Life*. London: Frances Lincoln.

Batchelor, S. (1997) *Buddhism without Beliefs*. New York, NY: Riverhead Books.

Bates, B. (1996) *The Way of Wyrd*. London: Arrow Books.

Battaglia, S. (2003) *The Complete Guide to Aromatherapy* (second edition). Brisbane: The International Centre of Holistic Aromatherapy.

Culpepper, N. (1952) *Culpepper's Complete Herbal*. London: W. Foulsham and Co, Ltd.

Davis, P. (1988) *Aromatherapy: An A–Z*. Saffron Walden: C. W. Daniel.

Davis, P. (1991) *Subtle Aromatherapy*. London: Ebury Publishing.

Davis, P. (2002) *Astrological Aromatherapy*. Saffron Walden: C. W. Daniel.

Eliot, T.S. (1986 [1943]) *Four Quartets*. London: Faber and Faber.

Farrer-Halls, G. (2000) *The Illustrated Encyclopedia of Buddhist Wisdom A Complete Introduction to the Principles and Practices of Buddhism*. New Alresford: Godsfield Press.

Farrer-Halls, G. (2001) *Meditations and Rituals Using Aromatherapy Oils*. Newton Abbot: Godsfield Press.

Farrer-Halls, G. (2009) *The Aromatherapy Bible* (second edition). London: Octopus Publishing Group.

Fischer-Rizzi, S. (1990) *Complete Aromatherapy Handbook*. New York, NY: Sterling Publishing Co.

Grieve, M. (1931) *A Modern Herbal*. New York, NY: Harcourt, Brace and Co.

Irwin, E. (1999) *Healing Relaxation*. London: Rider.

Lawless, J. (1992) *The Encyclopedia of Essential Oils*. Shaftesbury: Element Books.

Lawless, J. (1997) *The Complete Illustrated Guide to Aromatherapy: A Practical Approach to the Use of Essential Oils for Health and Well-Being*. Shaftesbury: Element Books.

Lawless, J. (1998) *Aromatherapy and the Mind: An Exploration into the Psychological and Emotional Effects of Essential Oils*. London: Thorsons.

Lawless, J. (2006) *The Fragrant Garden: Growing and Using Scented Plants*. London: Kyle Cathie Limited.

Mailhebiau, P. (1995) *Portraits in Oils: The Personality of Aromatherapy Oils and Their Link with Human Temperaments*. Saffron Walden: C. W. Daniel.

Maury, M. (1989) *Marguerite Maury's Guide to Aromatherapy*. Saffron Walden: C.W. Daniel.

Mojay, G. (1997) *Aromatherapy for Healing the Spirit: A Guide to Restoring Mental and Emotional Balance Through Essential Oils*. London: Gaia Books.

Rhind, J. (2013) *Essential Oils: A Handbook for Aromatherapy Practice* (second edition). London and Philadelphia: Singing Dragon.

Sargent, D. (1994) *Global Ritualism*. St Paul, MN: Llewellyn Publications.

Sellar, W. (2005) *The Directory of Essential Oils*. London: Ebury Publishing.

Tisserand, R. (1997) *The Art of Aromatherapy*. Saffron Walden: C. W. Daniel.

Worwood, V. A. (1987) *Aromantics*. London: Pan Books.

Worwood, V. A. (1990) *The Fragrant Pharmacy*. London: Macmillan.

Worwood, V. A. (1998) *The Fragrant Mind: Aromatherapy for Personality, Mind, Mood and Emotion*. London: Bantam Books.

Worwood, V. A. (2012) *The Fragrant Heavens: The Spiritual Dimension of Fragrance and Aromatherapy*. London: Bantam Books.

CPI Antony Rowe
Eastbourne, UK
October 20, 2023

remarkable, and I received similar help at the archives of the Affaires Etrangères. Again at the Conservatoire National des Arts et Métiers, I was able to see records with great facility through the efforts of Dominique Ferriot, Directeur of the Musée National des Techniques, adding to earlier kindnesses. Again at CNAM, Alain Mercier helped my studies and has recently taken great trouble with the provision of illustrations for this book. Access to the archives of Saint-Gobain was granted many years ago by the kind offices of Dominique Perrin, and he and Maurice Hamon have allowed me to use an illustration from that source.

It is impossible to record all the help I have received from British librarians and archivists. But I would give particular thanks to Gaye Blake Roberts for access to material owned by the Wedgwood Museum, to John Powell of the Ironbridge Gorge Museum Library, to David de Haan at Ironbridge for advice and help with illustrations and the use of material from the Elton Collection. Penny Pemberton and Len MacDonald, former Pilkington archivists, always made new acquisitions known to me, while Dinah Stobbs has made illustrations from that archive available for this volume. Over may years Ben Benedicz of the special collections department of Birmingham University Library lent generous polymathic expertise to every enquiry. His successors have helped with last-minute problems, while the staff of Birmingham City Archives have solved others and aided my search for illustrations.

In the task of co-ordinating material on technology transfer gathered over many years (not always with industrial espionage as the prime element in the research), of dealing with archive centres in Britain and abroad, helping to identify and, if possible, fill gaps in the information I had gathered, I had the help of Sarah Blowen as research associate during 1990–91. Her immediate perception of the nature and purpose of the project, her flair for research, and her tolerance of the eccentricities of an elderly colleague, have all contributed to a more complete and balanced survey than I could otherwise have achieved. My former colleagues, Rick Garside and Adrian Randall, have provided me with valuable resources in my retirement, and Leonard Schwarz has always been ready to talk over the most abstruse topics.

Finally, I have to thank Paul Harris for taking time off from his own researches to read much of the book in draft, providing the viewpoint of a different kind of historian, and much improving the muddier passages of my writing.

The Nuffield Foundation originally enabled my first forays into technology transfer, and again assisted at a later stage; SSRC and later

ESRC provided funding which enabled a substantial book, and not only specialist articles, to result from my studies. They have my sincere gratitude.

This book has been longer in the writing than I would have wished. My wife Thelma, who had been the source of comfort and strength for forty years, became mysteriously, but apparently not seriously, ill in 1993, but was found to have brain cancer at the beginning of the following year, and died within a few weeks. We had looked forward together to dedicating the book to her, and no one could have deserved it more. After some inevitable delay I now have to dedicate it lovingly to her memory, and I have joined to hers the names of those she most loved.

J. R. H.

Foreword

It is a sad duty to present the work of a late friend, especially when it is such an outstanding book. It is sad that John Harris did not see this masterpiece in print, although he had completed it to the last comma when he died suddenly. He had originally planned to dedicate it to his wife, Thelma, 'a source of comfort and strength for forty years', and a delightful person. Actually, she died three years before him and he could only dedicate his book to her memory. Still, this volume will be a lasting memorial to both of them.

It embodies an enormous amount of research, carried out over almost thirty years. However, one can perhaps be surprised that John Harris (1923–97) devoted so much of his time to French industrial espionage. He had grown up in Lancashire, and his first book, written with his school and university friend, Theo Barker, dealt with the growth of St Helens during the Industrial Revolution; it was followed by a biography of 'the Copper King', Thomas Williams. Then, in 1970, after teaching at the University of Liverpool, John Harris was appointed to the Chair of Economic History at the University of Birmingham. He might – to borrow the words of another late friend – have continued to exploit 'the gold mine' of the Industrial Revolution heartlands' history.

However, he was led, by questions such as the copper sheathing of ships, to take an interest – which continued to increase – in transfers of technology between Britain and France in the eighteenth century. This problem had been studied by Charles Ballot (who was killed in World War I and whose book was posthumously published), and later by W. O. Henderson. But John Harris soon discovered that massive archival sources remained unexplored, especially in France, where an interventionist state had left detailed records of its attempts to discover England's technological secrets. With the modesty which was so typical of him, John Harris mentions his 'limited and bad French', but this handicap – if it indeed existed – was overcome, and he made an amazing range of *trouvailles* in French archives from Lorient to Le Creusot, and, of course, in Paris. His inaugural lecture of 1972 proved how well he had mastered the subject.

After writing a number of articles, which are collected in *Essays in Industry and Technology in the Eighteenth Century* (Variorum, 1992), John Harris undertook to write the present book, which puts together, in a continuum, the results of his research and reflections, and which includes several completely new studies.

To some people, who only like macro-economics, industrial espionage may seem a trivial topic. Actually, readers of this book will find some cloak-and-dagger stories, but first and foremost an in-depth understanding of eighteenth-century economies. When following both French inspectors of manufactures in the French provinces and French spies in English manufacturing districts, they will find many insights into the two countries' industries, and also into the working of the French bureaucracy which managed economic affairs.

John Harris has also brought to life again many craftsmen, engineers, manufacturers and adventurers (such as Le Turc, in Chapter 17): the kind of people from the 'middling' or 'lower orders' who are elusive and too often absent from history books. But he also presents much new information on his leading characters: the Holkers, Trudaines, Wilkinsons, Milnes etc. In his hands (to use his own final words), the history of industrial espionage was 'one means of restoring the thoughts and activities of human beings to the centre stage of industrial history, from which a generation of writing dominated by economic analysis had largely banished them'. Indeed, he stressed the role of individuals: 'The remarkable thing is how few men, if well chosen, could impart a major technology'.

A careful and rigorous scholar, who was not keen on grand theorizing, John Harris was nonetheless ready to generalize from a solid factual base, as is obvious in Part 6 of this volume, especially in Chapters 20–22, where French efforts to acquire British technology and their results are critically appraised, with clear-cut conclusions. Industrial espionage was of 'overwhelming importance' in eighteenth-century transfers of technology. Thanks to spying, the French obtained – and often quickly – 'whatever technology they wanted'. But the results were disappointing to them: some transfers totally failed, while in other cases only a sub-British standard of technology was operated in France. John Harris carefully analysed the reasons for this failure, with brilliant pages on British *techniciens* and workmen who were suborned to work in France, but were often restless and too fond of the bottle. He also stressed that good craftsmen demanded good tools, which were not available in France, largely because they were related to the new and unfamiliar territory of coal-fuel technology (a concept which was Harris's crucial contribution to the understanding of the Industrial Revolution).

It is rarely that a work of history can be called 'definitive', or almost so, but this monumental book fully deserves this designation.

François Crouzet
The Sorbonne

Abbreviations

Introduction

In the late 1960s I made some studies of British industries in the early eighteenth century in which coal-based technologies were a novel element, and critical in their development. It occurred to me that it might be worthwhile to look at French industries of the period, to see how far a much lesser experience with coal-fuel technologies might have set them at a comparative disadvantage with those of Britain. If this seemed to be the case, it might by reflection further emphasize the importance and singularity of these technologies to Britain, as she advanced towards industrial revolution. Dubious as to whether I could resurrect a mere reading knowledge of a language which I had neglected for quarter of a century, and equally dubious as to whether French archives contained really relevant materials, I received the most friendly and heartening encouragement from two eminent French historians, François Crouzet and François Caron. Originally only intending to write a single paper, I was led deeper into the comparative study of French and British industries by two influences. One was that a concurrent study of the regional origins of industrial revolution in Britain was inhibited by causes beyond my control. The other was the fascinating, compelling richness of French industrial history sources, primarily the records of the Bureau of Commerce in the national archives.

It now seemed possible to write some papers which should be case studies of the transfer of industrial technology between the two countries, in which the theme of coal-fuel technology could continue to have a place. This was done over the next few years for several industries where the archival evidence, particularly the French archival evidence, was very rich. The industries selected were the plate-glass industry, the Birmingham hardware industry and the steel industry.

1

As these studies progressed, and inevitably evidence for other industries was found by the way, it became increasingly obvious that industrial espionage was extensively employed, mainly (but not exclusively) by the French, to achieve technological transfer between the two countries. In the case of the French this was an activity encouraged, but also commonly undertaken, by the state. In this it was paralleled by some other European countries. In the 1980s I used the opportunity presented by the giving of an L. T. C. Rolt memorial lecture to make a first general overview of the importance of industrial espionage in the transfer of technology in the eighteenth century, and particularly that carried out by France.

French industrial espionage was overwhelmingly concentrated on Britain, and by mid-century the first response to learning of British inventions was to acquire them by covert means, rather than 're-invent what had already been discovered by the English'.[1] While the French operation might have been the largest and the most broadly targeted as compared with those of other European countries, it was certainly not isolated, let alone unique. The concentration of industrial espionage on Britain was a clear indication that other nations believed that a technological lead had now been established there, in contrast to past centuries in which Britain had been predominantly a technological debtor. Similarly the effort made by Britain from the early eighteenth century to put legal restrictions on the transfer of technologies abroad by forbidding the free emigration or the foreign recruitment of those possessing critical skills, indicated a consciousness that the nation now possessed native technologies which it should reserve to itself as long as possible. There may have been cases in particular countries where there was not immediate reaction to attempts to take their technologies abroad,[2] but certainly from the mid-eighteenth century, possibly a little earlier, the resistance to industrial espionage was a fair barometric indicator of a British consciousness of growing technological superiority.

Industrial espionage had considerable coverage in two classic accounts of technology transfer, those of Ballot[3] and Henderson.[4] Nevertheless from the late 1950s it rarely justified specific treatment either in works on the British industrial revolution, or in those of foreign nations endeavouring to industrialize on the British pattern, and it is hard to find a listing even in their indexes. But there were papers in the mid-to-late 1970s in which industrial espionage in Britain was a substantial, even a central theme, and in 1981 the subject was treated in a classic work on technology transfer. Major conferences have subsequently arranged workshops or panels on the topic, and a French conference devoted its entire proceedings to the subject in 1996. Scandinavian scholars have been particularly important in the renewed study of industrial espionage, as two books published in the last few years make clear.[5]

Industrial espionage has of course continued, and is still with us, though there will be no attempt to give an account of it here. Much of the intelligence effort of the Cold War era was devoted to military-industrial intelligence, often by the bribery or suborning of those having access to the secrets of military technology in potentially enemy countries.[6] As we will see, espionage on military-industrial technologies was strongly present in the eighteenth century.[7] In modern, primarily civilian, technology there has been much attention given to massive attempts at industrial espionage like those in computers carried out by Hitachi at IBM and recently in the automobile industry by Volkswagen at General Motors. Intelligence agencies in the countries formerly arrayed in opposite blocks in the Cold War might have been expected to face a reduction in influence and funds as the threat of military confrontation dramatically receded. However, this has not necessarily been the case. To take one example, it appears that in France intelligence services have moved into a higher gear. The emphasis there now is on economic intelligence, which entails a mixture of commercial and technological espionage. President Chirac is said to have set up a special economic and technological intelligence coordination body, in part inspired by Japanese intelligence achievements. The USA is a particular target, and the CIA has accused the French of 'launching intelligence operations against US military contractors and high technology firms', and of having 'recruited agents at the European offices of three US computer and electronics firms'.[8] The ghosts of the Trudaines and of Tolozan, whose eighteenth-century ministerial activities we will be examining, no doubt approve Chirac's initiative.

The First Legislation: Causes and Implementation

PART ONE

The First Legislation:
Causes and Implementation

1 John Law, the Suborning of British Workers, and Legislation against Industrial Espionage

Towards the end of the second decade of the eighteenth century there was a sudden and unprecedented attempt to take British technology to France. This had the effect of shocking the nation into realizing that it now possessed technologies which it would be very undesirable to lose to a foreign competitor, and into going further and setting up the first important legislation to protect its technologies from international robbery. The concern about the French theft of British technology by suborning skilled workers was briefly associated with fears about the possible transfer abroad of British skills by our allowing foreigners to be placed as apprentices here, the main interest being in Russian apprentices. Though in the end no laws were passed about such apprenticeships, the two worries reinforced each other, so that there was a new awareness of the dangers of losing British skills to foreign countries.

The existence of British legislation against the emigration of skilled workers and the export of machinery is perhaps still most remembered for the debate at the time of abolition, and the apparently incontrovertible arguments of the free-traders who successfully campaigned for its ending. But the circumstances of its first introduction seem largely disregarded, though they throw very interesting light on early eighteenth-century attitudes to the transfer of technology abroad. In effect the legislation marks national recognition of Britain's change from being a debtor to becoming a creditor nation technologically. The chief

7

incident which prompted the legislation of 1719 was remarkable for the scale of technological transfer it encompassed, the range of skills involved, the measures government was prepared to take to repatriate emigrated workers, and some of the people who played leading parts.[1]

There were two reasons for the agitation which arose early in 1719 against the emigration of English skilled workers. The most important was a large movement of workers to France in a considerable number of trades, which was specifically organized by the French controller-general. The second derived from Russian efforts to learn English technology in England. In January 1719 the Master and officers of the Company of Cutlers in the Sheffield district (Hallamshire) petitioned the Commons that action should be taken against those whom they believed threatened a nationally valuable industry and one which was an important employer. They declared that 'ill disposed persons' collaborating with foreigners to 'transplant the Cutlery, and other Branches of the Iron Trade', had shipped several workers and their families overseas from both Newcastle and London and in particular had built 'Furnaces for the making of Steel' abroad. There had also been an attempt 'to ... place Foreigners Servants and Apprentices into the Manufactories of Iron and Steel' in Britain, but the main concern was the efforts to entice the Company's cutlery workers.[2] The Commons appointed a committee to investigate and report, adding to named members all those for the counties of Yorkshire, Shropshire, Derbyshire, Middlesex, Northumberland and Warwickshire 'and all the Merchants of the House'. Warwick may well have been included because of advance knowledge of another petition which was reported to the House ten days later from the ironmongers (i.e. inland merchants in iron and iron goods) cutlers, smiths and artificers around Birmingham. They complained that 'there hath been several foreigners, which as the Petitioners are informed are Muskovites' recently apprenticed in the district to learn trades practised there, for whom unusually high premiums had been paid. Once trained they intended to return to 'his Czarish Majesty's dominions' to train others. This, it was extravagantly claimed, would be 'of unspeakable Prejudice to our Iron Manufactory, and tend to the ruin of many Thousand Families' in the area.[3] The complaint was directed to the existing committee, which was shortly afterwards required to consider a further petition from London ironmongers and others against the enticement abroad of workers in iron, steel, tin, brass and other metals 'by offering excessive Wages, large promises, and other Arts'.

The Commons Committee examined two witnesses, one of whom was a man of much importance in the iron and steel trades, John Crowley (given as Crawley) whose father, Sir Ambrose, had established on the Derwent, a tributary of the Tyne, a great range of works for the making of goods in iron and steel, and for the making of cementation steel.[4] The witnesses confirmed both the inveigling of British workers abroad and the apprenticing of foreigners here, and a Bill was to be drawn up to deal with the two problems.[5] As the Bill, prepared with urgency, was read for the first time a few days later, a further petition came in from the Master and Company of the Clockmakers of London. Their petition resembled the previous one, it included watchmakers as well as clockmakers and it claimed to represent not only the London company but 'Hundreds more in Great Britain'. It made clear that their complaint was against the enticement of workers to France. At the point of third reading the Bill was directed to problems of iron and steel manufacturers and to apprenticeship as well as enticement.[6]

As it reached the Lords the enticement section seems to have broadened to include manufactures generally and the apprentice element was still there. At the Committee stage in the Lords a clause was added to make the statute operable in Scotland and another was proposed by way of amendment. This would have provided that foreigners should not be allowed to become apprentices in Great Britain without surety that they should not leave the country for seven years after completing the apprenticeship, unless given official permission, while British subjects who broke the law by apprenticing foreigners without the proper security should be disbarred from practising their trade for a similar period. However, this clause was lost on a vote and the apprenticeship provisions seem to have disappeared at this point, perhaps by virtue of the fact that it was felt that this clause would be very difficult to enforce if applied to the citizens of all countries. The Commons accepted the revision, the Act receiving the royal assent on 18 April.[7]

The first major Act against the transfer of British technology abroad was thus concentrated upon that aspect which related to the enticement of skilled workers and affected both enticers and enticed, so that an activity which was a common constituent of what would now be called industrial espionage became illegal. Henceforth anyone who enticed or tried to persuade any skilled worker in wool, iron, steel, brass or metal, or any clockmaker or watchmaker 'or any other artificer or manufacturer of Great Britain' to go abroad, and was convicted of it at quarter sessions or assizes, could be fined up to £100 for a first offence and imprisoned for three months, to be continued until the fine was paid. Second offenders could be fined at the court's discretion and imprisoned for twelve months, continuable again until the fine was paid. But prosecution had to begin within a year of the offence. Any workman going abroad to work at his trade or to teach it to foreigners, or anyone already abroad, was to return in six months, once warned to do so by a member of the diplomatic service or a secretary of state. Failure to respond would prevent the emigré from inheriting property in Britain or exercising control of it, and his landed and personal property in Britain could be forfeit to the Crown and he deemed alien. Those accused of enticing or being enticed could be required to provide bail until their trial or be held in prison if they did not provide it. Artisans convicted of an attempt or intention to go abroad to work had to give security against their repeating the attempt in future.[8]

Although trade organizations were instrumental in 1719 in instigating and maintaining the Commons' investigations into the migration of skilled labour from Britain, the Government was already aware of the problem. The Commissioners for Trade and the Plantations had realized that there was an outflow of valuable workers to France as early as November 1718, when they had had correspondence from Sir William Blackett in Newcastle, who enclosed a letter, which was almost certainly intercepted or provided by an informer, from a certain 'Sally' [Sully] at Versailles about English ironworkers going to France. It was this correspondence which had made commissioners enquire whether the king had legal powers to stop his subjects emigrating and employing their crafts abroad, or any right to require their return. By December, well in advance of the parliamentary petitions, they had been considering how an effective preventative clause could be put into an Act. The impetus to legislate had, therefore, arisen in government circles, and had not just been the response of an unknowing administration to vigorous proddings from provincial and London manufacturers.

However, once moves were afoot, they did not lack support. A broadsheet, possibly of the kind commonly printed to be handed to members of both Houses of Parliament and other influential persons, 'Reasons for Passing the Bill', stated the case more sensationally. It proclaimed, 'there are already great numbers enticed, and gone out of the Kingdom, and strenuous endeavours are made to persuade great numbers to follow them, and some of those enticed by them are worth near £1000 which they got by their trade'. Not only would this be disruptive to our foreign trade, but, where men went by themselves 'the Wives and Children of the Artificers ... will be a heavy burden to the parishes to which they belong'. There was some inconsistency here: wealthy tradesmen would be well able to take their families with them, or arrange for them to join them once the expert was established in a new country. Was it in fact the wealthy, or those in embarrassed circumstances who would be most liable to be enticed? Another representation, in the form of a parliamentary petition from London metalworkers and clockmakers, was made – in stronger terms than those in the *Commons Journals* – claiming 'that above 2000 Working men of Several kinds [in these trades] have been lately drawn into France, Russia and other Countrys', and supporting the representations of the Sheffield cutlers, who would not want the expense of a private Act, and backing the idea of a public one. The number of emigrating workmen was probably exaggerated and, given government interest, the need for a private Act seems unlikely. Even the passing of the Act in 1719 did not end the lobbying which now turned to its enforcement. In July traders in iron, steel, clocks, watches and other goods complained of the continuing problem of the seduction of workers. They still went abroad in numbers despite the Act 'in order to teach foreigners their several callings to the manifest prejudice of their native Country'. Within the last four or five weeks twenty had left the Thames on one ship and forty on another, and, despite the Act, clear instructions had not yet been given to the Customs officers to inspect ships and bring suspected tradesman emigrants ashore and demand security against departure. This petition was clearly of substance for it was presented by twenty petitioners and included the names of around eighty emigrant workmen, nearly all listed according to their trades.[9]

The legislation of 1719 against enticement of skilled workers overseas was extremely broad in its wording when it came to the destination of such workers. In effect, however, it was at the time specifically aimed at two foreign powers, France and Russia. Although the activities of the Russians caused alarm in official and industrial circles for a short period, this soon subsided, for the real problem lay with the French. In their case there was a substantial seduction of workmen even though the figure of 2,000 given in the broadsheet was obviously alarmist.[10] Closer proximity made migration easier to France than to Russia, and continuous political and commercial rivalry throughout the eighteenth century led to the French threat being treated very seriously at all levels. While all other artificers and manufacturers were

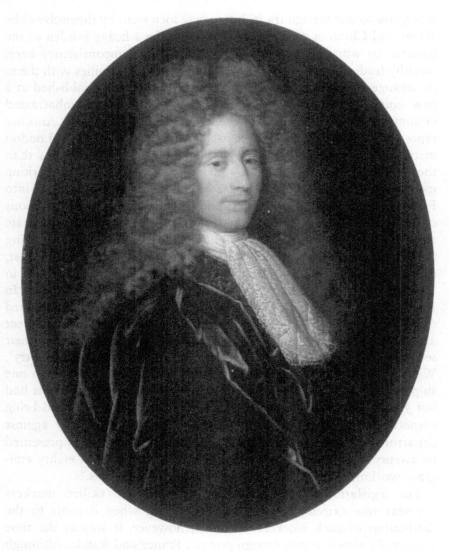

1.1   John Law by Alexis Simon Belle, 1720

included in the Act, the specific mention of wool, iron, steel, brass and horological tradesmen fits very closely the type of workmen who were currently being enticed to France. The French with their more developed industrial sector and better educated workforce presented a greater challenge than the Russians.

The seduction of British workmen was part of a grand scheme, not without some echo of the vaster financial schemes of the celebrated John Law, and it coincided with the peak of Law's influence under the Regency of the Duke of Orléans, with his final advancement to the position of first minister or Controller-General of Finances and, in its collapse, with the collapse of the Banque Royale and Law's disgrace and flight. As early as 1703, when he was travelling in Europe, Law had made proposals to the French government about industrial development in the districts of Lyons, Forez and the Beaujolais.[11]

There seems to have been a conscious concentration by Law on the enticement of workers in industries in which there was a British technological or skill advantage, for instance cementation steel production, watch-making, lock-making, one branch of glass-making (presumably flint glass, the only one where there was a distinctive British process) some kinds of iron manufacture (in which foundry work was prominent) and some aspects of naval design and technology, in which the new technique of bending timbers by steam heat was important. For a time John Law employed his brother William as a main intermediary in Britain. This may partly be due to his own difficult legal status in England following his conviction for causing a death by duelling, but is likely to be more concerned with his increasing and intense involvement with French finance and government in these years and the consequent need to devolve responsibility to his brother. There were two particular areas in France where the immigrant industrial workers were located. In the Paris area watchmakers were concentrated at Versailles and to some extent at Saint Germain, and there were foundry workers at Chaillot. In Normandy there was a group of works for several trades around Harfleur and in Honfleur, the names understandably leading to some confusion in contemporary English sources. Some of the industrial sites were on a private estate recently purchased by John Law. This may have been more a matter of patronage than the pursuit of personal profit; a number of prominent French ministers fostered infant industries on their properties during the eighteenth century.

The masters and workmen who emigrated to France before the enactment of the 1719 statute had, of course, committed no offence, though they may have been liable to the loss of certain rights of property and citizenship if they did not return after being told to do so. There were two serious difficulties in the way of their return, however. Some of them had no means to travel because of the collapse of the concerns in which they were involved, whether due to the fall of Law and the depreciation of the paper money with which they were paid, or to the debts they owed to local creditors. Secondly, many of them had been readily recruited for French service because they had contracted large debts in their home country, and it was largely fear of the pressure of their creditors or of debtor's prison that had led them to leap at the proposition of free travel to France and security of employment there. Hard as their situation was in France, prospects of penury and prison hovered over many if they returned. As a result, the Crown took the remarkable step of making available the sum of £3,000 to assist their return, and to help them to come to acceptable arrangements with their creditors. In itself this is a strong tribute to the importance the Government attached to the repatriation of these skilled workers.

How many workers were involved, and in what trades? It is difficult to be sure, but a rough estimate would indicate that about seventy watchmakers went over to France, a figure that has backing from both French and English sources. English lists would give fifty-three, if we try to avoid double counting on the one hand and include anonymous relatives and apprentices who are mentioned on the other. At least fourteen glass-makers are listed. Metalworkers number over thirty. Primary iron production is not mentioned, which is not surprising, for apart from the novel and hardly more than embryonic coke-iron process, it is hard to see what British ironmasters would be able to teach French ones at this date. Other trades which are mentioned are lock-making and file-making, steel-making, hinge-making and grinding. There are two smiths for ships' work, an anchorsmith, as well as founders. The founders who were at Chaillot are not clearly numbered and might considerably extend the total. Finally there was a woollen manufactory at Charlaval which seems to have been important, but only seven workers there are specifically named, though there may have been over eighty persons involved. The very minimum is therefore around 120 workers and managers, and it is likely that the total emigration, if we include some wives and children, would be well over 200. Some very important emigrants, like John May mentioned below, do not appear on lists but are obliquely or anonymously mentioned; for instance there was at least one tobacco worker. Law's scheme was certainly a major operation carried through with some of the ambition and grandeur that characterized his financial plans.

Much can be learned from the papers relating to the British government's attempts to recall and repatriate the workers from France. These attempts seem to have already begun under the embassy of Lord Stair, but were completed under that of Sir Robert Sutton. For instance, we know from Henry Sully ('the chief enticer') that when living in Paris in February 1718 he had been approached by Law who already had the idea of starting some 'Manufacturys' in France. Sully was a very clever watchmaker, of French ancestry, but brought up in England, who had achieved some prominence through his technical, mathematical and linguistic abilities. He gave Law his 'lights' on the matter and was sent to England next month to 'lay the Foundations of these Establishments', finding someone to head each, as well as workmen to make up the numbers required. He was specious, adept at self-promotion, willing to turn his coat rapidly, and noticeably lacking in loyalty or gratitude for past favours. His statement that he quickly realized that Law 'had no other view in these establishments, than to augment his Credit and render himself popular' must be taken with caution. It is more credible, however, that as 'Law's honours and dignities increased upon him, perhaps faster than he expected, his attention for his Manufacturys grew much slackened' and more was left to his brother William 'who is a man of a mean genius, and with whom the being a Scotsman or a Jacobite, or both, were the best titles to favour'. Sully mentions his own dismissal as head of the Versailles watch concern as if it were part of a conspiracy to sack the best managers of the English works, saying that it led to trouble, particularly for the workers, at all of the concerns. However, he had the grace to admit that Law had generously compensated him for the loss of his post.[12]

An interesting letter came from Lewis Douglas, who was probably an intelligence agent of Stair's in France and later was employed by Sutton. This states that he had given information to Stair which, Douglas claimed, led to the 'Destruction of all the English manufactures in France', and that he had gone to Rouen to help English workmen imprisoned there. He warned Lord Townsend against a group who had lately returned to England and been recommended by Sutton to the authorities back home though they had been 'Directors of English Manufactures' in France. Sutton did not know them in their true colours as Stair had done: 'there are not greater Enemies to the Government in the Kingdom than these men are'. They had started the English manufactures and kept them going as long as they could, and the four principals had only gone to Sutton to proffer their help in repatriating the workmen after they themselves had been without work for six months following the collapse of Law's affairs. In France they used 'in Publick Company ... to impose the Pretender's health on others and drink confusion to King George'. They were now conspiring to prevent the successful English prosecution of a man called Briggs (who had taken to France the English workers later imprisoned at Rouen) and to intimidate witnesses at his trial. These men, who boasted that they had tricked and fooled the British government, were being trusted with its money in the payment of compensation to repatriated workers.[13]

For his part Sully did not point out that he and his associates had hung on to their manufactures as long as possible, but rather hinted that he had been an innocent victim of Law's bubble: 'having been a great sufferer in the ill turn the affairs of France have taken this last year 1720, and nearly ruined as many thousands have been; I began to think of quitting a country so unhappily governed', overlooking the fact that 'the shipwreck of the year twenty' had been pretty severe in England too.[14] Henry Sully presented himself, his brother Richard and William Blakey, as men wrongly dismissed from their expatriate manufactures (though he had headed a subsequent concern, the existence of which he played down). Blakey had originally run the iron and steel works at Harfleur, while Richard Sully, after being the English agent for Law's French industrial concerns while they were being set up – no doubt, therefore, an 'enticer' of workers – had subsequently been inspector of the glass and ironworks at Honfleur.[15] All three went to see Sutton and a plan was concocted between them which led to a successful application to the Government for funds to supply a repatriation operation, a main feature being the money to pay the men's debts on their return. The operation was divided between the former managers. Henry Sully, who had been in close touch with the watchmaking colonies at Versailles and Saint Germain (his own second venture) and the Chaillot foundry, exerted influence on the workers there, and had the main liaison with the British ambassador. His brother went to Normandy where John Pagett, director of the Charlaval woollen works, was won over, sent all his workers home, and went to England himself. Blakey crossed over to England to negotiate with Craggs, the Secretary of State, who secured the Privy Council grant of £3,000 for the repatriation and debt redemption costs. Henry Sully was able to claim that his brother and he had ensured that 'there remains now not the shadow of any one of the manufacturys established by English hands in France'.

There is some surviving correspondence which further illuminates these letters of Douglas and Sully.[16] As early as the middle of 1719, a Paris embassy official had written to ask for a copy of the recent Act 'to be shown to Mr. Law's watchmakers here there's a good many of them begin to grow weary of the country and apply daily for papers to go home. I'm convinced when others see this Act they won't stand the penaltys contained in it'.[17] Stair himself took action, sending to Honfleur to persuade the journeymen and artificers of the glass manufactory to return to England.[18] At a higher level Stair made direct representations to the French Regent, the Duke of Orléans, 'that it is looked upon in England as an unkind proceeding to give countenance to the enticing away of so many of our Workmen of all Kinds'.[19] The embassy found the woollen works being set up by Law on his own estate at Tancarville near Honfleur particularly worrying. They reported that Spitalfields weavers in some numbers had already been attracted to Honfleur, and the coastal position encouraged the smuggling in of English wool as well as workers.[20] German workers with a new secret were being added to the steelworks; a 'famous workman from England' had joined the ironworks; English workers were being attracted by being allowed religious freedom and a Church of England minister and the *droit d'aubaine* (the reversion to the Crown of the estate of a non-naturalized alien) was being set aside. Countermeasures must have seemed all the more timely to the embassy, for Law had just begun his short incumbency as controller-general.[21] A kind of tug of war occurred over a dozen English workers whom Stair had given a passport to return to England but had been arrested and imprisoned at Rouen and Dieppe, and threatened with transportation to Mississippi, as Stair's passport had not been considered valid. Stair saw the Regent who declared the workers free to go home. However, Law sent a certain Jones, presumably the Chaillot founder, to try to re-engage them. Three succumbed, but at least eight were still determined to return to England.[22]

Sutton, in station by July 1720, continued Stair's work. He eventually secured the release of the English prisoners in Normandy, by now in the hands of the French Navy and intended to be transported to Canada rather than Mississippi. The collapse of Law's scheme 'the Disorders occasioned by the loss upon the Bank Notes' had enabled him to send many of the 'debauched' workers home, but he had to supply them with money to enable them to travel, some having wives and children with them. The best workers he thought had left Chaillot and he believed only a very few clock and watchmakers remained in Versailles, who would go home if they could be protected from their creditors. Jones, the head of Chaillot, would need more inducement. He had been well treated; a special foundry had been built for him by the French; he would try to bring over more workers and the French would put pressure on him to teach them his skills.[23]

By the time that Sully and Blakey came to negotiate with Sutton, the tide of British artisan emigration had probably turned, but the ambassador believed he had underestimated how many men had remained in France and so were open to their plans to act as intermediaries. The account of negotiations between Sutton and the three agents (the two Sullys and Blakey) has its amusing side, there seems to have been an exaggerated striving after secrecy and undercover operations. The original plan the three put to Sutton had a code system incorporated in it, by which the works involved were numbered 1 to 6, English and French seaports were numbered 7 to 12 and letters A, B and C were assigned to Blakey and the Sullys. Law, Sutton and others were assigned other letters, while chief workmen at different places got a designation of number and letter – for instance Jones at Chaillot was 1A.

The leader of the three was clearly Henry Sully, who was able to give the English government 'Information about the said Manufactories and the means to Destroy them, which he is very capable of, being a very ingenious Man, and well enough qualified for Business besides that of his Profession (watchmaker) but he is not without a good deal of Presumption of his own Abilitys'.[24] Not only the losses on paper money, but demands that they should teach their trades to French apprentices, were now alienating the English workmen. Sutton offered the three money, as they were best able to influence the workmen 'because they are the very men who seduced the principal and Greatest number of Artificers into this Country'. The key managers at the Charlaval cloth works should be a main target as French improvements in woollen manufacture were bringing them close to English standards. Blakey was to come over to England to explain the plan and the extent of Law's industrial operation which had cost the French 'a good many millions of Livres'. Richard Sully would do most negotiations with workmen being 'a very faithful, trusty and bold fellow, as well as crafty and cunning'. He should be rewarded by a pardon for his enticement of workers, and the poacher should be turned gamekeeper and rewarded with a Customs job on the Kent and Sussex coasts. The full complexities of the operation cannot be gone into, but the three were to avoid committing in any manner the British ministers either at home or abroad 'or hazarding the least misintelligence on that Account between the two Courts'. To this end Blakey was to write to the most likely workmen as if in Britain a 'Society of Persons out of Pure Affection for their Country had formed a Purse' for repatriating and settling the home country debts of the expatriate workers. Henry Sully was to be taken under Sutton's protection 'under the Title of one of his Secretarys'. Sutton proposed that 'they may be Gratified in some proportion to their Services, when they shall have succeeded in their Enterprises'.[25]

The return of the directors of the French works and their workmen was remarkably successful and there seem to be only a few cases of men with important skills remaining. However, the changed conditions in France after Law's fall, the absence of working capital and the lack of cash to pay wages, may have been as important in driving men out as was the financial aid promised by Sully and his group in making a return home more attractive. The disbursement of that aid led to a good deal of bitter dispute. There were complaints of partiality and favouritism by the disbursers, and of desperate problems of poverty and inability to resume their crafts from some returned masters and workmen. In an age when a certain amount of peculation and jobbery was regarded as inevitable too much should not be made of the accusations, but the surviving accounts of expenditure suggest that Sully and his friends looked after themselves well. Sully, of course, claimed that he had done an efficient and humane job, and had dealt with the creditors of returned men and settled their debts by compositions from 2*s.*6*d.* to 5*s.* in the pound, getting some out of difficulties they could not have surmounted themselves.[26] On his first return before help came from the Secretary of State, he had been 'followed every Hour by numbers of our poor workmen some of whom and their families are actually starving for want and loading me with reproaches for bringing 'em into misery when I promised them better things'.[27] However, when the money arrived he initially had only £2,000 to disburse of the £3,000 promised by government, probably because of queries about previous payments which Sutton had made through the Paris embassy.

Sully insisted that the other £1,000 would be needed if the debts of the ablest artisans were to be settled. There was clearly hatred between Sully and Stair's former French agent, Lewis Douglas, who wrote attacking the characters of the directors and renewing his argument that their plan to assist the government had made 'a merit out of necessity' and that their disbursements had been governed by favouritism. Douglas was bitter because he felt his own services had not been suitably rewarded, but he must have been regarded as trustworthy because Carteret ordered him to enquire about the money paid out by the Sully associates. A group of workmen acquainted with Douglas complained that the payments had been put into the hands of men of the 'utmost partiality and injustice'. Sully, Pagett, Blakey and another suborning watchmaker, Reith, had cheated them over money paid out both in France and in England, while at the woollen manufacture where some were employed they had been badly treated by Pagett, whom they charged with treasonable activities. Elias Barnes, one of the more influential repatriates, accused the Sully circle of being papists and Jacobites, and indicated Sully's involvement with Law and the French state. The moneys he believed should be 'equally disposed of by Proper Persons appointed for that purpose' and he considered himself cheated. Round sums of 50 guineas apiece were certainly paid out to Blakey, Pagett, and Richard and Henry Sully, the latter getting a further £40 for his family in France, and these were followed by other sums to the group as 'Directors' or as individuals. A John Sully received £120. Henry Sully got £230 for his French debts, William Blakey £50 for his English ones and there was a query about £215 paid to Richard Sully for bringing 'several of the Artificers from France by way of Dartmouth'. A statement by Henry Sully of debts which he claimed were agreed to be settled and for which the last £1,000 from the Government was needed, amounted to £3,000 and included £499 owed by the watch-maker Brabant, £159 and £280 respectively by the watchmakers Ackers and Cartwright, £108 by a 'hot-presser', £137 by a woollen manufac-turer and £226 by Sully himself. We know that £1,725 worth of these debts were settled for £431.[28]

Some accounts survive in which debts are particularized and a sign of the indulgence of the Directors to each other may be reflected in the settlement of the debts of John Pagett, which includes the item 'to sundry small affairs which I can't recollect at present ... £50'. He received £200 altogether but had declared his own and his father's debts to be £800 of which his own were £433.[29] He said his French job had been worth £300 a year. However, his former workmen declared that Pagett, who had operated under the alias of 'Brown', had kept most of the money the ambassador had allowed for the party's return home, so that they were 'starving for want of bread'. One of them also separately petitioned for himself, saying that he had been virtually kidnapped; Pagett had undertaken to take him to Scotland, not France, had used him barbarously, not given him what he needed when sick and frightened him with prison 'if he Stir'd from the Factory'. Another of the 'Directors', the watchmaker Reith,[30] was attacked by his workmen because he had persuaded them when 'under unhappy circumstances' (i.e. in debt) to go to France, but had demanded receipts from each of them for the money he had advanced them, to be returned to them when they got to Versailles. He had not given the receipts back and after repatriation they believed he would demand the money again.

From the correspondence of the returned emigrants we can gather background information about their earlier lives and scraps of information about the French works. Francis Moate, like so many others, had been under 'necessity' and 'constrained' to go abroad, that is, in debt. He had gone to the 'English facture [*sic*] of Smiths' set up by Law, where he and his apprentices had been greatly encouraged to develop brass lockmaking. He claimed to have returned to England for patriotic reasons, but once returned he faced poverty and creditors. Unable to make progress, he was invited back by Henry Sully to a works under the Duc de Noailles at Saint Germain in Paris, where English watchmakers were installed. There he got a well-equipped shop, the promise of free housing and 'extraordinary prices' for locks. Sutton succeeded in sending him back to England again, but once back he found it hard to get any of the money allotted to the returned men and had been given only 3 guineas. Curiously he attributed his first misfortunes to having worked for 'Gun' Jones, the Chaillot founder, when the latter had been blacksmith to St Paul's Cathedral, but had failed to pay Moate for locks supplied. 'Gun' Jones seems to have been much more than an ordinary blacksmith. He had been involved with the works of the York Buildings Company where he was associated with the natural philosopher John Desaguliers. He built a model Newcomen engine in Desaguliers's garden at the request of the King of Spain. He was 'another of those artisan-engineers who consorted with philosophers'. Among other skills he claimed to be able to assay ores for silver.[31]

James Reith, the watchmaker, had some tangles with customs officers. William Law had sent him to France with money and three gold watches, one a repeater, for his brother John. These were seized and William Law had to petition the Treasury to get them back, pretending there had been an error in declaring them for Customs and saying nothing about Reith's role in recruiting workers and setting up works in France. The watches were possibly patterns for imitation. When eventually he came back after employing more than seventy workmen at Versailles, Reith had been assured by Sutton that he would be allowed to bring with him large quantities of unfinished watches to be made up in England. In the event the goods were seized by the London customs officers as having been secretly landed, of French manufacture and worth £557, all of which added to Reith's problems. He had to pay workmen to retain their services without being able to make any watches and had to borrow £600. However, the Secretary of State obtained a *nolle prosequi* warrant from the king, and Reith got his property back without paying duty.[32] There is also a little more information on 'Gun' Jones at Chaillot. An Elizabeth Britain wrote on her husband's behalf (perhaps she was the literate spouse) that he was 'a very expert man in his trade' and that 'Gun' Jones had 'deluded' him into going to his Chaillot foundry whence his wife 'fetched him home ... and she is very confident he will never more engage in any such adventure'. She said that a Charles Green had been active in recruiting Chaillot workers and she had seen him there as Clerk of the Works. She revealed that, presumably following the collapse of Law's schemes, there was now the idea of a similar concern in Spain, for which Jones had tried to recruit her husband. An informer declared in April 1721 that, armed with a passport from the Spanish ambassador in France, Jones had gone to Spain to set up a works in Barcelona, while it was expected that Green would return to England to obtain more workers, a description of Green being given to assist in his arrest.[33]

What of the 'chief enticer', Henry Sully? We are able to set him in context from two pieces of evidence: first, the autobiographical details he gave in a memorial to Carteret in 1721 and, second, from a brief biography appended by his friend the great horologist, Julien Le Roy, to a posthumous edition of Sully's *Règle Artificielle Du Temps* (*The Artificial Regulation of Time*) published in 1737. Of French extraction, Sully was apprenticed to a London watchmaker and soon gained a reputation for great skill. He became interested in problems relating to longitude and Le Roy thought this was why he emigrated first to Holland and then to Vienna. Given the debts he needed to settle on his return to England in 1720 or 1721, he may have been running from his creditors. He quickly learned German. He seems to have first met with the publications of the French Academy of Sciences in Prince Eugène's library and claimed to have been an interpreter for Eugène, the Maréchal de Villars, and the Duke of Aremberg, 'so well known to many persons of quality and learning in Germany, France, England and Holland', at the making of the Treaty of Baden. Eugène had taken Sully into his forces and given him the maintenance of the army's watches. He read a paper to the Académie des Sciences in 1716 in 'mathematical mechanics' which 'tho' done at that time for amusement only' attracted the attention of the Regent. The latter wanted to meet Sully and Stair presented him at Court. The order of events is not quite clear, but Sully seems to have lived at two Paris hotels of the Duke of Aremberg when the latter took up residence in that city, the second being in Saint Germain, and while living there Sully married. Aremberg gave him a pension of 600 *livres*.

Sully began to gain acquaintance among notable watchmakers there. The Englishman Blakey first introduced him to Le Roy who became convinced of the superiority and cheapness of English watches and of the quality of Sully's tools, particularly his wheel-cutting machine. Sully wanted to set up as a watchmaker in Paris and, though a foreigner, to be a master workman. To this end he submitted a specially designed watch to the Academy and wanted to obtain a mastership by their favour, but the Paris watchmakers opposed it. Le Roy joined the opposition, for he had executed the watch and felt Sully was not giving him proper credit. A coolness over the incident did not long disrupt their friendship, but the watchmakers' opposition caused others to approach the Regent in Sully's favour, who made him a gratuity of 1,500 *livres*. This was handed over to him by Law in February 1718 and this acquaintance led Law to approach Sully about his schemes for English manufactures in France. Sully, as we have seen, advised him, found persons to head the enterprises, and himself at first headed the Versailles watch-making colony. According to Le Roy all the nobility went there for their watches. Sully was in clover: he had good apartments, a butler, servants, a coach and the management of large funds – in material terms he was at the peak of his fortunes.

Sully considered himself secure and gave up Aremberg's pension. He had brought about sixty watchmakers from London, paid their debts and compensation for their lost time, and 'made their condition so good that their wives did not murmur at having come to France'. Sully and his deputy director, Reith, had high salaries. Despite Law's great concern to establish valuable manufactures in France he decided Sully's regime at Versailles was too extravagant and dismissed him, replacing him by Reith. Sully moved into Paris in much poorer circumstances, where he fell ill. Le Roy felt Sully was so depressed that his recovery was retarded. However an aristocratic friend spoke to Law on his behalf and the controller-general gave him shares which according to Sully were worth 15,000 *livres*. Sully's statements about his successor, Reith, are at variance with their apparently ready collaboration in bringing back the workmen to England. Sully described the original directors of the French works as being supplanted by 'the vilest and ignominious practices of new and flattering aspirants to employments'. Reith was apparently the 'very worthless Person' who received £200,000 capital promised to Sully by Law and the Regent.

On receiving the shares from Law, Sully perked up at once and invited Le Roy to dinner within the hour! He now resumed his horological plans and persuaded the Duc de Noailles to set up a watch manufacture under his protection and Sully's direction at Saint Germain. Le Roy says it was set up to rival Versailles and create emulation between the workers – we may suspect that perhaps Sully saw it as getting his revenge. The wheel of fortune spun again; Sully took a large house and brought in watch and clock makers from London, Amsterdam and Paris. He had an excellent wheel-cutting machine made, turned out fine watches and pendulum clocks and traded in keen rivalry with Versailles for over a year. Reith at Versailles seemed to be getting very rich; Law discontinued further investment in that enterprise and withdrew, but allowed Reith to retain the existing capital. But now disaster loomed for both Sully and Reith. John Law's financial schemes collapsed and he fled from France; William Law was arrested and imprisoned. The monetary crisis hit consumption, especially of luxury items. Sully ran out of money to pay workmen and he and Reith were undecided what to do, while the French government took no interest in the fate of the English watch-makers at Versailles. At this point, therefore, the attempt which Sutton was making to repatriate workers under the Act of 1719 must have seemed like outstretched hands to drowning men to Sully and his fellow directors of English manufactures in France.

We have seen how they presented themselves to Sutton and took advantage of the situation. When the final payments were made to returned masters Sully claimed to be disappointed as he himself had only had 350 guineas, one-third of what he hoped for. In other words he had expected to receive well over one-third of the whole sum the Government had earmarked for the repatriates! For a time Sully continued in England, but as we shall see he was one of the active participants of the Law scheme who, once they had their debts discharged by the British government, returned once more to France.[34]

The correspondence about the returning workers throws a little light on an otherwise mysterious English technologist. John May erected the first steam-engine in France, but nothing else was known of him. However, a deposition about him survives from an E. Richardson, another British emigrant, though we do not know whether he was part of Law's scheme. Richardson had set up a large sailcloth factory for the French East India Company. He claimed that the Company had tried to buy suitable vessels for the trade from England, Holland and Hamburg, but that he had recommended them to obtain English experts for themselves. So 'Mr Laws [*sic*] sent to England to have one of the ablest constructors in the Kingdom, with three of the best Carpenters'. These men were sent to Lorient but, though excellent workers, were not honestly treated and had become dependent on Richardson. As in the case of 'Gun' Jones, there was now a plan for them to go into Spanish service.[35]

The shipbuilding expert revealed himself in a letter in the French foreign office archives. John May memorialized the Regent in June 1722. He said that he had been a naval constructor in England for fourteen years, had been involved in making and copying drawings of some of the vessels with best sailing qualities, and knew their dimensions and the best methods of construction. He was also in possession of the method of bending timbers by steam of which the English had the secret and had seen the plans of the necessary machine. He begged for a job in the French yards where he could demonstrate better and cheaper shipbuilding methods. He stated that Law had got him to come over in 1719 and had sent him to Lorient, but he had not been allowed any independent role there and returned to Paris only to find Law about to depart in disgrace. May had gone back to London but had been induced to return to France, where he had presented a ship model to the Regent. At this point May was apparently being considered once again for the East India Company service as the Regent did not wish to employ him in the French navy itself. Law had promised May 4,000 *livres* a year, but he was now asking for 6,000 and very substantial pay for two English carpenters he would bring over. There is no question that the timber-bending process was tried out. The British Embassy in Paris reported:

> a person is come over hither from England by encouragement from Mr. Law who has the Art of bending timber for the Bows of Ships and other uses; the experiment was made on Tuesday last to the satisfaction of the Maréchal d'Estrées, Mr. Law and others ... the manner of doing it is the same with that now used in our Docks of Deptford, Woolwich and other places.

At the time of these trials, in 1720, May was making out that he was the real inventor of the process, which had been stolen and presented to the British Admiralty by someone else. This must be specious, for had May been the inventor of the important process he would certainly have alluded to it in his petition to the Regent in 1722.[36] What happened to May between the middle of 1722 and the onset of the building of the Passy steam-engine is unknown.

What can we make of this remarkable episode? It seems to be the first occasion when there was a large and well-designed campaign to take English technology to Europe. It anticipates by thirty years the better known plan of D.-C. Trudaine at the Bureau of Commerce in which a principal element was the elevation of Holker, the Lancashire Jacobite and textile expert, to be 'Inspector General of Foreign Manufactures', that is, industrial spymaster with the chief function of enticing British workmen to France. While there is limited detail on the workmen and the processes of the Law schemes, and as yet no papers which elaborate Law's thinking have been discovered, it is obvious that this well-informed man believed that there was a range of industrial activities in which England had something to teach France. In woollens it included wool-combing, some kinds of weaving and hot-pressing; it is relevant that it was in preparatory and finishing stages of textile manufacturing, particularly hot calendering, that Holker established his reputation. We probably lack the full list of the making-up trades in metals which were involved, but anchor-smithing, lock-making, hinge-making, spring-making and file-making were certainly included, while the iron foundry at Chaillot was obviously regarded as very important. It might be interesting to see what element of continuity, if any, there was between the premises provided for 'Gun' Jones and the later engineering works of Périer at Chaillot. As Berthoud testified,[37] the English watchmakers arrived in France close to the peak of their European lead and Sully's influence was important. Blakey may have had two roles, as first director of the metalworks and as a springmaker supplying the watchmakers; it was he who introduced Sully to Le Roy. The watch-wheel cutting machines which Sully brought in, or had made, are indicated as being a central element in his techniques. These had been made by Lancashire toolmakers since the last quarter of the seventeenth century, and they were to be scaled up in the later eighteenth century as an essential of textile-machinery manufacture and other kinds of 'engine making'. Whether May had any chance of influencing the lines or construction of French East Indiamen is doubtful, but the steam-bending of timber was important and he stayed on long enough to see the first steam-engine in France to the point of operation.[38]

The steel-making incident is interesting because it confirms that English steelmakers had advanced to become among the European leaders, as admitted by Réaumur in his famous work of 1722. It fits in with the other intense efforts made by the French to master steelmaking at this time, particularly Réaumur's large and disastrous ones.[39] It suggests that if Law had very correctly identified areas like steel and watch-making as being ones in which the French were clearly deficient, his identification of others may have been correct. If flint-glass making was the branch of glass-making he was trying to bring from England, that would have been another bulls-eye. Neither flint-glass making nor cementation steelmaking were developed in France with real success before the Revolution. The Law scheme of technological transfer as a whole would show that the view advanced some years ago[40] that the balance of technological indebtedness between England and the Continent had shifted decisively in England's favour by 1710 was not maverick, but justified. Similarly, the list of processes – steelmaking, glassmaking, foundry work, hinge, file, spring, watch-tool making, hot-pressing of textiles, steam-heating of timber and the making of the steam-engine – would exemplify the extent to which the new favourable English technological balance was based upon coal-fuel technologies.

2 After the First Legislation: Emigration and Intelligence

Emigration

It was clearly unlikely that after the collapse of the great scheme of John Law for the attraction of British technologies and skilled artisans to France there would be another comparable flow of industrial immigrants for some time. On the French side Law's precipitate fall from favour was naturally accompanied by a ban on all his projects, not simply his paper money and company ones, but the technological project which involved giving privilege and status to British subjects, even if they were sometimes men of an apparent Jacobite persuasion. While some of the Britons involved in his industrial plans had no pressure put upon them beyond a reasonable requirement to pay their French debts before they left, for those workmen briefly threatened by forced emigration to Mississippi or Canada, or the director of the Lorient shipyard who was thrown into the Bastille, the end of John Law's spectacular years of influence must have been painful. They were unlikely to have wished to enter French service again, and they must have influenced other compatriots who learned of their experiences.

On the British side of the Channel a remarkable lobbying campaign had been swiftly consummated in legislation, and its chief target was, and continued to be through the century, the enticer or suborner. The warnings given to workmen by diplomats abroad had been successful in bringing home the British artisans in France. It was to be expected that the future emphasis would be on seizing men and their equipment at British ports, or in the regions where they were suborned, rather than sympathetically helping home men and their families who had gone abroad before any legislation had opposed such emigration.

28

However, though the climate had become so much less favourable, and though a considerable segment of industrial espionage was legally inhibited, and open transfer of technology condemned as undesirable, movement of skilled workers from England was not entirely stopped. Again, by the 1730s some knowledgeable Frenchmen were persuasively putting a case for the renewed acquisition of English industrial methods, of which they had acquired intelligence, directly or indirectly.

The first resumption of the movement of technology between England and France in fact came from the return to France of some of those who had been the chief organizers of the suborning under Law's scheme. On the whole their return seems not to have involved renewing their large-scale suborning efforts, and they thus did not open themselves to the main penalties of the 1719 Act. In the case of two experts, Henry Sully and William Blakey, they had already been resident in France when the Law scheme was initiated. Henry Sully, as we have seen, had been living in Paris since 1715, and Blakey was certainly there about that time, for he had introduced Sully to the great French watchmaker Julien Le Roy before the Law plan was implemented. As both Sully and Blakey had large English debts which, as manipulators of the government resettlement fund, they made sure were paid before those of the other returned masters and artisans, it is likely that it was debt more than Jacobite principle which had first driven them to France, though their Jacobitism may have been genuine enough, as some of their enemies claimed.

Once Sully and Blakey had got all they could from the British government they may have been very conscious that they had previously experienced a period of great prosperity in France, and believed that their skills would still be at a premium there. At the same time they probably lived in considerable discomfort under the anger and accusations of those whose expenses they were supposed to have defrayed, and whose debts they were supposed to have discharged, but whose cases they had treated with much less care than their own. The death of Craggs, a secretary of state who had been well disposed to Sully and his associates, and the succession of the less sympathetic Carteret, also seems to have discouraged them. The new legislation was very circumscribed in its application. Anyone wishing to travel to Europe in time of peace, who could present himself as pretending to gentility, or to merchant or professional status, or appear credible as a traveller in search of culture, the picturesque or a gentler climate, was going to find little to prevent him.

William Blakey's introduction of Sully and Le Roy would suggest that he was, like them, a watchmaker. He was, however, certainly for eighteen months director of the Harfleur works, which under the Law scheme was involved with the manufacture of goods in iron and other metals, and in steel-making. This combination is perhaps not too surprising, for Benjamin Huntsman was a near contemporary English horologist who had the invention of crucible-cast steel to his credit in the 1740s. There is no doubt that William Blakey returned to France. According to his son, also called William, the elder Blakey had 'uncommon experience in the mechanical arts and understood the making of steel and its nature as well as any man in Europe'. The son said his father returned from England to Paris in 1727 and set up a factory for clock and watch springs to which in 1733 were added mills for forging and polishing. The younger Blakey claimed to have been working at his father's factory in 1730. In 1730 he was by royal *arrêt* appointed master watchmaker of Paris, and he was subsequently naturalized French. There is difficulty in separating the activities of father and son. The son said that it was he who obtained a privilege for drawing pinion wire for watch and clock pinions, and for making steel bandages for hernias at the beginning of 1744. The pinion wire would have different numbers of 'leaves', to use the English term, which would produce the cog-like form of clock or watch pinions when subsequently cut up into short sections. The pinion wire was examined by the Academy of Sciences in the same year. They reported that there had been several fruitless attempts to discover the process in France, but it had been employed by the English, and them alone, for forty years. Plans were developed for a specialized water-powered mill for these products. There were petitions to obtain a second adjacent water-power site in 1755 and 1756, one mill being already at work. In 1760 a William Blakey approached D.-C. Trudaine, the head of the Bureau of Commerce, for additional privileges for his operation, and the title of *manufacture royale*. But a Mrs Blakey put in a more modest claim for privileges in the following year, which suggests that the father had been active in the business until then, and his widow had succeeded him. The son's later career was dominated by his energetic promotion of an ultimately unsuccessful steam-engine he had invented.[1]

Elias Barnes was of some importance in the Law schemes, and he and his son were wool-combers by trade. At the time of his return to England in January 1721 he is said to have come from Saint Germain, not either of the Normandy textile establishments, and this may connect with a mention of the Duc de Noailles having an English-type woollen manufacture there, as well as a watch-making one, probably in conscious rivalry to Law. While Barnes and his associates did receive some of the money which Sully had to dispose of, it was not much, and Barnes was clearly angered, accusing Sully of making off with the rest.[2]

On his return home Barnes became an informer to government about suborning and about offences against the legislation prohibiting the export of wool. He carried a letter of introduction from Sir Robert Sutton, the British Ambassador to France, to an official in London who was informed that Barnes 'will be able to make some useful Discoveries concerning several Practices us'd here to entice over our Manufacturers, and to carry our Wool into France'. Craggs, the Secretary of State, might, it was suggested, give Barnes some 'encouragement'. Barnes proceeded to give the government further information on wool smuggling between Britain, Ireland and France in 1723.[3]

In May 1721 he submitted to the Board of Trade and the Plantations a great scheme for the employment of child labour in spinning linen and cotton, which Wadsworth and Mann describe as 'a queer mixture of philanthropy and company promoting', involving the establishment of charity schools with women teachers at a rate of one to twenty pupils. It seems that spinning cotton of a fineness suitable for muslin was his aim, and that he thought that it could be profitable in such schools. This scheme had apparently some inspiration from French, and particularly Dutch, practices. Ignored by the Board, Barnes dropped the matter until 1724, when he claimed to have invented a new and improved spindle usable both with wool and cotton, though the latter was clearly the main target. Three women from each parish should be taught to operate the new spinning system by him and then return home to teach it locally, together with the use of improved attachments for spinning-wheels the cost of which would not exceed 15 shillings a wheel.[4] The Board interviewed Barnes but was in no haste to follow up his proposals. He went abroad and from Hamburg wrote to the Board that he would have 'to settle in some foreign part and teach his art of manufacturing wool, cotton, silk and thread, without he received some encouragement to return home'.[5] As he had not apparently taken workmen abroad the Board could not invoke that part of the 1719 Act against him, but they could demand his return home within six months, and did so. At this point he was at Amsterdam, he had previously gone from Hamburg to Berlin, and subsequently removed from Amsterdam to the Hague.[6]

Whilst at the Hague in 1725 he opened negotiations with the French ambassador, the Marquis de Fénélon. Barnes offered to bring to France both a new spinning-machine and a wool opening and mixing machine. The French government sought the opinions of their East India Company, of the entrepreneur of the fine cloth manufacture at Abbeville (a member of the famous Dutch immigrant family of Van Robais) and of Julienne, the entrepreneur of the cloth manufacture in the Gobelins. The East India Company sent in a short but pointed set of questions, an interesting one being whether Barnes's machine was multi-spindled; Julienne wondered whether the machines would cause unemployment; Van Robais sensibly said he could not pronounce on the machines without seeing them, but was willing to go to the Hague to do so. The French naturally wanted to know why Barnes had not been able to establish his invention in England or the other countries he had visited. He said the British East India Company was opposed to him, presumably from the idea that he might be able to make a muslin thread which could be turned into a British-produced muslin cloth, and so harm their imports, while the wool-opening machine, being better suited to coarse wools, would be more advantageous in France. But he did admit to Van Robais that he had handled his business affairs badly in England. The initial examination of his wool-opening machine by Van Robais at the Hague, and Barnes's own evidence about it, indicated that two men could prepare 500 *livres* weight per day with such a machine. Barnes claimed that even with a microscope – a rather remarkable appeal to the technology of the scientific revolution – it was impossible to differentiate the colour of wool of varied origins once mixed.

Barnes was encouraged to set up his machines at a Paris charity where the curé of Saint Sulpice had girls at work spinning linen and cotton. In April 1727 two deputies of the Council of Commerce, from Rouen and from Lille respectively, made visits to see his machines at work. They were accompanied by some members of the Julienne family previously mentioned. Having demonstrated the machines on the first day, Barnes said he would be perfectly happy to repeat the trials in the presence of Van Robais. Barnes's spinning-machine differed in two ways from French practice. It was in effect a spinning-wheel with a 3-foot instead of a 2-foot diameter main wheel and with a bobbin the diameter of which was smaller at the point where it engaged the cord from the wheel, and so turned faster. The bobbin was made of well-turned iron and attached very firmly to its spindle, avoiding vibration as it turned. The result was that a finer and more even thread could be produced much faster.

The wool-opening machine consisted of two wooden rollers mounted on iron axles and covered in lead sheet through which projected a set of bent iron points, each roller being turned by a crank handle. Mounted one above the other the points on each roller overlapped slightly, and as they rotated together they opened and mixed the wool. With different arrangements of the metal points Barnes had produced two versions of his machine, one for fine wools like Spanish, and one for coarse wools which corresponded to some French ones. The deputies concluded that Barnes's machine was useful for coarser wools, but of no value, perhaps even detrimental, for finer ones, and Julienne and Van Robais agreed.[7] However, the spinning device was regarded as important for muslins and Barnes was eventually awarded a very worthwhile grant of 1,000 *livres* a year.[8] We know that his operations at the Saint Sulpice charity proceeded without difficulty, and it is said that his spinning methods were taken up at Rouen and Lille.[9] Nothing seems to be known of the date of Barnes's death, or of the later use of his machines; possibly their saving of labour was a main obstacle to their adoption at this period, as it was to the adoption of Kay's fly-shuttle both in England and France. Barnes seems mainly to have claimed that his machines would be a mechanical method of raising French production to the speed of English hand production.[10]

John May, as we have seen, was brought over by John Law as a naval architect for Lorient in 1719. After a brief period there he returned to England, but reappeared in France with a steam timber-bending process, and in 1722 memorialized the Regent asking for further work in French naval yards. His activities between June 1722 and early 1725 are not known, but in that year he was a partner in a most remarkable venture. He was in fact the engineer who first erected a steam-engine – a Newcomen engine – in France. This we will discuss in detail when the story of the introduction of the steam-engine to eighteenth-century France is looked at as a whole.[11] He is mentioned here simply to establish him as one of the Law scheme immigrants who returned to France – indeed he can be regarded as the most important of them all.

Henry Sully, whom we have met as the main architect of John Law's project for the seduction of English workers, the 'chief enticer', did not long remain in England after he had scooped up for himself a generous share of the Government's grant for the returning workers. For the time being he continued his horological experiments concentrating on a lever-action clock and a marine chronometer. But with the death of Craggs as Secretary of State and his replacement by Carteret, Sully realized that government favour was over, and he returned to France. He worked initially as a mere watch repairer at Versailles, where he had once been so influential and affluent. He did persuade some English watchmakers to come over, and with them pursued plans for a marine chronometer, and for a new watch escapement which enjoyed some temporary success. He again read papers to the Academy in 1721 and 1723, but there were difficulties with the new escapement. Despite his efforts to secure favourable trials of his marine watches and clocks he had little success, and he found himself in the hands of his creditors, who seized his goods, including his watch tools. He died in 1728 still struggling under these difficulties. His friend the great Le Roy took a perhaps partial and indulgent view of him at his passing, suggesting that he was perhaps as much a martyr to his craft as others might be to their religious faiths.[12]

Another suborner who seems to have operated both during and after the Law scheme was John Harrold. A John Tyrer petitioned Lord Pelham early in 1725. He had been seduced to France five years earlier by John Harrold, but Harrold had failed to pay him for the work he had done there. Harrold was stigmatized by Tyrer as 'an old knave that has inveigled many of his Majesty King George's subjects hither to their ruin'. He was now in London 'to inveigle workmen from this nation as also to recruit men for the Pretender'. We have a description of an 'old bulky man aged about four score, with a grey head but weareth a wigg, vast white eyebrows commonly cut with scissors'. His normal London lodging was known, where a King's Messenger could take him and one of his sons.[13]

An English artisan who appears in French Flanders in 1730 is one of the first heard of in the years after the Law scheme who had not originally had a connection with it. George Gwin was originally living with an English watchmaker at Lille, who is unnamed among the immigrants of that period, though the watchmakers are generally well listed. Gwin was a metalworker who had set up an English textile finishing press which was working on materials for wall-hangings, plush, ribbons and other textiles. He had nearly finished another machine, but was awaiting the arrival of a set of rolls which he had ordered in London. The second machine, however, would be sent to Spain.[14]

At the end of 1730 the British ambassador (Waldegrave) wrote to Gwin ordering him home within six months under the 1719 Act, and the letter was sent to him by King's Messenger, so that there could be no doubt of his receiving it.[15] Gwin indeed received it, but did not submit without question. He pointed out that he had been an apprentice in London and was a Freeman of the City. His trade was to turn and engrave 'all sorts and compounds of metals after which my ingenuity led me ... into new Arts and Inventions' which were useful for manufacturing industries, and he had tried to get employment under various engineers in the King's service. He was *au fait* with hydraulic machinery and fire engines[16] of the latest kind, and the working and engraving of hard metals 'being master of most Mechanic Arts'. But, 'finding myself disappointed of getting my Bread in England' or at any rate obtaining only the wages of a common workman, he had emigrated to Lille. At the point where he had used up all his resources his talents were recognized by the magistrates and merchants of Lille, who had commissioned him to build an English-type fire engine for the town. If he could only be assured of a job in England by which he could maintain his family, he would be willing to go before the British ambassador in Paris (if his expenses were paid!) or alternately be examined by Colonel Lascelles, an English military engineer at Dunkirk. If a salary was guaranteed, 'I will return on sight, for I humbly assure your Lordship that it was perfect necessity that drove me out of my country and it deeply concerns me that I should show the people of this country any curious or profitable Arts that I am capable to perform'. Whether this reluctant transferer of technology did come home is unrecorded. However his attempted importations of English machinery into France meant that the Commissioners of Trade and the Plantations looked into the legal position on the seizure of machinery intended for export, and found that neither the 1719 Act or any other made provision for it, 'which is a defect in the said Laws'.[17] However, the pressure to rectify it was not yet strong, and a couple of decades were to pass before anything was done about it. During the 1730s the active suborning of English workers to France dies away, though the situation with respect to Europe as a whole is more complex.

French Intelligence of English Industry

Nevertheless, this does not indicate a decline of interest in English technology by French officials. There were important French observers in England during that decade, at least two of whom made analyses of the industrial scene which were highly original. Ticquet, who wrote in 1738 what seems to have been an 'inspired' letter to help connections in France who were seeking to supply coal from their mines for industrial purposes, provided a remarkable account of the place of coal in English economic life. He was in fact a French inspector of manufactures. He said that he was daily learning of the new uses to which coal was being put. 'Coal is one of the great sources of richness and abundance in England, and I regard it as the soul of the English manufactures. They have many different kinds of it which have different qualities'. He mentions some of the ways in which cannel coal could be shaped into objects for various uses, and he found it remarkable that some coals burnt with a clean enough flame for cooking, and said it could not only heat rooms, but be used in the kitchen and the laundry. It was used both by bakers and pastry-cooks. Beyond domestic purposes brewers, sugar refiners, dyers, hatters, confectioners, distillers (very common in the England of that period) vinegarmakers, soap boilers and bleachers all heated their various working vessels with it. Window glass, better than French, and very white crystal (this will be flint glass) as well as mirror glass, was made with coal-fuel. Planks, though they might have been cut for years, and apparently seasoned, were dried in a kind of coal stove, and not only planks but the thick beams for building ships could be curved as necessary in such stoves. He had been through some of the districts where iron and copper were worked with coal. He noted the good housing and diet of the industrial villages, which might be favourably compared with the most prosperous villages of Flanders.

Ticquet had made notes on British workmen's practices which were unknown in France, and which he would communicate to his correspondent on his return. Through an English friend who was a Member of Parliament he had been able to visit the thriving workshops of the Midland hardware industry; more remarkably he had seen high-quality Swedish iron converted to steel in Birmingham in coal-fired cementation furnaces provided with chests of Stourbridge fireclay. He would bring back specimens of the steel, not only for his correspondent but for 'M. Hellot'. This is Jean Hellot, the important Academician, who was employed over many years by the French state to report on various industries and their materials, including coal-mining, dyeing, ceramics and steel manufacture.[18] Ticquet went on to describe the latest iron-making techniques, the preliminary roasting of iron ore with coal before its use in the furnace, and coke-smelting, which he had seen at the very heart of technical change at Coalbrookdale. There he had seen coke-iron cast into large pots and into steam-engine cylinders which were 36 inches in diameter and 9 feet long. The polishing of these large iron objects had attracted his attention, particularly that of the insides of the Newcomen engine cylinders which would be used in draining coal-mines. He gave a long and detailed account of coke-making. His correspondent was apparently involved in lime production. Lime was a valuable fertilizer in agriculture, and agriculture was taken seriously in Britain by all wealthy and educated people. The use of lime was further advanced than in France, and Ticquet was interested to see practices which he had read about in British authors actually carried out on the land. When writing he was still in Shropshire, where he was surrounded by machines to roll iron, slitting-mills, polishing machines and machines for boring cannon. If his correspondent wanted he could let him have drawings of them, as he would spend a further two months in England.[19]

This letter was included with a memoir to a minister on 'Details of the different methods to be introduced and tested for reducing wood consumption in France' apparently a document of the 1740s. This in turn mentions a company which had set up coal-fired brick and lime furnaces in the Paris region, and seems to connect with the firm of Martin and Playette. There is a letter in the same file of about 1740 which advanced that firm's claims for brick, lime and plaster production with coal, and drew attention to works the firm had established or were expecting to establish at Fontainebleau and Marly (or in their vicinity) using Flemish workmen. They claimed their products were better than those from works fired with wood, from whose owners they were encountering opposition, and they sought contracts from the officials organizing building work at royal palaces. Possibly Martin or Playette was the recipient of Ticquet's letter.[20]

Other instances show that French inspectors of manufactures in the first half of the eighteenth century were not all mindless cogs in a system of Colbertian regulation, but had enquiring minds and were interested to travel in search of technological enlightenment. In 1771, at the end of a long life of service to the State, Marc Morel petitioned

Terray, the controller-general. He pointed out that Trudaine had known and appreciated his acquaintance with British industry.[21]

Morel said that he had gone to England in 1738, fired by zeal to get hold of the knowledge necessary for the kind of industrial set-up which had subsequently been established in France. His patriotism and wish to earn the favour of the Government had blinded him to all the dangers he ran and the troublesome and risky work he undertook. He had brought specimens of goods from many different English firms, and the knowledge he had gained was now embodied in French manufactures and was its own justification. He then recited his various acquisitions of technology for France, mainly from England, in dyeing, the currying of leather, and the manufacture of webbing. But he clearly regarded as his great coup the transfer he had organized from the French army of the Jacobite and former Manchester textile expert John Holker, which had been founded on Morel's understanding of the superiority of the Lancashire over the Norman cotton industry. Morel's discovery of Holker and its consequences will be a major theme in this study. As he felt death approaching, the old inspector besought the Government to allow his widow the same generous pension rights as it had been agreed to allot to the wife of Holker (now vastly more powerful, but once the recipient of Morel's patronage) if she outlived her husband.[22]

We normally think of the French silk industry as one in which there was an unquestioned European predominance over most of the eighteenth century. But Jubié, an inspector at Tours and a member of a family which had been very important in acclimatizing Italian techniques in France, made a reconnoitring and intelligence-gathering tour of the English industry in 1747, bringing back some unspecified ideas for his own family's manufacture near Lyon. This may have a connection with the arrival of Badger, with the important British invention of 'watering' silk, a few years later.[23]

Ticquet, Morel and Jubié were not the only Frenchmen closely associated with the Bureau of Commerce to have travelled in England, and to have a strong interest in developments there. The scientist Hellot, already mentioned, who was in charge of much industrial testing and implementation, and an Academician who was a long-term commissioner for the vetting of industrial schemes involving new technology, had travelled in England himself before (as we have seen) he sought further information through Ticquet's reports in the 1730s. Vincent de Gournay, an inspector of commerce, knew England fairly well, and was knowledgeable about English economic writing, translating Sir Josiah Child's work into French. Much of his earlier life had been spent in mercantile rather than in industrial activities, and this principal founder of physiocracy was clearly more interested in economic theory than technology, but it was valuable to the work of the Bureau to have a member who had devoted much thought to France's main economic rival. As an economist he certainly had a close influence on the thinking of the Trudaines and of Turgot.

The collapse of Law's financial system, and the anathema under which all his ambitious plans fell, meant that his great scheme for British technology transfer was not continued by the French government, even if they were willing to welcome particular technologists. But with the arrival of D.-C. Trudaine as the head of the Bureau of Commerce in 1749 there was a strong, purposeful and continuous effort to attract English technology to France, very different in style from the hectic, almost frenetic, and short-lived campaign of the Law years, or the intermittent and rather unfocused acquisitions of the two intervening decades.

PART TWO

Holkers and Trudaines

3 John Holker and his Patron

John Holker, Catholic, Jacobite, political and industrial spy, administrator and industrialist, had a long career, much of which seems more likely material for the historical novelist than the historian. He had great bravery, a talent for deception and undercover operations, but also common sense, shrewdness, diplomacy, and a power of judgement and a width of knowledge in industrial matters which amounted to genius. His career has been known in outline, and a useful French biography of 1946 is available[1] but the time must be approaching when a fuller life would be welcome which sets his career against the background of the contemporary industrial history of both England and France.

Holker's early life and social circumstances are still obscure. He was born at Stretford, at that time outside Manchester, on 14 October 1719, son of a father of the same name, probably a blacksmith, who had married a daughter of a John Morris. While his father died early, his mother certainly lived on into the 1760s.[2] Late in life he claimed gentry descent, but this claim is only heard once he sought ennoblement in France in the 1770s and is almost certainly specious, though he apparently tried to obtain an English College of Arms pedigree in evidence. In his mid-twenties he was a skilled cloth calenderer in Manchester, and the wide knowledge he later demonstrated not only of calendering, but of all the finishing trades, and of fine spinning, makes it clear that he was not a common workman, but a master tradesman, a partner in a calendering business. The great turning-point in his life was the rebellion of 1745. When the Young Pretender reached the town on his march south, Holker joined the Manchester Regiment raised in the Jacobite cause, as did his partner, Peter Moss. The regiment was heavily over-officered, and it is said that only a couple of the

43

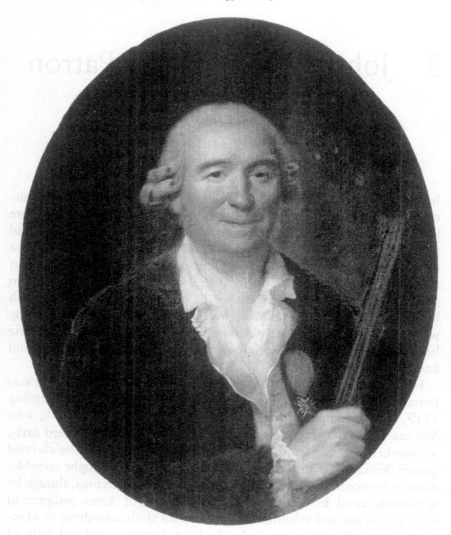

3.1 John Holker, Rouen manufacturer and subsequently Inspector General of Foreign Manufactures

officers were real gentry, most of the others were master workmen, small manufacturers and businessmen, but able to purchase a commission.[3]

Holker was made a lieutenant. Virtually nothing is known of his actions in the campaign until he was left in Carlisle with the rest of the Manchester Regiment as the Prince and the rest of his army crossed back over the Scottish border on 20 December 1745, leaving the garrison to their fate. The Duke of Cumberland quickly procured heavy cannon and resistance was hopeless. Holker and virtually all the garrison were captured on the 30 December. A curious inconsistency arises at this point; Holker's family and important friends in France later stated that he was at Culloden, but this was not the case. Holker's military record in France does not say he was at Culloden, but that he served as captain under the Prince of Wales in Scotland in 1745 and was taken prisoner at Carlisle. This may mean no more than that he joined the army which came from Scotland, and became a *capitaine en second* or lieutenant.[4] The only clear statement that he was at Culloden is in Condorcet's obituary eulogy of Mignot de Montigny to the Academic des Sciences in 1782. There he was simply recording his friend's important service to France in obtaining Holker's release from the army to establish English-type manufactures. Condorcet may simply have assumed that it was at Culloden that Holker was captured. Holker, as we will see, had some acts of remarkable bravery and daring to his credit, and had no need to make false claims. On one occasion, in the most distinguished company, he clearly stated he was taken at Carlisle, and a pamphlet written on his behalf by a friend at the beginning of the 1780s makes an unambiguous statement to that effect.[5]

Thus the available evidence indicates that Holker was a prisoner at the end of December 1745. Later he was certainly in Newgate prison with Colonel Towneley, Peter Moss and other officers, and he went for trial at Southwark on 23 June 1746, when true bills were found against thirty-six officers taken at Carlisle. The main trial of seventeen officers of the Manchester Regiment began on 15 July, nine being executed on Kennington Common on 30 July.[6] However, Holker did not face trial or execution. In late June, within a few days of the bills of indictment, an embarrassed official was reporting to the Duke of Newcastle 'Two of the Rebel Prisoners in Newgate, Peter Moss and John Holker made their Escape last night. 5 more had filed off their Irons and Coll. Townley [*sic*] had half filed of [*sic*] his'.[7]

The details of the escape were given by Holker thirty years later when he told the tale at the dinner table of the Duc de Choiseul where guests were vying with remarkable anecdotes. 'If you only want a story fit for a novel', he said, 'perhaps I should tell you one of my own.' In Newgate he and Moss had been allowed visitors, and they got them to gradually smuggle in ropes, files and a description of the prison and its environs. Their plan was to file through their leg-irons and sufficient window bars. One night, being on the top floor of the prison, they hoped to climb into the gutters and along them to a point where there was a gap between the prison roof and that of an adjoining merchant's house. They would cross the gap with planks taken from a tabletop in their cell, bound together to make a bridge 8 feet long but only 8 inches wide. On the night chosen Holker, a big man, had great difficulty in getting between the bars and Moss returned to extricate him. The merchant's dog was aroused, Holker descended into a water-butt and the two men became separated. Refused entry at one supposedly Jacobite house, Holker was eventually sheltered at another, and then smuggled into the countryside, whence he made his way to France by way of Holland.[8]

Lord Ogilvy, one of the most important survivors of the '45, formed a Jacobite regiment in the French army and Holker joined it as a lieutenant (*capitaine en second*).[9] Later in the year he took part in the Flemish campaign, was at the battle of Lawfeldt, where the defeat of Cumberland must have given him great satisfaction, and subsequently at the sieges of Bergen-op-Zoom and Maastricht. Holker again demonstrated his personal courage and his devotion to the Jacobite cause in 1750. In September of that year Charles Edward Stuart made his way to Antwerp and thence to Ostend, where Holker joined him. The prince wanted to go to England to confer with Jacobite leaders, and Holker went over with him as his sole companion and minder. For a man who had escaped Newgate and execution only four years before this was extremely brave. 'It is a tribute to his sterling qualities that he was willing to accompany Charles on such a perilous mission' writes Charles's biographer Frank McLynn.

Charles's arrival in London took the English Jacobites by surprise, and, though he addressed a meeting of fifty prominent supporters, there was clearly little enthusiasm for a rising unless accompanied by a foreign invasion. Whether Holker knew that Charles had abjured the old faith and entered the Anglican one during his visit is unclear. He would certainly not have liked the prince's abandonment of Catholicism. He joined Charles for the journey back to France which they reached safely on 23 September. It had been a brilliantly accomplished journey of political espionage, however negative its results. Curiously Holker seems not to have made any subsequent overt reference to it, though Charles Edward gave him a sword of honour in recognition. Perhaps the long quarrel between Charles and the French after their forcible arrest and expulsion of the prince in 1748 under the treaty of

Aix-la-Chapelle made it impolitic for Holker to refer to his close association with the prince once he obtained an important post under the French state. It did not end his loyal services to the cause. In 1752 he correctly identified to Charles the spy in his personal circle, young Glengarry, code-named 'Pickle' to his English spymasters, who betrayed the Elibank plot of 1752–53. With his strong allergy to good advice Charles refused to believe Holker.[10]

Holker might have remained in the French army but for the intervention of three men who were devoted to the improvement and development of French industry, an inspector of manufactures, an Academician who frequently advised the Government on industrial matters, and a minister of outstanding ability. Marc Morel had been appointed an inspector of textiles at Rouen in 1741, and had held an appointment there from 1738 according to his own statement. At the very end of his life he wrote to the controller-general of the period sadly contrasting his treatment and promotion with that of the Englishman he had 'discovered' and brought to the attention of the great. Morel, the son of a Calais trader, had a good knowledge of English and in 1738 he went to England, presumably with government approval and financial support, for a junior inspector is unlikely to have paid his own way. He went there to gain the necessary information to set up new industrial enterprises in France. 'The wish to be useful to my country and to earn the favour of the government' had 'blotted out for me all the dangers I ran.' The specimens and samples he brought back from a wide variety of English firms still existed and were proof of the 'hard and dangerous task' he had undertaken. Like many other Frenchmen who carried out even very limited espionage he emphasized the perils of his operations to the Government. How far he really believed he was at great risk from the English law is hard to tell. Unless he had been caught suborning English workers it is doubtful if he would have been in serious trouble, at worst he would have been sent packing back to France.[11]

However, he returned to France with a high respect for English manufacturers and their products. In 1753 he managed to get a manufacture of webbing on the English pattern set up, and was given supervision of it in 1754, and also a manufacture of English coverlets at Pont de L'Arche. About the same time through his English information network he enticed over two leather curriers, father and son, to establish that skill in France as well as it was practised in England. But at the head of his achievements in the transfer of technology he put the enquiries which had discovered the talents of John Holker of Ogilvy's regiment, and the efforts which had succeeded in getting him out of the army and enabling him to set up a manufacture of cotton velvet at Rouen.[12] Morel had later moved from Rouen to Caen and Trudaine had made his post there well rewarded, securing him a retirement pension of 1,000 *livres* a year. But when fatally ill in 1771 he wrote to beg a continuing pension for his wife after his death. She would have nothing, while Holker's widow would have a special pension of 2,000 *livres*; this he felt hard when they 'had pursued the same career'. It is easy to sympathize with his feelings at the way his protégé's fortunes had outstripped his.[13]

So far no one has been able to discover exactly how Morel got in touch with Holker. We know Holker visited Rouen in October 1749,[14] but it was the beginning of 1751 when Morel wrote to Daniel-Charles Trudaine, who had recently taken over the direction of the Bureau of Commerce. This must rank as one of the most important introductions ever made in the history of technology, for Trudaine stands out as one of the most successful and enlightened administrators of eighteenth-century France, and perhaps the most universally admired. Morel briefly sketched Holker's Jacobite sympathies and military record and said that he had been an important textile industrialist in Manchester. Many conversations with him had convinced Morel that he could be very useful, especially because he was familiar with the manufacture of fustians in Lancashire, and this implied a knowledge of cotton velvets. Holker was also an expert on all sorts of calenders, and these were essential for finishing these cloths. He had offered to go back to England and get workmen and involve himself in ensuring that, once established in France, the Englishmen would train French workmen. Though Morel wanted to take Holker to Paris to see Trudaine, explaining that Holker had only a little French, Trudaine decided to see Holker in the first instance without Morel in attendance.[15]

Holker's appearance on the local industrial scene at this moment was well timed. The French cotton industry had started to gain momentum at the end of the seventeenth century, particularly in Rouen. Using silk warps originally, linen warps were soon substituted to carry the cotton weft, and the manufactures at Rouen and Evreux began to put out much of the spinning in the countryside. There were attempts by the inspectors of manufactures and by the municipal and trade officials of Rouen to confine the new trade to the town, for instance on the specious plea that it would dangerously divert country people from farming, though one of the merchant members of the Government's

Council of Commerce put in a forceful and lucid case for untrammelled manufacture.[16] Eventually the strength of demand allowed the industry to continue to spread into the countryside, though yarn and cloth were brought into the cloth hall at Rouen for inspection. By 1732 there were about 60,000 people working in the industry in the Rouen region, and the trade continued to grow. In Rouen there was conceived a plan for a highly capitalized unit with large premises. The main architects were the merchants and shipowners d'Haristoy and Dugard, the former already prominent in a new concern for rolling lead. Their venture was centred on the production of dyed cotton yarn, particularly red. They believed, mistakenly, that they would be able to produce the famous 'Adrianople red', a dyeing process not yet successfully imitated in Western Europe.

At the end of 1746 d'Haristoy, Dugard and others formed a company with a local man who believed he could tackle the problem. D'Haristoy discussed the project with two intendants of commerce, de Montaran and Rouillé, and they referred him to Hellot, the important academician who was already a regular technical adviser to the Government, with a considerable specialization in dyeing. He still has an honoured place in the history of this branch of technology.[17] An exclusive privilege and the grant of a *manufacture royale* from the Government were regarded as essential for setting up this venture, but matters were complicated by a privilege obtained for 'Adrianople red' dyeing by an entrepreneur of Aubenas, Goudard. However, d'Haristoy wanted a privilege for his own firm's production, while being willing for Goudard to operate as a dyer of other people's cloths. D'Haristoy and his associates were very dependent on Hellot's opinion; he was the expert whose views the Government would accept. Eventually Goudard was brought in to the d'Haristoy project.

Once in business in 1748 the associates found it difficult to sell enough of their dyed yarn. They set up fifty looms to use it, but still found little sale. Financial difficulties grew, though Hellot encouraged Dugard that there would be eventual success, and there were hopes that Mme de Pompadour would give the firm her influential patronage. But the commercial problems of the firm went on increasing, despite additional capital, and poor yarn was one reason for them. There were more problems with the supply both of dyestuff (madder) and fuel, and attempts to use English imported coal ran into the difficulties common to French industrialists when first trying to use an unfamiliar fuel. When dyeing was done on a small scale with skilled and well-motivated workers results were adequate, when larger-scale operations were undertaken poor quality control, and labour which was idle and uninterested, spoiled operations. An important partner, Fesquet, withdrew, and set up a privileged manufacture of his own at Darnetal with the support of inspector Morel. D'Haristoy died in 1757 as did another important partner in 1761, and the enterprise then fades from view.[18] The true Adrianople process was only copied successfully in France just before the Revolution.

However, the d'Haristoy scheme is important in showing how Rouen industrialists were now thinking big, and were keen to bring in new methods. It was some of the key partners in this firm who helped the introduction of Holker into large-scale industry in Rouen. This was to have immense consequences. Holker was turned to in order to help in the creation of a cotton velvet industry, in which there had been earlier unsuccessful attempts, particularly associated with the Havarty brothers, British immigrants of the 1730s.[19] They are said to have been supported by d'Haristoy but to have eventually returned home.[20]

The meeting of Holker with Trudaine had obviously been most successful. Morel, as we have seen, had been excluded, possibly because Trudaine wanted to make a dispassionate appraisal of a man Morel seemed to be over-enthusiastic about. But Holker wanted someone with technical knowledge there. He wished the interpreter to be 'au fait' with manufactures and acquainted with the relevant technical terms, 'and a man acquainted with the English language, even himself an Englishman, may be ignorant of them' – just the kind of penetrating perception of one of the essential problems in transferring technology that marked Holker out as exceptional. He also wanted a secret interview 'if it became known in England that he had made known several secrets concerning the manufacture of his native country, without that gaining him employment in France', he would not be able to return home if there was an amnesty for Jacobite rebels, 'as he would be regarded as a traitor to his country'.[21]

The association with Trudaine, so fortunately made through Morel, was to be the dominating factor in Holker's career from 1750 until the minister's death in 1769. The Trudaine influence did not cease then, for his son, Trudaine de Montigny, succeeded his father in office and continued the fruitful relationship with Holker until his own fall from office in 1777. Trudaine came from a family of lawyers and administrators, ancestors having occupied the high legal office of *maître des requêtes*. His father, Charles Trudaine, had enjoyed a high reputation

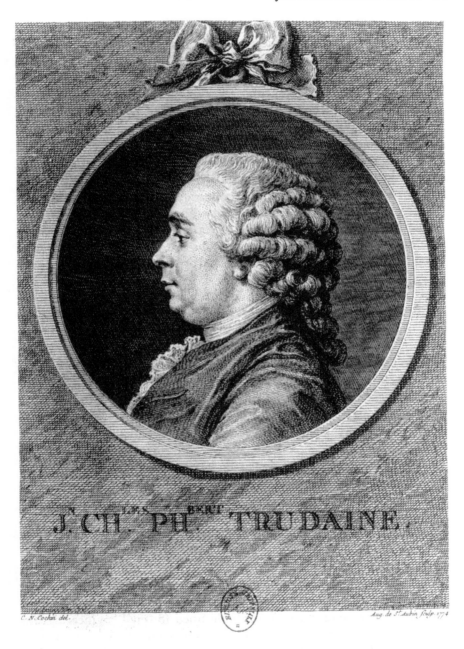

J. CH.^{LES} PH.^{BERT} TRUDAINE.

C. N. Cochin del.   Aug. de St Aubin Sculp. 1774

3.2 Daniel-Charles Trudaine (1703–69), Director of the Bureau of Commerce from 1749 until his death

for probity. Charles had also risen through the same essential office of *maître des requêtes* to be successively Intendant of Lyon and then of Dijon, a councillor of state, and from 1716 to 1720, *Prévôt des Marchands* (provost of the merchant guild) at Paris. However, he had refused to involve the municipal revenues in Law's scheme for a national bank at the time of Law's ascendancy and the Duke of Orléans was forced to dismiss him – 'we have taken away your place because you are too honest a man'.

Charles Trudaine's eldest son, Daniel-Charles, 'Le Grand Trudaine', born in 1703, had enough patronage to have become a *conseiller* at the Parlement of Paris at the age of seventeen. Next he became *maître des requêtes* and would have been content with a legal career. But in 1729 Cardinal Fleury, who had known his father well when they were respectively Bishop of Fréjus and Intendant of Lyon, had him appointed Intendant of the Auvergne.[22] There he proved that he was no mere placeman, but a gifted administrator, particularly in creating a road system to improve an impoverished province. Five years later Fleury recalled him to Paris as successor to De Gaumont as an Intendant des Finances and Conseiller d'Etat, and he soon became director of the *Fermes Générales*. But his name is perhaps most associated with his direction of the Ponts et Chaussées (the roads and bridges administration which carried out major civil engineering works) which a new controller-general, Orry, had decided needed reform. Trudaine provided inspiring leadership in this department for 30 years, but leadership which went hand in hand with strict economy and financial control. He identified and promoted the best experts, the outstanding example being Jean Rodolphe Perronet (1708–94), whom he appointed principal engineer, and who became perhaps the most celebrated civil engineer in Europe in the eighteenth century. Under Trudaine's direction 8,000 to 10,000 leagues of road were surfaced and raised to high standard, and great bridges built of outstanding architectural as well as engineering quality. Perhaps his most important contribution was his concern for the practical and scientific training of young engineers, for whom he established in 1747 the Ecole des Ponts et Chaussées, the first great institution for engineering education, attended by gifted students some of whom were not necessarily destined for civil engineering, for instance the great metals technologist Gabriel Jars, to whom Chapter 10 is devoted. Similarly he influenced French mining by the mining law of 1744 and the creation of a school of mines.

In 1749 Trudaine added to his responsibilities the direction of the Bureau of Commerce. In this office

> he was comprehensive and realistic in his understanding of the French economy, of its needs and resources, and of the means to improve it. He was almost unerring in his ability to perceive the essence of a basically simple problem and to prepare a single, practical solution. At the same time he was ingenious, intelligent and flexible when it came to devising a complicated and multiple policy to meet complicated multiple needs ... [In particular] he knew how to choose men, industrialists as well as administrators, and to enlist them in the execution of his policies.[23]

While fully aware of the growing differences in ideas on commerce, the rise of new economic theories and the 'kind of excitement' caused by new writing and by French concern with international rivalry, Trudaine remained a pragmatist. But he was tough on old traditional institutions and practices when they impeded newly developing trade and industry. Privileges and bounties continued to be granted, but sparingly, critically and for limited periods. After restoring the Bureau's finances 'he found himself by this means able to call into the kingdom, those branches of industry which were most flourishing abroad'. An illness in 1759 left him deaf and with some deteriorating bronchial affliction, but he was able increasingly to hand over the commerce administration to the son whom he had trained in it, Trudaine de Montigny. By his death, early in 1769, he had effectively given up all but the Ponts et Chaussées department. His commercial policies were largely continued by his son until he was driven from office in 1777.[24]

This was the man who summoned Holker to Paris in April 1750. Trudaine was joined in interviewing Holker by Mignot de Montigny, an Academician who was unrelated to him, but whose name is readily confused with that of Trudaine's son (Trudaine de Montigny), who in fact did not join his father at the Bureau of Commerce until 1754. Mignot de Montigny was one of those scientists whom the Government successively called in as regular advisers through most of the eighteenth century, and was one of the most effective. Holker must have impressed Trudaine at once, for he was brought to see Trudaine again in August, this time accompanied by Morel, and he was quickly sent to England on a three-month expedition of espionage and the seduction of workers.

Fortunately we can learn a little of this trip from some surviving accounts of Holker's expenses. He had been allotted 7,000 *livres*. He had travelled from Paris to Dunkirk late in 1751, and sailed thence to London. There he had bought a horse and made two trips north, one to Manchester and another to unspecified parts of Lancashire. He had also bought clothes, probably to replace ones which might have been too French in style, and included in his expenses the cost of three months' food, which nicely fixes the length of his expedition. He spent the large sum of £23 on cloth samples, which would serve to show the French the quality of Lancashire products as well as serving as patterns to be imitated. Three machine models were sent, but they must have been fairly simple, as they only cost 35 shillings for the three, together with their boxes. Holker had employed agents in London and in Manchester to make payments to men who were to follow him back to France. This establishment of agents, some used for years, was to be a feature of his subsequent espionage activities. He brought back some specimens of English cotton weft yarn, some loom parts and a number of tools for cotton velvet looms. We know that his mother was important in helping to identify the workers he wanted. The members of the Morris family he recruited were almost certainly her relations and one man is specifically referred to as Holker's nephew.[25] But he had not wholly relied on her to identify suitable workers for seduction to France, for his expenses included an item 'to two persons I employed in Lancashire to find the men whom I needed' who together received 5 guineas. Very remarkably he had provided for a further worker to come over when properly trained, this was Peter Morris 'whom I put out apprentice to cut and shear fustians' at a premium of 8 guineas. The apprentice is said to have turned up at Rouen in the summer of 1755.[26] While he learned fustian-cutting he was to have 1s. 6d. a day, which Holker arranged. Money was sent to pay the English debts of two of the workers, and maintain their families until they could join the men in France. Holker had also used his wife in his operation. The £50 he had left with her was spent by the time he submitted his expenses claim.[27]

The operation had thus been a considerable success, largely due to Holker's being able to return to his home district and recruit among relatives, friends, Catholics and men personally recommended, and by his careful measures to ensure the welfare of the workers and their families. While a party of about twenty-five English people arrived in Rouen, only around half of them workers, the others were wives and children. The English workers were carefully selected. Two, Hall and Leatherbarrow, were able to direct the preparation of cotton to the point where it was ready for the loom and to set up looms for all kinds of fustians and cotton velvets. Wild was a joiner who could make looms and also – critical in Holker's eyes – the 'dévidoirs' or clock-reels which could check the correctness of the count of yarn spun. There was a carpenter, Matheson, who was a specialist in calender building, and several men who were expert in finishing including the operation of calenders. These were Toyra,[28] Knowles and Partington, later joined by James Morris. Specialist fustian-cutting was provided from 1754 by an Irish recruit, Mulloy, and by Peter Morris, after he had learned the trade in Lancashire. It is interesting that two of the principal workers originally insisted on pseudonyms. Hall was said to be really Guy Hutin[29] while his brother-in-law, Leatherbarrow, took a name variously spelled in the archives as Andson or Hampson. This suggests that these superior workmen, described in 1752 as 'having their salaries paid by the king', either wished to cover their tracks in case they decided to return to England, or had property there which they did not wish to put at risk under the 1719 Act. Hall had been responsible for bringing over James Archer, a skilled silk worker who was a French speaker. He would at first be responsible for explaining the English processes to French workers. Here we can see Holker putting into practice his belief that it was essential that an interpreter should know perfectly the technical terms in either language. Once he had fulfilled his translating function, Archer would be retrained in the cotton velvet manufacture.[30]

D'Haristoy was quick to offer to form a company which would use the English workers' skills, 'a company of merchants capable of undertaking the new manufacture of English cloths which M. Trudaine has so much at heart'. Typically he was thinking big, proposing a capital of 300,000 *livres*. As was common with French capitalists, he wanted government support, but sugared the pill by asking the king simply to pay the interest on the capital, so as to inspire confidence in the investors. Having got provisional consent from an administrator, Machault, he had the English workers mount three looms at his own expense, which were to be tried out for six months under Morel's inspection, but with the workers paid for by the State. When the English workers arrived no arrangements had been made for housing them. D'Haristoy had to give them some subsistence money, provide them with bedding, and then lodge them at a cabaret, which was more costly than ordinary lodgings, but there was a shortage of local accommodation. Holker and d'Haristoy were hopeful of finding sites both for cotton velvet production and for a calendering works. In the first stages one of the barriers which national worker culture put in the way of technical transfer had to be overcome; the Englishmen were buying wood and making their own tools 'being quite unable to employ tools made for the use of French workers'. Holker had from the outset insisted that the first essential for high-quality cotton cloth lay in a closer control over the regularity of spinning-cotton yarn. This was done by use of the 'dévidoir' or clock-reel and by determining the fineness of the spinner's yarn by weighing her hank against one of standard length.[31]

Some months later Mignot de Montigny was being sent to Rouen with instructions to look into the viability of Holker's schemes for new manufactures in Normandy: 'he will inform himself on the skill, talents and behaviour of the English workers brought to France by Sr. Holker and assess the work they have done at the King's expense over the last four months'. The proposed site for calendering was to be inspected for suitability for manufacturing and for handing over to a group of entre-preneurs and 'he will negotiate with the entrepreneurs on the nature and the distribution of the payments which the King is willing to make to help set up this concern'. This would not be a subsidy paid in advance, but one based on the number of pieces manufactured per year, or the number of looms actually at work, and would be paid for in ten years. 'He must not listen to any proposal which seeks to establish an exclusive privilege, the King's wish being to create a very free trade.' While signed by Machault, this document seems to be a classic example of Trudaine's policy. Montigny was to discuss with Holker whether it was necessary to get any more workers from England, and if so how to get them, and to keep Trudaine informed of his findings. Another letter on Montigny's visit of inspection already talks of the enterprise to be set up as not merely privileged, but a *manufacture royale*. Emphasizing the potential export markets, particularly America, if a cotton velvet manufacture could be established, it puts special importance on the calendering: 'I am also informed that that which contributes most to the profitable sale of the cloths from [British] manufactures is the skill in giving them the fine finishes particularly by means of calenders which we have never imitated perfectly'.[32]

While some caution had to be observed in the subsidies and induce-ments offered to d'Haristoy and his associates, there were to be two contracts. One would be embodied in the usual *arrêt de conseil* (State decree) authorizing privileged concerns, but there should also be a secret contract, those agreements 'which are to be made public should only contain the conditions which they should publicly enjoy and the others should set out the pecuniary terms of which it is pointless that the public should be informed'. By September matters were reaching a conclusion. The Intendant, La Bourdonnaye, had been to inspect the pilot production of the proposed firm at Darnetal whose success Trudaine 'had always shown him to have very much at heart'. He agreed with Mignot de Montigny that the dual firm with its English calenders could 'encompass a rebirth of our Rouen manufactures ... you saw this before I did and you understood the whole importance of the two works' which were 'capable of changing the face of our manufactures'.[33]

There are some interesting comments in the notes on the draft *arrêt* for the new firms, some being Trudaine's. The cotton velvet manufacture was dealt with first. The text must not call the ventures the '*Fabrique* Angloise *de Rouen*', and Trudaine doubted if Holker should be explicitly named because of diplomatic relations with England. Similarly the products should be described as ones 'which are not yet made in France' and not 'in imitation of English'. Similarly with the exemption from all taxes to be given the English workers 'a general clause should be made for the *arrêt* ... for all foreign workers without talking about the English in particular'. An important aside dealt with Holker's position. He was necessary at Rouen, and would have to leave Ogilvy's regiment with his captain's pay of 1,200 *livres*, and an equivalent should be transferred to him as a civilian at Rouen. This should continue for four years, after which his profits from the works should maintain him, though 'extraordinary gratifications' were hinted at. He should now be able to bring over his wife and son from England to join him in Normandy. As further English workers arrived (three weavers, a shearer, a fustian cutter and a dyer), 500 *livres* should be paid to the entrepreneurs on account of each, presumably to cover the cost of their recruitment, maintenance and travel.

Holker's reward was certainly not confined to his 1,200 *livres* pension. In the cotton velvet firm he was to have a one-fifth share, valued at 20,000 *livres*, without investing any funds of his own, and there was to be a similar arrangement for the calendering business.[34] At certain points other partners could be required to produce additional funds to provide increased fixed capital but Holker was to have his share in the enterprise maintained without any further personal investment. Montigny would not countenance a draft *arrêt* for the calender concern which potentially restricted Holker's liberty to be involved in other calendering works. This was against the wishes of the Council of Commerce which wanted Holker to make calenders for wool and silk, as well as linen and cotton, in many parts of the country, while the firm now being set up could not fully provide all the calendering for Normandy.

In the secret version of the *arrêt* Holker was named as one of the five partners. The others were Pierre d'Haristoy, Louis Paynel, Robert Dugard and Claude Torrent.[35] Torrent was a very important businessman, whom Chassagne calls 'cet agent de Trudaine'. He had been involved in the West Indies trade, was currently Dugard's Paris representative, and was subsequently involved in an important rolled lead manufacture, in the lead mines of Lower Brittany, and not only in the Saint Sever works at Rouen but in the English-type textile manufactures of Sens and Bourges, as well as in insurance businesses, and in the manufacture of cotton velvet and other new cotton cloths. Holker was to have a cost-free one-fifth share. He was jointly, with an Inspector to be appointed, to produce an annual return of cloths made and calendered. The Crown turned over to the partners nine looms and other tools and machines already made by the English workers in the preliminary trial period.

The company was to receive a 60,000 *livre* subvention spread over ten years. Over 3,500 *livres* would be paid annually for the salaries and perquisites of Hall, Andson and Wild, as agreed with them when they were recruited in England by Holker. Hall, the foreman weaver, now teaching trainees, would get 1,610 *livres* a year; Andson, similarly employed, 1,150 *livres*; Wild as loom, mill and calender builder, 800 *livres* a year. There would be a bounty on English-type cloths produced of 4 *livres* apiece up to 1,200 *livres* a year, and up to 1,000 *livres* a year for all the pieces of cloth calendered by the English machines at the rate of one *sol* each. A fall-off of production in any year would not prevent the whole sum designated from being paid in respect of later production. There was also to be a bounty of 30 *livres* for each of the thirty looms the partners were contracted to build, and provision for payment for the other workers who were to be brought over. Four calenders were to be built, three being of English type with copper cylinders, the State paying 10,000 *livres*, being half of the estimated cost. The machines when completed would belong to Holker and would effectively constitute his investment in the firm. To guarantee the services of Hall, Andson and Wild, and allow Hall and Wild to bring their families to Rouen, they were to be allowed an annual retirement pension of half their present salaries, and they would be allowed a similar amount if they became ill and unable to work during a ten-year period, while their pension would be continued to their widows. If they were able to work after ten years and willing to do so, the pensions would be continued, but end if they refused to do their jobs without good reason. In the case of all other English workers already employed, or to be employed in future, they would be paid by the entrepreneurs on whatever terms they judged proper. Any difficulties or disputes arising on these agreements would be referred to and dealt with by the Intendant. The public version of the *arrêt* constituted the works of the partnership a *manufacture royale*.[36]

Almost immediately the partners purchased for 1,200 *livres* a walled plot in the Rouen suburb of Saint Sever. Within six months two calenders were at work, and 500 cloths had been processed. An additional 590 handkerchief cloths were calendered by way of trial. The Rouen cloth producers were being very careful and deliberate about deciding to commit their cloths to the process. As was only too often the case, the English dyer and the three English calenderers were over-fond of their drink. At Darnetal the partners were also performing their contract to the Government, twenty-nine looms were at work on plain and cut velvets and fustians. In the following year Mignot de Montigny came to Rouen to see how far the Government's measures were successful. He objected to a clause in the agreement which had slipped through which would allow partners, apart from Holker, to be involved in other calendering enterprises. The Government had not wanted that to happen. Equally Montigny did not want Holker to have to pay interest to his partners on the (in fact fictitious) sum of his investment. His partners were presumably making this claim on the grounds that they had in fact advanced this sum by giving him a one-fifth share in the business. The partners would not receive their subsidy until they had put these things right, a remarkable testimony to the way Holker was esteemed by the administration.[37] This was also shown by an additional bonus paid him in August 1753 for his care in establishing the manufacture, bringing his total remuneration for the year to 2,000 *livres*. Trudaine also felt it right to give 'some little reward ... to the English and French workers who have been most successful in the operations on the new cloths so as to excite more and more emulation, I have very much at heart the success of these establishments and the augmentation of the English colony'.[38]

An important accompaniment of Holker's Lancashire recruiting expedition was his collection of a mass of cloth samples, particularly from Manchester and the surrounding country. On his return he and Morel co-operated to gather these into a 'Livre des Echantillons' (sample book), mainly of Manchester textiles, but with some from Norwich and Spitalfields. The samples comprised linens, cotton linens, silk and cotton, wool and cotton and all-cotton cloths. The care and detail given to the collection by Holker were remarkable. Linen thread from Scotland, Ireland and Silesia was distinguished in the samples and, as well as silks from the famous Derby factory, they illustrated ones from Spain, Piedmont and Italy. Fortunately this collection of 115 swatches survives in nearly pristine condition in the Musée des Arts Decoratifs in Paris, and it has been expertly described by Florence Montgomery. It must have been of great importance in giving empirical proof to the French authorities of Lancashire superiority, convincing them of Holker's profound knowledge of textiles and particularly cotton, and confirming their support for him.[39]

Morel's dying claims on the Government in 1771, citing his importance in the launching of the Holker concerns, seem to have had good foundation. From September 1752 Trudaine required that Morel should 'watch over the manufacture very closely, which has as its objective the employment of a number of English catholic workers' and that he should encourage and reward them so that other Catholic workers would be attracted to France, knowing that they would be well received and paid. Morel did in fact visit, report on and check the returns from the manufactures until 1761 at least. In 1754 he went over to England and brought back with him the English currier Wilson, with the important skill of making the leather covering for the best hand cards for carding textiles. He also brought back samples of dyed cloth. He may also have been responsible for the arrival of further workers at Saint Sever, including a mechanic, Richard Smith, the calenderer Noah Hallowes, and a group of Irishmen, Thomas Davis, Neil Davitt, John Mulloy (all weavers), and Charles Smith, a dyer. By the end of the year the partners had entirely concentrated their operations at Saint Sever, where they had fulfilled their undertakings by setting up over a hundred looms. Holker was in direct control of the whole enterprise, while beneath him the two English foremen, Hall and Leatherbarrow, oversaw the production side. English workers were divided up and carefully associated with appropriate numbers of French workers, so that skills would be passed on. In some cases the fear that their own jobs would be at risk once they had passed on their skills worried the British workers; this emerged strongly with the fustian cutters, so Trudaine dealt with the problem with his usual generosity and good sense; they would have an annual pension of 300 *livres* and 100 *livres* for every French workman trained.[40]

While they had their commercial ups and downs, the large-scale cotton velvet and calendering ventures continued until the 1790s, and Holker and his son added the perhaps even more important large-scale production of sulphuric acid in the mid-1760s, of which more later. However, by the end of 1754 the industrial operations which Holker had undertaken had been set up with technical success and great commercial promise, and within the proposed timetable. There can be no doubt that Trudaine was immensely impressed. He had already shown that he was keen for Holker to spread his cloth finishing techniques far outside Rouen, while the successful use of the English workers whetted the minister's appetite for further transfers of technology.

In late 1754 or early 1755 Holker put forward a remarkable document.[41] Startling in its boldness, it was on the one hand well directed to Trudaine's desires and preoccupations, while on the other Holker's existing successes in undercover operations in Britain and in setting up Saint Sever gave it credibility. The document began by reciting his achievements in the Rouen textile industry. Then came the proposition.

> If one plans to bring to France foreign skills, and principally those of England, where industry has made more progress than anywhere else, one can first use Sieur Holker to establish and keep up a secret correspondence with England to get thence certainly and quickly all the models of machines and the samples and tools one needs.

Examples of trades where the English had the lead were those of currying leather, the shearing of woollen or cotton cloths and particularly the manufacture of the light metal goods of Birmingham and Sheffield. Holker alluded to the British legislation now coming into existence against the export of tools, though he did not say how limited it was.[42] This could hinder the transfer to France of new English processes. Holker gave as examples of new English industries in France the watered silk works of Badger at Lyon and a white earthenware works at Montereau.[43] Men, as well as equipment, might be brought over, especially if Dutch rather than French ports were used as 'ships loaded for Holland are not inspected so rigorously' and carefully chosen agents should be appointed in London and Rotterdam. At London it would be sensible to employ three or four agents to avoid having a solitary agent setting a monopoly price on his services; competition between agents would hold down the costs of clandestine operations.

London was the best port for the dispatch of equipment and workers because of the vast movement of trade through the port, Rotterdam was the handiest staging post on the Continent.

Where French entrepreneurs wanted English workers to improve their methods of manufacture and products 'one may bring them over for them by the intervention of Sr Holker, but by using other means'. Because of the threat of fine and imprisonment under the English legislation any English merchant approached to entice men would charge a high price for his services. 'The surest and cheapest way to succeed is to send over an English worker employed in a French works so as to choose the workers who are needed, make an agreement with them, organize their passage to France and stay with them until they reach their destination.' This would help to avoid their desertion while still in England after they had been contracted for, and the 'difficulty these people find themselves in when they have landed in France without knowing the language' which led to increased expense, as well as the danger of the immigrant workers hiring themselves out to other employers for more money once they were abroad. The travel expenses of the workers should be paid by the Government, and they should be contracted with for so much a month for one or two years, on the basis that French firms would take them over on the conditions which had been fixed with them in England. 'This method seems to me the quickest and cheapest to transfer skills from one country to another.' Sometimes things were accomplished expensively in France which were done cheaply in other countries, because successful innovators demanded exclusive privileges. Even where this was not the case the entrepreneurs made a great effort to conceal their working methods, so that others would not enjoy the benefit of their new processes. Even when they only asked for modest help in setting up their concerns, this would often be far more costly than bringing over two or three English workers who could be circulated between the relevant works in France until the point where they had trained sufficient workers. If clever and useful, the Englishmen would eventually find employers who would be keen to retain them in French service.

This would also avoid difficulties which were sometimes not fully apparent. Many of those who tried to copy foreign expertise in France by trial and error and succeeded in small-scale trials hastened to set up large concerns without having mastered all aspects of a trade in which they were newcomers. Others, even less knowledgeable, but avid for profit, invested in these concerns and all were quickly ruined.

If the Government agreed with Holker's proposals and was prepared to spend something to attract good workers, he thought they should show preference to English Catholic workers, because it would be less costly to attract them and easier to retain them. It would be better to find unmarried workers who could be kept in France by offering dowries if they married Frenchwomen. They should be exempt from the taxes on foreigners and from all public dues for their lifetimes, and sometimes pensions should be given to Protestants who turned Catholic. Another useful plan would be for Holker to visit the bases where Scottish or Irish troops in French service were stationed, and arrange that when these regiments recruited soldiers in Britain, they could sometimes covertly engage artisans, intending them for French industry, and the Government could buy them out of their regiment on generous terms when they reached France.

If Holker could be given some remarkable recompense as a reward for his services to date, this could have important consequences. For instance, he could be given a commission as an inspector-general of manufactures concerned with foreign manufactures set up in France, with a salary which could partly go to his widow and children after his death. The news of this would persuade some of the Manchester manufacturers he knew to offer their services, especially some of his Catholic acquaintances, and this would enable him to extend his present concerns and start others elsewhere, with an emphasis on cloth finishing.

Again Holker could visit other cotton manufacturers including those making cotton velvet, whose works were less efficient than his own at Rouen, and show them the best English methods which would allow them to produce as well and as cheaply as his own *manufacture royale*; as yet they could not make the strongest velvets or the full range of varieties which would satisfy the market, and they were deficient in fustian-cutting, shearing, and various dyeing and finishing processes not yet fully practised even in his own works. Better looms and twisting and winding mills were needed if the English were to be equalled.

A plan was mooted for setting up a parallel enterprise in Brittany to the one now active in Normandy, with a similar 'colonie angloise', but this time two English spinning-mistresses would have to be specially recruited. To meet English competition more English calendering machines should be set up, including one at Paris, at 4,000 *livres* each. Equipment to heat plates for hot-pressing woollens should be set up in several textile centres, including those competing with the English in the Levant trade, which explains why it was thought important to start operations in Languedoc. To establish English finishing methods need not be highly expensive, it needed only one English finisher for each press erected. It would merely be necessary to pay their travelling expenses and arrange small pensions, which might only apply to their widows and children: 'Otherwise it might be difficult to keep them in France, and even hard to attract them, when they are well-behaved and skilled in their trade, two highly essential qualities.'

Finally Holker suggested that he could be sent on tours of inspection into all the provinces of France where there was wool or cotton production, so that he could see where there were defects which could be corrected, and help by improving poor quality cloths or introducing new types of fabric. He would work to create new manufactures in all places where they would be useful to the State.[44]

The memoir has an air of assurance about it, as if previous discussions with men in power had virtually invited it, or at least given it a green light. This is confirmed by Holker's rapid appointment in August 1755 as Inspector-General of Manufactures[45] 'et principalement de celles qui sont établies à l'instar des étrangères et des ouvriers étrangers' (and principally those using foreign methods and foreign workers). Trudaine now brought him out of the army. Having prolonged his leave from Ogilvy's regiment and obtained his back pay in 1754[46] he now asked for his discharge on the most favourable terms because of his use to commerce. This was done by giving him a 600 *livre* army pension as it would 'attach him more firmly to France'; the possible award of the military Order of St Louis was already suggested.[47] Holker's commission from the controller-general stated that Moreau de Sechelles had been told of his 'good lifestyle and morals, ability, and intelligence in relation to foreign manufactures'.[48]

Holker was to get the high official salary of 8,000 *livres*, a great increase on his officer's pay, and to visit, encourage and report on textile manufactures much as envisaged in his own proposal, and with the same emphasis on the finishing processes. Quite exceptionally he was tacitly permitted to carry on as an independent entrepreneur and, indeed, to add further ventures to those he was already engaged in at Rouen, while remaining a generously salaried public servant who was able to advise the Government about firms which could be in rivalry with his own. He must generally have been tactful in his official dealings, and it was only towards the end of his career, and after a generation in office, that he was seriously attacked on this potential conflict of interest.[49]

Almost immediately he began tours of French regions, which he carried out vigorously for well over a decade. He was introduced by letter to the intendants and inspectors of industry in the different provinces, who were required to give him all the information and facilities they could so that he could carry out his appointed tasks.[50] In communicating with Trudaine he did not take a narrow technical view of things, but commented broadly on deficiencies in French trade and industry and on the state of the population. In one of his first reports[51] after his appointment he regretted the lack of manufactures in the countryside, a theme he frequently returned to, and the extent that this meant poverty and hunger for the population, especially in winter, and the way that this could be mitigated by employment. France's West Indian colonies could provide cotton to be spun in the home country. Too often cotton was imported from foreign countries as yarn. He suggested sending out not merely agents to distribute raw cotton into new districts, but skilled spinning-mistresses who should accompany them, each to take on ten learners at a time, and to be provided with suitable wheels, cards and reeling equipment. Once taught the pupils could go off to their home villages and spread the best spinning techniques among relations and friends, a kind of monitorial system to achieve distance learning.

Holker outlined some elements of a putting out system for spinners, including weekly visits by an employer's agent to the districts around a textile centre to give out raw cotton and collect yarn. This was probably based on the Lancashire practice he was familiar with. He also advocated setting up cloth manufactures outside the main towns, with the aid of a short-term government subsidy, as a means of avoiding shortages of spinners and high costs. Here as always he insisted that the range of counts should be firmly controlled and standard hanks fixed according to the *tarif anglois* (English scale). Once the cloth producers got yarn of the exact fineness they required they could 'bring into existence textile products of every kind, and put France on an equality with England in foreign trade'. Holker listed towns he had already visited, including Provins, Saint Dizier, Villefranche and Auxerre. It was possibly on this early trip[52] that he made his first and helpful visit to Badger's calendering works at Lyon. Particularly notable was his picking on Sens, 'the most beautiful town in the world for the spinning industry and for clothmaking'. Some spinning and stocking weaving was already begun, but its meadows were well suited as bleaching grounds, and the frequent watering and the stretching out of the cloths could be carried on by a mixture of English and Flemish practices. Sens, as we shall see, was shortly to be a centre of his proselytizing of new industrial methods.

In 1756 he reported on St Quentin, Valenciennes and Cambrai and generally on the Lyonnais, Dauphiné, Picardy and Champagne, and of course the textile techniques with which he was most familiar and on which he was most expert are repeatedly emphasized. But this was not merely a matter of his own preoccupation, for instance the Government specifically asked him to see if English hot-pressing methods would improve the 'Londrin' (London or English-type) cloths of Languedoc, so important for that focus of Anglo-French commercial rivalry, the Levant trade. His reports on textile manufacture, which after all was dominant in industrial production, ranged over a wide technical territory, from his criticisms of French failure to use hot water and fuller's earth in degreasing cloth, and to employ the English fulling mill with its hammers, to the lack of sheep breeds which could provide fleeces of the quality of their English counterparts. It is surprising enough that a man who had undergone hardly a decade as an apprentice and master in the Manchester finishing trade should be able to comment so broadly and effectively over such a range of textile manufacture, even if one makes allowance for the fact that the finishing trades gave an excellent perspective point for a view of textile manufacture as a whole. South Lancashire, home to considerable linen and woollen, as well as cotton, production would have given a particularly profitable experience. One has to admire the sensible bounds Holker set to his expertise; he did not pretend to teach the manufacturers and workmen of northern France how to make fine linens, nor those of the south how to make silk, though he has the odd observation on finishing or 'watering'. He gave high praise to some of Vaucanson's silk throwing machines at Aubenas.[53]

What does astonish is his ability to make important observations on industries which one would expect to be closed to him. As early as 1756 he reported and advised on the great centre of metal manufacture at Saint Etienne. He was able at once to fasten on to serious defects in the gun trade, and on the heavier end of hardware manufacture. The barrels of muskets and sporting guns were badly welded for instance, which he attributed to the badly forged iron supplied to Saint Etienne. Hardware was crudely produced. When goods had to be polished it was done by hand, whereas the English had moved to powered polishing equipment which did the job much better and with ten times less

labour. Where power was employed, for boring and some other operations, it was inefficiently used because the water-mills were poorly
installed, and often built in places where they did not have sufficient
water to work throughout the year. There was insufficient provision
for an overnight build-up of water in reservoirs to ensure work through
the day. Holker met Carrier de Montieu, an important manufacturer,
who clearly was greatly impressed by him. They discussed the question
of the large illegal import of English hardware, already a major problem, and Holker undertook to supply Carrier with English samples and
prices. If Carrier could not successfully imitate the goods without a
transfer of technology, Holker would get for him the most appropriate
English workers.

Carrier soon wrote to Trudaine, clearly following up Holker's advice,
and asking for English workers. His analysis of Saint Etienne's deficiencies was clearly inspired by the inspector-general; the workers operated
in individual isolation at their forges, while the English usually worked
in small teams at workshop or forge; the English employment of power
gave far superior polishing; they used powered rolls to laminate metals
exactly in one operation rather than by resorting to battery, and did the
job four times quicker; the French used files when they could grind with
a powered wheel at a hundred times the speed. As far back as the
memoir to Trudaine proposing his inspectorate, Holker had emphasized
the importance of English hardware methods to France. At the time of
his Saint Etienne trip Holker had been touring extensively and was much
away from Paris; there is no indication that he had had any dealings with
Michael Alcock, the important Birmingham manufacturer who had come
to France at the beginning of 1756, and he is not mentioned in the
report.[54] The views expressed in Saint Etienne seem to have been entirely
Holker's own, which gives a remarkable example of the extent and
width of his industrial interests; few textile men could have given such a
trenchant criticism of the shortcomings of the metallurgical industry.
Holker also examined the calendering and goffering (making crimped or
wavy with hot irons) of the Saint Etienne ribbon manufacture. He indicated that the use of machines and heat there was uneconomical, and
undertook to send machinery from Rouen.[55] He severely criticized the
operation of ribbon looms.

At the same time he voiced general views on French industry which
penetrated into issues of enterprise, competition and industrial culture.
At Saint Etienne he believed that work was done without any spirit of
competitiveness. They kept on turning out the same old products

without innovating or creating new designs and tastes. He was surprised by their lack of drive in continuing to rely on manual labour without introducing inventions which might substitute for it. But this seemed almost the norm among the *bas peuple* in France, in contrast with the English artisan class, who were imbued with activity and industry. Clearly Holker thought that industrial improvement derived from the skilled workers as much as from the entrepreneurs in England. Like nearly all contemporaries (though not always modern historians) he thought that taxes and dues contributed to poverty among French workers; they and their products were charged with government duties and there were a thousand difficulties over the circulation of the products within the country and dues to pay both within the country and on export. Anxieties about these things lowered men's spirits, torpor became an infectious disease. The English workman was in relative comfort, well fed, working in freedom and able to dispose of his produce freely: 'These amenities in life can have a greater influence on the spirits than either air or climate.'[56]

There were two parallel aspects to Holker's career in France. On the one hand he helped create and develop new firms in which he himself, his son, relatives and long-standing associates were involved. In some of them, notably the heavy chemical industry, he, and increasingly his son, had a financial interest. But in all cases there was an introduction of English technology. For the present we will pursue the other aspect, Holker's more diffuse and general activities as inspector-general, and subsequently return to the enterprises in which he had a close personal involvement.

Holker continued to try to get additional workers from England, but after the outbreak of war in 1757 he seems not to have repeated his earlier personal espionage expeditions, but to have relied on contacts. In 1760 he told Trudaine that Torrent, his partner in several textile ventures, had asked him to obtain an English dyer:

> consequently I wrote to my mother, but I have to warn you that I can't perform a similar commission in the like circumstances without there being great risks to my family, and perhaps even you cannot believe the way I am regarded in England because of all the different tasks I have performed [in France]; those people who are associated with me and have to continue living in England consider [my French operations] as a misfortune for them.[57]

In the early 1760s Holker was much pressed to try to help French woollen manufacturers, a main reason being that the French wished to

take advantage of the wartime break in trade between England and
Spain and to replace Spain's former imports of English woollens by
French goods.[58] The obstacle in many cases, however, was the poorer
quality of French woollens. In 1762 he obtained a range of English
samples which he boxed and sent to Amiens so that the manufacture
and finish could be understood; from Amiens they could go on to Lyon
and Montpellier and from those regional centres to other wool manufacturing places that Intendants thought useful.[59] Already Holker was
talking about composing a kind of instruction manual.[60] At Sens and
elsewhere he was pursuing a favourite project of obtaining cotton-
spinning mistresses who would then send their trainees out to educate
others. He was prepared to do this for woollens, but would need to get
hold of a knowledgeable woollen spinner and provide her with a
special wheel for spinning woollen yarn. Cotton clock reels would
serve for wool as well, though specimen hanks of wool spun in the
English manner would be needed for examples. In any case Holker
insisted on the limited expenses he would need to set up a spinning
school and to buy in the raw wool. He thought the perfecting of the
manufacture of baize was worth taking a great deal of trouble over,
and dyeing was important here.

> I think it would be well to employ an English dyer in the present
> situation, because they dye cloths in deep colours much better than in
> France and much more cheaply: but it is no small matter to find a
> good dyer who would suit; men of talent and good behaviour don't
> readily agree to leave their country; moreover it is not possible to find
> a dyer who can make himself understood when he gets to France, and
> sometimes the people to whom one entrusts this kind of worker [i.e.
> the employers] when they have got hold of their secret and can man-
> age without them, try to find improper tricks to get rid of them. This
> is so revolting to an honest man that one would not care to get
> involved with it – however there is nothing I would not do to fit in
> with M. de Trudaine's designs and the good of the State.

The job could not be done cheaply, because he would need to send
someone (presumably English) to choose a person who would be suitable, or get his London agent to come over to Ostend to talk the matter
over with him. Holker could not write directly to the agent to do the
job, because of the severity of the English laws – he was presumably
worried about the English government's opening of foreign letters,
particularly in wartime, and the agent's possible conviction for suborning. The dyer, if procured, should be tempted with funds to set up a
firm or be given a pension, a worthwhile man could not be got without

such terms. Holker said he would like to send over someone to learn dyeing in England, but though a young relative of a Rouen dyer was willing to go over he had no English and English workers would not work with him (particularly in wartime!). However, when his own son was old enough he would train him in dyeing and other textile processes and send him over to bring back English methods. As yet he was a few years too young.[61]

In another letter about getting an English worker for the bleaching of bayettes, Holker thought an outlay of 700 to 800 livres might be needed. The worker would need good pay and even a pension, 'because it is not possible that after he has worked over here he will be able to return to his country'. Whether Holker was simply concerned about the 1719 Act or expected the war to continue and affect the worker's situation if he wished to return is unclear.[62] To some of his neighbours and connections at Elbeuf in Normandy who were trying to develop baize manufacture so as to break into the Spanish market, Holker was recommending the fly-shuttle, and drew up a memoir on the subject. Goy, the inspector at Elbeuf, trusted it would be printed, so as to be spread to other woollen manufacturing centres: 'I am going to devote myself intensively to help him in his work, and thus to profit increasingly from his wisdom' [ses lumières].[63]

The French efforts to break into British cloth markets in Spain during the Seven Years War continue to be reflected in Holker's tours and in his efforts to help French woollen manufacturers. Over 1762–63 a Beauvais firm, Ruste, Garnier and Le Brasseur, approached him about problems in making baize and *sempiternes* to replace British goods in Spain. So far they had not succeeded well.[64] Le Brasseur had toured the Spanish market, and the firm had put twenty looms at work for it. They were following the example of another local manufacturer who, with the encouragement of the Council of Commerce, had worked with the local inspector to produce cloth of a suitable quality for Spain. However, these efforts were frustrated by imperfections in the finishing, particularly of the white cloths, which constituted three-quarters of the market, and where the Spanish were adamant about quality. There had been experiments in bleaching in Paris and Rouen as well as at Beauvais, but while one bleacher, Verité, had achieved some success, the return of peace meant that the Spaniards would simply resume their old patterns of English trade, while the French were still struggling with weaving the cloths on new looms which still had to be paid for. New equipment would be needed for bleaching, and the opposition of the Beauvais guilds, which forbade the use of fulling mills, had to be overcome. Early in 1763 Ruste was exploring a further market for baize, and trying to obtain specimens of the English versions which were exported to Guinea. As Ruste was consulting with an eminent French scientist (Duhamel de Monceau) about information he was supplying for one of the prestigious *Descriptions Des Arts et Métiers* volumes which was to be devoted to bleaching, he must have been thought of as very knowledgeable.[65]

In April of 1763 Ruste was still hoping that Verité could solve the bleaching problem. As so often in industrial experiments he could succeed well with smaller samples, but not with whole cloths. He was also trying to get French friends in London to get from English experts the answers to questions about baize production for which he needed information, including degreasing, fulling and bleaching, and arrangements were being made to have the information sent in the ambassador's diplomatic bag. However, at about that point[66] it was decided to give a modest bounty of 600 *livres* to Verité and send for Holker, who promised to demonstrate the very latest English practices in finishing. Ruste had already visited Rouen to see Holker. He had also been impressed by the work of one of the English spinning-mistresses whom Holker had brought over, 'Mlle Genny' (Jenny Law) who was teaching the use of the large spinning wheel.

Early in July Holker was with Ruste and Company at Beauvais, and attracting fervent praise, 'M. Holker est un homme inimitable, grace à ses talens nous tenons enfin le blanc Anglais. Les bayetes qu'il vient de travailler chez le Sr. Verité sont d'une blancheur et un éclat que l'Anglois ne surpasse point, nous sommes tous ravis et enchantés' (Mr Holker is an inimitable man, thanks to his talents we can at last produce English white. The bayettes he has just worked at Mr Verité's are of a brilliant white which the English themselves could not surpass; we are all delighted and enchanted). Manufacturers, merchants, finishers and other people crowded hurriedly in to see the 'present with which M. Holker has pleased us'. On his 'lumières' the success of the 'bayettes' could be established. The cloth, though rough before Holker treated it, was soft to the touch afterwards, and gained 'infinitely in respect to appearance and quality'. Apparently Holker's use of urine in the degreasing of cloth before bleaching for white goods, or dyeing for coloured, was an innovation to Ruste and his Bayeux colleagues. After Holker's demonstrations there was 'intense emulation' and the observers were loud in their praise. There was similar interest at the other end of the production process as Miss Law established good order in a local charity institution where a public spinning school had been set up, and the places for students were continually filled. So many were attracted by the new spinning methods that Ruste thought the older ones might soon be abandoned. If all the changes in production were implemented 'no English cloth can any longer intimidate us'. Holker advised the partners to stop or recall their first intended exports to Spain which had been manufactured before his arrival, so as not to spoil their reputation in that market.

A further letter from Ruste said that 'Mr. Holker surpasses himself daily' and he was producing perfectly white cloths for them without the blue tinge which had previously been present. The finisher, Verité, who had previously experimented and had 'worked through so many nights only to arrive at mediocrity' was now wholeheartedly seconding Holker's efforts. Holker's cloth, unlike that finished previously, could be washed and remain perfectly good, while the former looked horrible once washed, 'the most pitiful thing in the world'. Like so many French innovating industrialists of the time, Ruste was keen to have spinning wheels, hand cards and shuttles supplied, and made enquiries with Holker for plans for English cloth presses. He seems to have wanted at least some of these things free or subsidized from government or the intendancy, and made skilful pleas to that effect, 'like the spinning wheels, the cards were made to be given to our poor spinsters who only live on bread and water, and who have not the money to pay the smallest part of the cost'. At the end of the correspondence Ruste acknowledged the receipt of twenty 'navettes anglaises' – Kay's flying shuttles – which he had distributed to baize weavers, and hoped to receive more.

Ruste seems to have been both an enthusiast and a skilful memorialist of the government, and his lavish praise of Holker should be a little discounted, but Holker's reception elsewhere was similar. An inspector of manufactures who was not critical in a merely negative sense, enforcing the letter of regulations, nor the purveyor of abstract and unspecific ideas of principle, but one who could on occasion roll up his sleeves and work alongside the local manufacturers, was a most refreshing change. The new methods Holker propagated emphasized the English technical lead which already existed. 'We seem today to be ... in an age of enlightenment' ('Siècle des lumières') wrote Ruste, 'in agriculture, the arts, and commerce; we take the English for our models, because they do things well.' He wished that French capitalists would support trade in the products of their national industries as the English did, rather than despising it as something beneath them 'ce commerce n'a rien de Roturier' (there is nothing plebian about this trade).

However, not every manufacturer was equally enthusiastic about Holker's inspections, though critical views were very rare in the early years. In 1759 he had trouble with Mainbournel, who was trying to develop cotton velvet manufacture and was bitter about the development of the privileged manufacture at Sens in which Holker was deeply involved, and strongly criticized the quality of the spinning there, especially that by children, and the early standard of the product. At the same time Mainbournel refused to allow Holker to inspect his own works. Holker was able to show Trudaine that good quality velvet was being produced at Sens, that the problems in recruiting and training young workers were well worth the trouble, and were now overcome. This meant that there was now a large use of French labour, while Mainbournel apparently imported his yarn from Utrecht. His works was virtually inoperative, and he was unwilling to learn. This problem of empowering Holker as inspector to examine the works of men who were actual or possible trade rivals was to recur much later, though here Holker insisted he was keeping strictly to his official duties.[67]

While it would not be possible to show the impact of Holker in every tour of inspection he made, one which is unusually well documented may be given as example. This was the month-long tour of Languedoc which Holker made in the summer of 1764 to Mende and other parts of the Gévaudan, Alès, Uzès, Nîmes, Montpellier, Castres, Albi and Montauban. Holker's detailed account of his tour as presented to the Archbishop of Narbonne survives in departmental archives and has been discussed by P. Vayssière,[68] while a very detailed account of that part of the tour which was through Gévaudan survives as it was written up on a day-to-day basis by the local *subdélégué* of the intendant.[69] This was not Holker's first visit to Languedoc which he had toured in 1756, early in his inspectorate.[70] Now he was well known from his circulated memoirs, one of which was published with illustrations of English hot presses and other equipment in the same year.[71] On this visit Holker was accompanied by his son John, whom he was training to succeed him in his post after a period of attachment, a practice well known in public office in France at that time. The example, at a more exalted level, of Trudaine and his son would not have been lost on him.

There was no question of Holker being an inspector sent from Paris to poke his nose into the affairs of provincial businessmen resentful of interference and criticism. This return visit to Languedoc was specifically requested by the Estates of the province which allotted him 6,000 *livres* – in addition to the 8,000 *livres* a year he was already receiving as inspector-general, not to mention his 600 *livres* army pension. This emphasizes Holker's pre-eminent position in an inspectorate whose basic pay was commonly 2,000 *livres* a year,[72] although it was to rise later in the century.

As Holker's visit was mainly targeted on the woollen industry, it is hardly surprising that his comments and strictures closely resembled those he had made on the production of light woollens in Northern France. Naturally he recommended the English practices he knew well, the slight oiling of the wool to improve its handling in carding, spinning and weaving, the need for greater regularity in spinning, for which Holker again recommended the use of a standard *dévidoir* and the setting up of spinning-schools, originally under English spinning-mistresses, with the use of the large spinning-wheel. In some places John Kay's cards should be turned to, now made by the Le Marchand brothers of Rouen. The use of the distaff was still practised by some Languedoc spinners – Holker had never met this piece of industrial archaeology before! Once taught, spinners should be paid according to the fineness of their yarn. Washing should be more thorough and fulling should be done with an attractive mixture of putrid urine mingled with pig dung, and the tubs and beaters should be redesigned on a lighter pattern than in the conventional fulling-mill. Holker did not merely advise, he had the equipment built and demonstrated it. He showed the importance of using hot water instead of cold in some finishing processes; here the difference between his native Lancashire with its cheap coal and Languedoc, much of which had a fuel shortage, would hinder the taking-up of his advice. Similarly he emphasized the importance of hot-pressing and the use in the presses of glazed cardboard (which ought to be made in France) as well as the introduction of calenders.

The amount of advice that Holker gave on sheep-rearing and shelter and on pasture was quite remarkable, and most of it seems good sense. He considered the local sheep well bodied and well tended on the whole, but thought that the quantity and quality of feed was more important than modifying the breed, though this was not to be neglected. But he particularly attacked the pens in which sheep were shut during the winter, in which there was no provision to get rid of dung or urine. This not only affected the health of the animals but caused part of the fleece to be discoloured and worthless. There should be ventilation at the top of the covered pens, to let air in (but not wolves!), and straw for the ground, to be periodically removed. Sadly, in many parts of the province the supply of winter forage was too poor to allow its use for litter as opposed to animal feed, and Holker discussed this. The local bishop and officials had recently tried cultivated pasture (*prairies artificielles*) planted with sainfoin, and then distributed this seed to farmers. In some places the cultivated grasses had been burned out in hot weather, and here Holker advised sowing the grasses with barley or rye which would protect them – agricultural advice new to the province.[73] Once again we realize the breadth and intensity of Holker's observation of the British scene, which (in his few adult years there) had taken in not only the skills of his own trade of calenderer, but the bleaching, dyeing and finishing of many textiles, and from that had gone on to an understanding of the basic production processes of several textile industries, and even to an intelligent acquaintance with farming practice and that of metal-goods production.

Holker was always alive to the situation of all ranks in society, and had a particular care for the poor. He was clear on the means to be taken to improve and increase the wool supply, but saw that the limiting factor was the poverty of the peasant. For the steps he proposed to be successful:

> It is necessary that the inhabitants, especially the country-dwellers, should be able to rise above their present poverty and enervation; he [Holker] was deeply touched by the general misery of the population, indeed he was so affected by it that upon his arrival he told us ... that he feared that his travels in the Gévaudan would come to nothing, as he saw no way that anything could be done in a province where all the inhabitants seemed so poverty-stricken.[74]

In comparing production costs in England and the Gévaudan Holker found that the cost of raw wool was lower than in England 'but the cost of labour is much greater'. Some English weavers could make over two shillings (up to 3 *livres*) a day while 15–20 *sous* was the going rate in the Gévaudan, so that wage rates could rise substantially without affecting competitiveness. But he was well aware that the local merchants were scared of extending their trade and taking it directly into foreign countries 'frightened that they might risk their fortunes'. In the large French towns merchants were not so timid, and the local merchants could follow suit, providing they chose their foreign representatives carefully.

In some places merchants were worried that Holker's recommendations for changes in working methods and the size of cloths could not be forced on the workers at once as they would not want to abandon their customary practices. The merchants anticipated disorder and a falling off in manufacture and in consumption. However simple the new methods were to implement, some manufacturers would not dare to use them initially, some merely from prejudice in favour of old ways, others because of worries that changes Holker recommended in the widths of cloths would bring customer resistance, or affect profit margins. Holker insisted that he did not want to put constraints on manufacturers, 'he agreed they should be left complete freedom to work in the way they had used to', it was dangerous 'to forbid them to use the old ways and compel them into new ones, that we ought to imperceptibly and voluntarily persuade them to follow the new ones and encourage them by example and get them to make experiments'. Once they saw the advantages of change they would adopt it of their own accord. Now he had seen the state of things on the spot, Holker would produce a supplement for local manufacturers which could be circulated with his existing pamphlet, and would take in their particular problems. The onus should not be left with the workmen, it was the local merchants who should set an example in promoting new kinds of cloth and exploring foreign markets. Up to now they only acted as passive commission agents for merchants in the great towns of France and were content with small profits, acting so as to augment the profits of the distant merchants by forcing down as much as possible the returns of the local manufacturers, who often gained little or nothing. If they would only act independently as merchants and deal directly abroad they would then be able to let the producers earn the wages their work deserved.

Similarly the merchant manufacturers, one tier below the merchants proper, paid too little attention to the spinners and weavers who worked for them 'the poor folk are slaves to the merchants who, in the main, have no other object but their own private interest'. Again he attacked the inspectors of manufactures at Montpellier and Marseilles as a source of trouble, unresponsive to ideas for less rigid controls over cloth types which had been operative since 1756, and needing a thorough shake-up.[75] For the workers themselves he believed that the only way to get them to change their ways was by practical demonstration:

'Good advice will make no impression on a workman, settled in his principles and work practices; it is only by example that one can convince him of the true situation'.

This account of Holker's tour of Languedoc in 1764 brings out many features of his work. He was sure that in many departments of textile production English practice was better than French, but technically he tended to stick to what he knew about; it was largely on cottons and light woollens that he pronounced most strongly, and he was very keen to improve the quality and regularity of spinning and the efficiency of the finishing processes by introducing English methods.[76] What is most impressive is Holker's ability to take an overview of the economic situation in the province, to allow for acute fuel shortages in some districts; to see the decisive importance of the forage supply in maintaining and increasing sheep flocks and the wool crop, and to suggest ways of managing the new sown grasses; to show the importance for wool quality of washing sheep and over-wintering them in good shelter. To the relationship between regional agriculture and industry he added, as we have seen, an understanding of the wider national and international trading of industrial goods. While prepared to advocate some subsidy from the national or provincial coffers for training, or the exemplary installation of new equipment in manufacturing (therein taking advantage of French governmental attitudes towards intervention in industry which had no English parallel), he was generally keen to advocate a liberty from controls typical of his native country rather than of France. In addition to those freedoms just mentioned he recommended that the Uzès Protestants should be allowed as much liberty as Catholics were allowed in England, which would double their efforts in trade. The Lyons authorities should be content with their domination of the upper end of the silk market and let the Nîmes entrepreneurs concentrate on the cheaper end, and the manufacturers should not be hampered by quality controls 'we have to clothe people of every condition who demand materials of very different styles'; there should not be any impediment to the spread of industry into the countryside, whatever guild officials might wish. The 1764 inspection should not be treated in complete isolation, it was Holker's second tour of the province, while his son made several later ones. But the *subdélégué* at Mende seems to have voiced a general appreciation

> after having helped M. Holker in all his operations, which he pursued with the greatest diligence, it is very much to be desired that the public, which has been extremely satisfied with the width of his

knowledge, the simplicity, exactness and success of his processes should also make haste to profit by the enlightened views which he has personally communicated to them.[77]

4 Holker, Kay and Badger

John Kay

Holker's duties as Inspector-General of Foreign Manufactures implied an overview not only of those manufactures which he and his family and close connections established in France, but of those established by other Britons, in some cases men whose arrival had been coeval with his own and his move from a military to a manufacturing life. Two of them had been much better known on the English industrial scene than he. One, John Kay, was established as a significant inventor and patentee since the early 1730s, the other, Michael Alcock, had been one of the largest manufacturers in the Birmingham 'toy' trade. Kay had come to France while Holker was newly commissioned in the French army; Alcock had arrived about the time when Holker was made inspector-general, but had certainly not been recruited by him. Both generally detested Holker's assignment to interfere in their operations or regulate their procedures: back home it would have been inconceivable to an English manufacturer in one industry that a man whose training was in another should tell him his business. That in a French context Holker was evidently a much more successful businessman than they were, and that his understanding of the broad industrial and administrative scene was quite remarkable, only served to increase their dislike. Neither of them had Holker's Jacobite credentials, or had risked their life in that cause, so their loyalty to France was more suspect. Though both died in France, and Alcock founded a family of some importance, both were tempted to return home to England when things did not go right for them in France, and Kay several times yielded to the temptation. Though both were men of high ability and were recognized as talented by the French administration, they were both men of whim and mood, and Alcock was also prone to periods of depression and acts of violence.

Much of the historical detail on the career of Kay has been clouded by mistaken evidence, provided by people who were related to, or connected with, the inventor. Few of these knew anything much about his long connection with France. However, the superb scholarship of Wadsworth and Mann, in their classic account of the rise of the Lancashire cotton industry, not only sorted the wheat from the chaff as far as Kay's English activities were concerned, but identified and examined the main French sources, and their work has only been supplemented here. Kay's English activities will only be summarized, while his relations with the French government and other Englishmen in France are discussed more fully.

Born near Bury, Lancashire, in 1704, Kay was apprenticed to a reedmaker, and practised the trade until 1733. His lifelong devotion to invention began with a patent for twisting thread in 1730, and in 1733 there was patented the famous shuttle, originally called the 'wheel shuttle', but later given the name 'fly' or 'flying' shuttle in England, which probably reflected the title of 'navette volante' which it had acquired in France. Much of the early employment of the shuttle seems to have been in the woollen trade – of which of course there was a flourishing branch in East Lancashire. But Colchester was a main early centre for the shuttle's introduction. The advantages of the shuttle were its ability to dispense with a second weaver when making broad cloths and, according to the inventor, an increased speed and regularity of weave. On the one hand the working weavers in Colchester protested vigorously at the dangers of technological unemployment, on the other, Kay and a group of partners were continually in conflict with the masters for copying the shuttle without permission, or using it without paying the modest licence fee. Attempts by the partnership to get redress in the courts were frustrated by legal difficulties and delays.

In the Lancashire woollen district the shuttle was objected to as too small and too light. Kay therefore made it longer and heavier, and also introduced an immovable rather than a rotating spool, which with the larger shuttle could carry far more weft. These improvements were made by 1735, but were not patented, and manufacturers took the risk of using the fixed spool without paying for licences from Kay, some claiming rather unconvincingly that the wheel shuttle itself was not new. Similar infringements began in the Colchester district, and Kay's legal position on the unpatented fixed spool was poor. There was another spate of legal actions by Kay against Lancashire men in the early 1740s, indicating that the shuttle's use was spreading in its improved form, and it was also taken up round Leeds. While there are statements that Kay was driven out of England by riots against the shuttle, and personal threats, they probably oversimplify the situation. The pamphlet which gives an account of the troubles, and was probably drawn up by John Kay and his son Robert in the early 1760s, seems to put the riots in the early years of the invention's diffusion.

It was almost certainly the approaching expiry of the patent in 1747, aggravated by his failure to derive worthwhile profit from it even when it had been in force, which drove Kay abroad in 1746.[1] Wadsworth and Mann may well have a point in suggesting that Kay's later reluctance to make solitary journeys on French government service to promote his inventions may have been coloured by an abiding fear of worker violence derived from his English experience. But his failure to speak or write French – he was scarcely literate in English – probably has a bearing here. And, if his business ability in early life was as poor as it seems to have been later in France, Kay may also have had bad debt as a reason for going to France, and he said as much in a letter to the Society of Arts in the 1760s.[2]

The time of his arrival in France can be fairly accurately tied to the end of 1746 or the first weeks of 1747. His French partner said in November of that year that Kay had been with him for nine months, while the news that Kay's wife had died in England after the birth of their thirteenth child reached France in the same month. Given the slowness of French bureaucratic processes, the facts that an *arrêt* was issued in November 1747 in favour of Kay and his partner Daniel Scalogne, and that they had applied for a privilege in the spring of that year, make it virtually certain that they were in contact from the moment of Kay's arrival in France. This suggests that his emigration was not opportunistic, but arranged. Kay went straight to Scalogne's works at Abbeville. Daniel Scalogne and his brothers were second generation immigrants of a Dutch family which had been in France for about ninety years. Their father had been the first foreman of the Van Robais firm, the famous manufacturers of fine woollen cloth who had been brought by Colbert from Holland in order to raise the standards of the French industry, but the brothers were now working independently of the original firm. Daniel Scalogne had spent seven years in England, and one source says Kay had already visited France in 1745.[3]

Kay had no modesty about his worth or that of his inventions. Offered a pension of 1,200 *livres* a year by the French government he demanded £10,000 as a price for the rights in his inventions, the fly-shuttle and the bobbin-shuttle. As late as August 1747 he claimed to be about to withdraw his offer in a highly typical letter, ill spelled and reflecting his native Lancashire speech:

> As you canot find out no wea to gratifi mee for what I have shoad you that will be of ane [any] survis to mee for that reason I will not sho you ane more, in four or five months time I could meack your shuttle meackers and weavers parfect so that the(y) might do as well without me as with me, my resolucon is this that except you can find some wea to rease me ten or twelve thousand pounds of the factres [factories, *sic*] that my invenchons will be of sarvis to [to] be pead me in five years' time at fore or five set times without that I will not meak ane bargain with you at all.[4]

The *arrêt* for Kay and Scalogne said that they were in partnership at Abbeville to make and diffuse the shuttles and to instruct shuttlemakers in producing them and weavers in using them. There was no intention to prevent weavers who took up their shuttle from reverting to the conventional one when appropriate. Trials had been made before Inspectors General of Manufactures, there had been memoirs from them, from the Deputies of Commerce, and reports from two commissioners, Machault and Leroy. Kay and Scalogne were to get a fourteen-year privilege of manufacture (exactly the time which would have been granted by an English patent) from the beginning of 1748 and any persons who counterfeited the shuttles or used them without the written consent of the partners were liable to have their shuttles confiscated and be fined, and any who were permitted to make the shuttles could only do so at a price fixed by Kay and Scalogne.[5] But Kay was not happy with the privilege arrangements and was at loggerheads with Scalogne by the following May. He was only reconciled by an inspector of manufactures on the understanding that Scalonge 'will leave of his sile ways'.[6] Kay set up a Paris workshop but by the autumn of 1748 was refusing to make more shuttles, even at high prices. A worry, which was to prove a lasting one for French administrators, raised its head in this instance: though Kay and Scalogne were at odds, Scalogne was said to be involved in the suborning of workers to go to Spain, and Kay to be thinking of emigrating there, all the more disturbing in that he was now working on a multiple-thread spinning device. Kay was prevailed on to sell the rights to use his shuttles to entrepreneurs of *manufactures royales* and to other manufacturers in Languedoc, payment to be divided with Scalogne.

In 1749 it was recognized that the shuttle had not spread as widely as was desired ('the majority of the manufacturers of the Kingdom have ignored the advantages which one can obtain from these shuttles'), that the partnership with Scalogne was not working, and that a new approach was needed. Now Kay proposed that all manufacturers in the kingdom should have the use of the shuttles, provided they were made by him and so marked, and he would increase production by bringing over one of his sons, probably Robert, and would himself travel to the main centres of production to make known the advantages of the shuttles. However, if anyone counterfeited the shuttles, or used them without payment, confiscation and a fine would still apply. From Kay's point of view perhaps the main provision was that Scalogne was no longer to interfere in his affairs and that he himself was now to become a royal pensioner at 2,500 *livres* a year as long as he and his son remained in France and produced shuttles.[7]

To the question of the pace and spread of Kay's invention we will return, but in the short term it was said to be spreading in Berry, Orléans, Vire and Caen in 1752[8] and Kay petitioned Trudaine to prevent it being counterfeited around Orléans in the April of that year.[9] Briefly in 1753 we seem to find Kay contented, even exuberant, about his treatment in France. The authorities asked Kay to look after Badger, the newly arrived English cloth-finisher, and first to write him a letter of encouragement. He stayed with Kay in Paris before setting off to Lyon to introduce his celebrated equipment for watering silk. Kay, who never seems to have written a line in French (his letters in that language were written by others and signed by him) and whose English, as we have seen, was execrable, told Badger that 'the sooner he could make the French perfect, the greater his benefit would be'. He assured Trudaine in the same letter that Badger 'had nothing to do but follow Mr. Trudaine's directions and make him his friend' Having got his pension just before Badger left, Kay 'let him see what a bag of money I received every three months, and it was owing to Mr. Trudaines's goodness'.[10]

While some interest still remained in the shuttles (though as in England they ceased to spread after a few years, and then were not revived for a long period) Kay now devised a method for making hand cards, the standard equipment for carding textiles, by new machines of his invention. However, he only did so, according to Bellefonds, after a brief return to England, and his promise of a card-making invention was a peace-offering to Trudaine.[11] In 1754 he built two machines, one of which punched the holes through the leather covers of the cards more regularly and smoothly than a leather worker could do by hand; the second machine bent the ends of the wire teeth of the cards more accurately than could be done with a hand tool and much more quickly. There seem to have been teeth on Kay's cards which were not only more regular, but more numerous and shorter than on existing ones. Trudaine decided that there should be a proper testing of these machines and their product and this was prompted by some first essays with them by inspectors of manufactures and master manufacturers of the Elbeuf district of Normandy. The cards were supposedly usable for different kinds of textile, and Trudaine had examples sent to the Van Robais firm at Abbeville in 1756, and even to manufacturers at Carcassonne in Languedoc. There, while the superior work of the cards was recognized – they had 126 rows of teeth in the length and 63 in the width – it was observed that they could not be charged with as much wool as the old ones and the carder could not earn a living from them. Much clearly depended on the fineness of the woollen yarn required and the fineness of the cloth to be produced, and there was little to be gained for coarse cloth.

Nevertheless, there were some sales of the cards in Languedoc, and the machine seems to have been taken up in several parts of France, but to make less exacting cards than Kay had himself produced. A Lyons cardmaker, previously endeavouring to imitate better foreign cards, probably Dutch, came to stay with Kay to learn his methods in the autumn of 1754.[12] His shuttle pension had been cancelled, probably because of an absence in England, but he received a new one for his card machines. By 1757, however, the Le Marchand brothers of Rouen had been empowered to set up in that town a workshop for the production of cards on Kay's system, but asked for a subsidy of 600 *livres* in order to establish their firm, and a bounty on each pair of cards produced. Holker had been asked to report on this scheme. He said that the cards were less robust than the ordinary ones, but equal in quality to English ones. The cards had been tested at the school set up with his co-operation to teach English spinning methods there. Feydeau de Brou, the local intendant, proposed to pay the Le Marchands the 600 *livres* for their loss of time and the investment to date, 400 *livres* a year for six years as a subsidy on the shuttles, and a bounty for each worker trained. They were to be bound to make at least 2,000 cards and were to keep a weekly register of sales for the local inspector of manufactures. Trudaine seems to have agreed and left the intendant a free hand.

The Le Marchand brothers seem initially to have been recruited by Holker to go to Paris to gain practical experience of the machines from

Kay himself.[13] They seem to have started well. Godinot, the Rouen inspector, reported on their output from May 1758 to June 1759, and on whether the cards were sold only in the generality or further afield. They had been welcomed at Amiens where seventy-two pairs had been sent. Thirty-seven had gone to Holker himself, and others to his associated cotton velvet concern at Saint Sever and to Sens. In all 379 pairs had been dispatched, all for cotton manufacture. Godinot added his reflections on the old and new types of card; the older did only half a job which in turn meant poor yarn and, of course, poor cloth. Trudaine praised Godinot for his efforts, and endorsed his suggestion that the cards should be sent to the inspector for the Beaujolais for the cotton industry of his department. But typically for him, while not completely forbidding the suggestion of an increased bounty for the Le Marchands, Trudaine believed that the intendant at Rouen should consider that if the cards were as good as they were made out to be, they would sell themselves once their superiority was seen, despite the initial prejudices caused by slower working and greater cost which Godinot had pointed out.[14] The Le Marchand brothers circulated a printed 'Notice to the Public' about their cards, clearly acknowledging them to have been 'Inventés par le Sieur Kay'.

Though Kay does not appear to have fallen out with the Le Marchands, he did with another cardmaker he had trained, and to whom he owed money, and who claimed to have improved on the Englishman's cards. Then there were further problems over his privilege because Kay was not himself making enough cards, and finally his refusal to train workers on a new card-making machine caused his privilege to be suspended in 1759.[15] Though he had already had 10,000 *livres* from the Government, he refused to make the card-making invention public without a large payment from the authorities over and above his pension.[16]

A quarrel Kay had with one of his sons which embroiled an inspector of manufactures caused him to return briefly to England in 1757–58. In 1757 Trudaine de Montigny wrote to his father that 'Mr. Kay is at times not an easy man to handle; if he returns to Paris, I shall endeavour to make him see sense'. He was not minded to send Kay's sons back to England as their father was demanding, they were of an age to manage their affairs as they wished as long as they did nothing that put them in the hands of the police.[17]

A 1759 rumpus was more serious and Kay returned to England under a cloud. Wadsworth and Mann thought that he continued in

England for most of the 1760s, but already in March 1761 Kay was back in Paris, and asking Feydeau de Brou, the Intendant of Rouen, to intercede for him with the elder Trudaine. De Brou met Kay and told him that Holker was the right person to sort his affairs out with the administration, and made it clear to Kay that he thought that he was 'a man who does not listen to reason any longer'. Kay soon wrote to de Brou however that 'it is the first time that I learnt that the Sieur Holker should be employed in my affairs, or meddle with them in any way', though it is inconceivable that he did not know that Holker was advising Trudaine. He declared that his dealings had mainly been with 'Mons. de Montigny l'academicien', that is Mignot de Montigny, not Trudaine's son Trudaine de Montigny, though he was an Academician too. In fact all these men worked closely together. Kay claimed that Holker had badly used a man called Falkener ('un homme de son pays') – probably meaning a fellow Lancastrian – even though Falkener had gone over to England for him to recruit the English spinsters now at Sens. Falkener was now destitute, having been offered only a workman's job at Rouen by Holker though 'he is a gentleman born and has never worked a day in his life'.[18] By his espionage Falkener had lost a valuable estate in England and was now unable to return.

Kay expected equally bad treatment if he was involved with Holker. Later, in 1779, he claimed that his departure for England in the 1760s was due to his distaste for a forced business alliance with Holker:

> I have been starved of(f) the kingdom twice the Reas(on) that I went to England the theard time Lord Trudean would forse me to go into pardener Shipe with Mr. Holker at Rouen to set up a factre to meak Cards at Rouen with the Engines [Kay's card-making machines] for all the wooling and Coton factres in france. I gave maney good Reasons aginst it.

But he was told that 'Lord Trudaine would not meak ane other agreement with me. I Reseved [received] Seven hundred and fifty Livres for six month's pension and set of(f) for England I could not think of a better wea to breack Mr. Holker plan'. But he accepted that this caused Trudaine's anger.[19]

In May 1761 Kay approached Trudaine in a singularly unfortunate letter. It began 'I have the honour to tell you that we have been quarrelling for eleven years past on the matter of the card machines'.[20] This itself raises a problem, for Kay is supposed to have first produced the machine in 1754.[21] It is unlikely that Kay, however intemperate, would make a statement which would be utterly at variance with

Trudaine's own knowledge; possibly there were difficulties before Kay made the machines public in 1754, and prototypes at least were on hand in 1750. Kay said there had been seven years of dispute with Jacques Chrétien de Fumechon, an inspector of industry who had become inspector-general in 1744 and was stationed at Rouen.[22] Chrétien had corresponded with 'three or four of my children who had bad dispositions'. Kay thought that it could only have been Chrétien who had blackened his reputation with Trudaine by false reports and by maintaining that Kay was a man who went back on his word. Clearly Kay's many quarrels began at home. Twenty thousand *livres* paid at the outset, the inventor said, would have made him more contented and given him more pleasure than 100,000 would do now. He was now ready, Kay condescendingly told one of the greatest men in France, to make an agreement with him to promote the card machines 'dans leurs derniers perfections' (indicating that improvements had been made). He wanted the arrears of his pension paid, which he had not received for a year and three months (this may give an idea of the length of his absence in England) and the return of his machines. While Trudaine was not a man to be influenced by fawning or adulation, Kay's letter was remarkably in contrast with the servile obsequiousness and elaborate stylistic etiquette almost invariably used by those asking ministers for favours. Kay had however written to an unnamed dignitary a couple of months earlier, and in a more suitable style, asking him to intercede with Trudaine, but his claims that Trudaine had not made proper agreements with him despite continual requests over eleven years were unlikely to have been listened to. He said that if he had been given 'reasonable' encouragement he would have invented and perfected other things of great value to France.

In Kay's absence Trudaine, with the help of Ballainvilliers, the intendant at Riom, had been attempting to spread the use of the cards round Le Puy because of the better work they performed, despite the problems of less durability and the costs of some preliminary working of the wool on traditional cards. At least the price of the cards had been substantially reduced by a Le Puy cardmaker.[23]

There seems to have been no accord reached with Trudaine because Kay once again went back to England, probably for the last nine months of 1765, and made considerable, but as usual, undiplomatic efforts to find patronage in his own country. On this occasion he seems to have got in touch with the British ambassador to France, the Duke of Bedford, following the Peace of Paris, and probably went through the forms of recall by diplomats abroad under the provisions of the 1719 Act.[24] This he apparently did in 1763, and it was also the basis of a letter to Arkwright who had been seeking information on John Kay senior's patents, and his treatment as a patentee.

John Kay's son Robert, himself the inventor of an important weaving device, the drop box, had apparently returned to England before his father, and had approached a relatively new body, the Society of Arts, with an improvement to his father's 'wheel' or 'fly' shuttle in February 1764. It was referred to their 'Committee of Mechanics' by April. Robert Kay seems in fact to have produced a shuttle largely of a brass construction. The committee seem to have been at a loss to know what to do about it, and to have displayed that ignorance of the mainstream of contemporary technology which meant that the impact of the Society on the Industrial Revolution was nearly negligible. Nudged into wakefulness by Robert Kay in December, they confessed that they did not 'know any person who understands the manner of using his Shuttle' and asked for full written instructions. Robert Kay sensibly doubted 'whether or no the Committee will be able by any instructions that can be given by letter to try the utility of the wheel shuttle'. He suggested that the improved shuttle should be tried in the Bolton area where the cotton weavers were now extensively using his father's wooden version. This correspondence seems to have got nowhere.[25]

In late 1765 John Kay himself was in correspondence with the Society. He was promoting his two machines for making wire cards, apparently for use with both wool and cotton, and claiming that their particular virtue was that 'children of twelve or thirteen years of age is more proper to work these Engines that I have made than grone up person's' and that even so they would produce as much work in one day as in twelve by the old methods.[26] The machines were examined by the Committee of Manufactures in January 1766, in his presence, and they found them 'very ingenious and well contrived'. They asked that six pairs of cards should be made by the machines and offered Kay 2 guineas for the materials. However the Society received an undated letter from Kay two days before the machines were to be examined, and nothing more is recorded. Items in French archives give Kay's side of the story and give his ostensible reasons for breaking off negotiations. He claimed in the 'Memoire du S. Kay, ouvrier anglais' that 'the Society had subsidized him and got him to make new machines while promising him a substantial reward'; this seems to much exaggerate their support. He said that he had made several trials of his card-

making machines, to which he had made some well-regarded improvements, but that he had been deeply offended by a member of the
Society's Committee on Mechanics who had strongly attacked him for
going over to France 'ou il avoit contre tout probité communiqué ses
decouvertes' (where he had, most dishonestly, made known his discoveries). Kay said he chose to regard this hardly surprising remark as
'mauvais traitement'. He was also 'frustrated' in his hopes, which
seems to mean that he did not think the Society would reward him. He
now sought to go back to France with one of his sons, but he wanted
to have his travelling expenses paid, and have some debts paid off
'which he had been obliged to get into in order to live'. He attached to
his memoir to the French government three models of the improved
cards he now made. In two of them the teeth were placed closer
together, which would make the carded wool finer.[27]

Kay had hardly allowed the Society of Arts a real chance to help him,
for he had broken off negotiations prematurely and wrote to Trudaine
de Montigny to support his return. He produced a few untypically polite
words by framing his letter as one of those New Year felicitations which
French subordinates or pensioners were accustomed to send to powerful
patrons (some of Holker's survive) generally in a distinctly sycophantic
style. Kay's to the younger Trudaine simply came 'to wish you and your
father a happy new year and many of them', and immediately got down
to business. He claimed that he had gone to England nine months before
because of encouragement from the 'Society of London', by which he
meant the Society of Arts, not the Royal Society. This really does not
square with his statement in the 'Mémoire' that he had himself approached the British Ambassador in Paris for help to get home without
penalty; but he repeated his dubious statement about substantial help
from the Society. The Committee of Manufactures which had looked at
his machine were (he said) 'most of them old *fabricans*', using the French
term. They had referred the matter to the 'Committee of Mechanicks'
but in the interval before that meeting the distrustful Kay took the
machine apart, took key pieces away in his pocket and locked up the
rest. When the committee met he faced the accusation about his unpatriotic behaviour, made 'to make it appear that I was a rogue' for going to
France. One member said 'that I might make my fortune with working
for them and I had not persuaded him but that I had instructed they [*sic*]
French in everything that I know'd and that I had stayed in the Country
as long as they would have anything to do with me'. Asked to withdraw
before the mechanical experts examined the machines, Kay again took

the key parts off them. The Society was tolerant enough to ask him to make some cards, as we have seen, and pay for the materials, and tried, according to Kay, to disavow those who had so strongly attacked him. Despite the Society's attempts to appease him, Kay took away as much of the machines as he could carry, and soon after brought away the rest, so that his touchiness had ended his chances.

The machines, according to Kay, now embodied both improvements he was envisaging before he left France and others 'that I have learn't by inspectin into the Cards that are made here'. Trudaine de Montigny was curtly informed that 'if your father is willing to make a reasonable agreement with me', the terms of which were to be made very clear before Kay left England, he would return to France. This, however, must ensure that he did not have 'any thing to do with such a scoundrel as Holker and his followers'. He wanted all the arrears of his pension, and warned Montigny that if he wished to have him back in France he should be 'Expedishus in your answer or else necessity will oblige me to take their money [The Society of Arts?] or apply to some other ambassadour'.[28] An invitation must be accompanied by expense money! This was hardly the language to use in addressing a French minister. The letter collapses into all the pathos of poverty at the end: 'I have borrowed a guinea of your ambassadour but he will not advance any more without your order'.[29]

The Trudaines now turned to Holker for his views, which can hardly have become friendlier if he had seen the original of the Kay letter just quoted. From Holker's reply to Trudaine de Montigny it seems that in the short interval before he wrote Kay had added the virtues of his shuttle to his claims about card-making. From what we have learned of Kay, Holker's observations seem both inevitable and judicious. 'Kay is a distrustful man who regards as his enemy anyone who wants to advise him'; but for this fault he could have been very fortunately placed in France with his pension of 1,800 *livres* and his exclusive right in the shuttle which he sold at a very high rate in several Generalities. Holker defended the value of Kay's shuttle, and dismissed the views of the inspector in Carcassonne who had denied its usefulness to Trudaine de Montigny. This opinion 'joined to Sieur Kay's bad conduct towards your father' [Trudaine senior] had lost Kay his pension. The card-making invention was being used by the Le Marchand brothers in Rouen who produced much the best cards for cotton, but Kay's insistence of having 100,000 *livres* for his invention had frightened everyone off. All the well-meant advice he had been given had flowed (to use a

Lancashire idiom for relations between those two redoubtable Lancastrians) like water off a duck's back, and Kay's demands for such a sum implied that the Government had given him nothing. Holker believed that he had sold the card-making machines to the Le Marchands for 1,000 *livres* before leaving for England, so that they now had possession of them. Kay may have done this to spite Holker and prevent him being involved with his invention. Holker did not think that Kay should be encouraged to come back. He had been ungrateful in attacking in England the character of his chief patron, the elder Trudaine, and those close to him; Holker almost certainly inferred that he himself was one. 'If he does come back you can never satisfy him, and so I would advize you not to concern yourself in the matter.'[30]

But the Trudaines were more merciful than Kay's fellow Lancastrian. Kay probably returned to France in 1769, and cards made by his machines were being sent for trial to several provincial intendants (Lyon, Burgundy, Languedoc, Champagne) in that year, probably with some satisfactory results, because in 1770 Kay obtained a bounty of 2,400 *livres* and a pension of 1,500 *livres* because of the card-making machine.[31] The plan for spreading the use of the machines seems to have become bogged down; the proposal that Kay should be granted 1,200 *livres* for taking six pupils (four for Normandy, one for Beaujolais, one for Sens) raised doubts when he was unwilling to give up his 'secrets'. In 1779 Kay recalled that ten years before the elder Trudaine had consulted Mignot de Montigny to provide a plan for spreading the manufacture and use of the card-making machines for cotton and wool, and securing their general adoption within eighteen months. Kay had recently seen the plan, now in the office of Tolozan, 'but this plan did not please Mr. Holker and his son'.[32]

However there is evidence that Trudaine de Montigny did send the card-making machines to the Rouen generality, the very home district of the Holkers, in 1771, on the basis that they were a major improvement on those produced by the Le Marchand's with Kay's earlier machines. The new machines had been officially tested and approved. If accepted at Rouen a reward could be paid to Kay, perhaps at the rate of 600 *livres* a set. But the officials did not get a favourable reply from the cloth workers who tried out the cards.[33] A reconciliation had taken place between the older Trudaine and Kay before the minister's death. '[He] was angre with me for sum time but he was frends with me before he dyed' and the minister had made arrangements that Kay's pension should be restored on condition that he taught clockmakers the art of making the hand cards. Thereafter Kay's movements are difficult to trace; though at Sens in 1771 he had subsequently another period in England from 1773 because of his refusal to give up his secrets. He returned late in 1774. He was setting up machines at Troyes in 1776, but was back in Paris in the following year.[34]

The French government, especially if we consider that the Trudaines, his original patrons, were no longer on the scene, was very generous to Kay. In the summer of 1778 he wrote that his payment from Troyes had tided him over, otherwise he would have had to leave France 'for want of bread'. 'I tack caffe twice a day wich is nine sous, six sous my diner and half a botel of wine at night and all is gon besids my Lodgins I Have not eat supers for above forty years past.' He was given a gratuity of 600 *livres* a year from 1 January 1779 'this artist is in an extreme misery and unable to continue his work'. But the first gratuity only cleared his debts, and once he had prepared a new set of tools he would need at least four rooms for workmen. In October he was asked by Necker to see Tolozan about money, and in November he was given an extra 600 *livres*, though of course his claims to have lacked help from the authorities for over twenty years were wholly wide of the mark.[35] While there have been different dates suggested for Kay's death, he was certainly alive in late November 1779 but probably died in the winter of 1780–81. In 1779 he promised a whole collection of inventions, one for silk-twisting, a water-powered ribbon-weaving machine, a warping device, a spinning-wheel for wool, cotton-carding and spinning machines, and a new fly-shuttle less likely to break thread, but the authorities seem to have recognized that age and poverty meant that he would not get very far with these plans. Nevertheless Mignot de Montigny, who had long known him, urged a generous view on the Government: 'cet artiste bien connu par son industrie a l'inconvenience d'être difficile à gouverner, mais qu'il est homme de génie et il est d'autant plus à propos d'examiner ses propositions que la dépense n'est pas bien grande' (this artisan is well known for his hard work but is difficult to control – he is, however, a man of genius, and therefore attention should be paid to his demands, which are not great).[36]

Kay's involvement with the French state prompts many reflections. Perhaps most remarkable is the extent to which he was supported; his genuine talent was recognized and continued to attract grants. This reflects great credit in particular on the two Trudaines and the academician Mignot de Montigny. There were times when he was out of favour and unsubsidized, but these coincided with times when his behaviour was outrageous, or times when, having pocketed the latest instalment of pension or gratuity, he took off without permission for England. It is not surprising that his fellow Lancastrian, John Holker, was frequently out of patience with him. His own fidelity to the French was in contrast with Kay's precarious loyalty, his own managerial efficiency with Kay's fecklessness and continual shortage of money (even in those periods when he had a good pension), his own self-help with Kay's profligacy. Kay's frequent flights from France and his regular returns holding out the begging bowl must have aroused in Holker feelings like those of the deserving towards the prodigal son. In a sense Kay's apparently unhindered comings and goings between England and France made nonsense of the 1719 Act. But this was really directed at the suborned workman, enticed by a British or foreign agent to go abroad and spread his skills beyond the seas. It rarely questioned the independent traveller or businessman as Kay would claim to be (he even called himself gentleman on a patent application) despite his provincial accent and low literacy. The workmen he took to France were mostly his sons, so suborning was hardly the word for their emigration to join their father.

There can be no doubt that, in common with some other emigrants, Kay's greatest enemy was his own character. He was fickle, irascible and, at times, treacherous.[37] He could not even retain the loyalty of his own sons. Perhaps his deepest trait was distrust, and it was just as marked when he was in England as when in France. The grass always seemed to be greener on the other side of the Channel, but France it was that received his final preference.

It has frequently been pointed out that, after his original success in demonstrating the flying shuttle, and the French authorities' strong efforts to promote it, its use died away for decades and only returned in the years before the Revolution. Perhaps too much should not be made of this as an indicator of a supposedly lower interest in technological change and innovation in France than in England. In England the original introduction had been in the woollen industry, despite the fact that cotton was by the 1730s more prominent than wool in Kay's native Lancashire, and a main attempt at its introduction had been in the Essex woollen trade. It had failed to take on. Only in the late 1760s was Kay's invention being extolled, and support being sought for its inventor, because of its recent rapid adoption in the cotton trade.[38] It was not reintroduced into some English woollen districts until the 1790s. Certainly the French evidence indicates that frequent breaking of yarn was a problem, the time lost outweighing the otherwise faster and more regular work with the fly-shuttle.

In France it is doubtful if its use persisted except to a small extent in the enclaves of English workers. It began to gain ground again in cotton before the Revolution, accompanying the new flood of English industrial immigrants in that industry who brought improved carding and spinning techniques, which perhaps provided a yarn more suitable for use with the fly-shuttle. The hand cards did not take off either, but were persisted with, large numbers being bought for the works where Holker had influence. Workers in France as in England always found reasons for not changing their ways; any new device would be damned as producing work of lower quality. Even when prejudice had been disposed of, French workers, often peasants scratching a few additional *sous* from by-employment in their homes, had a point in claiming that the cards, intended to do better work on fine wools, were of no great utility for the more common coarse ones. Even where they were technically appropriate, the early need for preliminary carding on the customary coarse cards before the finer new cards (with their greater number of exactly bent and accurately ranged wires) were employed, meant that the cost of maintaining the two kinds of card and the slower production time had to be set against the superior quality of the product. The introduction of the new English cylindrical carding machines in the more important cotton regions before the Revolution took the new technology past the immemorial use of hand cards, and meant that Kay's invention was no longer potentially of critical importance.

John Badger

One of the most interesting English industrial immigrants of the middle years of the eighteenth century was John Badger, a finisher of silk goods. He arrived in Paris in 1753 after lengthy negotiations with the Duc de Mirepoix at the French embassy in London, in which a M. Destouches was intermediary and interpreter. How Badger was recruited is a little controversial: Bussière, who gives the fullest account of Badger and his family, and Bellefonds, who gives a good succinct account, are the only scholars who have looked in detail at the massive file[39] on the English finisher. Bussière says that Holker drew the attention of the embassy to Badger as a result of information gained on his espionage and recruitment trip to England in 1752, on the basis that he was a great expert on the watering of silk. Bellefonds tends to believe that Holker's effective connection with Badger's operations really began in 1754 when he organized the obtaining of materials and machine parts from England on his behalf, and that Badger was anticipating meeting Holker in person for the first time in 1755. The accounts are compatible if Holker, himself a finisher and thus well situated to know the personnel and gossip of the trade, learned in 1752 that Badger was a good worker in desperate poverty and yet one of the few people knowing the secrets of making good 'watered' silk. He could have passed his name to the embassy without meeting him, and Bussière's and Bellefond's views could virtually be reconciled on that interpretation.[40]

Badger, a native of Oxfordshire, had been working in London, but was unemployed. He was about forty years of age, married with two children and with his wife expecting a third. He seems to have negotiated straightforwardly with the French ambassador, and without excessive demands. He did not ask for a shilling for himself until he was on board ship – perhaps the French had experience of English workers who took their money and then ran – but only subsistence for his family. In fact he was given 1 guinea a week. Rather optimistically he believed that if he was recommended for work in France he could quickly discharge his debts. He agreed to go to France ahead of the rest of the family on the supposition that their separate journeys would attract less attention from the British authorities but, according to Bellefonds, the French apparently wanted to be sure that he possessed the skills he claimed before they took the whole family over. His wife lived secretly in Portsmouth for some months after he left in August 1753, fearing arrest if she stayed in London. There she lost a baby in childbirth, and complained that she had been refused any assistance, but she was given money for her passage in January 1754, and was met at Paris by John Kay, as her husband had been a few months before. While there may have been delay in getting money to Mrs Badger, one would not expect niggardliness from Trudaine without good cause, and he assured a correspondent that he was in touch with the London embassy about her welfare, that she was to be paid the guinea a week, and that he had provided the embassy with funds for the purpose. He would get Kay to write to Badger to reassure him. Badger himself was temporarily tided over with small sums and even given new clothes. A letter of August 1753 had requested care when Badger was taken from the public coach on arrival in Paris, because he had no French and there would be English people on the coach, and he must not be given away to them. This may have been because of the danger that his family could be detained in England if discovered.[41]

Badger's rapid removal to Lyon is understandable, it was after all a main centre of the French silk industry. The superiority of the English in the technique of making the 'watered' silk that they had developed was a worry to the Lyons merchants and manufacturers, as this was then a highly fashionable product on the international market. In 1752 and 1753 the Abbé Lemaire had been negotiating with an English silk finisher in Copenhagen who, after getting imported tables from England, almost certainly cast-iron ones, was now equalling the home product. He wanted 1,000 Danish crowns for expenses in coming to France, a fourteen-year exclusive privilege and 3,200 *livres* to set up at Lyon.[42] Presumably the contract with Badger short-circuited these arrangements. The attention of the great mechanician Vaucanson had been directed to the silk industry, and some celebrated inventions resulted, if ones more important for mechanical perfection and indicating future technical direction than for their immediate commercial significance. He had been consulted in 1753 about the possibility of developing a better calender for the Lyon industry. He had received 1,200 *livres* from the town for partial coverage of his costs in building one, but it does not seem to have been taken up. Badger was thus directed to Lyon not simply because it was the main centre of the silk industry, but because there was a felt need for his exact expertise, for despite all these efforts it had to be admitted that 'la moire française, malgré tout, restait au second plan'[43] (French watered silk, despite all efforts, remained second-rate).

Badger's operations in Lyon were based on a contract with the Government. His provisional agreement at the point of emigration to France was that he would be supplied with all necessary premises, tools and machinery, and once he had produced watered silk equal to English he would get an exclusive privilege for fourteen years and a pension.[44] Once he reached Paris he had had further discussions; for a short time other centres were considered as well as Lyon, and new contractual elements were proposed which had not been discussed in England with Mirepoix. This is understandable, for the embassy staff could not possibly have had all the technical and commercial information necessary to make a detailed agreement, but it is also understandable that new conditions would have worried Badger. However, Badger was again promised a 4,800 *livres* grant from the Crown, and a pension, and his equipment was to be provided free, but it was not made clear whether it would be made his outright property. There was now a requirement that he would teach a pupil his methods. This demand frequently upset English industrial immigrants; they were willing to sell themselves to practice their skills abroad, but were not willing to teach them for it was on this property in skill that their economic value depended, as they well knew. But Trudaine insisted that Badger's pension depended on his training a pupil. Kay got into Badger's confidence while he stayed with him in Paris, at least partly by taking him out to the French equivalent of the pub, but rather treacherously relayed their discussion to Trudaine's associates:

> he has been all a long obstenested [obstinate] and sead that he would tack care to kep his seackret to himself and that he would have his wives father to com over agenst the meshen [machine] was ready in order that no person should larn ane thing from him often in the Evning him and I went to the Cabre [Cabaret] and I Reasoned with him that if he went on in that wea [way] that he could not Expect to do well.

In fact, of course, Kay himself had hang-ups about allowing others to make shuttles and cards, and it is amusing to see him accusing another of obstinacy.[45]

These enforced changes in his terms of operation clearly rankled, because nearly forty years later a pamphlet published by Badger and his sons carefully recited them. On the other hand the Trudaines were fundamentally generous, extracting from the Conseil de Commerce a pension of 1,200 *livres*, payable to his wife if he predeceased her, and a pension of 600 *livres* to his children, presumably after her death. Badger by December was concerned to be conciliatory, to show gratitude and emphasize his loyalty. He assured Trudaine that he had no thoughts that he would be off home once his 'afeaiers was maied up in England'. His English business was long settled up, and the promise of a pension to his family had been conclusive. He promised Trudaine 'not to Faile of Doing all that is in my Powewr to Ples him and to Sarve the Country, not Dawting in my Self of his Doing Honorably bie me'.[46]

Arrived at Lyon, Badger lodged with an English tailor, Scot, who had been living there for some years, with whom he had excellent relations, and whom he brought into his business. His main discussions were with Flachat, the *prévôt des marchands*. He had been promised state funding for his calendering machines, and rent-free accommodation, but he had expected both to be in his full possession. The State, however, insisted that the machines should be its property, while the town in fact rented him an empty site in the convent of the Feuillants, erecting wooden buildings in it, while Badger wanted stone-built workshops, and he only got cramped adjoining rooms for living quarters. French officials found that they had another difficult customer to deal with. Flachat told Trudaine how hard it was to get Badger to moderate his demands: 'Il est d'une méfiance sans égale et d'une charactère des plus violentes qu'il y ait, la moindre opposition le met hors de lui'[47] (He is singularly full of suspicion, and has a very violent temper – the slightest opposition sends him into a rage).

Some of Badger's irritation was due to his anxieties about his family's safety; once they arrived in Lyon he wrote to thank the Trudaines 'for all Favers – in Partikeler this of Sutch Tender Cear of my Fammely' in their journey. Now he was losing no time on the building for his workshop, on the stables for the horses to work the mill which powered the calenders, and on the framework for the machines themselves. One problem was obtaining sufficiently large timber for the calender frames; he wanted Trudaine to know of his diligence and have a good opinion of him. Again, there were problems about the production of the iron plates necessary for the working surface of the calender; iron-casting in France was less developed than in England, and soon the important iron roller, which needed exact turning as well as casting, was creating a problem, and there was little hope of having that made in France, while other rollers had to be of lignum vitae.[48] Holker was certainly involved at this point, and as a calenderer himself he would know what was wanted. He used a Samuel Parsons in London as his agent. There was a fault in the first roll cast. The second, though well turned, was slightly under the specified diameter. It was not shipped until this had been reported to, and cleared by, Holker and Badger, though this involved unwelcome delay. But iron plates and lignum vitae rollers were ready.[49]

The lignum vitae caused problems; its use was almost unknown in France, but Kay suggested to Badger and the Bureau of Commerce that it might be found in naval yards, for the British were certainly using it for pulleys. There were various difficulties both in the procurement and the technical quality of the parts of the calender. Rolls which had air holes had to have them filled with 'screws' before turning, much as was done with guns, some of the lignum vitae had to be discarded because of woodworm damage, and replacements shipped from England. Badger wanted to furnish his calender with its 'burden', the enormous box containing weights, by filling it with cast iron, and pleaded with the Government for the free supply of broken cannon to provide the iron, though he later found some other cheap source.[50] Delays and technical problems dragged on, and even by June 1754 had not been obviated. Meanwhile Badger's regular remuneration was dependent on his successfully setting up the manufacture, and he had to plead with Trudaine to send him further subsistence money for his family and himself. Holker made sure he did not over-charge the Government.[51] The timber for a second, smaller, calender proved of disappointing quality, some locally cast iron plates were poor, and would want more work done on them if they were to be usable, and ones on the way from England might have to be awaited before real progress could be made.[52] However, all the materials needed were on the site by August.

We know from later correspondence that Badger had problems with local workmen, beginning with the making of a model of the calender and continuing with the large-scale version. Badger apparently had no ability to make a comprehensible machine drawing, he simply had a mental picture, and was only capable 'de s'annoncer qu'en anglais que [the workmen] ne comprenait point et l'interpreter ne pouvant même expliquer les termes distinctes en menuserie, il n'avait pu par consequent l'amener à un succes aplaudit qu'après des opérations infiniment multipleés' (of speaking in English which [the workmen] did not understand, and the interpreter could not even explain the basic carpentry terms; as a result the much vaunted successes were only arrived at after numerous repeated attempts). An ironmaster complained that the supply of iron for the calender had similar difficulties; the costs increased as work had to be done over and over again if the job was to be done well, in order that the silk-watering process could be done as efficiently in Lyon as in England. Badger had never previously built a calender himself, and was unsure in his instructions.[53]

Calenders had been constructed by the following year, and Holker went to examine them as part of a long tour of industrial inspection. As a calenderer himself his opinion would be a very knowledgeable one. He thought the calenders capable of much improvement, and not quite right in proportions and in movements 'which could hardly be otherwise with workers who were ignorant of such work, and did not understand the person who was directing them, and though a model had been provided, the same work had to be done over and over again' which bore out very well the later statements of the French carpenter and metalworker.[54]

The first specimens of watered silk sent to the Bureau of Commerce in September 1754 do not look good even to a layman's eye, and are clearly not the 'magnificent' items described by Bellefonds;[55] there is probably a confusion with later samples which are good. Seeing these early samples one can understand Holker's view that perfection was a long way off, but Badger made continual efforts at improvement. The cloth specimens of September were almost certainly first trials, for the calenders were not officially put to work until mid-November 1754.[56] In December Vaucanson went to see the machines, and the visit was all the more important as he was accompanied by the new intendant, Bertin, a protégé of Madame de Pompadour.[57] Early in his intendancy Bertin took an interest in sericulture and silk-spinning. Bertin's support for Badger must have required great forbearance. Badger had acted almost incredibly in refusing the intendant entry to his works earlier in 1756. Bertin was naturally enraged, and had to be calmed down by Flachat, the *prévôt des marchands*. He explained to the intendant that Badger had been upset by Vaucanson's presence:

> He is by nature suspicious, and has always insisted that the skill which he brought over should be kept secret, knowing that there have been many attempts to acquire it, and that it could readily be carried off to Italy or Germany if precautions are not taken to prevent it.

Flachat reported to Trudaine on 9 December 1754 that Vaucanson had now seen the calender and continued to praise it and admire its construction and simplicity and smoothness of operation.[58] Though a great mecanician, Vaucanson would not of course have the expert critical trade view of Holker, himself a calenderer, and certainly after Holker visited Badger six months later he set himself to help Badger with improved lignum vitae rollers from England and improved iron plates.[59]

In 1756 and 1757, however, there is clear evidence that the Badger operation was producing good work, and in the former year Holker drew up an agreement with Badger on behalf of the Government, the opening sentence recording 'The success of this establishment and its usefulness to commerce require many precautions that its secret may not be divulged and it may not be carried abroad'. This meant that the knowledge of it should only be entrusted to a few persons, but they should be so treated that they would wish to remain in France. Badger was to train two people, so that there would be three people capable of directing operations. The firm so formed would receive 8 *sous* per *aune* for black cloths and 6 *sous* for all others, and from this Badger would pay the running costs including the provision of horses to power the calenders. Badger would teach the two trainees all aspects of the craft. The first was Scot, with whom he had been associated since his arrival in Lyon, and who had acted as interpreter for some time.[60] The other was Seguin who had also been working with him previously. Seguin had previously been *valet de chambre* to Flachat, the *prévôt des marchands*, so Flachat was going to retain a close connection with the business. The trainees were to live with Badger during his life, not to work elsewhere and to make a sworn oath to the city government not to betray secrets entrusted to them. But, if the Conseil de Commerce eventually decided that more trainees were needed, or the secret should be confided to additional persons, Badger and the other two would have to comply.

Badger had to give the trainees a sixth share of the takings and an additional maintenance payment, and after four years there was to be a more equal division of the returns. In the event of Badger's death his widow would take over his proportionate share, and a third of her share would devolve to her children after her death. The king, to encourage this useful enterprise, would grant the free use of the calenders he had paid for to the firm, while the *prévôt* would arrange that the rent of the premises should be paid by the silk manufacturers' guild of Lyon. The silk manufacturers showed their appreciation of Badger's work by asking Trudaine 'to encourage this man and tie him even more strongly to France' by implementing the 1,200 *livre* pension with reversion to his family, as originally promised. As he had only had the food of his family paid for and the cost of necessary furniture, and enough to keep his workforce together, Badger should now receive the promised 4,800 *livres* in two annual parts – to make sure his zeal did not diminish![61] These arrangements had the support of Bertin, as Intendant of Lyon.

Thus by 1756 the technology of producing watered silk had been effectively transferred to France. We will not follow in full detail the subsequent career of Badger and his family. For some time after Holker drew up his draft agreement there was debate between the various authorities involved. Bertin for instance wanted more trainees to be taught and wanted the associates to take their oath of secrecy not before the municipal authorities but before himself as intendant, which he thought would be more impressive. There were disputes about how much the whole concern had cost to set up; eventually it was recorded as 47,000 *livres*, including Badger's gratuity. There were squabbles with the community of the Feuillants who found the Badger household and the little industrial community distracting and irreverent neighbours, and wanted their rent arrears paid up by the guild and future arrangements regularized. But Trudaine de Montigny confirmed the Council's willingness to pay Badger his pension and a gratuity, the whole arrangement was accepted by the Crown and La Michodière, Bertin's successor as intendant, was officially so informed.[62]

For some years the enterprise seems to have been very successful, profits over a ten-month period in 1760–61 were 30,000 *livres*, 100,000 *aunes* of silk were treated by the calenders, and even operating the machines 16 or 17 hours a day they could not keep up with the work which was coming in.[63] There was an evident opportunity to set up additional works. Seguin was the favourite of Flachat, who had the ear of Bertin; the latter now, with Mme de Pompadour's support, had reached the summit as Controller-General. Badger tried to retain Seguin as partner by increasing his remuneration once he had learned the trade thoroughly,[64] but a break-up became inevitable.[65] There was competition between Seguin and Badger over attempts by the authorities of Nîmes, the rival silk town to Lyons, to have a calender built there. Seguin now wished to leave Badger and build a second calender nearby. Badger, likely to be deprived of much of his trade and with a large family to feed, showed great reluctance to go to Nîmes. However, despite Holker's support,[66] Badger could not prevent Seguin's being permitted by the local authorities, without any obstacles from the central government, to establish another large calender. This seems to have been costly but well constructed, and operated profitably for some years. Having failed to get support for building a new calender for himself at Lyon, Badger eventually involved himself with calenders at Tours and at Nîmes. However, by the late 1770s Seguin sought to withdraw from business, and both old age and a decline in the fashion for watered silk were apparently motives. Seguin finally gave up business in 1789. Badger had retired himself, but two of his sons were now effectively monopolists of the watered silk business in France.[67] During the early period of Seguin's defection Badger had claimed that he could not support his large family without his pension, and he was now able to extract a further 600 *livres* pension from the Government,[68] to compensate for Seguin's breaking of his contract and his competition, and another 500 *livres* from the Lyons silk guild. For a time Badger tried to extract a permit to import English hardware duty-free, but gave this up when the additional 600 *livres* came. For some time in the early 1770s there seems to have been overproduction from all three calenders.[69] Seemingly the family was doing well in the years just before the Revolution, with the father getting the healthy total pension of 2,300 *livres*, and the watering business picking up after the early 1780s.

Badger's involvement with the Nîmes silk industry has now been investigated, but it does not seem to have been a good example of technology transfer. While Nîmes was a very successful centre of the cheaper end of the silk trade, particularly that in silk stockings, the trade was largely in the hands of the local Protestants, compensating for their exclusion from the professions and many public offices, while municipal affairs were in Catholic hands. The Nîmes silk merchants were resentful of the privileges of the Lyon silk manufacturers who had exclusive rights to make the superior kinds of silk product, while they themselves had to sell some of their produce through Lyon or Tours. A Protestant commercial pressure group, 'Le Commerce', fought to break through to the upper end of the market, from motives which were more driven by social and religious dissatisfactions than by an objective assessment of profits. They resented that to get the best finishes, including watering, they had to pay high charges for the use of Badger's calender at Lyon.

Holker was consulted and agreed to promote the building of another Badger calender at Nîmes, and Trudaine required Badger to make his secrets available to the 'Le Commerce' associates. These proposals took two years to bring to fruition, and the results were expensive. Badger was to get a payment of 6,000 *livres*, with additional pension rights for his family. The site and the construction of the calender would require a further 24,000 *livres* to be paid to Badger, but he was to provide some financial guarantees. However the municipality made difficulties, the intendant wanted Badger to commit his 'secret' to paper for the provincial archives, and the local authority eventually insisted that a local calenderer, Jullian, be taken into partnership. But though the calender was supposed to be finished by 1767 and the secret communicated, Badger demanded additional money from the city and the Estates of Languedoc. Despite agreeing to spend three months a year at Nîmes it seems that Badger wanted to make himself scarce, while there were complaints of serious faults in the machine. Eventually after an enormous fuss, amounting to virtual 'comic opera', Badger was able to separate himself from the enterprise after pocketing 9,000 *livres*, Jullian was set aside in a flurry of lawsuits, and the enterprise was handed over to a Protestant entrepreneur, Renouard, who seems to have operated the calender with limited profits and much below capacity. The Estates had to pay heavily to renovate it in 1788. Overall,

> it seems clear ... that the Calandre Anglaise never equalled its counterpart at Lyon, neither in the volume of its production, nor in its profitability to those who operated it, nor in its relative importance within the municipal manufacture ... The venture never fulfilled the dream of making Nîmes a centre of fine silk production.[70]

In 1784, when already in his seventies, Badger saw another opportunity of imitating English finishing processes. The French could equal the shine and brilliance of English satin finishes, but only by making a stiffer and less supple cloth: 'le secret a toujours été impénétrable'. Badger made a brief visit to England, but was betrayed to the English authorities by someone from Lyon and came back hurriedly. However, he claimed to have returned with the secret, and tried to obtain 20,000 *livres* for machine-building. But he retired in the following year, having made over his new secret processes to two of his sons. How far the process ever actually worked is uncertain.[71] In 1791 Badger memorialized the National Assembly for the continuance of the pensions, and the retention of the reversions to his widow and male children. The ecclesiastical buildings which contained his working premises should not become 'biens nationaux' (nationalized property) but be given to him, together with other parts of the whole site and additional living quarters, while the State should put them in repair as well as the wooden part of the calender which was due for a major refit. For good measure, his apartments should be refurnished. He claimed that if he had to move to another site removal and refitting costs would be high.

The Badger family had become French citizens in 1760 after solicitations from Holker on their behalf, and the names of one of the sons born in France, 'Louis-Benoit', indicates that they had made a degree of cultural transition, though for some time at least they remained Anglican in religion. A brother of Badger had apparently joined them, though Choiseul had resisted his immigration during the Seven Years War for fear that the British might be sending him over as a spy.[72]

The Revolution brought disaster to the family. One son, Justin, was a senior officer in the national guard at Lyon, Pierre a captain, and most of the family were associated with the counter-revolutionary insurrection. Peter and Louis were captured and executed in 1793. Justin escaped and returned to refurbish and carry on the family business until 1800 when his father died at a great age. In 1802 Justin apparently emigrated leaving the business to Faye, a former apprentice of his father, who had married Louis Badger's widow. The firm still existed and prospered under one of the Faye family in 1844.

Badger's move to France and his activities there bring out some interesting points. First, in recruiting him the French had very correctly identified an operative with the knowledge and skills that were wanted. While there is no evidence that he was directly recruited by John Holker, it is possible that Holker, formerly in another branch of the same trade, and on a suborning trip to England at the right time, was able to provide the embassy with the name of a man who was down on his luck. On several occasions after Badger's move to France we find Holker willingly helping Badger, both before and after he was commissioned as Inspector-General of Foreign Manufactures.

The French administration, which effectively means the Trudaines, was generous in support, but clear that Badger would have to show that he could work the watering process successfully before he would get the reward that had been promised in terms of gratuity and pensions for himself and his successors. With Badger, as with other British industrial immigrants, the question of his being able to continue in possession of his 'secret' was a serious one. The privilege was, though not equivalent, the nearest thing the French had to a patent grant, but in the end Badger did not get one. There was clearly a struggle of wills over the teaching of the process to others. Badger tried to keep it within his own circle, and to involve only his sons, a brother, and his compatriot, Scot. But local influence in Lyon forced him to include Flachat's servant Seguin among the trainees; how far this was an attempt to break the English monopoly is not clear. When Seguin broke away it was hard for the Trudaines to resist the powerful support he had obtained, particularly as they were known advocates of competition as against exclusive rights, and freedom of industrial information as against secrecy and craft mysticism.

It was only around the time of the worst period of strong competition and poor trade after 1772, when he had run up a number of local debts, that Badger threatened briefly to 'go away and take his talents elsewhere if no one would come to his help', but the Government did come to his assistance. He seems to have been trusted to return when he made his expedition to England to learn the satin process in 1784. The fact that fear of betrayal and arrest brought him back prematurely indicates that the 1719 Act, while frequently infringed, did have some deterrent effect, as many other instances show.

5 Other Industrial Ventures: Textiles and Vitriol

Holker's activities were not confined to the Saint Sever works, to tours of inspection, and to keeping an eye, benevolent or reproving, on some of the more important of the independent English industrial immigrants. He took an active part in developing other textile enterprises with English associates, particularly at Sens and Bourges, and he himself also spread his own manufacturing interests (sometimes involving his son very closely) into the making of glazed cardboard for cloth finishing, hitherto unknown in France, and much more significantly, into chemical manufacture, involving two successive English sulphuric acid processes. He has thus a role of the first importance in establishing the heavy chemical industry in France.

Textiles

First let us consider the textile manufactories. These cannot be examined in full detail, but it is useful to see the extent of the business created by the early wave of English immigrants, that which came before the arrival of the new spinning and rotary carding machines in the last three decades of the century. These new works of the 1750s and 1760s were very dependent on the group of twenty or so workers whom Holker had brought to Saint Sever for the cotton velvet and calendering and dyeing enterprises. These he continued to watch over, to be 'the soul of', in Bellefonds' words;[1] he was able to use his government influence to have their privileges renewed, while leaving the day-to-day direction to men who were hand-picked by him for their technical skill and steadiness, a central core being bound to him by ties of their Lancashire and Jacobite origins, some also by family relationships. To his relatives James Morris and James Hope, dyers and calenderers, he largely handed over the finishing side of the business in 1763, though both the enterprises he had started in the 1750s continued to be called Holker and Company, they were in fact separate entities.[2]

The two main textile enterprises which Holker was instrumental in founding at a distance from Rouen were at Sens and at Bourges. We have seen that Holker in his first tour report had an almost lyrical passage on the potential of Sens for cotton finishing and manufacture. How far this was spontaneous and how far prompted by the fact that Trudaine's own estates were nearby is not clear. Holker had the strong belief that high-quality spinning was the foundation of successful cotton manufacture, and he began by sending an associate, Falkener, over to England to recruit two skilled spinsters to act as teachers and set up a spinning-school. Miss Heyes and Miss Law were recruited and promised an annual pension, and set up a spinning-school at Sens. The full-time manager was a man from Lyon, Gouttenoire, but Holker effectively pulled the strings. The spinning-school opened in 1757. For some time the yarn was of indifferent quality. Gouttenoire initially could only recruit child spinners who spoilt much cotton daily 'but it is not easy to find adults willing to enter this kind of school'. This problem had been overcome by getting Cardinal de Luynes to put pressure on the *curés* of the local parishes to persuade their parishioners to work there! In January 1759 Holker sent the Englishman David Hall to work with Gouttenoire. Hall was one of those whom he had originally brought over to Rouen and who had been one of the supervisors of Saint Sever for five years. 'He is a very steady fellow with a lot of experience. You may be assured', Holker wrote to Trudaine, 'that with Gouttenoire he will leave no stone unturned to bring this manufacture to the peak of perfection.' Holker claimed that he was putting 2,000 *livres* of his salary each year into sustaining the Sens concern and paying the wages of English workers.[3]

Now Trudaine assisted Holker to find men of capital who could back the business effectively, and by the end of the year a group of moneyed partners had been got together including Claude Torrent, already mentioned (see p. 58), who also backed other enterprises in which Holker was involved (Saint Sever and Bourges). To these were added Holker himself, Hall (his real name of Hulme being made known in the documentation) and the fustian cutter Peter Morris, a relative of

Holker's and brother of the Rouen calenderer. The capital was 60,000 *livres*. In the following year the firm received official recognition as a *manufacture royale*, with provision for relief from the taxation on foreigners for workers who were not French nationals, exemption from many other taxes for the principals in the firm and for the chief workmen, permission to contract workers for a six-year period, and duty-free circulation of their goods throughout the country. They now had 200 spinners at work and twelve looms set up. By 1765 Holker could proudly report on 130 looms at work, with thirteen spinning-centres in the adjacent countryside within a radius of 50 kilometres, making Sens, as Chassagne puts it 'an urban centre of rural proto-industrialization'. Miss Law (Mme Robion), now married to a French weaver, was still teaching her skills; for some time she operated from Montigny but then went back to Sens.

In 1769 the ownership of Sens was altered and we know that Prévost, the treasurer of the Ponts et Chaussées, came in, while a Sens merchant, Richard, now shared the management with Hall. The Holker family interest was still strong, but it was John Holker junior who was now a shareholder, for 24,000 *livres*. It was at Sens that he first assembled a jenny, having brought an early machine back from an English espionage tour of 1770 (see Figure 7.1, p. 149).[4] In the late 1770s the firm was a major source of employment and prosperity in Sens. The preparation of raw cotton and spinning employed 426 people, mainly women and children, weaving employed 137 men, and there were fifteen dyers. One point where there was a danger of bottleneck in production was carding, and in 1778 one of Kay's last commissions was to install his machinery for making hand cards at Sens. Carding engines were also tried out. First the proprietors brought William Hall over from England to construct them, probably his was one of the several types which preceded Arkwright's,[5] but it operated badly and the Arkwright type came in almost at once. This was brought in by the Milnes as part of their introduction of the range of Arkwright machinery. The first of the family to emigrate had entered France at Rouen, approaching John Holker senior as his intermediary with the French government.

There was a further revision of the Sens partnership in 1778 with a capital of 210,000 *livres*, the two Holkers and Morris being substantial shareholders. Another 120,000 *livres* was to be borrowed. Hall as manager was not financially involved. The firm was seriously affected by the problems caused by French involvement in the American War of

Independence, and in 1782 had 300,000 *livres* worth of unsold stocks; it sought a 50,000 *livres* loan from the Government early in 1786. That year of course brought the Eden-Rayneval commercial treaty. The proprietors had urged the Government to pursue the very opposite of the treaty's policy, and to return to the strict enforcement of the prohibition of the entry of English cottons. By the following winter the firm, like many others, was demanding large subventions from the Government to help meet English competition. They made their case in part on the need to alleviate the desperate plight of starving workers, but they seem to have had little response. However successful Sens had been as a well-capitalized firm attempting the English methods of the middle of the eighteenth century with assistance from the French state, it clearly was not able to sustain English competition of the 1780s and 1790s which was swiftly adopting new and continuously improving textile technologies. By the firm's ninth year only 60 weavers were at work and the minister, Chaptal, was being unsuccessfully appealed to for subsidy. An enquiry into the product found the chief problem to be one of excessive prices. Sens was less competitive than cotton velvet manufactures at Rouen and Amiens, and the firm was liquidated in its thirteenth year.[6]

The Bourges manufacture is always associated with Holker, but while he was very important in initiating it, his personal involvement was not so deep or long lasting as in that at Sens. It was initially based on three of the English workers previously brought over by Holker – Davis, Porter and Morrison. That they were encouraged to set up in Berry is probably another example of the direction of new industrial ventures to provinces which were particularly impoverished and lacking in manufactures. It fairly closely coincides with Alcock's establishment of English hardware production at La Charité in the same province.[7]

Already in 1756 the Intendant of Berry at Bourges was making payments to Davis for the setting up of a textile firm there.[8] Holker submitted a large expenses demand, 4,320 *livres*, for money he had borrowed on behalf of Davis from Torrent, the investor in other concerns Holker was involved in. This had been spent to cover the expenses of Davis in getting English workers. It was Davis's wife who had been sent to England to find them just as Mrs Alcock, at almost the same time, had been the recruiter for her husband's La Charité works.[9] Once again Holker solicited Trudaine's interest in finding capitalists to invest in the new concern. In 1757 an *arrêt* was obtained from the

Government to set up the firm as a privileged manufacture, with a wide remit for light woollens, silk mixtures and canvas, as well as cotton. That cotton was not concentrated on to the extent it was at Saint Sever is probably related to the precariousness of supply in the Seven Years War. By 1757 Davis had received over 15,000 *livres* in subventions to set up the business. Already Lesage, later to be very influential, was associated with the direction of the firm.[10] It was given the highest status of privilege as a *manufacture royale*, together with exemption from import and export duties in the major tax area of the Cinq Grosses Fermes, permission to set up a Paris warehouse, various tax concessions and the right to refer any disputes to the local intendant. Further subsidies were due when 120 looms had been put to work, or were to be paid as a bounty on output at 2 *livres* per cloth.[11] Another bounty, derived equally from the State and the province, was to go to the English workers, at that time nine men and three women.

In fact all this subsidy was not paid; by 1762 some of the workers were dead and others had left France, probably to return home. The names of newly recruited workers which are on record would suggest that few came from England; four of them, Casey, O'Connor, Ryan and Cusack are clearly Irish. Possibly some of them may have been recruited, as Holker had proposed, from the Irish regiments in the French army. Certainly it was Holker who induced the Kelly family (who seem to have come to France independently, and had unsuccessfully tried to make English woollens at Rheims) to join the Bourges project. Other men who had already worked with Holker in Normandy were attracted to Bourges: Thomas Clarke, Richard Smith and yet another Irishman, Garrity. Clarke [sometimes given as Clark, later calling himself Lecler] was to be an important industrialist in his own right, and soon moved out of Holker's shadow. The Irish influence was briefly increased by the arrival of Robert Balfe from Tours where he had been working for the manufacturer Chedreau, but he returned to Tours to set up a production of English silk handkerchiefs. It was again an Irishman, MacCarthy, whom Holker had certainly brought from an Irish regiment in France, who installed hot presses at Bourges.[12]

By 1762 a group of seven Paris capitalists increased the invested capital to 230,000 *livres*, but much poor cloth was being made and the new investors wanted firmer direction and increased Lesage's influence. This seems to have led to trouble between the three English principals and Lesage, and in 1764 the three seem to have made a partial retirement from the business, though Holker and other Rouen participants retained their interest, being represented by the investor Pierre Godefroy. Clarke seems to have withdrawn and set up a rival weaving firm in the town, which led to Lesage protesting to Trudaine about the competition. It was probably this that induced Clarke to go off to set up a more substantial firm at Brives.[13] This period of change was marked by a shift of market orientation: without abandoning either silk and wool products it was decided to concentrate on production of cotton for calico-printing, which had recently been freed from government restrictions. During these alterations Torrent, the important investor and ally of Holker, withdrew. Holker was nevertheless asked by the intendant to provide samples of small Manchester piece-goods designed for the West African market (in which the French ambassador in London had agreed to help) and he was to give full descriptions and explanations of the samples. He had a Mr Drumgold and a Captain Tarbuck send some via the London embassy as requested, but thought that the exercise need not be repeated: such cloths were already successfully made at Rouen, whence samples for copying could readily be supplied.

As at Sens, a large number of spinning-schools were set up both at Bourges and at a number of accessible centres; 'sans filature on ne fait rien qui vaille, c'est le fondement de la manufacture' (without (good) spinning nothing worthwhile can be done, it is the foundation of the manufacture) Lesage wrote to Trudaine, wise advice which had been continually urged by Holker for a decade. Trudaine applauded the spread of spinning into the countryside and wanted all the cloth sold to be printed. In 1766 too, the privilege of the firm was renewed, compensation was paid for the expense of setting up the spinning-schools and bounties were given on production. Part of this was to go to the workforce – providing a hundred looms were kept at work. Lesage emphasized to Trudaine de Montigny that Berry was a hundred years behind the times,[14] a province without roads, canals or communications, and the inhabitants plunged deep in idleness, timid, enervated by a misery which was only alleviated counter-productively by plenty of bad wine. However the firm by employing 1,700 men and women and with 170 looms operated by outworkers was doing its best to invigorate the region.

From now on Holker's connection with the firm seems to have been intermittent. Lesage pressed on strongly. The privilege was again renewed in 1767, and accompanied by a large loan from the Government, the total capital now being over 300,000 *livres*. But there had to be a continuous and disquieting search for more capital which was eventually unavailing – clearly the enterprise did not generate enough from profits for adequate ploughing back, and Lesage's repeated attempts to expand operations were at the expense of opposition from large investors, and two of the largest left in 1770. Over the next few years Trudaine de Montigny tried to help the firm by leaning upon wealthy merchants and capitalists, including the occasional farmer-general, to encourage them to invest, but to little effect. Though the existing investors had never seen more than 5 per cent interest on their money, the company was renewed for fifteen years (from 1777) in 1773, but Lesage foresaw the dissolution of the firm at the end of the period. The company was socially valuable, it employed 300 looms and 3,000 workers in a poverty-stricken area. Intense efforts to increase sales were made. Holker visited Bourges and reported that Lesage was very active and unusually talented in finding markets. The latter managed to bring in some more wealthy investors in 1774 and claimed that demand exceeded output, but that the works was becoming ruinous for lack of maintenance. At the renewal of the association in 1777 Trudaine de Montigny got an augmented group of associates to raise their investment to 800,000 *livres* in return for the Government granting 100,000 *livres* towards rebuilding, and 15,000 *livres* a year towards maintenance.

In 1775 Holker came to Bourges at Lesage's request to arrange for the installation of a new calender to replace one he had set up many years before. He assured Trudaine de Montigny that the manufacture was still worth supporting and commended the employment of many spinners, weavers and printers, most of the printers being children. The design and colour of the printed cloths were good as was the teaching. Holker believed that as the works he had visited were 'the work of your father, I think you will learn of their progress with pleasure'.[15] Early in 1786 the firm believed it was the biggest in the country, having then 2,500 employees, and it tried to reject the new directives which subjected the cloths they produced to being sealed by officials. Like some other producers they deprecated this 'absolutism' and supported 'liberalism', while stressing their success in 'vivifying' Berry at the Government's behest. The shareholders had no desire themselves to be manufacturers. They had been persuaded into supporting the concern by the Council so as to give life to a region which had 'fallen into the most frightful misery'. To treat these pure capitalist entrepreneurs like common manufacturers would make them throw their hand in and leave the business. Losses during the American War were followed by low returns after it, and one may guess that the Eden-Rayneval treaty further depressed the investors. The firm began to fold-up, printing of cloths was ended, and Lesage only engaged in spinning and weaving, though almost 900 'unfortunates' were still employed in Year II. The loss of raw cotton supplies from San Domingo seems to have been a serious blow and Lesage abandoned Bourges for Paris soon after.[16]

While Holker's personal involvement with Bourges was not as close as that with Sens, it is important for his record that he supplied the key workers and much of the relevant technology in the important initial stages, together with the organizational pattern. The concentration of the weaving, bleaching, dyeing, calendering and printing elements, and their close links with dispersed but closely supervised and controlled spinning-centres, made Bourges, even more than Sens, a remarkable example of what it was recently fashionable to call proto-industrialization. It would be hard to find examples of any British merchant manufactures of the period so developed within the meaning of that term. But of course these examples did not lead on to deep mechanization, to extensive use of power and to a true factory system, as opposed to the mere concentration of many workers in large buildings and the employment of great capitals. The most sophisticated and large-scale proto-industrialization did not in itself induce the decisive technical change to the factory system, or become a significant element in an industrial revolution. It had to await the arrival of new technology of cardinal significance, none of which came from French firms and virtually all from British. Existing centres of developed and concentrated industrial production in the proto-industrial style were often, in terms of water-power, fuel, and access to metallurgical and mechanical skills, ill placed for the new system. Thus proto-industrialization did not easily roll on into the new industrial order, but stopped in its tracks.

This was certainly the case with Sens and Bourges. However their eventual failure is not wholly to be ascribed to the limitations of proto-industrialization: their capacity to survive in a more competitive era was affected by their deliberate siting for social reasons in districts which had a very stagnant or nearly non-existent industry. Neither their economic geography nor their worker culture was ideal; their investors were often reluctant, and recruited by government arm-twisting, while their adherence was partly secured by privileges and subventions received by the companies.

Vitriol

As we will see, the Holkers, father and son, were not inseparably tied to proto-industrialization, but continued, as long as they had influence and relevant authority, to welcome new technological advances without any inhibition in favour of the existing industrial order. But before considering their welcome to the new wave of textile machines of British origin, their achievement in setting up a key chemical manufacture on the English model deserves attention. This was important for textiles, but in the long term it was also the basis of the heavy chemical industry of the nineteenth century. Chronologically it fits usefully between the first group of English-based improvements brought in by the senior Holker in the 1750s, and subsequently spread through his influence as inspector-general and as government protégé, and the Holkers' later interest in the English technical advances which had occurred since the father had left for France, and which became available in the 1770s and 1780s.

Already by the 1760s Britain had established sulphuric acid production on a greatly increased scale. The first important practitioner was Joshua Ward, who developed a variant on the 'bell' process where sulphur was heated in the presence of nitre and over water and the vapour condensed under a glass bell. Ward and his partner White operated from the mid-1730s at Twickenham using large glass globes. Ironically Ward may have learned of the basic process during a residence in France, but it had only been used on a very small scale and largely for apothecaries. The use of globes depended on the skill of glass-blowers, which is understandable when we realize Ward was eventually using globes capable of holding 40 gallons or more. While the pollution caused by his works caused its removal to Richmond in 1740 – thus showing that a pollution problem the Holkers later met was encountered at the very start of the large-scale manufacture of vitriol – Ward created an industry, because he reduced the cost of sulphuric acid from around 2 shillings an ounce to 2 shillings a pound. It was already realized that sulphuric acid could be used to speed up bleaching, for cleaning and pickling metals, and in precious metal recovery, and that price was the sole hindrance.[17]

In both Britain and France the rapid development of the cotton industry was creating new markets for sulphuric acid at this time, in the pioneering of new indigo-based blue and green dyes, and in providing important chemicals for calico-printers, this trade being freely permitted for the first time in France in 1759. Here dilute sulphuric acid was used to clean cloth of residual bleachers' materials before it was printed, and, in the popular blue-patterned cloths, to remove dye-resistant materials after cloths had been printed by a resist process. Again successful experiments in Scotland in the mid-1750s encouraged the large-scale employment of sulphuric acid as a 'sour' for bleachers,[18] though there are established instances of its earlier use.

The economics of employing sulphuric acid for this wide range of uses were greatly improved by a new Birmingham invention of the 1740s by Samuel Garbett and John Roebuck. Instead of glass globes they used lead-lined chambers, which allowed production on a much larger scale. This depended on the ability of leadworkers to make tight joints without solder. Three years after setting up their first (and long-lived) works in Birmingham in 1746 the partners built a very large and famous works at Prestonpans in Scotland. In the cases both of Ward and of Garbett and Roebuck the inventors did not originally patent, but tried to protect their inventions by secrecy. Eventually Ward did patent his method in 1749 and Roebuck and Garbett theirs (in Scotland) in 1771. In neither case did either secrecy or patent prevent industrial espionage and the copying of the processes. But in 1765 the French spy Gabriel Jars found elaborate measures still being taken to protect the Ward process,[19] and the scientist and inspector Faujas de Saint-Fond found security tight at Prestonpans in 1784. The lead chamber process eventually held the field as it was able to reduce the price of sulphuric acid to 4*d.* a pound.[20]

The original role of John Holker in the foundation of the sulphuric acid industry in France was an intermediary one, but initial failure in that respect led to a much more direct involvement. The first approach to the French state came from Brown, a man of British birth but by the early 1760s holding a profitable position in the Austrian Netherlands as an Inspector-General of Taxes to Maria Theresa. There is a presumption that he had learned of the process from another Englishman, Thomas Murry, who had left England under a cloud in 1759. Murry proposed a manufacture of sulphuric acid with glass globes, of nitric acid, and eventually of copperas. The backing of the Austrian government was obtained in 1762 and a state factory founded, but Murry had abandoned this by 1770, after which he turns up in France.[21] But the Murry–Brown connection is by no means simple, as Brown apparently recommended a lead chamber process to the French, while all Murry's schemes seem to have been glass-globe ones.[22]

Brown offered his services to Trudaine in 1764. He indicated his responsible position in Brussels, his willingness to come to France, and the importance of his project, based on the existing costs of the products to France. He would produce sulphuric acid, copperas and nitric acid and he said that the importation costs of the first two from England were considerable, while nitric acid, though home produced, was expensive and could be made more cheaply. He knew there was a state saltpetre monopoly in France[23] and would want to have it at the existing price. He believed he had identified a sulphur source in pyrites found on the Normandy coast at Fécamp. He listed a large number of uses of his proposed product in industry, giving prominence to textiles.

Brown believed he could find friends with the necessary capital, but wanted privileges and grants for land, buildings and equipment. His partners were two men with Irish names, Connely and Tierney.[24] Rights to extract pyrites and copperas deposits were demanded, and bounties on the copperas and sulphuric acid produced, together with the rights of untaxed circulation of the final product in France, while there should be the usual exemptions from taxes and services for senior workers and managers given to privileged manufactures, and Brown and Tierney should avoid the economic penalties on foreigners of the *droit d'aubaine*. Of particular interest is the request for 1,500 *livres* to obtain an English leadworker able to make joints in lead without solder 'which ... is unknown in France and which cannot be managed without'.

By the middle of October Holker had been turned to for advice. He supported the scheme because of the avoidance of imports, pointing out that 'it not infrequently happens in wartime that one pays three times the value'. It is both interesting and ironic in view of his own later sulphuric acid project that he insisted 'one should without scruple refuse the exclusive privilege' which Brown had asked for. Brown was now in Paris and could be dealt with direct. Trudaine endorsed the letter to the effect that his son, Trudaine de Montigny, should see Brown, while the technical side of the project should be vetted by two scientists regularly employed by the Government, Hellot and Mignot de Montigny. He did not think that trade in the chemicals was so large that the Government should put its hands too deep in its pockets. But with his usual perspicacity Trudaine noted 'I don't know ... if English workers who are engaged in this type of manufacture would not be the best to establish it in France'.[25] Within a few days Hellot's report was in. As so often with contemporary scientific-technical reports by academicians, there was a mixture of the relevant and the misleading. Hellot knew much about the use of the chemicals in dyeworks; as we have seen he was regarded as an eminent authority on dyeing. But he emphasized nitric acid as more important than sulphuric which 'is only employed in some chemical operations [i.e. laboratory or pharmaceutical ones]. This article is not a considerable item in trade'.[26] This shows he did not appreciate either the acid's potential use in bleaching or its recent employment in calico-printing.

The reliance placed on Holker is shown by Trudaine de Montigny asking for a further memoir from him before approaching the controller-general about Brown's proposals. Holker clearly supported Brown. Nevertheless over two months later nothing significant had been done, and Holker wrote to the elder Trudaine in some agitation. Brown 'awaits with impatience the Arrêt de Conseil which M. (Trudaine) de Montigny has promised him'. Brown had been away from his Brussels job for nine months, and though Holker had tried daily to reassure him, he seemed to have made up his mind to return to Brussels unless he received definite news that his enterprise would be supported. Holker asked to be told of any problem which hindered the *arrêt* – he himself did not know of any – and the privilege had been so drawn up that the Government did not have to pay Brown anything until he succeeded in making his process work. Holker felt that his own honour was at stake, it was only through his encouragement and support for the French scheme that Brown now risked losing his job at Brussels. Trudaine at once had a check made that the *arrêt* had been sent off; if it had been delayed it should be sent immediately. Action was now taken, and by 1 February Trudaine de Montigny was writing to Holker that *arrêts* in Brown's favour had been signed by the controller-general. One gets the clear impression that Holker had to go over the head of the dilatory younger Trudaine to his father, the more expeditious and decisive man, despite age and ill-health. Even so, this belated activity was nearly too late. Brown had already left Rouen for Paris on his way to Brussels, but John Holker senior said he could get his son to intercept him there so that Brown would be able to see Trudaine de Montigny, send in his notice to Brussels, and alert his French financial backers, including Connely, who was a Dunkirk merchant of Irish extraction.[27]

However, the plan was not implemented despite the *arrêt*. By the following January Brown was again petitioning the Government, but this time with two new associates, Garvey and Norris, the former an Irish merchant in Rouen. They had tried hard to find a suitable site at

Fécamp, and at another place on the banks of the Seine in Normandy, but had failed.[28] They proposed to combine their coastal works with the smuggling in of English East India tea! Next year they were proposing to embark on brandy smuggling too, presumably in the opposite direction. This hardly seems to fit with their wish to be regarded as serious industrialists. They now wanted to build their works at Saint Sever near Rouen, where of course Holker's main works was, and were arranging to buy land there. With this modification they wanted to have the *arrêt* of the previous year confirmed. However it was noted, probably by Trudaine, that Brown's final parchment version of the *arrêt* had never been sent to him. It was June before arrangements were in hand to reissue the *arrêt*.

The works was then described as something proposed by, rather than just supported by, Holker, and the previous search for a site was said to have extended to Brittany and the environs of Nantes. Possibly Holker had appreciated that the scheme was losing impetus, and that the only way to support it effectively was to site it where he could keep an eye on it – and where a textile industry market would be close by, important when a commodity as difficult to transport as sulphuric acid was involved. Correspondence shows that it was he who had negotiated the purchase of land at Saint Sever; the far end of that suburb is mentioned as the site more than once, possibly indicating that a pollution problem was already in the minds of the entrepreneurs. Brown and Holker were to go to the glassworks at Mancomble to see to the making of the globes required for the works. No explanation is given as to why the more modern, large-scale, and cheaper lead chamber process had been discarded, possibly the necessary leadworker had not been obtained from Britain, or if one had been obtained, he had not succeeded. Brown was to arrange the obtaining and transport of the Fécamp pyrites, while leaving directions for the speedy erection of buildings for the new works at Saint Sever.[29]

Unfortunately there is an annoying gap in the archives for 1767. By the following year two important changes had taken place. Holker had replaced Brown as the chief entrepreneur; apparently he believed Brown had let him down in some way, as he describes himself as Brown's 'victim'. Secondly his son, John Holker the younger, was now taking an important part in the establishment of the works and had become the technical man, as well as having a part in the general negotiations with government. The younger Holker had been carefully trained to work alongside and eventually succeed his father. From 1764 he studied in Paris. J. G. Smith points out that chemistry was prominent in his education and that he was a pupil of notable scientists like Rouelle, Nollet and Cadet. His father supervised his practical industrial studies, keeping him by him in Rouen for a few weeks at a time, teaching him to spin and card both wool and cotton under the supervision of an English forewoman spinster, and putting him out to a woollen dyer of Darnetal to learn the operations of dyeing woollen cloth. 'I see him frequently, and I always find him with his sleeves rolled up, in his waistcoat with an apron in front just like a workman.'[30]

In 1767 Holker junior had begun to make tours abroad under the orders of the elder Trudaine, who sought not only the advice of Holker senior but that of Montigny, the academician. In that year young Holker was to take in the northern French textile towns on his way to Dunkirk or Calais, whence he was to take passage to London. There he was to stay several months.

> He will try to get himself taught the secret of fine waxed cloth, of the distillation of oil of vitriol [sulphuric acid], he will make himself familiar with the great vessels used in this distillation, with the working methods of manufacture of green copperas [a mordant], and all that concerns these important subjects; if he cannot get himself taught them, whether by an agent [manager] or other means, he will get acquainted with someone who is knowledgeable and do all he can to get him to France.

This list is enormously extended, and embraces many trades, and there were supplementary requests from many other officials. But it is interesting that sulphuric acid is so prominent, and that young Holker was to investigate it during his London residence. It may well be that he had been informed of the results of the relatively recent English visit of Gabriel Jars, a very important French scientist and technical expert.[31] Jars had been able to enter, but only briefly, a glass globe sulphuric acid manufacture near London. This trip preceded the visit young Holker made to Brussels the following year, in which he used the alias of 'Hilton', which he had used in England, taking his mother's surname. He made a stay of some length and his father sought for him a formal accreditation to the French envoy there 'so that he may claim him back in case of accident'. While in Brussels the young man was to seek information on several matters 'above all that of vitriol'.[32] According to Smith he did this by purchasing the secret from Brown[33] but he may have already picked up much information in England. In any case he does not seem to have learned anything about the lead chamber process, either in England or Belgium. His work was, however, well regarded by the Government, and he was named 'adjoint' or assistant to his father at the end of 1768, with an enhanced inspector's salary of 2,400 *livres*.

During the course of 1768 the two Holkers had been straining every nerve to get sulphuric acid manufacture established on their own account. In a letter probably very early in that year Holker senior approached Trudaine de Montigny for his support, saying he was always conscious of the favours done them by the two Trudaines, but was concerned at asking the younger Trudaine anything likely to cause the slightest trouble – an early indication that he did not expect the drive and attention from the son that the father had given to schemes he favoured. He excused his forceful advocacy on the grounds of his 'attachment éternal' to Trudaine de Montigny. They had both long wanted to develop vitriol production in France. Holker's devotion to this end had led to his victimization by Brown.[34] He had taken every step to ensure that his son had a thorough knowledge of the business, even getting him to take risks which were well known to the younger Trudaine, which may refer to the English rather than the Brussels espionage. Most French industrial spies emphasized, even over-emphasized, the dangers in England, while diplomatic protection had been obtained for young Holker in the Austrian Netherlands. The necessary knowledge now secured, Holker père pressed for privileges to set up his own manufacture.[35]

For this a subsidy, a site and a specialist globe-blower were needed. The last problem was under control as a man had been contacted in London and was coming over. Holker's son was not yet in a position to provide his own share of the capital, and this was needed if he were to find partners, and his father claimed he could not help him 'sadly, despite all the good I have done in France I have not enriched myself by it', and he would remain of limited means unless assisted further. Given his basic salary of 8,000 *livres* a year and other pensions Holker was certainly not poor. We have no good information on his income from the projects at Saint Sever and Sens, but even if he only got interest on his investment (partly a free-gift from the Government!) he got a significant return.

At this point Holker introduced a proposal which was difficult for Trudaine de Montigny to accept, and inconsistent with his own previously expressed views on industrial policy. He asked for an exclusive privilege for vitriol manufacture in Normandy. He knew that Trudaine fils had already been informed of his request, and that it had caused him great anxiety. Exclusive privilege had been a *bête noire* to the elder Trudaine and in one sense the son was only carrying on the father's policy, but he was very much a member of the physiocratic circle, and perhaps in him the mixture of ideology with empiricism made his opposition to state-conferred monopoly stronger than that of his father. Holker's argument was that the firm he was sponsoring would have to carry out much expensive development work, and train workers. As soon as the plant was viable anyone could start up a rival firm next door, recruiting the workers the Holkers had carefully trained, and able to acquire the *ballons*, the great glass globes, with no development costs. The company was designed to be able to supply the whole national market; if rivals could be in business soon after they were operational themselves, their own enterprise could lose half their initial outlay 'and I would have ruined my son and his partners'. Holker believed that investing in a company so dangerously exposed to competition 'would be carrying imprudence to excess'. The Holkers were not asking for a national monopoly; it would be possible for rival establishments to be formed in Nantes, Paris, Lyon, Mantes, Marseilles, Bordeaux and other places. Holker also believed that the British would not readily lose the place they were building up in the French market, and would even be willing to supply the French market at a loss for a few years in order to break any French rival and secure that market; the only remedy for this was an increase in the import duty on sulphuric acid.

There was a further and distinctly peremptory letter from Holker to Trudaine de Montigny on 11 April 1768, demanding to know his views on the vitriol manufacture, because of the need to acquire a building site, to bring in a glass expert and to fix terms for partners and capital. He had pressed his views in conversation and in memoirs,

> but it seems to me that you have no trust in me, that you do not take my word about what I have put to you and that moreover you do not have any plan to set up the firm concerned. I therefore ask you to tell me your firm intentions, because there is nothing more annoying than to stay so long in suspense.

Holker said he had overcome a problem about a loan by going to a private source 'as you have always made great difficulties for me on the business of a loan'. He also brushed aside the objections to a Normandy monopoly on rather specious grounds. Could he have an answer to confirm the project or to abandon it? This was not the way in which officials, however important, addressed government ministers, and Trudaine de Montigny was taking over the important group of departments which his ailing father had long and powerfully dominated. Two reasons may be suggested for this remarkably tough tone. One may have been that Holker was worried that the delay and lack of decision that had plagued Brown's original scheme might wreck his own. Another may well have been Holker's dependence for the essential expertise on his son, and his son may already have been displaying the almost manic drive and overambition that were to prove disastrous later. Holker seems to have idolized his only son, and to have lacked his usual discretion and good judgement where he was concerned.

However, Holker gradually backed away from conflict with Trudaine de Montigny. He sent him an extract from a British newspaper where someone had tried to exculpate him from some accusation made by Brown. A claim had been made that Holker fils had bought the secret of sulphuric acid manufacture from Brown, and that a works was being built in France. 'They are not deceived' wrote Holker, 'for I have just purchased a large site' in Saint Sever. He does not however give any indication that there had been a deal with Brown; if there had been one the payment would have been considerable and there would have been an attempt by the Holkers to recoup the money from the State, as necessary in obtaining the process for France. After all, obtaining British industrial secrets was a central element in Holker's official duties.

Holker informed the minister that he had arranged with an Englishman, now on his way to London, to get a glass-blower for the globes. Talks had already taken place with the workman. He ended his letter however on a touchy note. He had begun expenditure on the works in the hope that Trudaine de Montigny would support him. Otherwise he would have to

> set up this firm on behalf of others, as I have always done in the past, without getting any gain for my own family. This does not seem fair to me, after my hard work for sixteen years under the directions of Monsieur your father, who always showed the greatest desire for my benefit, and I hope that you would act towards me in the same way; unless this is so I will have much to complain about.[36]

Within a few days Trudaine de Montigny had returned the English newspaper cutting to Holker, glad that it had done him justice, which implies that the story of the acquisition of the process from Brown was untrue. He would gladly support Holker in setting up the vitriol works. 'You know that I have full confidence in you and how great is my inclination to do what you want.' However, he still had an 'extreme repugnance' to the exclusive right to manufacture in Normandy, but made a friendly invitation to talk over the issue in Paris 'and hope you can bring yourself closer to my ideas'. However reluctantly, Holker did give way, and early in July sent Trudaine de Montigny a short summary of a revised request. Under the name of Chatel and Company a vitriol and nitric acid works would be set up at Saint Sever as a privileged manufacture. There was a customary group of exemptions from certain taxes and services, mainly for key workers; local taxes were to be moderate, there were to be no duties or restraints on movement of products within the country or on export. There was to be a custom-free entry of saltpetre up to 30,000 *livres* a year and, most important, the firm was to secure a bounty of 10 *livres* per quintal on acid produced up to 3,000 *livres* a year, while there was to be a subvention of 6,000 *livres* for expenses already undertaken. But there was no exclusive privilege for Normandy, nor would there be an immediate extra duty on foreign imports of vitriol, though this would be reconsidered once the new concern was properly established.[37]

Early estimates of the costs of the works were considerably increased during the negotiations with the Government, one reaching nearly 88,000 *livres*. There were huge sheds to house the globes, of which 400 would be used at a time (fifty spares would be needed in case of breakages) and these two sheds would each be 360 feet long. Together they would cost 24,000 *livres*, the works site 25,500 *livres*, and a horse-mill for grinding materials 2,400 *livres*, while another 2,400 *livres* were needed to obtain the foreign glass-blower. To concentrate the acid more glass vessels would be needed, and more large sheds, though these were a mere 130 feet long.

The *arrêts* needed to be registered in the Parlement of Rouen, but there was strong local opposition to the step. However, sufficient senior officials of the Parlement were persuaded to support Holker so that the registrations were completed by May 1769. At this point the younger Holker, who had only recently married, fell ill, and his father too was out of sorts, worried about the son's health and still affected by the anxiety he had felt over the Rouen registration. But he wrote to Trudaine de Montigny 'I nevertheless expect to come and see you immediately when requested, whether before or after the holidays' – in other words he made it clear that he had resumed the role of the obedient official.[38]

The works, once approved, swung rapidly into production, selling 45,000 lbs of acid in its first year, and to markets as distant as Lille and

Marseilles. Despite the refusal of exclusive privilege, perhaps even in some attempt to soften that refusal, not only were the import duties on vitriol raised, as the Holkers had originally asked, but the large government loan which had not initially been granted was implemented by an advance of 20,000 *livres* in 1770 when Holker needed to refund an investor hurriedly. The works, large at the outset, was further expanded in 1771 and 1772. The expansion of 1772 seems to have involved conversion to the lead chamber process.

In the early 1770s 130,000 to 140,000 lbs of acid were made annually; by the mid-1770s there was a doubling of output and production at the end of the next decade was 300,000 lbs. The management of the works was entrusted to Jacques Chatel, a clerk of Holker's and the nominal entrepreneur, until he left to set up his own works in 1792. The younger Holker's appointment as a full inspector-general in 1777 on a salary of 8,000 *livres* a year would in any case have prevented his day-to-day supervision of the works, but he was almost immediately sent on a commercial-diplomatic mission of importance to the newly created United States and was never again active in French industry. It was his son, John Holker III, destined to be an important figure in the French chemical industry in the next century, who took over from Chatel, and it was in that industry, rather than the textile trades in which the grandfather had been so prominent, that the long-term family influence was to be felt.

The Holker contribution to the French chemical industry was very important. While their Saint Sever works was the major Normandy supplier for many years, their fears that it would be impossible to keep the secrets of the process to themselves, or defend it against industrial espionage, were well founded. Smith gives an excellent account of the imitative lead chamber plants of Fleury in 1774 and Anfrye in 1777, influenced by the local amateur scientist de la Folie, as probably was the works of Stourme in 1778, which was also aided by the bribing and seduction of Saint Sever workers. From Normandy the lead chamber process went to the famous works at Javel near Paris in 1778, and then to Montpellier, Nîmes, Agen, Marseilles and other centres. By 1782 Chaptal wrote that few chemists were now ignorant of the lead chamber process. French industrial success was substantial; by 1793 between produced. The demands of war, however, where the need for sulphur and saltpetre for gunpowder manufacture was imperative, enormously reduced the productive capacity of the industry, and some works closed. Coal supplies for use in concentrating acid were also affected. But once

Coal supplies for use in concentrating acid were also affected. But once the military situation had eased the industry resumed its successful course. There was a proliferation of works round Rouen. There were major new developments at Nancy, in the Strasbourg district, and at Lyons. Chaptal, scientist, minister and propagandist for the application of chemical science to industry, founded an important Paris works just before 1800.[39] In addition to that of Chatel, a Rouen merchant, Jacques Payenneville, and his partners set up one at Honfleur. Some shares were sold in 1791 and by 1810 the firm belonged to Edward Chamberlain, an English immigrant who was involved with several enterprises in Normandy. Chamberlain rented it to the Delahalles, uncle and nephew.

In many industries the French tended to remain parasitic on advancing British technology. Even after acquiring the primary breakthrough inventions, they failed to produce significant incremental improvements themselves, and had to await their arrival from Britain. Smith however shows that this did not generally apply in the chemical industry.[40] The pioneering of soda production under the Leblanc process was to result in technology transfer in the opposite direction, from France to Britain, but this falls outside our period. In sulphuric acid production there was extensive experimentation by Chaptal, Clément and Desormes and others, and even if this did not always lead to immediate dramatic technological improvements it made advances in knowledge which were important to the long-term development of the industry.[41] But there were major practical innovations by the French right at the end of our period, the employment of furnaces external to the lead chambers for the combustion of the raw materials, the use of injected steam to promote reaction in the chambers, and methods of continuous process rather than intermittent operation, though these only came into practical use *c*.1810. Here one of the important innovators, possibly even the originator, was John Holker III. The first two innovations entered the British industry about the end of the first decade of the nineteenth century, probably learned of from Chaptal's *Chimie Appliqué aux Arts* (4 vols) of which there were French and English editions by 1807. The British picked up 'the French plan' of continuous working after the collapse of the Empire, in the same way that there was a rush by the French from 1814 to raid Britain for the industrial improvements of the war years. At this point France's sulphuric acid production was larger than Britain's, stimulated by their growing Leblanc soda industry (which had hardly started in Britain), and technically superior.[42] However, the original basis of the French sulphuric acid production was in technologies derived from Britain, which had been successfully naturalized in France by the Holkers.

While to pursue it fully would take us too far from our central theme of industrial espionage as it relates to the transfer of technology, one problem encountered by the Holkers' vitriol factory at Saint Sever should be mentioned. We know there had been opposition to their letters patent for the vitriol manufacture being registered at the Parlement of Rouen in 1769, though the substance of the opposition is not known, and it was overcome by the influence of Council of Commerce and the controller-general. However, by 1771 a legal campaign began in Rouen which attacked the Saint Sever works as a source of pollution. A group of local worthies, headed by an army officer and a priest, gathered evidence of alleged damage to the health of some humans and to that of animals. There was said also to be great harm to flower gardens and vegetable gardens, and to dyed cloth stretched on tenter frames. Eventually an examination of the district was carried out under the authority of the controller-general and of Trudaine de Montigny. The party of inspection was headed by a noted doctor, and included apothecaries, chemists, merchants, and the secretary of the Royal Agricultural Society of Rouen. They reported that damage was very minor and those employed at, or living close to, the chemical works were very healthy. The local opposition naturally wanted the case to be pursued only in the local courts, while the Holkers wanted any dispute to be referred to the Royal Council. The whole episode has a considerable interest as an early and detailed case of industrial pollution by the heavy chemical industry, and one which long precedes the bitterly fought contests between South Lancashire landlords and the great alkali manufacturers in the early nineteenth century.[43] It deserves a fuller study as an episode in the history of the environment.

The Holkers, with some justification it would seem, counter-claimed that their opponents were mainly acting as an ill-motivated cabal, simply jealous of their success and influence; here we have an interesting indication of dislike of these Englishmen as government favourites. 'These complaints can have no other basis than that of jealousy' wrote the younger Holker to Trudaine de Montigny:

> these people are always disposed to be at odds with me and I am liable to be continually troubled in my manufacture ... I think it is sufficient for me to recall to you, in order for you to make a decision, that it was in 1767 that I made a journey abroad on your orders so as to gain

knowledge of manufactures and particularly those of oil of vitriol. You are aware of the toil I had to achieve this.

In the end the liberal establishment of that era, in the persons of Turgot as controller-general and Trudaine de Montigny as director of the Bureau of Commerce, came down heavily on the side of the Holkers. John Holker senior wrote to Trudaine de Montigny:

> my son has just told me that you have given us an *arrêt* which removes the demands of our enemies concerning the oil of vitriol works. Allow me to offer my sincere thanks and declare how recognisant I am of all your kindnesses; I ... wish with all my heart to have you know how deeply I am attached to you.

The king had declared that the *arrêt* of September 1768, registered at Rouen in May 1769, should be enforced, and that the operation of the chemical works should be unimpeded, while the complaints of the Rouen inhabitants were referred from the local courts to the King's Council. Needless to say, no more was heard of them. But local feeling against the Holkers cannot have been assuaged by this strong response from authority. Under Turgot and Trudaine criticism of the Holkers could be silenced, but when Turgot was dismissed in 1776 and Trudaine de Montigny followed his friend and mentor and left office in the following year, the Holkers were more exposed than before.[44]

6 The Successful 1770s: John Holker II, Tours and Reports

The careers of the Holkers from the late 1760s have an interesting complementarity. The son took on the arduous duties of the fieldwork, whether industrial espionage in Britain or tours in France. His father was increasingly an elder statesman of the industrial administration. We have the detailed plan of the son's first visit to England in 1767, and it must be remembered that he was only 22 at the time. On his way from Rouen through northern France he was to spend time at the textile manufactures near home at Louviers, Elbeuf and Andelys before going to Amiens and Abbeville, where he was to see the MM. van Robais and their famous works. Thence to St Quentin for a look at fine and ordinary linens, to Lille and Tourcoing for an examination of wool preparation and degreasing, before making for a port to take ship for London. These French inspections were perhaps to fill in gaps in the younger Holker's experience, so that he had a better background against which to look at English practices.[1]

At London he was to spend three or four months, visiting dyeworks and others involved in finishing woollens, especially those intended for export. His other main object in the London region was, as we have already seen, to look into vitriol and copperas manufacture, to learn about them from a manager or to suborn an expert to go over to France. But John Holker II seems only to have picked up information on the obsolescent globe process, and may have had to supplement even that by his Brussels visit. After leaving London he was to travel to the West Country to study the making of fine woollens, especially ones for export to the Levant, Spain, Portugal and the British colonies, and the production of some main types of cloth sold for home consumption and export. Perhaps it was for this part of his journey that he had been previously sent to pick up a background knowledge of French woollen production.

From the West Country he was to go north, endeavouring to take in Birmingham on his way. There he was naturally to concentrate on the Birmingham toys (*quincaillerie fine*), but also on steel-making, and he was to find a skilled worker in that industry who could be induced to come to France if need arose. Birmingham was of course an important and early centre of cementation steel-making, while there remained a grave deficiency in both the quantity and quality of French steel. A Birmingham man, Michael Alcock,[2] basically a hardware manufacturer, but with steel interests, was currently experimenting with steel-making in France, but not successfully. The Trudaines may have been looking for a replacement if he did not succeed, which may explain the proposal for deferred recruitment. From Birmingham young Holker was to go to Yorkshire where he was to look into the making of narrow cloths – 'petits lainages'. But he was mainly to concern himself with the production of thin cardboard which the French believed was concentrated in Yorkshire, and was mainly in the hands of two entrepreneurs. This matter was of 'the utmost importance'. He was to do everything possible to achieve this object, to examine the different kinds of card, to see if some new machinery had been devised to improve manufacture and to secure either a drawing or a model of it and take the necessary steps to get it to France. This part of the instructions was almost certainly inserted by his father, with his great personal knowledge of the calendering operation in which the shiny card would be used. The expertise of John Holker senior would mean that he would be able to build machinery from a plan or model, especially given additional eyewitness evidence from his son, no greenhorn when it came to the textile trades. Here the enticement of workers would not be necessary.

Naturally young Holker would go to his family's home territory in Lancashire, to look at cotton and fustian production and also fine serge production, and then survey the whole Manchester scene. He had a particular brief to examine ribbon manufacture. Bolton, Blackburn and Rochdale were to be visited. The Holker works at Rouen were no doubt again in mind in a directive to look at cotton velvets including machinery, prices and the remuneration of workers at each stage of production. He was to make drawings of any useful machinery in the cloth trade, as well as paper-mills, fulling-mills, mills for grinding dyewoods, and windmills and water-mills generally 'all these will be subjects which he will examine and describe'. Mines and knitting machinery, especially anything new, should be looked at before he went to Scotland, the working of the coal-mines round Newcastle being emphasized. There was no detail given as to what might be looked at in Scotland, and this part of the journey seems eventually to have been abandoned – hardly surprising considering the complexity and extent of the young Holker's commission. Among things to be examined on his return journey through England were the heavier side of the Sheffield iron trade, and silk manufacture in Derbyshire – no doubt the famous Derby silk-mill. At Nottingham stocking manufacture in both silk and cotton was to be viewed and also the type of earthenware for which the town was well known.

More broadly Holker was to make 'a detailed study of the practices of that country'. French administrators could never quite believe in the untrammelled freedom of British manufacturers, so he had to look into the regulations which were in force and the means of preventing abuses and of encouraging the arts and commerce. This may have some connection with the Society of Arts, to whose limited and marginal industrial bounties the French tended to ascribe a disproportionate importance. He was also to strike up an acquaintance with families of young farmers and ploughmen to see how commons were converted into pastures and the flocks of animals bred and managed, and, if need be, make contracts with some men to follow him to France.

The younger Holker must have fairly staggered under these initial responsibilities, but more were added. He was to go to see the making of Staffordshire pottery and its firing and the use of salt in glazing, collecting specimens of the clays used and sending them back, and checking whether wood or coal was used in the furnaces. He was also to pay attention to finer pottery and white crystal [flint glass]. Tanning, wallpaper manufacture (which was done much better in England), and glue manufacture were mentioned in passing. He was to keep an eye open for small enamelled metal jewellery, in which the English had a good trade, but this was to be looked for in London – Birmingham and the Bilston area were not mentioned in this context. If he were to go anywhere near the Cornish tin mines he was to check on the stone, fossils and other minerals which accompanied tin, which could help in discovering French mines. There was no point in bothering about the working of the mines, the French thought they knew all about that – no doubt founded on the evidence of Gabriel Jars's British metallurgical expedition a few years before (Jars was himself from a family involved in metal-mining).[3]

While in London Holker was to make note of the street lighting at night, what sort of oil was used in the lamps and how the service was paid for. Also he was to find out about the city's water supply and the provision of water to public fountains and to private houses, which was thought to be efficient and cheap. While the use of steam pumps is not specifically mentioned, this enquiry clearly looks forward to the later Paris water schemes of D'Hérouville and Périer, in which there was a key English technical contribution. As we shall see, such public services were regarded as part of benevolent administration, knowledge of which international opinion believed should be freely shared between European states; there was no hint of industrial espionage here.

Weighted down by all these instructions, young Holker received yet further supplementaries – steel-polishing machinery for which both plans and machines should be seized upon, and metal button manufacture. Here we encounter the common situation that some of the government officials and advisers were apparently unaware of what other men had already helped establish and encourage; both of these were trades established in France with some success by Michael Alcock.[4] Sawmills should be seen, they were used in England as they were in Holland, and were desirable in France, where it was recognized that trees from French forests were floated down the Rhine to Holland, sawn by the Dutch mills and subsequently sold back at high prices to the French. This was later a subject of investigation by the French observer and spy Le Turc.[5] Printing on cloth could well be looked at – the composition of the colours, and the manufacture both of wood blocks and the copperplates which the English were now using. English earthenware was increasingly fine, decorated with bright colours and enamel. It was selling well in France and should be looked at; perhaps the first wave of exports of the newly invented printed pottery is involved.

Again the limited French knowledge of the British scene is shown in this part of the instructions; Holker was not only to find opportunity to talk with merchants but also those persons in the British administration concerned with the policies for promoting manufactures. He was to report on the amount of liberty allowed to each manufacturer, on inspections and 'marques' [presumably meaning taxes on particular manufactures], on the guilds and on the regulations and laws governing manufactures. Once again we have French incomprehension of the freedom of British industry. But of course there were exceptions and nuances which confused French observers who had never resided long in England. There was the emergence of a highly complex system of excise laws with intricate rating and measurement of materials and commodities; a rudimentary patent law, with a rapid rise in patents from mid-century;[6] some export bounties or drawbacks on exports; a few restrictions on manufacture, like the Fustian Act of 1736; the powers of the City Companies within London, which might induce ideas of more general guild importance; prohibitions of certain exports, like raw wool, often smuggled to France, particularly from Ireland. These examples could readily convince French administrators that British industry must have a host of regulations not dissimilar to their own.

Another person who provided instructions for young Holker illustrated these confusions and misconceptions when he asked for two copies of the British official collection of printed regulations on manufactures – if there was such a thing! If there was not such a compilation he conceded it would be too difficult to collect individual regulations for serious study – which Holker, by now inevitably reeling under the great mass of his instructions, may have regarded as a small mercy. Failing such a compilation, confusion could be avoided by talking to those who knew about these supposed regulations. Were quality of materials, the lengths and widths of cloths, and their finishes regulated in England? Were faulty producers fined and their goods confiscated as in France? Effectively this enquirer wanted to know whether or not England had a true Colbertian system. Were there regulations 'to raise every piece of cloth to the highest possible superiority by the excellence of the materials and the spinning, and consequently thereby achieve the highest possible price, or is the greatest perfection possible for commerce thought of as everything which sells well and abundantly'? Was lower quality thought of as a good thing if it fitted in with the tastes of the consumer? There were then detailed enquiries about supposed official controls.

From what he would have learned at his father's knee about his native country, young Holker could have answered most of these questions without leaving France, and one may suspect that some of these requests for enlightenment were struck out of his final instructions, especially if his father had the opportunity to look them over. But the last enquirer must have been a senior government official or adviser, and this illustrates areas of profound ignorance of British practice in high places. However, even here one must not pass by with a dismissive smile. At the very end the enquirer directs Holker's attention to an important matter. In England was the fly-press confined to use in mints or allowed to be employed freely? The free use of this and other machines (often confined in Europe to mints for fear of counterfeit money) was an essential element in the rise of the light engineering of Birmingham and the growth of the 'toy' trade. What metal manufactures were the presses applied to? Was counterfeit money common in England as a result? This was no silly enquiry; Birmingham had a bad reputation for counterfeiting, and of course it was the great centre of production of a widespread token coinage of rather indeterminate legality.[7]

Though the Trudaines were very ready to pay for the acquisition of technology from the great rival, England, they were not in favour of lavish travel expenses and expense accounts. Holker was instructed:

> Throughout this journey he will be as economical as he can in his expenses, and as he will be bound to give small tips to the chief workmen of the manufactures and workshops which he needs to visit, [he] will be allowed three hundred livres a month dating from today for the time he is in France and four hundred livres per month while he is in foreign countries (counting from the date when he informs us of his arrival there) for all travel costs and emoluments until he returns.

He was thus to live, travel and bribe in Britain on about £17 a month. He was to use an alias while abroad, taking (as we have seen) the name of Hilton, that of his mother's family.[8]

The young Holker, appointed as 'adjoint' to his father in 1768, made another visit to England within a few years; he seems to have spent much of 1770 in England, returning home by the end of the year. His father wrote to Trudaine de Montigny in October 1770 regretting that he had been unable to meet with the minister either in Paris, or Amboise where the inspector-general now was, and where Trudaine had been expected to visit Choiseul on his estates. He had wished to discuss with Trudaine topics arising from his son's English tour. His son had already traversed five or six English counties and was very pleased with what he had been able to see, and he had managed to get several reports back to Holker senior.

There was one discovery of great importance. He had learnt about a new kind of cotton-spinning machine. It was very simple, and one operator could produce as much as fourteen spinning women. It was going to be of great use to the English and enable them to produce cloth much cheaper than the French could. Holker senior wanted Trudaine to consider this and plan to prevent the import of English cloth, without which restriction French manufacturers would suffer.[9] The machine was of course the jenny, the first of the famous Lancashire cotton machines to be received in France (see Figure 7.1, p. 149).

Holker said his son had just been through Derbyshire to look at the lead and copper mines there, and would then go to Yorkshire and thence through the North Country, but he would not go into Scotland on this trip because the end of December would be very unpropitious for travel there, and he would set off back to France. While in England he had heard the harshest complaints against his father but that would not, said Holker senior, hinder him from doing his duty for his French masters, for the Holkers had no reason for caution in the face of these criticisms. Once his son was home they would select the discoveries arising from the trip which were most important and which most needed to be brought to Trudaine's attention. They would then devote themselves to establishing these things in France. Interestingly Holker asked Trudaine to burn the letter – which its survival shows he disregarded. Holker had obviously become concerned over any possible carelessness at the Bureau which might leak information about his son's travels, and about any attempts by him to inveigle workers or bring back prohibited models or plans, before he got back to France. But in fact the younger Holker was back in Rouen by New Year 1771, and writing at once to Trudaine de Montigny to convey the unctuous New Year good wishes which officials customarily sent to their heads of department, and favoured subjects to their patrons. He told Trudaine with some complacency that he had been able to pursue his English travels 'completely undisturbed and without any awkwardness whatever'. His travels, he believed, had been profitable, but he had not stopped for any length of time anywhere and he had only been able to make notes, and so he could not immediately give a full account to Trudaine. Nevertheless he was keen to see Trudaine in Paris very soon.[10]

The younger Holker made yet another journey to England in the following year. Though referred to as his second, it perhaps means his second since becoming officially attached to the Bureau, or the 1767 journey was perhaps disregarded as being concentrated on sulphuric acid technology. Before the 1772 journey Guines, the French ambassador in London, was officially informed and asked to receive young Holker favourably and give him any help he needed and he was told that Holker would be using the Hilton alias.

Before setting out young Holker wrote to Trudaine de Montigny at the beginning of June. He first assured him of the total success of the vitriol works. He simply awaited Trudaine's final orders to set out, having previously thoroughly discussed the general purposes of the expedition with him in Paris. He wanted his latest instructions as to what to concentrate on, and at the same time he wished to have a code with which to correspond with one of Trudaine's officials.

> 'Whatever troubles I create for myself I would be willing to take on any risks which would gain the objective of the cardboard [for cloth pressing] which is so important to our manufactures of narrow woollens, so as to prove to you that I desire nothing more than to further your greatness's desires for the public advantage.'

Despite Holker's minimizing of the difficulties of his previous journeys, his precautions for this one were serious and carefully taken. He wrote to Trudaine's nominee, Bruyard, enclosing a letter for his chief stating that it was essential that his journey should be known only to Bruyard and Trudaine. 'So I commend myself totally to your discretion, on which my success and my personal safety depends, for neither my wife (he had married Elizabeth Quesnel in 1769) nor my family know of my departure for London.' Bruyard wrote by return that Trudaine wanted him to concentrate on the cardboard process, otherwise he left it to Holker to seek information on whatever he thought important. He had been made responsible for arranging a code for communication between them. One idea was a book code 'each of us having a copy of the same book', but Holker could choose any other kind. On 19 June Holker sent Bruyard a cypher system with an example of its use. He thought that a simple inspection of the code would be sufficient for Bruyard to grasp it, otherwise he would send a more detailed explanation. He thought the code should not be too easy to break.

The only thing about which he thought he might need to send intelligence from London was the 'secret of bending timber, whether for naval or other purposes'. Only if Holker thought this process worthwhile[11] would he contact Bruyard and ask for a payment to be made, which suggests that someone at London had offered the process to the French government in return for a specified sum. Apart from this he would investigate the cardboard process for cloth-pressing, the making of white lead (where he would try to obtain sufficient enlightenment on the technology to induce a company to organize itself in France in order to produce it within the year), the production of flannels at Welshpool, and the making of fine woollens in the south of England. He would willingly go to Scotland and over to Ireland, particularly to look at their linens, and inform himself on the price of labour, and the cost of provisions and raw materials there. His father, now at Paris, was insistent on seeing him before he left for London; once he had conferred with him he would take post for Calais. From London he would travel night and day to Yorkshire to learn the secrets of cardboard manufacture.

A few weeks later his father wrote that he had news from his son who had seen the French ambassador in London, where he had spent a few days, and then gone to Leeds via Sheffield. There he had investigated an English method of making cloths with a waterproof finish, but the cloths had in practice been found to leak where they rubbed, so that the inventor no longer had any desire to communicate his secret! His son would tell Trudaine the story when he got back. However, young Holker's wife had also had a letter from him written at Halifax where he had attained complete success in the cardboard investigation. He was now on his way to Scotland and northern Ireland. One wonders whether the famous lead chamber sulphuric acid works at Prestonpans was included in the tour, and helped to convert the Holker works to the same process.[12] Again Holker senior wanted Trudaine to burn his letter, though obviously the request was again disregarded. Why was his son able to write so readily to his father and his wife when such a fuss had been made about code communication, and with Bruyard alone? It may well be that the Holkers felt secure in using their regular contacts and agents in England to convey their letters to ships' masters at the ports, rather than entrusting letters to the ordinary post, and that they believed their own methods were less leaky than the official channels via the London embassy. Perhaps, like Le Turc later, they believed themselves at greater risk of being betrayed to the British authorities by French enemies than by British contacts, hence the desire that even ministers should destroy evidence of Holker II's movements until he was back in France.[13]

As well as his visits of observation and espionage to Britain, the younger Holker made reports on French districts. One must be very early in his career, perhaps at his first nomination as his father's *adjoint* in 1768,[14] for he refers to 'the little experience I have' and the task being beyond 'my capacity and my age'. Nevertheless he had already submitted a report on Rouen and now prepared one on Aumale, Amiens and Abbeville where he had been asked to examine the reasons for their languishing and decadent state and propose means to remedy serious commercial abuses in each town. However inexperienced, his views were forceful. Regulations were attacked and the remedy (he said of Aumale) was 'to give to the manufactures the liberty which is completely necessary to expand trade, to stimulate industry, to remove the penury which the greater part of the regulations involve'. Later in the report are some observations which seem to have a physiocratic bias.[15]

The reports of Holker II cannot be followed further here, except where they refer to English practice translated to France or where there are notable reflections which are influenced by his knowledge of England. Following his investigation of the English use of glazed cardboard in pressing during his visit of 1772 he was involved the following year in helping to set up at Aumale the important firm founded by Flesselles and the Englishman Price. The latter claimed to have previously been at the head of a large firm, presumably in England. They had some difficulty with the local intendant, who thought their claims for subsidy exorbitant, and felt that their installation of sophisticated finishing equipment for woollens was merely a way of covering up the defects of slack manufacture and inspection. Holker II seems to have made cardboard in Rouen by the English methods and to have provided this, and presses of his father's design, to the entrepreneurs. There are specimens of Holker's cardboard in the French national archive files. However, as late as 1775 the Amiens firm was still importing cardboard, and apparently also the cast iron plates for the presses. When major local bankruptcies threatened to drag down Flesselles in 1777, the cloth printers of Amiens petitioned the Government to support this concern, which had been launched under Holker's auspices. Flesselles survived and was petitioning for further government support in 1779, on the ground that he was about to increase the number of his English cloth presses from eight to sixteen, saying, with some unintentional irony, that his works had been shown both to Holker II and to the local inspector, Roland de la Platière. In fact Roland was about to launch a bitter attack against the Holkers.[16]

In May 1773 Holker II was ordered by Terray, the controller-general, to make a tour of central France and the Midi, where he was to be mainly concerned with textiles, with the means of improvement of existing manufactures and with suggesting potential areas for development. There was a strong concern that some manufacturing districts were declining and that there was considerable unemployment. Imbert de Saint-Paul, the inspector at Nîmes, wanted an inspection of a new works to produce English cardboard for the textile industry, set up by Gentil near Uzès. The intendant had done much to encourage the works and had visited it himself with the inspector of manufactures of the generality. Holker II had been sent some of the cardboard in 1772, which was then being employed in the finishing presses of Colson, whose works both Holkers had previously visited. Some of the cardboard the younger Holker had then seen was not strong or shiny enough; he had doubted if some which was as good as the English was actually made by Gentil, and he wanted a much more rigorous testing of Gentil's product. But in his 1773 visit he was very favourable to Gentil, and surprised that he had made such progress but, unlike the inspector, he considered the card remained inferior to English. It was not equally shiny on both sides, the paste from which the board was made was not consistent enough, and Gentil certainly could not have sold his cardboard in England. His production costs were such that one might as well have imported English cardboard. Gentil was now using his own pressing and calendering equipment, but some of it, particularly the cylinders, was poor. However, Holker went to the Bishop of Uzès and secured support for Gentil. He would get new cylinders made, and provide other equipment to make the works profitable, and apply to the controller-general for some relief on duties for the manufacturer.

On the same tour Holker II visited Lyons, including the works of the hardware manufacturer, Le Cour. He had lived many years in England, probably working as an engraver, had an English Protestant wife, and had been partner in Michael Alcock's famous English hardware or 'toy' works at La Charité. While Le Cour was having problems he was also making important advances. He faced high raw material costs and opposition from the Lyons goldsmiths, because he wished to make plated and gilded buttons, buckles and similar products. Though Holker does not mention it, there was also a bitter quarrel with the button-makers guild. But Le Cour was now building an enormous fly-press which could stamp out buckle chapes from steel blanks, and had devised a machine to shape the chapes. By these means Holker thought he would be able to produce chapes as good as English ones. This was important, because while Alcock had largely naturalized the processes of the Birmingham toy trade in France, he had not really succeeded with buckle chapes, and his sons, who had a works at Roanne, not far from Lyons, imported English ones.[17]

In 1774 Holker II visited coal workings in Languedoc, and was often depressed by the low quality of the mining techniques. But his English experience led him to write a short panegyric on coal, not unlike the one Faujas de Saint-Fond was to make in 1784 after seeing the coal-based economy of Birmingham. Holker wrote:

> 'I cannot help saying that it is with the greatest satisfaction that I heard of all the discoveries of mines of this kind made in recent years. There are certainly few things which are so useful to humankind, given that it provides the means of setting up nearly all the different kinds of manufactures.'

If good coal supplies could be found in Languedoc the results could hardly be imagined. 'Fire is so greatly needed for the arts that they only thrive in those places where it can be obtained plentifully and cheaply. Now it is the arts which give affluence, affluence which determines the population, makes landed property more valuable, and causes waste land to be cultivated.' The Estates of Languedoc should work to encourage a coal industry, and to ensure that mines were competitive and thus produced cheap coal.

Cheap coal, it was again emphasized, was not only a basis for a more comfortable life for the poor, but a basis for new industries. Holker cited steel production, for which France was dependent on Germany and England, and emphasized the gains which could come from production of the English type cementation steel, made in coal-fired furnaces from Swedish bar iron, which after forging would be used for cutlery and similar goods. Such works had to be near coal because of the huge quantity of coal consumed. Holker perhaps helped to set French government advisers on the wrong track by suggesting that high-quality iron from Roussillon or other French districts could be used, 'but this can only be decided on the basis of ad hoc trials' he prudently added. England, thanks to works at Sheffield, Rotherham and Birmingham, annually produced 4,000 tons of this steel which sold widely abroad, and it was much used at Saint Etienne. If in future it seemed possible to set up the industry in Languedoc, Holker would be willing to set it up himself 'or to bring over workmen from England if necessary to direct cementation furnaces'. Once coal was available it would be possible to follow the English in expanding the heavy hardware and cutlery industries. There were good water-power resources for mechanized grinding and polishing in the English fashion, while fine hardware in imitation of Birmingham was, he thought, perfectly possible to establish. All this of course depended on the successful exploitation of coal, and he conceded that most other raw materials would have to be imported, but felt that Languedoc's communications were good and that with local effort and government support the province might 'compete with all the industrial nations'.

Holker overestimated the effects of coal-mining in Languedoc, forming too optimistic a view on the basis of recent attempts at large-scale exploitation, and the mining entrepreneur Tubeuf whom he admired was to fail in his ambitious schemes.[18] But Holker warned local industrialists that coal which had a great deal of sulphur could eat away the bottoms of copper boilers, as the calico-printers of Orange had discovered when boiling up dyes, and advised the industrialists of Languedoc to have lead bottoms to their boilers, for lead was resistant to sulphuric acid, and so lead bottoms would last much longer. This problem and its solution were new to the Orange manufacture, as he believed they were to Languedoc men 'where the use of coal being very new they have not made the investigations necessary to deal with these difficulties'. Here we have a good illustration of the way in which the gradual, long-term, nature of technological change based on coal in Britain had led to many alterations in equipment, which had to be assimilated by other economies desirous of basing themselves on coal fuel.[19]

One new industry Holker thought should be set up in Languedoc was of English coal-fired earthenware. He was about to set up an earthenware manufacture in a Rouen suburb. Once well established he would have very skilled and intelligent workers whom he could spare for Languedoc. This pottery had great advantages over that ordinarily used in France, the English now sold it extensively in Europe and it would be coming into France too if it were not prohibited. One main advantage was its extreme cheapness: you could have a dozen plates for 3 *livres*. It was attractive in colour and of a harder and more solid body than ordinary earthenware and less liable to have the pattern removed when the pottery was rubbed or knocked. It was not red and porous like that which the French were accustomed to; and it was both lighter and more durable. Once the first works of the kind were established in Languedoc and others began to imitate them a competitive market would exist, and its prices would make it possible to export the new earthenware.[20]

After this display of enthusiasm for potential developments, Holker II carefully fed in cautions. One could only achieve a significant industrial development over time. Such gradual development would slowly create a class of men who had a sufficient standard of life and possessed sufficient wealth to have the courage to take risks, and the good sense to see that they performed a service to society by their industrial initiatives. They would fully understand that it involved putting some of their wealth and their peace of mind at hazard. In other words Holker looked to a steady growth of wealth to induce an increasingly entrepreneurial attitude, and it may be presumed that he believed this to have been the English experience.

Another advantage of 'major importance' could come from cheap coal. This was lime-burning. Cheap lime would greatly increase its use in agriculture where it could be applied to arable lands, particularly on clay. He pointed out that the wide distribution of coal-mines made lime cheap for many English farmers, but the proof of its value was that even where lime and coal had to be brought from a distance, and the treatment was dearer, the English still employed it on their ploughlands. Holker emphasized that lime was often an excellent fertilizer for pastures as well. Finally, if Languedoc could once manage to produce all the coal it wanted for its own needs, there was always the possibility of exporting it, and Holker waxed lyrical about the extent of the English coal trade, both coastwise from Newcastle and to many European ports, and its great employment of shipping. In view of the future history of the region some of Holker's advice and encouragement may now seem over-optimistic, but he was urging the industrialists of Languedoc to take every advantage of new coal-mining developments whose extent, quality and cost were still to be discovered. His whole emphasis was on the need to move France to a coal-fuel technology like that which the British had already largely achieved.[21]

In 1777 Holker II was very active nearer to the family base in Rouen. In that year the manufacturers of Louviers wrote to Tolozan appealing for help. They were short of spinners and wanted to save their labour by using machinery. They wanted the best machinery available and specialized help with it, and they believed that Holker (apparently they meant the father) would assist them with his expertise and models of his machines. But it was the younger Holker who replied to Tolozan in September. He would soon be at Rouen and there would organize the dispatch of 'my spinning machine' (that is a copy of the jenny he had brought over from England), as well as a spinning-mistress who was skilled in using it.[22]

He was using his English contacts in the same year to bring over to France, on Trudaine de Montigny's orders, a range of samples of the goods which Britain exported to her North American colonies. These would be then sent round all the manufacturing towns of France so that they could be imitated and supplied to exporters and shipowners who could thus take over the trades which Britain had formerly enjoyed with her rebellious colonies. As so often happened Holker II had to put in a plea to Necker for repayment of the large sum he had expended, while the bales containing the samples had become stuck in transit at Paris and had not reached him.

The Bureau highly approved both the industrial espionage which the younger Holker carried out in Britain and his spreading of good industrial practice, mainly on the English model, by his tours of inspection in France. Next, as we shall see, they directed him to important liaison work with the rebellious American colonies, with whom the French were about to become allies in a successful war with Britain. This effectively ended his work as an inspector of industry, though he continued the rank and emoluments for a few years longer. At this point we must resume the story of the father's career until his death in the mid-1780s, only dealing with the son's fortunes as far as they affected the father's.

7   The Difficulties of the 1780s

In the late 1770s John Holker senior seemed to be approaching the end of his career in a position of power and influence, and with his reputation with government assured and unblemished. But there were increasingly poisons within the cup. One important disadvantage was the loss of powerful ministers with whom he had had good relations. The co-operation with the elder Trudaine had been long and remarkable, and lasted from the early 1750s to Trudaine's death in January 1769. Trudaine's great ability, his unrivalled knowledge of a number of important aspects of the State, like transport and mines, as well as manufacturing matters, ensured that he was indispensable. He avoided promotion to any of the few more important offices of state, perhaps on the grounds of his persistent bronchial ailments, but more probably because he knew only too well that some of the other offices of state were more vulnerable to the fickleness of factions and courts than his own. His loyalty to those whom he esteemed and who served him well, therefore, was able to continue down the years and remain effective because he himself remained in office. This unbroken patronage of 'the great Trudaine' was of inestimable advantage to Holker. While his son and successor, Trudaine de Montigny, is thought to have been less decisive and less diligent, and more devoted to social life, he generally followed the same policies as his father and continued the patronage of his father's protégés. He was less discreet in his own political alliances, and was more openly partisan towards the physiocrats and particularly close to Turgot. The opposition which was eventually successful in destroying Turgot, and was able to feed on wide popular distrust of his liberal policies, profoundly affected Trudaine de Montigny. He resigned in 1777, effectively dismissed by Necker, dying a few months later, aged forty-five.

The problems John Holker senior began to encounter in the 1780s were all the more galling because of his considerable social elevation in the 1770s. At the beginning of the decade as a Jacobite ex-officer[1] of distinguished service he had been appointed a Chevalier in the military Order of Saint Louis. In November 1774 he had obtained letters of nobility. To do this he had to 'prove' noble ancestry. Here Holker's claims were probably as spurious as those of many others in contemporary France who managed to obtain such letters from the king, or of the many families in England who laid claim to gentility and a coat of arms after rising through trade, industry or the professions.[2] The document conferring nobility on Holker states the real reasons for the elevation:

> the progress of the arts has in all periods merited the attention of wise
> governments, and we, following the example of our royal predecessors, have encouraged them by suitable rewards, and our desire is to
> give them particularly to those who have employed their talents to
> contribute to the advancement and happiness of our people by finding
> for them new means to help their industry.[3]

It was for this motive that the signal favour of nobility was to be conferred on him. He had been to the trouble of getting an English College of Arms pedigree in 1770, no doubt as concomitant to his obtaining his military Order. This evidence was certified by the then ambassador in London, and supported by English Jacobites in France, including three heads of English or Scottish seminaries in Paris who put their tongues in their cheeks to testify to Holker's gentility. The conferment of nobility on Holker was a reason for the jealousy of one of his principal traducers, Roland, who fruitlessly sought that distinction.[4]

The animus against the Holkers, which surfaced after their protectors were dead or fallen from power, began at the end of the decade. In 1779 an Amiens merchant, Pailleux, was concerned at excessive liberty given to manufacturers. His representations were part of the intense current debate on the subject, as the Government tried to find a compromise position between those who wished to retain the controls of guilds and inspectorate over the type and quality of goods produced, and those who wanted such restrictions removed. There was a strong note of Anglophobia in Pailleux's correspondence. He believed that foreign merchants, mainly English, had large stocks of goods in France which had come in illegally, and that these imports were continuing despite the war. Like many who favoured controls over French manufactures, he took a very pessimistic view of French products: 'the

English have always prevailed over us in the making of all woollen and cotton cloths'. Though they might be inferior in some basic manufacturing processes the English always won out by their superior finishing.

He delivered an impassioned attack on the Holkers. He believed, mistakenly, that Holker had been responsible for sending his son to the United States of America and that his real function was to set up manufactures there. This would mean that the former colonists, with plentiful raw materials, would develop successful manufactures and trade, and become rivals to the French, rather than useful co-operators. He claimed that Molard, Holker's Paris agent, had explained this to an Amiens manufacturer. Pailleux regarded the supposed Holker plans as treasonable, and likely to cause ruin to the country's manufactures, and wanted Holker senior arrested until his son returned to France. A supplementary and confused complaint concerned the importation of English cardboard and the efforts to manufacture it in France under Trudaine.[5]

The Roland Affair

A distasteful and extremely hurtful episode towards the end of Holker's career was his quarrel with Roland de la Platière.[6] Roland was an embittered inspector of manufactures who had failed to advance his career as he thought his merits deserved. Humourless and a workaholic he achieved great position only late in life, at a time of political chaos in the early stages of the Revolution. Even then his office was gained largely through the machinations of his much younger, attractive and ambitious wife. He tried to do a good job as Minister of the Interior, but his wordy and legalistic approach and lack of political acumen left him an easy victim to the Robspierristes and the Paris commune, and he had ineffective support from the failing Gironde faction.[7]

His miserable death as a fugitive, by his own sword, conscious that his wife was already executed by the guillotine, invokes our sympathy for Roland, but his conduct towards Holker shows him at his worst. From a Villefranche family of bourgeois and small land-owning background, which had largely lost its money in his father's time, Roland had apparently rejected the priesthood which his other brothers had turned to for a living.[8] He tried to find a career in business, but with little success. He tried to use the influence of a relative, Godinot, who was an inspector of manufactures at Rouen, to get him a trainee post in the inspectorate there. But in fact it was Holker's support which was decisive. Roland worked hard to cultivate local magnates and the Chamber of Commerce who might support his further promotion. He also produced long memoirs on local industries, the first of many, to the same end. Yet it was ten years before he obtained advancement, when Trudaine appointed him a sub-inspector at Clermont de Lodève in Languedoc. In Roland's Rouen period Holker appears to have been friendly and helpful to the young man.

Roland regarded the Lodève post as small beer. He told Trudaine shortly after his arrival that 'you have sent me among a population of ferocious animals ... beyond the reach of anything that is decent'. Though he thought well of some of the local cloth manufacturers, he was bitterly contemptuous of others. However he got on well with the intendant, who generally supported him. But a furious quarrel with a powerful and disreputable manufacturer, Jean Martin, who at several times threatened him with violence, may have resulted in representations by Martin in Paris and at Court, leading ironically to Roland's removal by promotion to an inspectorate at Amiens in 1766.[9] There he quickly came to dislike the official attitudes, and that of the intendant, and regarded the town as a centre of economic, and particularly industrial, reaction. In this he may have been right, and in attacking the old Colbertian system which the locals were happy with he believed he was propagating the new liberalism of the Trudaines. But there can be no doubt that he was spiny, tactless, self-righteous and aggressive in manner. He particularly attacked the reluctance of the Amiens guilds and manufacturers to see the free movement of industry into the countryside, though this was now legal. In some cases his policies were justified, but they were offensively presented. His continual going behind the local authorities to get the backing of the Trudaines was resented, as were his lengthy absences on French and foreign travels, and time spent in study and writing rather than his basic duties.

Roland seems to have added the Holkers to his enemies by quarrels which escalated over the years. He claimed to have asked Holker in 1767 for samples of English cloths to make in Picardy and instructions how to make them, but without co-operation from the inspector-general. Holker probably resented the idea of Roland getting the credit for his expertise; had Roland asked for Holker's help through Trudaine he would probably have got it.[10] In the 1770s two further causes of deep friction can be traced. One related to Flesselles, an Amiens woollen manufacturer who, unusually for a local industrialist, became a close friend of Roland. Flesselles was interested in adapting English cloth finishes. In 1772 he approached the younger Holker to help him after he had completed his second secret mission to England. Holker fils came to Amiens and, as we have seen above, tried to help Flesselles both in respect of the English cardboard for glazing cloth which he had been at such pains to study in England, and the provision of presses of the type his father used. While the testimony of other Amiens manufacturers in favour of Flesselles when he ran into difficulties a few years later suggests that Holker's assistance was important, Roland claimed that improvements were due to Price, the English finisher who worked with Flesselles, and not to the Holkers.

The other, and very critical, cause for quarrel lay in one of the publications by which Roland desired to spread his fame and so circumvent the frustration and lack of advancement he experienced. As we have seen Trudaine de Montigny had been driven from office in 1777, and died shortly afterwards. The revised administrative arrangements at the Bureau of Commerce did not favour Roland, as Tolozan who disliked him became increasingly influential, and eventually sole intendant and the head of the Bureau. Roland's application for a post as inspector-general had been rejected. Then, trying to compensate by his writings, he secured a commission to write a volume in the celebrated but much retarded series, the *Descriptions des Arts et Métiers*. The volume was to deal with the craft of making cotton velvet. This was very likely to be a cause of offence to Holker in itself. It was he who had introduced the successful production of this important and fashionable material; unless he was to get very full and exact credit for his contribution he was going to be angered. Together with English finishing and controlled quality spinning this had been one of his main contributions to the French textile industries. He must already have been incensed by Roland's claim that Price had first brought in English finishing when he had himself introduced the methods twenty years before. This had been followed by statements that he, Roland, had introduced and improved the jenny.[11]

Roland in seeking material for his short book wanted to examine the Holker factories. It is understandable that the Holkers refused him entry. Roland, being the obstinate man he was, sought letters from Trudaine de Montigny to give him official entry, but then did not take advantage of them. He later taunted the elder Holker that if he had not been 'more of a manufacturer than an inspector he could have published the *Art* himself, it would have been a good way of revenging himself'. Of course the Academy of Sciences would not have agreed to two works on the same craft being commissioned simultaneously. Roland's many critics in the administration doubtless considered that if he had been doing a thorough job as an inspector he would have little time for the long travels at home and abroad, which brought little result, and for his increasing volume of writing.[12]

The outrage caused by *L'Art du Fabricant de Velours de Coton* (The Art of Making Cotton Velvet) was primarily due to its introduction, where a very personal attack was made on Holker, without naming him, but in such a way that the target was unmistakable. This was both bizarre and wholly out of place in a work which was supposed to carry a state of the art account of an important technology under the aegis of the Académie des Sciences, perhaps the most august scientific institution in Europe. While Roland tried to claim the contrary, he certainly would have had the publication heavily censored if Mignot de Montigny in particular had really read the introduction, and this is possibly true of other Academicians who were supposed to have approved it. That he got away with publication in the short run seems due either to official readers skimming or skipping the introduction, or to Roland adding to it at the last moment before publication.

He accepted the English origin of cotton velvets. But he went on: 'One only sees in France four or five specialized manufactures of this kind, and the entrepreneurs hold up the price of their goods so high that the result is the introduction of a large contraband trade from England.' The restrictive practices of the French producers prevented any competition with the foreigner. The English raw material came, like that of the French, from their own colonies and must have been equally costly, while English labour was dearer than French. He charged the supposedly monopolistic group of French producers with confining the cotton velvet industry to only three or four places in the country, and restricting the looms to a mere 300 when even a single town like Amiens could have had thousands. This was the outcome of 'the favour, the distinction and the privilege which have been given to these Manufactures'. He accused the group of preventing the Academy of Rouen from disseminating memoirs which would have extended useful knowledge of the processes involved.

In his passage on the origins of the industry in Normandy he gave favourable mention to the Havard brothers who had first introduced the English methods, but unsuccessfully. D'Haristoy too got credit for setting up the Darnetal manufacture. Holker without even being named

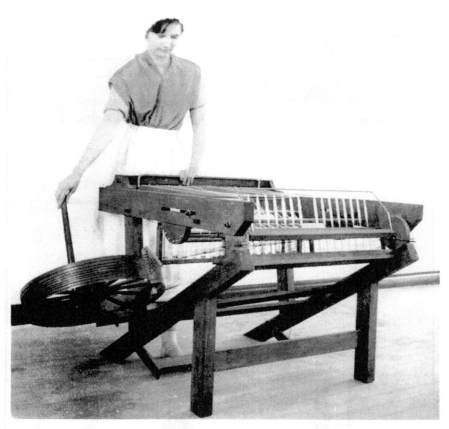

7.1 A spinning jenny reconstructed from James Hargreaves's patent specification of 1770

was treated scornfully, 'a calenderer from Manchester ... having es-caped and fled,[13] brought workers, his relatives and others' to France. There he had 'rapidly made one of the most outstanding fortunes of the age'. The Saint Sever manufacture was alluded to as 'the basis for new projects for the administration, which having poured out subsidies with a great abundance' now regretted concentrating them on this enterprise. The problem had been the mixing of private and public interest, the interest of a private person having prevailed. Turning to carding, Roland made much of Kay's card-making machinery (though he did not get his name right). Kay detested Holker, Roland may have

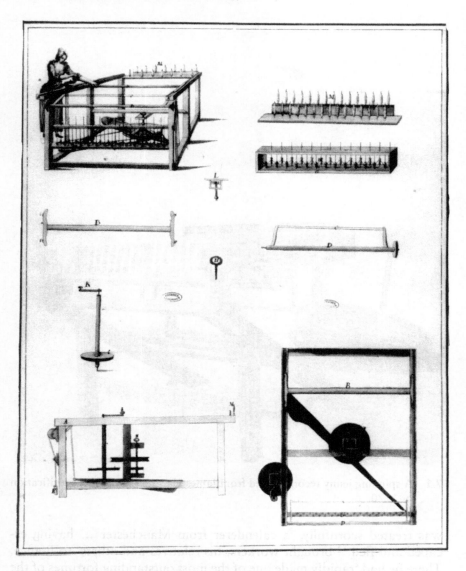

7.2 A jenny as illustrated by Louis-Casimir Brown, Inspector of Industry, in an Archives Nationales document of 1779

hoped to needle the inspector-general. The younger Holker got no credit for bringing the jenny to France 'for some years it was an object of mystery' wrote Roland, trying to tar the Holkers with the secrecy brush; the 'first known and publicly used is that which I managed to

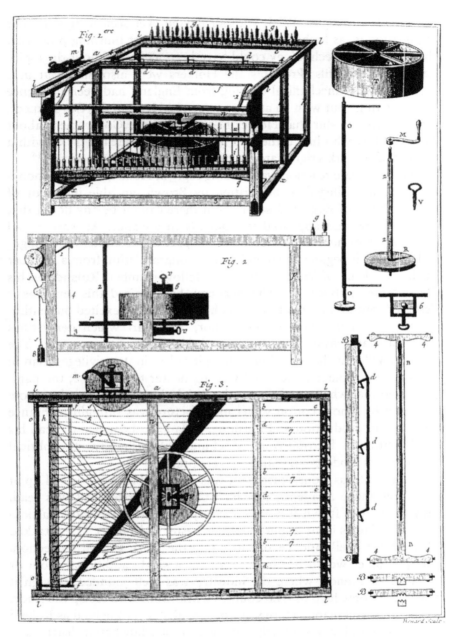

7.3 A jenny as illustrated in *L'art du fabricant de velours de coton* by Roland de la Platière, 1780

have made in August 1775, without having ever seen it myself'. The implication is, as he had insinuated with the latest finishing processes, that the English technology could have been gained without the espionage of Holker fils. Probably the Holkers were also hinted at in a suggestion that mechanical carding from England had been in France for some time, but with an attempt to conceal it from the Government. This carries the slur that Holker had not told the Government about James Milne, who had turned up to see him at Rouen in 1779 with a version of the Arkwright carding engine. This was utterly untrue.[14]

The immediate reaction was a telling reply in Holker's favour. Anonymous, it was alleged to be written by Brown, an able inspector of manufactures of English descent,[15] but there cannot be any doubt that Holker knew and approved its contents in advance. At least it had some traces of humour, which Roland's part of the controversy singularly lacked. It began as a spoof letter of congratulation from a member of the Academy of Villefranche to his fellow-member, Roland, on his *Descriptions* publication. The Academy had praised this series as it deserved 'but that on Cotton Velvet has particularly excited our enthusiasm'. Especially, mocked the author, 'that part which demystifies these dark and mysterious workshops' deserved public gratitude. The town of Villefranche would in future glory less in its privileges than in being the birthplace of Roland! Getting nearer to the bone, the pamphlet said that whereas a lesser author might have simply tried to show how and by whom cotton velvet manufacture was brought to France and explain production and finishing, Roland had decided to head his work with the Introduction. Mockingly, its urbanity, its political economy, its modesty and fairness were praised.[16]

But a fictitious Rouen merchant was supposed to have turned up at the Villefranche Academy, to which the Roland pamphlet was read, only for him to frown furiously at every paragraph and most particularly at Roland's irony about the 'Manchester Calenderer'. He attacked 'this odious libel', and set out to refute the work section by section. The pamphlet would not help to set up a single additional loom or machine in France, where the industry was well founded, though it might give some help to rival countries who wanted to set up the trade.

Cotton velvet manufacture was not spread all over England as Roland had supposed, but was closely confined to the Manchester district and was intensely developed, firms with 1,200 looms being known. While in France there were indeed only three or four firms which were *manufactures royales*, Roland was deliberately concealing what he knew perfectly well, that numerous independent producers made cotton velvets in many places in Normandy as well as at Sens, Amiens, Bayeux, Gisors and elsewhere, though business had fallen off recently because of the high price of raw cotton during the American War of Independence. Holker, far from trying to act to the exclusion of others, had set up English-style cotton spinning in many parts of the kingdom, and new varieties of cottons were being made in many places as a result. There could be no price maintenance in the cotton velvet industry because the many separate manufacturers would have undercut the *manufactures royales* if they had attempted it. The French price was low enough to make English contraband imports unlikely; what happened was that the commercial supposition about English superiority in quality was such that Paris dealers sold French cotton velvets as English, pocketing a large price differential for themselves in the process. Until the French producers had been able to imitate English velverets and velveteens well, there had indeed been a contraband trade. There had been a route for these goods – as apparently there was still one for narrow woollens – through Boulogne and Amiens where they were illegally sealed as being local manufactures. Roland as inspector at Amiens should have done something about this, had he not been so taken up with his literary labours![17]

Holker, said Brown, had effectively introduced cotton velvets, and by hands-on demonstration, not by writing books for dilettantes rather than for those really concerned with the trade. Saint Sever had been the great example, and many manufacturers had resorted to 'debauching away' the workers when, had they applied to Holker, he would have been ready to show them the best methods of making cotton goods, and he had done this even before he had any obligation to do so as inspector-general. Brown claimed there were up to 1,400 cotton looms now at work, but many of the smaller makers were ignorant about fustian-cutting and backward in their knowledge of dyeing, while some lacked finishing equipment. Holker had offered the Chamber of Commerce of Rouen to take in trainee fustian cutters for four-month training periods. He had not been able to make a similar offer on dyeing 'for the English dyers were so dissolute, that no sooner had they set to work than it was necessary to dismiss them'. But Trudaine had endeavoured to get over this by posting learners to the best dyeworks, two of whom had been trained respectively at Saint Sever and Sens.[18]

Holker had established heating stoves for burning off the loose surface of velvets, of his own invention, together with other finishing machines, on the premises of a good dyer at Rouen. This was intended to assist the small manufacturers. There was no way of keeping secrets in the finishing processes for there were seven or eight men in this department at Saint Sever who could leave the works at will. Brown believed, whether correctly or not, that an English shearer had taken back to Manchester – where it was previously unknown – a machine which Holker had devised for singeing velvet; it was later used in England for narrow woollens.[19] Price's machine at Amiens, so vaunted by Roland, was just the same, and if Roland thought it so significant, why had he not disseminated it throughout his area of inspection?

Brown instanced many cases where Holker had spread the whole gamut of cotton manufacturing techniques to new districts, for instance the Bordeaux area, where he had sent spinning-mistresses and foremen. Brown claimed that Lancashire labour costs were not significantly dearer than those around Rouen, being reduced by the low local costs of butter, milk and potatoes, and the great use of apprentices and child labour. Coal was extremely cheap there, and of the greatest importance for heating the houses of the poor as well as for finishing and dyeing. At the same time machines saved labour costs in Lancashire, and water power was coming into use. While he did not make a clear distinction between labour costs and wage rates in Manchester and Rouen, Brown's argument may have had some relevance. But the great advantage the English had over the French, according to him, was in the free circulation of goods within the national borders; in France 'at every step one finds barriers where one has to pay duties', though new national policies now formulating under Necker might some day alleviate the problem.[20] Brown argued that, far from there being a limited number of looms in the hands of a few privileged men, there was a wide distribution of looms making cotton velvets and related cottons.

Brown showed by quotation from the original that the 1776 report of the Academy of Rouen concerning the coming of the cotton industry to the province indeed gave full credit to the Havard brothers and to d'Haristoy and his associates, but it had clearly stated that 'M. Holker brought us the art of making velvet and other English cotton cloths', calendering by cylinders, both hot and cold, as well as a new blue dye, the sulphuric acid manufacture, and the manufacture of baize. He had introduced a thousand improvements in woollen finishing and in dyeing and spinning equipment, while women taught by him were spinning nineteen threads at once (on the jenny). The 1776 report expected yet further advantages to Normandy industries from both the elder Holker 'and a son who is worthy of him'. Roland was thus thoroughly convicted of *suppressio veri* on a massive scale.[21]

Brown said that Roland was either ignorant of Holker's arrival in France or had deliberately misrepresented it. He had taken part in the '45, was captured at Carlisle[22] and had avoided execution by escaping to France, where the Young Pretender had given him a commission in Ogilvy's regiment at its formation. After the Flanders campaign he had visited Rouen in 1749, met several merchants, and had been taken up by Morel, as we have seen earlier. He had then entered into negotiations with d'Haristoy, who got Morel to write to the administration, which led to Ogilvy's introduction of Holker to Trudaine, early in 1750. This in turn had led to Holker's perilous journey to England on behalf of the Government, the obtaining of English cotton workers, and their establishment at Darnetal. The contemporary attempts by others to establish the relevant branches of the cotton industry in France, cited as critical by Roland, had all been failures.[23] As for Mignot de Montigny, he would willingly back all the statements which Brown had made, and both he and his fellow Academicians, who had together formally approved Roland's work, were horror-stricken at its untruths and at having 'given credit by their respectable authority to what was a libel in every sense of the term'.[24]

Brown argued that the subsidies given to Saint Sever had been related to the cost of obtaining and installing English machinery and workers and to limited bounties on the early output, well justified by the foundation of many parallel firms at Rouen and elsewhere. Roland's attacks on Holker's origins were discreditable. Had his parents not apprenticed him to the textile trade, to which Roland directed such scorn, France could have not received immense benefits from him. It was in fact this calenderer who, as Inspector-General of Manufactures, had obtained for Roland the place of *éleve* in the inspectorate, which the influence of his relative Godinot, the senior inspector at Rouen, had up to then failed to secure. Holker had again helped Roland in opposing his dismissal from his job as inspector at Amiens when he had aroused deep enmities in the business community there, and this was fully established by letters of thanks which Roland had written to both Holkers at the beginning of 1773, 'in the strongest and even servile terms'.[25] As late as January 1773 Roland wrote to Holker père in confidence of 'your friendship towards me, and your good offices with M. de Trudaine, which have always been a source of inspiration to me' and begging Holker to intercede for him to get some of his emoluments for 1770 which he had not yet received. Holker did so with success, for Roland later sent Holker a copy of the letter of thanks he wrote to Trudaine de Montigny.[26] It was after these many kindnesses that Roland had tried all kinds of underhand tricks to get information out of Holker for his projected *Art du Fabricant de Velours de Coton*, and when Holker had remonstrated, had written him a haughty and inappropriate letter, and then taken revenge by his slurs on Holker in the pamphlet.[27]

As to Holker's low birth, he had been regarded as of gentry origins when nobility was conferred on him by Louis XV in 1774 – no doubt Brown knew how much Roland himself coveted ennoblement. If the publication under discussion had been of great practical significance it would have been entrusted to Holker who had brought the relevant processes to France and employed them successfully for thirty years, rather than to Roland, who knew nothing much about them. Brown regarded Roland's remarks on Holker's wealth as pure jealousy. On the other hand he had himself made claims to inventing or introducing various industrial improvements, all meretricious. Of course the claim to introducing the jenny was singled out as wholly false, for Holker fils had brought it over as part of his industrial espionage expedition of 1770, and there were now around 1,200 in France. The Holkers had not kept the jenny to themselves, but invited all provincial intendants to send spinning-mistresses to Sens to learn to use the jenny and had undertaken to send them back home with a model of the machine.[28]

In carding, Holker had first brought over Hall, and then Holker's English contacts had sent Milne to him, in fact to demonstrate the new Arkwright method of carding. Two machines were set up at Holker's Oissel works in 1779, and were visited by Tolozan who had ordered one for the Government (probably for the permanent exhibition at the Hotel de Mortagne) whence Roland had got his description and engravings. So much for Roland's imputations that the Holkers had tried to keep the new carding methods secret for a time. In his remarks on dyeing Roland had plagiarized a report of 1756 on the methods of a Rouen dyer, and his account of dyeing in blue in the English manner would have proved disastrous if followed, while many of his supposedly novel methods were known to all dyers.

Roland had been made a fool of by his own unjustified hatred of the Holkers, which he had voiced under the pretext of producing a work for the public advantage. He should employ his literary gifts on something more suitable.[29] Lest there should be any doubt about the libellous nature of the publication he was attacking, Brown attached a copy of Roland's introduction to the *Art du Fabricant de Velours de Coton* to his own text.[30]

The controversy now continued, with a friend of Roland's providing a reply to Brown's pamphlet, similarly acting as a mouthpiece for Roland.[31] He said that Brown had been provoked that Roland rather than Holker had been invited to write the work on cotton velvet manufacture. It had been perfectly proper for him to write it, as it was commissioned by the Academy of Sciences (with material deriving from the Academy of Rouen) and approved by the Academy.[32] Most of Holker's unjustified fury came from the perfectly correct references to him as a Manchester calenderer. It was not denied that Holker had helped Roland to get his first trainee job. But it was emphasized that his later posts in Languedoc and Picardy were not due to Holker's influence – though there had never been any suggestion that they were. There were restatements of Roland's claims that he had unfairly been denied entry to Holker's works, though travels in Italy were made an excuse for his subsequent failure to present himself there after he had received letters from Trudaine de Montigny authorizing such visits.[33] The situation of the Holkers was of course a difficult one in respect to their own trade practices; while willing to spread basic English techniques through many parts of France in co-operation with the Government, they and their business partners nevertheless wanted to retain some technical leadership over their local rivals and were not willing to throw their works open to them so as to make instantly available every knack in the trade. Roland's supporter was able to make capital out of this, and out of Brown's suspect claims that French production and product costs were as low as English. The writer said that Price at Amiens had not been willing to show his methods to Holker fils on the grounds that he was a rival businessman as well as an inspector of manufactures. Many other manufacturers were said to have taken this attitude to the Holkers.[34]

The English expedition of Holker fils was derided and the dangers of the industrial espionage ridiculed, while it was misleadingly suggested that Roland had travelled to England after war had already broken out in 1778. The pamphleteer claimed that if Roland had been given money from the Government as Holker had been he could have brought back all Manchester technology![35] But in fact the Bureau of Commerce would never have trusted La Platière's judgement on textile technology, and young Holker had brought back the jenny. The contributions of the Holkers to many branches of textile technology were ridiculed by the pamphleteer, a dangerous line of argument considering their major achievements. Even their introduction of vitriol production was rubbished.[36] While not wildly intemperate in tone the pamphlet had, though making some hurtful personal attacks, failed to disprove what was not really controvertible, the outstanding importance of the Holkers in the development of the French textile industry, and particularly cotton velvets.

Much more offensive were a set of printed letters, the first supposedly from a member of the Academy of Rouen to a member of the Academy of Sciences at Paris.[37] Their tone was sneering, claiming for Roland a place as a member of the cultivated and literary world, deriding Holker as common fellow. Given Holker's important and honourable position and Roland's reputation as a boring author whose works sold badly, this was not an approach likely to create sympathy. It is obvious that Roland was either the author, or at least a very substantial ghost. Holker, the writer says, had written like a stable-hand or a lackey, thus asserting that Holker rather than Brown was the real author of the *Lettre d'un Citoyen de Villefranche*.[38] The writer was clearly disturbed that the Introduction to the *Descriptions* volume and the *Réponse* had upset some members of the Paris Academy, and had made them regret commissioning and approving the work on cotton velvet. Though claiming to support literary and civilized values against those of the crude and unliterary Holkers, the piece quickly descends into a trough of vulgar abuse which must have lost Roland's cause any remaining support. Holker could hardly read his Prayer Book, he had never read a book; with wealth he had become insolent, he had lived in the depths of poverty in England 'his origins are lost among the meanest of Manchester's inhabitants', his wife (presumably his first wife Elizabeth Hilton) was illiterate;[39] he had been a mere workman rather than a substantial tradesman in Manchester, and only followed the cruder range of the calendering business.[40] He had known nothing when he came to France; he brought with him only 'a capacity for intrigue which turned into impudence'.[41] He lied when he talked of his services to his adopted country. He lied when he talked of a price on his head in England after the '45 – he was too mean a subject.

At this point Roland had clearly become demented by hatred. For Holker had been greatly honoured for important services to France. He had (as we have seen) been the personal companion of Charles Edward

Stuart in England in 1750. Roland, himself a rather unsuccessful inspector of industry, was stupid enough to sneer at Holker as 'A knight of industry, such as it is rare to see'.[42] Holker as an ex-officer with considerable active service had been made a Chevalier of Saint Louis, the main military order; normally businessmen could seek only the Ordre de Saint Michel. Nevertheless that order was strongly coveted, and was for instance a matter of great pride to one of the most successful business managers of eighteenth-century Europe, Delaunay Deslandes.[43] Given his attitude it is no wonder that Roland's own campaign to be ennobled was turned down without ceremony. He ironically illustrates the passion for nobility frequently cherished by subsequent revolutionaries.

Roland had to admit that the Academy had removed his Introduction from all subsequent copies of his *Art du Fabricant*, but tried to squirm out of the obvious implications. He published a letter in his support from the anonymous Academician he had written to, but while the correspondent wrote that Holker 'held forth in Billingsgate (en style des Halles) to an Academy which promotes culture',[44] there was much more crudity in this and the Roland-inspired pamphlet than anything in the Brown/Holker *Lettre*. A third letter was published which Roland had written to Mignot de Montigny. Again there was a great deal of wriggling, but Montigny, he had to admit, had informed him that the Brown/Holker pamphlet had been 'a critical work which proved troublesome for me'.[45] Roland's further excuses that he had not actually named Holker in an attack which was admittedly aimed at him, and that there was no significance in his failing to mention all the important firms 'which they attribute to him', as being irrelevant to an account of the industry, could hardly have been feebler. His attempts to justify his giving credit to the Havards and d'Haristoy for technical success in the industry rather than to Holker were wholly unconvincing. He sheltered behind source material he had carefully misinterpreted, for as a junior official he had lived twelve years in Rouen at the peak of Holker's influence, and would have to have been blind and deaf to be unaware of the extent to which he had transformed the industry. It is clear that Montigny had reproved Roland for his condemnation of Holker for gaining wealth in business, and for his ingratitude to a man who had helped him to obtain his career.[46]

For Roland the work proved a considerable disaster: 'M. Tolozan has made for me a devil's vespers of the [Holker] affair and the tone of my correspondence ... he gave me a great tirade on inspectors who were academicians, who wrote, etc.',[47] and he lost for some time any credit he had with the administration. He was certainly not earning any credit by his current work as inspector. He failed to make a proper report on his Picardy area in 1782, on the excuse that he had made a full one in 1781 and that a locally published almanac would update it. A series of annoyed and reproving letters from senior administrators had a cheeky reply from Roland who simply dodged the real task. 'Roland, without appearing to occupy himself greatly with details demanded of him, has simply sent back an extract of the heads of the same letter in the margin of which he has permitted himself to set down some dry and laconic observations.'[48] Neither nobility nor real promotion was offered, and he turned increasingly for reputation to writing, particularly to his *Dictionnaire des manufactures, arts, et métiers* (1784–92). His sideways promotion to Lyon was mainly important as a means of enabling his dangerous involvement, first in the provincial politics of the Revolution, and subsequently and fatally in national politics; in both his wife was a key influence. The last meeting between Roland and Holker in the early 1780s shows the inspector-general trying to make casual conversation and to propose a discussion, only for Roland to carefully snub him, so that Holker left saying he had still not forgiven him.[49]

The American Involvement

Much more dangerous to Holker's position than the Roland quarrel was his son's involvement in the affairs of the infant United States of America – the Roland controversy merely dented dignity and raised blood pressure. From 1777 the two Holkers, with French government support, had been involved in commercial and financial dealings with the American rebels; initially they helped their commissioners in Paris to obtain supplies for their army. In 1778 the French government sent the younger Holker to Philadelphia. He had originally two roles. The first, to convey indications of support to Congress in advance of a French alliance and a declaration of war, was initially frustrated by the refusal of Vergennes, the French foreign minister, to give him full diplomatic accreditation. The other, to promote French–American trade, build a commercial network and open avenues for French investment in America, he entered into enthusiastically. The merchant and financier Robert Morris agreed to act as his managing agent, a move all the more fateful because of Morris's enormous influence as Superintendent of Finance in the American government during 1781–84. Once the French and Americans became overt allies Holker was officially appointed agent of the French navy in American ports and in July 1778 consul at Philadelphia; soon after he became consul-general for Pennsylvania, Delaware, New Jersey and New York.

The problem was that he was not yet officially forbidden to carry on private trade, which he had originally been encouraged to foster. This problem was exacerbated when the original team with whom he operated changed, and Gérard was succeeded by La Luzerne as French minister in America, and Sartine, an ally of Vergennes, was succeeded as navy minister by Castries. Neither of them would have been concerned with Holker's original political-commercial remit, and both would think of him simply as a servant of the French state – after all he was still an inspector-general of industry and enjoying the perquisites of that office. Yet he was being importuned by merchants and bankers of the first importance back in France to execute commissions for them and, with his father's assistance, fortified by his great knowledge of France's industrial products, to fill the gap left by the shortage of British goods in American trade, in the hope of supplanting the British in American markets not merely during, but after, the war. The affairs of John Holker junior in the United States do not concern us in themselves, except in so far as they led to serious difficulties and anxieties for the father in his declining years and in so far as they carry reflections on the industrial work which the Holkers had accomplished in France.[50]

It is clear from correspondence at the highest level in the French government that the Holkers were expected to advise on the potential of French trade with America. In November 1779, Tolozan, the important intendant in the Bureau of Commerce, wrote to the father, at the express direction of Necker, about information he had given a few months before on the different goods which were best for the American trade. He requested a further memoir on possible trade connections, and on those industries which were already in existence in America. He was invited to get such information from his son if need be, and forward it to Tolozan, or direct to Necker. A very similar request was made by Montaran on behalf of Necker in the following February, particularly asking what alterations or adaptations would need to be made to existing French products to fit them to American tastes and purses. What were foreign nations currently providing America with, and could the essential details be supplied with samples wherever possible? Furthermore were there any such goods the production of which was unknown in France? Which districts of France were likely to make the goods most successfully?[51]

Important French businessmen were soon importuning Holker fils for an opportunity to get into American trade through his good offices.[52] His father was involved the following year in organizing exports of cloth from Decretot of Louviers and Grandin of Elbeuf, amounting to 30,000 *livres*, in which the Holkers would take shares. Their Saint Sever firm was preparing to send a venture of high value, even with the risks of a winter voyage. Cottons, some printed, would follow from the Sens firm in the spring. Holker senior discussed the proportion of those exports which father and son might take on at their own risk. A prominent Irish merchant in Rouen, their friend Garvey, was involved with a large earthenware export. Unfortunately it is only rarely that the American papers of the younger Holker afford any information on the Holkers' industrial activities in France.

The younger Holker wanted his wife to join him in Philadelphia, but her own family and Holker senior were against her travelling in winter, and indeed during the war at all. Sound advice from father to son was regrettably not followed, that he should be more careful in his business affairs, not get involved in American politics, and that he should remain an 'honnete homme'. There is no clear evidence of blatant dishonesty, but there is evidence of deals and trading ventures on a scale so vast as to be reckless, and of a group of American associates at least equally dangerous and gigantic in their uninhibited speculations, several of whom died insolvent.[53]

The businesses in which the younger Holker was involved are numerous, and my superficial survey of the sources will not have unearthed all of them. They included dealing in bills of exchange, speculation in United States funds; shipowning (one of his ships was the *Holker*); privateering; the West Indies trade in provisions, sugar and rum; whaling; at least exploration of possibilities in the fur trade; land speculation; and eventually investments in the iron trade, including the first Pittsburg ironworks. He was deeply concerned in the first American China voyage, that of the *Empress of China*.[54] In 1781 the French authorities became concerned that Holker fils was making a personal profit out of exchange dealings made on government account, and that their affairs were not getting precedence over his private business. In August 1781 Robert Morris had reassured some of the senior French army commanders.

> They complained of Mr. Holker's conduct towards them, and as I was
> well acquainted with Mr. Holker's transactions I took occasion to
> explain the same and to assure them over and over of what I do most
> sincerely believe, that Mr. Holker is as honest a man, and as zealous
> for the King's service, as any that ever came from France.[55]

Holker was given the plain choice between acting in the capacity of
a French consul, or that of an American businessman, and chose the
latter. He then, of course, had to settle his accounts with the French
government, and particularly with the navy. From 1782 he ran into
grave problems in settling his private agency accounts with Robert
Morris (rather than his official ones with Morris as Superintendent of
Finance) and finally he came to believe that Morris had deliberately
delayed settlement in order to take advantage of currency depreciation. Yet at times when Morris's private affairs had been difficult,
Holker had helped him with money and credit.[56] By 1784 the two
were quarrelling bitterly. Holker was put under great pressure by the
French government to settle his accounts and return to France, or lose
his office as inspector of manufactures, but he found it impossible to
return as he could not settle the accounts. Worse, he continued his
own speculative trading, and particularly, in partnership with Daniel
Parker, took on large contracts for the supply of the American army
with clothing and provisions. There was also the question of the
profitability of the French trade with America as organized and invested in by the two Holkers.[57] Within a few weeks the younger
Holker was being asked to contract for officer's clothing.[58] As late as
1783 he had entered into large private contracts for the supply of
naval stores to France as a member of Parker and Co., in which
Robert Morris was also involved. He was shipping masts to France in
the following year and naval stores were again being dispatched
towards the year end, but as early as July 1784 Daniel Parker's affairs
were known to be in an 'alarming situation' and his goods were being
seized by former trading associates as security.[59] While other creditors
were seizing the property of Parker and Co., the firm itself, perhaps
as a pre-emptive measure, seems to have been selling off ships and
goods. Meanwhile the firm of Turnbull and Marmie in which the
younger Holker was a partner, and had carried on trade with France,
had its bills under suspicion, and as early as June and July 1784 they
were only accepted after they had been guaranteed to major French
business houses by Holker senior. These guarantees were thought to
be more than he could sustain.

The father's health was being seriously threatened by his anxieties. A letter of June 1784, probably from a member of the family, told his son how all this was lacerating his feelings. Each letter from French creditors was now 'a twist of the dagger as it entered his bosom'. All these disagreeable events so upset him that for eight days he was struck down by an illness so severe that his life was despaired of. His son was reproached: 'all this Sir should convince you of the necessity to hasten your return, so as to relieve the anxieties of a person so dear to you, and console him in all those problems which your absence has occasioned him and still daily affect him.'[60] But matters did not get better. In July 1784 Daniel Parker was preparing to flee America and his creditors, leaving his partners William Duer and John Holker to face the music, while the settlement of accounts between Holker and Robert Morris had broken down and deteriorated into pamphlet warfare and legal wrangles. A further problem in the French trade was a quarrel, now before the American courts, between Holker and an American merchant, Samuel Wharton, who had been exporting goods from Nantes and Lorient which had come from the Saint Sever Company and other French firms. Again, a fire at Holker's Philadelphia house in 1780 meant that American Loan Office Certificates were destroyed and could be replaced only with difficulty.[61] While Holker the younger seems to have temporarily returned to France in 1790, when he was pursued by some of those who had received guarantees from the Holkers about cargoes they had dispatched to America over a decade before, he was apparently unable to return before his father died in April 1786.[62]

Holker senior's declining years were thus troubled by the attacks of envious rivals and the unbridled speculations of his son in America. In other ways, however, there was testimony to the importance of his achievements, and the regard in which he was held by famous men. An interesting, if oblique, testimony to his work as a conductor of industrial espionage comes from attempts to entice him back to Britain in 1780, effectively a British attempt at counter-espionage. While taking the sea baths at Dieppe for his health, Holker received letters from Marsh, one of his old London friends who had long acted as his agent, '(he) has always fulfilled my commissions though often difficult and often dangerous for him, but his attachment to me has always made him overcome the difficulties'. Since the American war began there had been an additional link inserted into the chain, Holker's friend the Rouen merchant Bunel, who received letters for Holker which were specifically marked. Marsh had been approached by a 'person of importance' in England who was aware of Marsh's acquaintance with the Holkers. The person would commit nothing to paper, but wanted to arrange a personal interview with Holker at Ostend or some other place agreeable to him, but insisted that the discussion would not be dishonourable to either Holker. Marsh could not go further, but said that if Holker wished to have his liberty in England, and rejoin his old friends there, that would be entirely up to him. Holker assured the French government, 'if they believe that either my son or myself are capable of such base conduct, they deceive themselves'.[63]

This had not been the first time the English government had tried to get him to betray his loyalty to France, twenty-five years earlier Fox had tried to get him to cross the Channel by offering him a pension of 12,000 *livres* a year which would descend to his family. The elder Trudaine had been kept in the picture by Holker, and had seen a copy of Holker's letter replying to the offer. The Bishop of Derry had more recently tried to win him over, and Holker had again informed the French government.[64] Holker thought that it was his son whom the British were now most concerned to seduce, but 'all the money in England would not entice him', and if he had not been sure of his loyalty he would never have let him leave for America. If keeping a rendezvous in Ostend or elsewhere would be useful in uncovering British plans, Holker said he would be willing to go and 'use all the dissimulation necessary, despite my character which is so opposed to it', but would await instructions. The permission for Holker to go was granted by Louis XVI in person. But the important man who was to have come over with Marsh had faced some delay because he needed to consult a member of the House of Lords not then in London, and it became necessary to fix a new date at Ostend. Holker had alternatively suggested a meeting at Amiens or Paris. Nothing further is known of this scheme to tempt the Holkers back to Britain, but it was a source of worry to Holker: 'it causes me tremendous mental torment'. Confidentiality at his end was secure, because his second, French, wife had acted as his secretary in the matter, 'so, no need to worry'.[65] The rewards given to Holker in France were already acknowledged to be a temptation to others to follow him there. A Mr Cramond wrote to the British government advocating the appointment of a consul-general in France, largely to prevent the settling of British artisans. He was afraid that the encouragement given by the French government to Holker would tempt others to follow his example.[66]

Holker in his last years was highly regarded by some of the most important American emissaries and commercial men in Paris, and in particular by two of the greatest men of the age, Franklin and Jefferson. He was particularly friendly with Franklin, who apparently was involved in some of the early Franco-American trading ventures of the Holkers. He performed small commissions for both, obtaining a copying press – presumably the new type invented recently by Watt – and chased up delayed consignments of books and other goods from London. When Franklin left France in 1785, his health giving much concern to his friends as he was plagued by both gout and 'the stone', he was carried in Marie Antoinette's state litter. He stayed with the Holkers for a couple of nights at Rouen on his way to Havre, 'when we took an affectionate leave of each other'.[67] Holker clearly wrote to Jefferson on a personal basis and in his own hand, and when writing in English his spelling betrays his limited formal education.[68] Matthew Ridley, a close business associate of Holker junior, spent some time in France in the early 1780s and wrote warmly to Robert Morris about the father: 'Holker has got a good Father here. I was going to say better than he deserves; and perhaps should did I not know him better than I do.' On another occasion, 'Nothing can be kinder than Mr. Holker is to me. He is a real good man'.[69]

John Holker was so wide in his influence, and touched the industrial and administrative life of France at so many points over four decades that any attempt to sum him up is bound to do him less than justice. He was a man of great courage, he would be of interest if only as an officer of the '45, the perpetrator of the daring and successful escape from Newgate, the Jacobite officer in the French army. While still in the army he made the remarkable journey into England as Charles Edward Stuart's sole companion in 1750. Once he was taken up by Trudaine, he again embarked on a dangerous programme of espionage, this time industrial espionage, in England. Even so this new espionage was not many years after the Newgate escape, and he was running the risk of recapture as a dangerous Jacobite rebel, not merely, like other industrial spies, the penalties for suborning workers under the 1719 Act, or organizing the export of certain machines.

His textile operations in Rouen involved the setting up of the cotton velvet industry as well as the manufacture of other cottons, and this was essentially associated with the establishment of new standards of hand-spinning and the setting up of a large and efficient finishing industry of which calendering was the single most important element, though fustian-cutting, bleaching and dyeing were improved. His technical influence was very important in other large industrial units outside

Rouen, like Sens and Bourges. He clearly had a great ability to recruit the right men in England, and to retain their loyal services in the long term. If he did not succeed with Kay and Alcock, he was dealing with men who were of extremely difficult character, who left a trail of discarded associations and partnerships, men who seem to have been impossible to satisfy, and involved in disputes within their own families as well as with the outside world. Their very real talents were made less useful by their great personality defects.

Holker's English was awkward and ill spelled, his spoken French limited and unpolished. Yet his letters and reports are remarkably clear, forceful and telling, which must mean that his selection of secretaries and amanuenses was as good as his choice of technical men, so that his meaning was conveyed with force and clarity. He had much to impart, as can be seen in the reports of his tours of inspection. If he had merely been a skilful emigrant calenderer, like Badger, that would have earned him a small corner in textile history, but he had a remarkable knowledge of the cotton industry from top to bottom. He inculcated best practice (generally Lancashire practice) in carding and particularly in quality spinning (which he regarded as the foundation of the industry), in weaving, where his own works seem to have persisted with the fly-shuttle when others did not, and of course in finishing processes. But in the finishing trades he did not confine himself to calendering and hot-pressing, he put effort into improving bleaching and dyeing. Remarkably he was well informed on woollens, particularly light ones, and commented critically on most aspects of manufacture. This was not destructive criticism, or the laying down of principles leaving others to master the practice. Not only, as we have seen, did he publish a guide to the manufacture of *bayettes* but he was to be found in the workshops with his sleeves rolled up demonstrating the technology in a basic hands-on way. Nor was he solely concerned with the manufacture of woollen cloth; he was interested to pursue the industry to its agricultural base in the care and housing of flocks and the improvement of grassland. Having left a specialized branch of Lancashire textile production while still in his twenties he was even able to give shrewd advice on metal manufactures and the hardware and gun trades, yet he never seems to have pontificated about industries where he was not able to give a worthwhile opinion. His son may have had a superior knowledge of the chemistry involved, but the industrial reputation and administrative strengths of the elder Holker were indispensable to the creation of a sulphuric acid manufacture in France, forming the essential basis of the heavy chemical industry.

The evidence of the tours, we have said, marks out Holker as one of the great observers of the eighteenth century, bearing comparison with Daniel Defoe and Arthur Young. He analysed the weakness of French industrial organization, but he did not condescend. He may have been strong on the defects of the practice of workers and small masters; but he was more critical of their superiors, merchant manufacturers, merchants, and the guilds; it seemed to give him genuine pleasure to see increases in employment, the spread of industry into the countryside, the introduction of new products. Industrial difficulties and opportunities were alike seen with a sympathetic eye for the workers' situation, and, as in the Gévaudan, he hated to see them miserable. He never despised the French worker, whom he believed was the equal of any other national, providing that he was properly trained. The policy of the Trudaines seems to have been entirely congenial to him, balancing the advantages of subventions and tax exemptions for desirable new industries against the dangers of long-lasting exclusive privileges and continual financial spoon-feeding.

Holker believed in the open mind, and lifelong learning. In 1760 he wrote of a pushy and over-confident young manufacturer 'if he has all the talents he boasts of, he is very happy, given his youth and the short working life he has had. As for me, though I have been conversant with manufactures for twenty-eight years, I find myself in a learning situation [dans le cas de apprendre] every day'.[70] While Saint Sever and the other textile works he was connected with had not maintained comparability with England as the revolution in textile manufacture gathered pace there from the 1770s, he was able to appreciate the value of machine carding, endeavoured to get early versions to France, and was thoroughly capable of recognizing the critical importance of Arkwright's new carding and spinning technologies. Had his son remained in France with his drive and his avidity for the new, but with his father by him for some years longer to restrain his frenetic ambition, they might have made the transition to the water-powered factory to complete their previous adoption of fly-shuttle and jenny. Holker's opinions continued to be sought by senior officials to the end of his life. During the final discussions on the Eden Treaty he provided an opinion for some vital debates within the French government about French industry's ability to respond to English competition.[71]

Holker was both a great servant of the French state and man of remarkable individual industrial and business achievements. That this remarkable combination was possible was largely due to the wise policy of the Trudaines, but if they were the enablers, he was the achiever. In him loyalty and faithfulness matched ambition and vision. He remained true to the religion in which he had been brought up in 'old catholic' Lancashire. His attachment to the Jacobite cause he risked his life for in 1745 and 1750. As late as 1768 he tried to bring together Charles Edward and English Jacobite representatives to plan an English rising, but Charles, disillusioned and debauched, was past such schemes, though he thought well of Holker. McLynn's judgements are very favourable 'unlike so many Jacobites in the diaspora, who put their own careers first and their rightful king a poor second, Holker never lost his fervid Jacobite commitment', even after 'many of his more vaunted friends of high rank had forsaken him [Charles Edward] ... Holker was a colossus of a man, possessed of immense abilities and able on his own to give the lie to those who assert that Jacobitism was only ever attractive to reactionary troglodytes'.[72] On his general attitude to affairs in France, Gillispie says 'Holker saw beyond the profits of the moment and the season. His was the spirit of adventure in industrialisation ... he thought to force the pace and revolutionize the entire French economy'.[73] Of Holker's achievements in Rouen, Chassagne writes, 'in a dozen years Holker ... set up with his associates a veritable manufacturing complex in which it is no exaggeration to see the basis of the growth and prosperity of Rouen in the nineteenth century'.[74] He was certainly the most important individual in the whole process of technology transfer in the eighteenth century.

PART THREE
Metals and Arms

8   The Hardware Industry

While no grouping of industrial sectors is perfect for the study of industrial intelligence, industrial espionage and technology transfer, there does seem to be a natural one which relates to the production and working of metals. In part it is concerned with the obtaining of British techniques by the French to make products for ordinary civilian consumption, in part it relates to demands for war purposes, almost entirely for the navy.

An industry for which technical transfer is well documented is the small metal or 'toy' industry typical of Birmingham. The other common name is the 'hardware trade', frequently referred to by contemporary Frenchmen as 'quincaillerie anglaise'. While these terms are notoriously difficult to fix with precision, what is clearly involved in transfer to France is the production of light metal goods, of which the most common are buttons and buckles. Also included are tinderboxes, snuffboxes, cane heads, sword hilts and a host of other small items, generally designed to be decorative, and often silvered or gilt, or made in alloys designed to be cheaply attractive, like pinchbeck. There are also a few products of a more sophisticated kind, like Sheffield plate. Already by the middle of the eighteenth century it is important to appreciate that much of the output of the 'Birmingham hardware district', to give it the standard description of the mid-nineteenth century, was made by specialized tools, often machine tools, of great variety. There were many kinds of lathes, drop-presses, fly-presses, rolls (some miniature, some quite large) boring, piercing and slotting machines, just to mention some of the most notable. At one end the trade elided into the true jewellery trade, and into silversmithing (as it did in the celebrated Soho works of Matthew Boulton), at the other into the lighter end of mechanical engineering, where the French description 'metallurgie legère' is very appropriate. While the palm certainly passed to the Americans in mechanical engineering around the middle of the nineteenth century, the world lead was very much in the Birmingham region in the latter half of the eighteenth century, and Birmingham's failure to continue and develop its lead has never been fully analysed. However, the world's 'metal bashing' industries of today are all in some degree its technological inheritors.

The transfer of Birmingham technology to France is largely associated with one man, Michael Alcock. As his operations have recently been discussed in detail, they need only be summarized here, and its espionage element brought into focus. He was born about 1714, and probably into a prosperous brass-founding family. By the 1750s he was in a very large way of business and among the manufacturing élite of Birmingham. He was in partnership with William Kempson. They both called themselves 'merchant' to make it clear that they did not belong to the common herd of small manufacturers. Both partners had substantial houses, and owned or rented land, Alcock living at Langley Hall, some miles out of Birmingham, while Kempson lived in a 'genteel and pleasant' house attached to a large and well-planned works in Birmingham itself. The works was called 'a big and famous manufactory' by a Swedish visitor of 1749, and was described by the partners as for button-making or pinchbeck manufacture, but snuffboxes and brass fittings for furniture were turned out as well as buttons. Alcock had a separate thimble-mill, and an investment in one of the Birmingham cementation steelworks, while both had an interest in a file-cutting invention and in a machine tool for the clock trade. It would hardly be possible to find a man more central to the operations of the Birmingham metal trades than Alcock, or a larger employer, for the partners employed 300 to 400 workers.[1]

Alcock astonished all his acquaintances by suddenly departing for France at the end of 1755 (or just possibly the first days of 1756), the partners being declared bankrupt in February 1756. The failure is said to have been needless commercially. What happened is that Alcock left with one of his girl workers, Sarah Green, but making sure that he took £1,000 with him. This led to a complex failure, which was not finally settled until 1779, probably after the visit to England of Alcock's elder son in 1778. As Kempson was allowed to continue in business by the creditors, the young mistress seems to have been the cause of Alcock's flight. There is so far no evidence of Alcock's having been in negotiation with the French government before his departure; if he approached their London embassy nothing is known of it. He would have been aware that, despite the prohibition of pinchbeck imports in 1740 and that of metal buttons in 1749, English hardware was being massively smuggled into France. The extent of the contraband was such that when ideas about a possible commercial treaty for improved trade with England were advanced in the 1760s and later, the French were ready as a bargaining counter to sacrifice their prohibition on hardware.

There was thus no question that when Alcock offered his Birmingham technologies to France that the authorities would know that there was a market for those products, and that establishing the technologies would save foreign exchange. The French failure to create an extensive 'toy' trade themselves is not fully explained, but some reasons can be found. They were very deficient in the non-ferrous metals, especially in tin, copper and zinc. But the machines used in the Birmingham trades were often in origin, as the French soon pointed out to Alcock (and to his successor and rival firms in their 'toy' trade) the same as those employed in mints, and mints tried to prohibit their use in outside commercial establishments for fear of counterfeiting. This was not unrealistic, it is no coincidence that Birmingham was a main centre of counterfeiting and of the production of the great output of token coins, permitted in practice, but of doubtful legality. The reasons why machinery associated with mints was freely allowed commercial operation in Britain are unanswered because historians have never thought to put the question.[2]

On his arrival in France, Alcock at once memorialized the French government on the goods he would be able to produce, some emphasis being put on the new fashion of using polished steel for buckles and similar items, and he included mechanical file-cutting and a new system of pottery decoration, probably the new methods of printing on pottery just developed in England. For a time he worked with a man called Cugnoni who had been an export merchant in Birmingham; whether this connection had been planned before his departure is not known. But this, like so many of Alcock's partnerships and business associations, proved very temporary. The French government quickly gave him a privilege, in May 1756, but it only covered the 'toy' manufacture and not other manufactures Alcock said he could develop, and gave him a choice of sites, including Rive de Gier and Roanne. But he was most interested in Vierzon in Berry. There was a primary iron industry of quality there, but a complete lack of secondary metalworkers. It was, however, a province which the French government regarded as being in great need of economic stimuli. Nevertheless there seems to have been in Trudaine's mind a feeling that the Saint Etienne area might both be the most suitable site, and one where existing metal trades could most benefit from the example of new English techniques. However, Michael Alcock finally settled for La Charité-sur-Loire in the first-chosen province, Berry. The Loire of course could provide navigation, but not always efficiently, and there was water-power for the kind of mill with multiple drives on several floors to a variety of metal-working or polishing machines which was now being used in some of the larger Birmingham works.

To set up a large concern Alcock needed capital and a core group of skilled workers. He was first joined by a skilled machine-maker, Adam Tinsley, who proved both expert and dependable, and remained the technical keystone of the works for more than thirty years, though he never bothered to learn French. Another essential technician was the die-engraver, and here Alcock was able to find a very skilled man, Paul Lecour, a former apprentice of the French royal engraver, but who had worked for fourteen years in England and had an English wife. With Le Cour as with Fresnais, a Paris notary's clerk who had found investors and become a partner in the firm, Alcock had managed to choose an associate who was about as difficult in disposition as he was himself.

However, Alcock and his wife were reconciled, and she brought his two young sons to France, where they began to learn the technology of the toy trade very rapidly. Mr and Mrs Alcock associated quite amicably with Sarah Green, to the bafflement of their French partners and connections, and she brought over her father and two brothers, and lived with them. They seem to have been expert founders and turners, while her own skills 'extended over all the branches of button making'. Mrs Alcock was now making trips to England to suborn and bring over additional workers, but presumably only brought over a few at a time, because, outside his own family, Alcock never seems to have had more than a dozen English workers at La Charité. This was clearly not what he wished, for attempts were made to get more. In addition to those wanted for La Charité, Trudaine pressed Alcock to obtain others for Saint Etienne. Unfortunately on her third recruiting trip to Birmingham Mrs Alcock and some of her workers were arrested.

The plan had gone very wrong. What actually caused the collapse of the recruiting scheme was a failure of liaison between Mrs Alcock in Birmingham and her servant and accomplice, Ann Partridge, in London.

Miss Partridge was not prepared to take over to France on a single trip the whole party which Mrs Alcock had sent down to London, but only to take over the wife and son of Adam Tinsley the machine-maker, presumably intending to make a separate trip for the others. There seems to have been an odd and almost comical collapse of communication between the participants in the suborning mission. After bringing the Tinsleys to La Charité Ann left without saying anything to Alcock. She seems to have gone straight to an Englishwoman, Dame Willoughby, living at Saint Omer, but Alcock had a suspicion that she would return to England and give evidence about Mrs Alcock's suborning of workers. The Lieutenant of Paris, a *lettre de cachet* and the mounted police were resorted to in order to arrest her, all quite needlessly. In fact Dame Willoughby had been involved in the seduction of Birmingham workers for Alcock since his first months in France. Holker had appealed to the controller-general in May 1756 to have her exempted from a recent order about the expulsion of foreign nationals, because she was useful to Alcock. She owned an estate near Birmingham and was able to help organize the movement of the workers he needed for France, and even send some of the materials he wanted.[3] However, four men left in London somehow gave themselves away and were arrested, and this in turn led to Mrs Alcock's arrest and the incarceration of them all in Warwick Gaol. No punishment of the men is mentioned in the press, presumably because the authorities were more concerned to punish their suborner rather than those enticed. Mrs Alcock spent three months in prison, while additional evidence was sought. She was released on the huge bail of £1,000. But when she came to trial she was acquitted, and indeed Alcock hypocritically wrote about her 'honourable acquittal', though both knew perfectly well that they were breaking the 1719 Act. If the statement is true that Mrs Alcock was congratulated by the court, and taken home in a coach and six by the foreman of the jury, this might well show that the Act was unpopular at that time in the Birmingham region, particularly if applied to people of substance and standing.[4]

The subsequent attempts to obtain more workers were unsuccessful, though Alcock was appealed to by the French authorities, particularly for Saint Etienne. For his own part he especially wanted workers for steel-making on which he hoped to concentrate after he left La Charité in late 1764. There had been another major drive to obtain workers in 1763 when sixteen workers who had been recruited were seized by the Birmingham authorities before they could leave.[5] The Green family at

La Charité became disaffected, first refused to persuade relatives and friends in the Black Country to join them in France, and finally went home themselves.

The story of La Charité is one of great complexity, and will only be touched on here as far as it relates to the transfer of technology. There can be no doubt that Alcock was difficult to work with, even though some of those he took on as working partners, especially Fresnais and Le Cour, were certainly men of an equal waywardness. But Alcock's capacity for quarrelling with those who worked closely with him was remarkable, and hardly equalled even by John Kay. Early in 1758 he, Fresnais, and another investor were furiously quarrelling with Le Cour and Tinsley. The latter, subsequently regarded as an ideal employee by his French masters when Alcock had left La Charité, had gone on strike and come to blows with Alcock.[6] The argument was patched up by Tinsley losing a small share he had been given in the enterprise but doubling his salary; Le Cour left the concern and set up on his own, which was an effective way of spreading the technology, if not one the La Charité investors had envisaged or wanted.

Holker had been asked by Trudaine to keep an eye on Alcock's enterprise but, given his main base was in Rouen, this was not easy to do and he and Trudaine were soon highly anxious about Alcock's performance. While good machines were mounted and workers trained, and new investors found, the day-to-day running of the works was not well organized. Fresnais and Alcock were soon at variance, so the investors brought in two young men from Paris to act as departmental managers and they did not fit in well either with Alcock or the people of the locality. Trudaine had reason to be astonished at 'the want of discipline that prevails in the internal administration of this manufacture'. Alcock protested his hard work and long hours, and that he tried to keep out of controversy, but the people of the district regarded him as 'without conscience or morals and unsociable'. He was said to be violent and to beat workers, and pay them irregularly, and while the rules drawn up for the works by the local intendant laid down many penalties for bad behaviour by the workers they significantly included rules against their beating and ill treatment.[7]

The bad relations with the local inhabitants led them to accuse Alcock of counterfeiting money, an attack which was clearly related to the use of machinery which in France had only been known of in mints, combined with the use of silver and gold in plating buttons and other products. Fresnais passed on slights about Alcock's morals to Trudaine.

Technically many of the problems were overcome, but with delay and much stress. The failure to seduce more English workers meant that Alcock had to train an entirely new workforce without help, including artisans from unrelated trades, peasants, boatmen, women, girls and children. Initially there was naturally a high wastage of materials, including those which had been silver plated or gilt, and here there was a layered monopoly of gild restrictions, both locally and in Paris, to be circumvented if the precious metal recovery was to be achieved which was normal in Birmingham.[8]

Alcock had grave difficulties with wealthy new investors who had been brought in by Fresnais, and with the two departmental managers, Sanche and Hyde, particularly the former, whom they had introduced. His own share of the profits was heavily whittled down, while the English workmen, and particularly his favourites, the Green family, were attacked by Fresnais and his allies. In a long and detailed discussion of 6 March 1760 on the problems of La Charité Holker suggested Trudaine should 'make Fresnais act a little more politely than he does to workers who have left their own country for the service of the French state, this is the best way to attract others when we need them'. Fresnais was detested by the workers in general and Holker was very angry about his harshness to the Green family 'for a foreigner who feels himself mistreated does more damage than one can imagine'. If Green wrote home to England he might seriously deter other workers from coming to France by telling them about his unfortunate plight.[9] These problems added to existing difficulties. One was the ease with which English buttons were imported, despite a prohibition of 1749, in Dutch, Swedish and Danish ships, so that not only the shops but even the hawkers openly sold buttons and other English toys. Button-making depended on a collection of workers with different skills. These skills had been passed on from father to son in England, and French peasants with no industrial background could not be expected to turn out work so good and so cheap. Alcock's own views on the training problem were rather contradictory.[10] Fresnais made continual demands that Alcock should teach him a key process, that of gilding. He seems to have been plotting to leave the firm and to master the different branches before doing so, while investigating several possible centres where he might set up production and attempting to suborn La Charité workers to help him.[11] This led to his dismissal in late 1760 at Trudaine's instigation.

Alcock for a time claimed that all was now well, that during 1762 the plant expanded and employed 250 workers, which probably did not include many outworkers, and that over 1762 and much of 1763 it was making a good profit. However, he and some of the remaining English workers were under a continual campaign of vilification by Sanche and some major investors. Alcock increasingly sought to get out of the firm and start manufacture somewhere else, but of course this was opposed by the outside investors, so that he now proposed to enter into the manufacture of cementation steel rather than 'toys' if he succeeded in leaving. Alcock's understanding with Holker and Trudaine that he would import Birmingham techniques into Saint Etienne was not consistently followed up. He may have been right in the very early stages that it was counter-productive to do much at Saint Etienne before La Charité was properly established; he may have been very much restricted in his capacity to initiate technical reform in that large centre of metal-working by the disasters which befell his attempts to suborn and bring over more English workers.

Certainly he did not achieve his promised boast of making La Charité and Saint Etienne 'Birmingham in France as good as that in England'.[12] Had he been able to bring over scythe-makers, saw-makers and file-makers things might have been different, and he might have been able to give more help in Saint Etienne. It was not that nothing was done; Alcock was sent over to see Saint Etienne industrialists as early as 1757; he took Tinsley over to that town, and some Saint Etienne workers were sent over to La Charité to be trained by them.[13] One of Alcock's machine tools was later used there in the early attempts to make guns with interchangeable parts, and it is said that the distractions of the Revolutionary period led to the abandonment of recently acquired improved techniques of the English type.[14] Nevertheless, a continual cause of concern to Holker and Trudaine was that Alcock did not give the time and effort they thought appropriate to Saint Etienne and to the appeal for technical help from the major arms manufacturer Carrier, which followed Holker's remarkable analysis of the town's production deficiencies of 1756.[15] Trudaine was probably right to have preferred Alcock setting up at Saint Etienne in the first place, and while Alcock continued to try to justify La Charité as a reasonable site for the lighter 'toy' trade, he had to admit that Saint Etienne was better for heavier work and the tool trade, 'if his Lordship (Trudaine) wishes to have the remainder of his views accomplished he must send me to Saint-Etienne, the only place where they can be accomplished'. An advantage for that town was its excellent supply of cheap coal.[16]

The Saint Etienne problem probably exacerbated the situation caused by the continual vilification of Alcock by Sanche and the La Charité investors, so that a visit by Alcock and Holker to Trudaine early in 1763 to explain Alcock's new plans to the minister led to a very unpleasant interview for Alcock, though Trudaine had relented by May and was prepared to accept Holker's new enterprise. But Alcock was thoroughly disgusted with his associates, he told the intendant 'really my Lord I would choose to live upon bread and water in a cottage, than have to do with such secret enemies, even though living in the highest affluence'. He would not put up with incessant quarrels 'even to gain a million'. In the end Sanche and Hyde were relatively co-operative in his departure, they had achieved their object by easing him out and supplanting him in the management.[17]

Alcock's new activities fell into two parts. One, to be covered later in this chapter, was his lengthy but unsuccessful attempts to make steel, the other was to set up another hardware works which was to be run under the names of his two young sons, Joseph and Michael junior. After some vacillation it was at the last minute decided to set this up at Roanne rather than in Languedoc.

La Charité continued under Sanche and Hyde, but they did not long give satisfaction, their administration being showy, expensive, and involving a costly building programme. Having done all they could to malign and expel Alcock, they now claimed to have been his trainees. They could not manage without Tinsley and got him a state pension to secure him to the firm. But some technical aspects outside his skills were disastrously managed. Alcock regarded the gilding process as his great personal trade secret, and a full description of the process, involving a considerable use of mercury, was carefully filed away with the La Charité firm's Paris attorneys.[18] It remained undisturbed until very recently under its original seals, so for some reason, though there was desperate trouble in this department after Alcock left, no one was sent to retrieve it.

The solution was to send Hyde to Birmingham. He had come to France with his family in childhood and was English-speaking. There survives a highly coloured description of the trip, possibly written by Sanche's highly facile propagandist pen. The memoir refers

> to those secrets of which the English are so jealous that they have cost the lives of all those enquiring foreigners who tried to penetrate the laboratories of Birmingham, either being denounced to the legal authorities to pay the final penalty [of course industrial espionage, even

suborning, was not a capital offence] or being assassinated on the spot
... a bold and enterprising man but also wise and prudent was needed
to discover the secrets and one whom a life continually in a thousand
dangers would not worry or deflect ... such a unique person was Sieur
Hyde.

Having reached Birmingham, Hyde set about finding a workman with
the trade secret of gilding, but weeks passed, and Hyde suffered from
bouts of fever. 'He had everything to fear from the men he had to
confide in, who willing to betray their masters, would betray him
without scruple.' However he eventually found a discontented foreman,
though kept on tenterhooks by the man's failure to keep appointments
at taverns. Eventually he was persuaded to part with the secret, but this
was to be demonstrated in London, where he would train Hyde in the
process.

They set out for the capital, 'but they were just 32 miles out of
Birmingham when Sieur Hyde was taken with a violent fever, stopped
his journey and retired to bed. They were soon joined by two men sent
after them at full gallop'. Hyde

> only had time to grab his pistols which he always kept under his
> pillow, and seeing two armed men approach his bed at such an un-
> seemly hour, for it was after midnight, he fired a shot which grazed
> the first man who appeared, and received a similar graze from his
> comrade which went through his nightcap and slightly wounded him
> in the head.

But he and the workman got away, and Hyde claimed to have learned
the gilding process in London. How much reality there is behind this
sensational tale is uncertain. However, many years later, in 1785, Hyde
certainly used the episode as an important element in his claim for the
Order of Saint Michel.[19]

While their skills in publicity and the memorializing of government
enabled Sanche and Hyde to obtain *manufacture royale* status for La
Charité, and the toll-free sale of products throughout France (two
concessions which enraged Alcock, who had never been able to obtain
them when he was at La Charité), they gradually became alienated
from many of the investors, while one large investor, Billard, whose
creatures they were, died insolvent in 1769. After quarrels with other
investors they were eventually thrown out in 1771. But from this
situation they made a remarkable recovery, ironically in part based on
their claim to have been trained by Alcock.[20] Despite the spirited
opposition of their former associates at La Charité they were favoured

by government officials (including Trudaine de Montigny and Holker) and allowed to set up a 'toy' works at Amboise under the patronage of Choiseul in 1771. This does not seem to have been successful, but was converted by Sanche into a vast bubble of a steel-making firm between 1782 and the Revolution.[21] From the point of view of the toy trade the Amboise works at least marks another transfer to a new district of the basic technologies Alcock had introduced.[22]

La Charité continued on its troubled, often tempestuous, passage. Despite new investment the assets were found to be grossly overvalued, the business was sold out to one of the larger investors in 1773, and the investors had lost 1.5 million *livres* by 1778. In 1785 the last remnants of the business were about to be closed, but now Hyde returned with a take-over scheme which he hoped would receive the backing of the controller-general, Calonne. With his weakness for vast projects Calonne was interested in buying La Charité for himself, but he soon fell from power and Hyde did eventually acquire it, no doubt very cheaply. But by 1809 it was, ironically, a poorhouse.[23]

We get two views of the technical state of La Charité after Alcock left it, both through Matthew Boulton. A business agent of his, Thomas Ingram, visited the plant and reported to him in 1774. He mentioned that he got inside 'by the assistance of money and some craft', that is, there was an element of the kind of industrial espionage which was experienced at Boulton's own works.[24] Ingram said the machines were exactly like those at Birmingham, but some small differences existed in the use of boxwood shapes for some kinds of button. There was a high proportion of production of cast buttons for military uniforms. But in some respects the technology was behind England. Furnaces used bellows where air furnaces would have been used in Birmingham, charcoal was used instead of coal. There was a mill, but a horse-powered one, used only for rolling metal, not for multiple drives to machines on several floors. These were deteriorations in practice since Alcock left: he had certainly been using coal, if complaining about supply and quality. One of the essentials when he was looking for a site in Berry had been a water-mill. The gilding of the gilt buttons, Ingham said, was good. In 1774 the number of workers employed was 300, apparently about half the number when Alcock left, though it is always difficult to be sure about the basis of statements made about employee numbers as there were outworkers as well as those in the factory.[25]

The second account of La Charité is by Boulton himself. He and Watt were invited to France by Calonne's government in 1786 on what was effectively an industrial consultancy,[26] a main item for their opinion being La Charité, which Calonne intended to take over. His brother, the Abbé Calonne, had industrial interests, notably in an early cotton factory and in steam-milling. It was clearly envisaged that he would have involved himself in the hardware manufacture, and he accompanied Boulton on a visit there. Boulton was critical both of factory organization and technique, but we must remember that his own 'toy' manufacture had been a financial disaster. He said that too much production took place in one vast hall. A managing partner with a share in profits should supervise the whole, there should be a good book-keeper, partly to check on the manager. A senior workman in each branch of production should hire and pay his own workers, the goods should effectively be sold on from department to department at set prices. This was Boulton's own system at Soho, he said. But La Charité should concentrate on long runs of stock items, high fashion goods should be made near Paris. Optimally the horse-powered rolling-mill should be replaced by one powered by water or steam; Boulton could alternatively supply ready-rolled metals to La Charité at less than the cost of those they rolled themselves. A man with real entrepreneurial qualities was needed to run the place – someone like the Abbé Calonne – or it would never succeed.[27]

It remains to make a rapid survey of the French hardware works outside La Charité, and see how far the techniques brought over by Alcock, or other techniques acquired from England, were employed. We have seen that on leaving La Charité Alcock founded a works at Roanne with his sons, the agreement concerning his departure from La Charité requiring the works to be in their names.[28] By June 1765 Alcock had trained about 200 workers, many of them youngsters now able to contribute to family income. Three years later there were 100 workers apart from many outworkers, and there was a concentration on buttons, and on the cheaper kinds. Again we have a very useful account by Thomas Ingram in 1774. By this time Michael Alcock senior had left the works. The sons refused to break their 'sworn rule' and let Ingram inside the works gate, but agreed to talk to him. 'These two young men' (Ingram wrote to Boulton) 'are such that you would admire ... I never saw men better calculated for the undertaking they are engaged in.' They produced wire buttons at a price below Birmingham and the 'best tin silvered buttons I ever saw', much in demand. They would be 'in time powerful adversaries' to Birmingham, and they were very inquisitive about developments in their native town. They had, unlike La Charité, inexpensive single storey works, which were at least as useful. They had embraced Catholicism, and took care that it was evident. Specialization was initially important, 'they have buttoned themselves to buttons was their phrase, as they sencibly [sic] observed their father's misfortune arose from pursuing too many things at once ... they seem to have all the knowledge, with prudence to shun the mistakes he fell into'.[29] A few years later, however, Joseph, the elder brother, was willing to branch out. In 1777 and 1778 he made visits to Birmingham. Partly they were private[30] and may have related to the winding-up of the Alcock-Kempson bankruptcy of twenty years before.

However, Joseph Alcock was also under directions from the Bureau of Commerce to look into developments in ornamental hardware, but also into rolling and slitting-mills for iron, tin plate and nail rod, where France was behind-hand. For his own purposes he concentrated on buckles, candlesticks and silver-plated goods. On his return he seems to have left the Roanne buttonworks to his brother for a time, and concentrated on the new lines of Birmingham goods he had investigated at a factory at Beaulieu nearby. Buckle chapes presented a problem, which he partly solved by importing them from Matthew Boulton, whom he had met on his visit. Coming in via Ostend they only had to pay a 1 per cent insurance, which shows how easy the entry of English hardware to the French market could be. The failure of the French government to enforce effectively the prohibition on the import of British hardware is interesting and not fully explained. In 1760 Holker suggested that officials of the *Fermes Générales* should inspect the premises of those selling hardware and levy fines and impose penalties. It was sometimes said that a prohibition properly enforced at the frontiers might prevent German and other high-grade metal tools which were greatly needed from entering France. One difficulty may have been the complex problem of definition of the many goods involved. As early as 1752 there was a discussion about whether prohibitions on clocks and watches and hardware should be sacrificed as part of a reciprocal tariff deal with England.[31] Joseph Alcock made strong representations in 1784 about the importation of English hardware and its effect upon his firm. Much entered by direct trade routes, the exporters paying a 5 per cent insurance against seizure (they presumably concealed the goods in some way), some by the relatively lax controls at Dunkirk, where they were passed off as coming from Holland, some via Ostend, whence they entered France as German or Dutch goods.[32] The Alcocks' works, flourishing during the American war, was adversely affected by the peace, and especially by the Eden Treaty of 1786, in which hardware featured prominently, though Roanne seems to have had a hundred workers as late as 1791, and the Alcock brothers still had a buttonworks at the time of their deaths in the early years of the nineteenth century.

The rapid departure of leading members of La Charité meant in effect an accelerated spread of the Birmingham technology which Alcock had introduced. Paul Le Cour left as early as 1758; a skilled engraver, with fourteen years of experience in England, he clearly had advantages. While it is sometimes said[33] that Le Cour had actually worked in Birmingham, this was not claimed by him as far as the present writer is aware, and he was not slow to cite his qualifications. In 1758 he obtained an *arrêt* to set up a works at Talende in the Auvergne, near Clermont, with investment provided by a La Charité man, Fournier. He was allowed duty-free exports, the right to employ both French and foreign workers, and to have his English wife naturalized. He set up water-powered rolling machinery, drop presses and cutting-out machines, but the partnership was in financial trouble within a year, the two partners quarrelled, and Le Cour proved as difficult and ill behaved as he had been at La Charité. They separated, and the authorities relieved Fournier from his creditors' demands for some years. He was still in business in the late 1770s, but again on the brink of failure.

Le Cour had moved to Lyon, first working as a craftsman for other button-makers, but then setting up his own privileged manufacture in 1764. He was allowed to build all needful machines, rolls, lathes, a drop press and so on, but the fear of contravening the regulations about minting was so acute that he got a separate special permission for a drop press in 1766. Though allowed, it was only permitted on condition of the inspection of his works by the local *Cour des Monnaies*, which was extended to include his stamping-out machine and furnace. Somehow Le Cour changed his spots, and from being an unsociable tearaway became a large and respected manufacturer and employer, making goods 'in imitation of English'. Though he had disputes with the local button-makers guild, he seems to have had a good case. He took large premises in an unoccupied public building and spent heavily equipping them. He brought in a local capitalist, who supplied funds in return for learning the art of manufacture; he himself provided the knowledge for powered machinery, but brought in others for metal preparation, casting and gilding. The Lyons works contained a horse gear with a drive to several floors to work machinery. He employed a number of foreign workers of whom we know nothing except that one was Saxon; he had large military orders for France, Switzerland, Sardinia and Naples. As early as 1772 he claimed to have given Lyons a new industry, for eleven other firms had been set up in imitation of his. This is interestingly paralleled by a statement by De Nogent, the entrepreneur at La Charité in 1782, who reckoned that La Charité had been the origin of an 'infinite number' of firms that followed their methods, but generally, he claimed, by making a cheaper and nastier product than the true 'English hardware'.[34]

Fresnais left La Charité after Le Cour, having investigated Paris, Talende and Saint Etienne as possible sites for his operations. His first works was in Paris, with a partner called Ricard; they split up and a second works was set up at Essone.[35] This may exhaust the works which had a direct connection with Alcock's operations, or were directly or indirectly inspired by his example. But there were other attempts, one certainly big, rash but unsuccessful, which derived from the Birmingham example.

This, the most odd of the firms, is that associated with Charles Emile Gaulard de Saudray. De Saudray had a remarkable career in which his venture into industrial espionage and the 'toy' trade was merely one among many adventurous and bizarre episodes. He was born in Paris in 1740, and seems to have been well connected and well educated. He entered the army when very young and served in the Seven Years War. By 1763 he was secretary to the French Ambassador to St Petersburg. How he acquired them is unclear, as he seems to have been an infantry officer, but he certainly picked up cartographic and engineering skills. While based at Saint Petersburg he was sent to make a survey of the Volga.[36] On his return to France in 1768 he was appointed as 'engineer in chief to the Foreign Office' and put in charge of the map room at Versailles, and then quickly assigned to a survey and demarcation of the French frontier from the coast to the Rhine. But by 1769 he was secretary to the French embassy in Berlin, where he made a study of Prussian light artillery of which he brought back detailed drawings – how far there was military espionage rather than mere intelligence-gathering is not known. For a time, in the absence of the ambassador, he was French resident or representative in Berlin.[37]

Returning from Prussia he resumed military service, but soon was posted as secretary to the London embassy. He claimed to have taken an interest in the industrial activities of the countries he lived in when on foreign service, and in Britain this became an obsession with the

Birmingham trades in their multiplicity and diversity. He believed that successful transfer of these trades to France would need the recruitment of a large number of men with different but complementary skills. What is unclear is how far he was aware of, and appreciative of, the degree of technology transfer which had been already accomplished by Michael Alcock, and by the other firms which had taken their technological lead from La Charité. His long absences from France may have left him ignorant of what was happening at home.

After eighteen months he was diverted from his British interests by a journey to Holland 'for the service of the King' as he cryptically put it, probably a job with an intelligence element. While Ballot says that Trudaine and Turgot backed de Saudray's investigations in England,[38] there seems little doubt that at this time he was primarily working under the Foreign Office, and that Vergennes was a powerful patron. When he returned to England de Saudray again visited Birmingham. He came to the conclusion that the highest manifestation of the Birmingham system was the creation of water-powered factories in which a powered drive was converted to a vertical axle from which gearing enabled horizontal drive shafts to run through several floors of a building, working lathes, small rolls, lathes, polishing and buffing machines and similar devices needing only light power.[39]

By 1777 he had decided that Matthew Boulton's works were the ones to be concentrated on, and that industrial espionage was the one way of obtaining its secrets.[40] Subterfuge was needed

> because over the door of Mr. Boulton is written in gold letters approximately these words "Entry to these works forbidden to all persons whatsoever, because of the problems that have arisen from it". I did enter, taking the greatest precautions; two hours after I made my drawings I was denounced to the British authorities, two of my [suborned] workers were arrested, and I would have been myself if I had not fled England to avoid it.[41]

While de Saudray may have been exaggerating in saying that his life, as well as his liberty, could have been in danger (and his liberty would doubtless have been secured by the French embassy to which he had been specially recommended by Vergennes, either by diplomatic representations or by paying his fine) we have another case where countermeasures do seem to have at least temporarily frustrated industrial espionage and suborning. De Saudray's obsession with the multi-purpose mill did not blind him to other things, he did recognize the importance of the relatively new crucible cast steel invented by Huntsman and its qualitative significance for cutting tool manufacture. However, though he believed he could suborn English workers to make crucible cast steel in France, his ideas about it were muddled (as was common with his countrymen) believing that it was merely melted steel, and that it was produced in a reverberatory furnace. He realized that there was something special about the iron from which it derived, but initially thought that English iron would have to be brought over to France, whereas of course the English used Swedish iron in their steel-making.

As early as 1775 de Saudray formed a plan for setting up a French company to be entitled 'Manufacture Royale à l'imitation de celle de Birmingham' and he approached the Government at the end of that year. He met some of the problems of those seeking permission, support and privilege, not to mention finance, in order to introduce new technology into France. He did not want nobles to be put off from participating by ideas of *dérogeance* (loss of status by taking part in trade) though this concept was declining in significance. He was not deterred, he said, by the general prejudices, and did not believe that an interesting technical discovery could ever become a sign of 'shame and debasement', a view that would have fitted well with the attitudes of Trudaine de Montigny and Turgot. His financial backers would want him to ask for privileges for the proposed company, on the other hand he knew that Trudaine and Turgot would not want to give exclusive rights of manufacture. It took about a year to get round to the application for letters patent, which may show some inefficiency or some carelessness by de Saudray in fitting in with the Government's commercial bureaucracy. But he had already obtained the greater part of the machines, matrices and tools. He had on tap those whose skills could provide a rapid-gilding liquor, make silver plate, enamel on copper, and produce pinchbeck and ormolu goods. There were machines he indicated whose employment had led to the labour needed for polishing steel and other metals being 'incredibly' reduced in Birmingham. By these methods a child could sometimes do in a day as much as four men without the machines, a new adult worker could produce almost perfect work on his first day. De Saudray said he could also obtain steelworkers, though we have shown that he understood crucible steel very imperfectly. However, he petitioned for no exclusive privilege, 'knowing the precious effects of liberty, and totally respecting the very estimable system the Controller-General seems to adopt'.

This did not limit his demands too seriously. He wanted to bring foreign workers over to build and set up machines, and to have them recognized as master workmen, he wanted to have a bounty on some exports. The only satisfactory coal for his steelworks was English, and he wanted to import it duty free. He wanted the King to give him a water-mill site near Paris. English iron for steel-making (as we have seen a mistaken need) should also be imported without duty, the works should be a *manufacture royale* from the outset. For travelling expenses, works site exploration, and bringing over an English master workman and twenty others he asked the 'modest sum' of 10,200 *livres*.[42]

From this point on de Saudray's rather extensive demands ran into grave difficulties from the rapid succession of ministers. Turgot fell from power in 1776 and Trudaine de Montigny was forced into retirement in the following year. However, the new controller-general gave his blessing and a new intendant of commerce began drawing up a very favourable letters patent. But the controller-general died and, as was customary, his successor took a fresh look at the scheme. This put de Saudray in a great difficulty. Thinking the letters as good as granted, he had gone to England to bring over twenty workers and their equipment, while his associates had started development work at Canon-les-Bons-Gens in Normandy, near Falaise. With the business in a terrible tangle, de Saudray got his old boss, the foreign minister Vergennes, to lean on the Bureau of Commerce to speed up the letters patent. Once more the grant was looked at anew; there was to be more subsidy but fewer privileges. But at this point the Intendant of Commerce involved, Fourqueux, resigned and a new intendant took over. This was Tolozan,[43] who eventually became head of the Bureau, a tough character. The letters patent failed to materialize.

The large group of English workers could not face more delays, they had been in France for eight months. At Canon-les-Bons-Gens they found the only optimism was in the place name. It was a spot where 'there was not a building ready for them, where they could not even find needle and thread, and were perpetually shut up in a room so as not to be buried in the mud'. Not unnaturally they set off back to the Birmingham hardware district, and their promises to return if things could be sorted out were probably in many cases not very sincere. They would be further dissuaded because a chief workman was arrested on his return and jailed for a year, presumably for suborning others. De Saudray, undeterred, returned to England to recruit more workers to operate the two consignments of tools and machines which had reached France. Some workers were obtained, but his investors ceased to back him, seeing no hope of continuing, for Tolozan and Necker had decided that Normandy was to be rejected as a site for a works. The plant was too near the coast, so that it might serve as an entry point for contraband English hardware, and Normandy was already too full of manufactures![44]

This adverse decision caused the dissolution of the company despite the pleas of de Saudray, and alternative plans of development which he proposed.[45] De Saudray claimed that he had already suggested to the investors that a site near Paris was preferable, and that he had leased land on an estate of the Duke of Orléans. It was probably here that he had already set up several branches of the Birmingham manufacture, but whether the expensive rolling-mill costing 60,000 *livres* had been erected here is not stated. The policy of the House of Orléans to involve themselves in important industrial ventures, often in conscious rivalry with the patronage of the State, would no doubt have created worries in the minds of de Saudray's investors in any case, and later, in 1782, the Duke of Orléans offered to take over the whole venture in return for making a share allotment to de Saudray.[46]

De Saudray's affairs varied from encouragement to depression in bewildering fashion. He had taken drawings of Boulton's machinery, based on a stay of only two hours in his works, but then set about making a scale model of the multiple-drive water-powered equipment. In so doing he incorporated some simplifications and 'perfections' of his own, but whether they were really improvements is unknown. However his patrons arranged a display of the 'superb model' before Louis XVI in August 1777, a good move in that the king's hobby was ornamental metalwork. The king was highly impressed by the machine, and recommended that the project should be backed to the tune of 250,000 *livres*. Vergennes wrote that he had again made representations to Necker on de Saudray's behalf because of the public interest in the machine and 'the feeling it has created in ... the mind of His Majesty, who has sensed all the advantages which can be obtained from it'.[47] This was all carefully ignored by ministers, but at any rate an official enquiry was activated, with commissioners named by the Academy of Sciences, and not only Vergennes but the Duc de Nivernois showed an interest in its results on de Saudray's behalf.

The commission consisted of prominent members of the Academy: Montigny, Abeille and Macquer, and Montigny, as we have seen, had been a great advocate of the obtaining of English technology since the early 1750s. The commission encouraged the employment of machines like de Saudray's which would assist in meeting English competition based on the 'low price and the perfection which results from the use of machines. These mechanical aids have enabled them to make with precision and few workers, and quickly, what was made before with many workers, in a much longer time, and less perfectly'. De Saudray, however, was offered no exclusive privilege as it would be ruinous to those who had already set up companies to manufacture English hardware. His propositions about steel-making would be examined once he was in a position to produce trial samples of his cast steel and they could then be compared with specimens of the English product. It was made clear that the individual machines his mill would work were already employed at La Charité and Saint Etienne. Moreover Le Cour was using at Lyon almost exactly the same kind of mill that de Saudray proposed, the Birmingham mill with low production costs, the only difference being that it was horse powered.[48] Le Cour's machine similarly worked rolling, boring, turning, stamping, cutting out, smoothing and polishing machinery, and the goods he turned out, including those in polished steel, would be those to be produced by de Saudray.[49] The Government therefore did not give de Saudray the wide group of privileges he asked for, but Necker and Tolozan proposed a 6,000 *livre* reward for his services, a 1,000 *livre* annual pension and the Order of Saint Michel, but none of these was implemented.[50] The death of the controller-general, Clugny, again set back the whole administrative process, though in 1779, 1781, and 1782 Vergennes again intervened on behalf of de Saudray.

For three years he struggled on alone, claiming to have employed up to eighty workers. Then in the early 1780s there was discussion about a take-over of de Saudray's operation by some powerful businessmen, the Orsels. The brothers Antoine and Joseph Orsel came from Lyon.[51] The elder had spent ten years as a merchant and manufacturer in Birmingham, where he had made a fortune. Like Alcock, he claimed to have an interest in a steel manufacture there. There seems no way in which Orsel could have spent ten years in Birmingham without operating in a period of warfare between England and France, while a French merchant importing Birmingham goods into France must inevitably have been breaking some customs regulations, and the Orsels glibly talked of the large amount of English merchandise that came in by way of Ostend.

In 1779 they very grandly informed the Bureau of Commerce of the great wealth of their father, a senior Lyon merchant, worth 1.5 million *livres*, their payment of 24,000 *livres* a year to the State in import duty, and the 40,000 *livres* a year they got from the invested capital derived from their English operation.[52] Now, however, they were setting up Birmingham-type hardware works in France, hoping to be favoured by the State for their work, besides having the satisfaction of being useful to their country, and of making war against the English in their own way.[53] They now operated from several centres, from Amboise where they had sixty workers in 1779, from Paris where they made buttons, and at Raucourt and Lamecourt near Sedan, where they employed child labour in filing and polishing steel objects. In all they had 600 workers. They said their buckles and buckle chapes were as good or better than English, but they had to get round the unfortunate prejudice of the market for English ones. By 1785 they employed over 500 in their manufacture of 'ouvrages d'acier à l'instar des Anglois à Lamecourt près de Sedan' (steel objects as those made by the English at Lamecourt near Sedan),[54] having bought the *seigneurie* of Lamecourt for 100,000 *livres*.

The Orsels offered to buy out de Saudray's defunct company for 60,000 *livres*, direct the firm jointly with him, and set up his water-powered machine. Whereas in 1779 they had wanted the elder brother to be given the cordon of Saint Michel at once, and the younger given it once their operation was running, they now demanded it immediately for both, they claimed an annual turnover of 400,000 *livres*, and talked about opening additional works in Champagne. But if they went in with de Saudray they wanted the existing debts of his firm discharged, and they also asked for letters of nobility for their father.[55] The deal with the Orsels seems to have been on the table when de Saudray renewed his petition to the Government, now in effect to Calonne as controller-general whose love of ambitious industrial projects was becoming known. De Saudray approached him originally on the basis that he would have a powerful merchant backer, unnamed, but seemingly Orsel. However, once Calonne seemed strongly interested in the scheme de Saudray dropped the Orsel connection. He now proposed to make a full-scale machine, to obtain workers from England – who were already on their way – and to develop cast steel production. Though he had proposed this five years ago he would be willing to forget the fact and give all the credit for its introduction to Calonne.[56] However, for trial purposes in producing cast steel he would want to import a certain amount of Newcastle coal and Swedish iron, though he would try to replace these with French coal and iron over time. De Saudray received a bunch of privileges in 1784, some of which seem to have been dependent on his operating the Birmingham mill properly, and at the same time a pension of 2,000 *livres* a year, for which the only condition was the deposit of his machine at the special repository where technologically important devices were exhibited, the Hôtel de Mortagne in Paris, begun by Vaucanson, now supervised by the scientist Vandermonde.[57]

De Saudray valued the pension highly, and because of it he did not get a military pension, though he received the Cross of Saint Louis. However, after only three years the Commerce pension was suspended, when he was again abroad 'on the King's business'.[58] The reasons for its suppression were that his model machine had been evaluated as unable to produce silver plate, or roll and polish steel like those in Birmingham – probably this was the opinion of Vandermonde – and that his Paris works employed few men, and they turned out little. The resulting row over the pension took on enormous proportions and consumed a vast amount of bureaucratic time and paper, its value to us is that it provides a main source for de Saudray's activities. Amusingly he was worried that his pension was in danger now he was turned fifty – he was not to die until the reign of Louis Phillipe! Once again his cause was taken up by his old Foreign Office bosses; after Vergennes's death it was the Duc de Guines, a former London ambassador, who took up the cudgels on his behalf.[59] While he was right in saying that his pension was not conditional on his industrial performance, he would not have had much chance of regaining it in the increasingly chaotic state of administration and politics of the last days of the *ancien régime*. But de Saudray was an important figure in the event which marked its collapse.

De Saudray was appointed second in command of the Paris militia on its formation in July 1789, and within a few days he took a prominent part in the capture of the Bastille, locating, procuring and directing the cannon used by the beseigers. He was wounded saving the life of a senior government official uninvolved in the defence of the fortress. He was honoured by the National Assembly in 1791, given a pension of 1,000 *livres*, and promoted lieutenant-colonel. Bailly, as Mayor of Paris, and Lafayette were prominent in gaining him this recognition. They also gave support (with de Guines) to the restoration of his Commerce pension, and after some bureaucratic dithering and confusion this seems to have been restored.[60]

Like many inventors and technologists de Saudray felt that there had been too great a cleavage between practical men and the scientific establishment under the *ancien régime*, he was much involved in a Société du Point Central des Arts et Métiers which made representations to the National Assembly and the Convention about the examination, registration and reward of new inventions, and this despite his active membership of the official Bureau de Consultation des Arts et Métiers. In 1792 he founded the Lycée des Arts, which would give public courses on scientific subjects, and honour inventors, but also encourage arts and letters. By this time he had inherited a large fortune. He obtained the lease of part of the Palais Royal, formerly the Paris palace of the Dukes of Orléans, and spent 400,000 *livres* on developing facilities for an ambitious college. While many scientific courses were given, de Saudray lectured on economics. In 1798 the buildings, largely wooden, burnt down uninsured, taking his fortune with them. The institution was revived in more modest form in 1802, the name being changed to Athenée des Arts. However de Saudray's sole additional contribution to technology was a fire-ladder. He died forgotten and in poverty in 1832.[61]

De Saudray's effective contribution to the development of English hardware technology in France was not great. He seems to have been operating in England very much as the servant of the French foreign office, though there was a ministerial commission, which must have been from Necker, for the 1777 visit, and earlier ones seem to have been sanctioned by Turgot. There was a continual see-saw in the support of his scheme from changes of controllers-general and of intendants at the Bureau of Commerce, which other innovators introducing foreign technology also experienced, for instance Le Turc.[62] But there is a feeling that many of his difficulties lay in inter-ministerial jealousies between Commerce and Foreign Affairs, and it seems that even so powerful a man as Vergennes could be frustrated in his patronage of de Saudray by the bureaucratic opposition of another ministry. The jealousies came to a peak in the affair of de Saudray's pension. The assiduous support of the Foreign Ministry may have to do with the non-commercial work of de Saudray, and not only in England; if his tasks 'on the King's business' mean as a secret agent, then the Foreign Ministry may have been trying to reward him indirectly for services they were not willing to specify openly.

On the other hand there is evidence that de Saudray was over-excited about the significance of the Boulton mill, he may have regarded it as a telling demonstration of power applied to a group of Birmingham technologies, but there do not seem to have been many such mills in the

Birmingham hardware district, and some of the operations could be carried out in disaggregated fashion, for instance in separate rolling-mills, and by other machines worked by human power. De Saudray seems to have tried to close his eyes to the importance of earlier infusions of English hardware techniques into France since 1756, and their spread beyond the works of the Alcocks, and to the operation of mills much like his own at La Charité and Lyons, though the La Charité mill does seem to have been of limited success and we do not know how many processes were powered by its water-wheel. Le Cour's horse mill at Lyon seems to have been little different in principle from de Saudray's. It is curious that he never advanced the argument of the greater power potential of a good water-mill and the greater number of machines it could potentially drive. Of course the limitations of water-power at Birmingham were the motive for the building of the first Watt engine at Boulton's Soho works. It seems likely that though de Saudray had grasped the general technology of the Birmingham industry he was much less knowledgeable about the detail of the skills of the individual trades. He does not seem to have understood much about the economics of the hardware industry, or its business side. Indeed at times he appears almost to have emphasized his detachment from the business aspect. 'An engineer is not a manufacturer, and when he has done his professional job it is not his fault if he is abandoned.'[63]

He was certainly dedicated in his industrial espionage and suborning of workers, and his activities show how complex and unpredictable the results of these activities were. On the one hand he did get into Boulton's mill and make drawings and recruit workers, on the other he was surprised shortly afterwards and had to get out of the country as quickly as possible, some of his workers being caught. Later he recruited more workers on at least two occasions, apparently in substantial numbers, and got tools out to France, though some of these were held up for a time by Customs. Many workers quickly returned home. However, some were then arrested and one imprisoned. The counter-activities of the British authorities were therefore at least partly successful, the legislation of 1719 to some extent effective.[64]

There is no comprehensive account of the operations of the Orsels, whom we have seen offering at one point to step in and save de Saudray's scheme. The elder, as we have seen, had been ten years in Birmingham as a merchant, and for some of the time at least as a manufacturer, and then returned to set up works to produce English hardware near Sedan, at Amboise, in Paris and in Champagne. The

Sedan operation was a large one. It began in the village of Raucourt but soon moved to Lamecourt, a league from Sedan. The Lamecourt works was one of the most ambitious factories of the age, with very extensive housing for workers, officials and the managers themselves. In 1783 the factory employed 150 workmen and sixty apprentices, paupers from the foundling hospital of Paris and the hospital at Metz. The Paris apprentices were housed and fed, but merely received a sum of 120 *livres* when they had completed their training. There was also a large number of outworkers in the villages of the principality of Sedan, largely employed in cleaning up roughly stamped or cut out goods before they were polished and buffed. A chapel had been built for the workers. The principal production was of English pattern hardware, but of low quality,[65] which was imitated by the extensive use of machines to increase precision and speed. There was a large water-powered rolling-mill, stamps for buttons and buckles, five presses for cutting out, and a particularly large one for buckle chapes, and a water-powered polishing-mill in which sixty children could be employed to polish and buff hardware, with a treadmill to use when water was short. Apart from buttons and buckles a wide range of 'toys' were made. Coal was imported from Liège, high-quality iron from the Duchy of Luxembourg. The works were managed by the younger brother, Joseph. The elder, Antoine, managed the Paris merchanting end, the goods when manufactured were dispatched to him and he determined business policy. In the early 1780s the firm was exporting extensively to Spain and Italy, and maintained travellers there.

However, local officials believed that the Orsels were using the Sedan base as a means of smuggling in English merchandise because of the special privileges of the principality of Sedan in foreign imports and in the passage of local goods into the rest of France. The works did not work at full capacity for long. An observer reporting to the local intendant in 1783 said that local rumour was that the 'manufacture is to a great extent losing its first splendour', and he questioned the size of its workforce; for instance, on the basis of the numbers of the internal workforce he queried the correctness of the supposed number of outworkers.[66] The powered polishing-mill seemed undermanned, many anvils were not being used, the rolling-mill was inactive, and the four forges were deserted. Soon the Orsels were claiming that without help the buckle manufacture would have to be abandoned and that only ten polishers remained at work. In some unspecified way letters of nobility for themselves, the exemption of the workers from the *taille*, and *manufacture royale* status would help. They believed that the low estimations by British manufacturers of the value of their imports under the Eden Treaty allowed them to evade duty and put French competitors out of business. They asked for 10,000 *livres* a year for a devious scheme to get round the problem, but their request was refused.[67]

The Orsels were generally regarded as tricky customers. The Sedan observer quoted above thought it suspicious that the Orsel's operations were inspected by officials of the Metz mint but were allowed to proceed unhindered, while others setting up a rival works were put out of action by having similar machinery stopped and put under seal by the same officials. Their treatment of workers was harsh. When in Birmingham the elder Orsel had introduced a German called Kern to come over to work for him in the inlaying of steel with gold and silver 'but when Orsel had lern'd all he could he wou'd not pay him according to Agreement but played him many dirty tricks' and Kern went to work for Boulton and Fothergill.[68] The sharp practice was continued in France. We know from the Sedan observer that one of the brothers had recently made a journey to England and had probably made contact with Birmingham workers; we also know that another emissary had been sent to Birmingham but, being discovered, the local manufacturers had taken care to exclude him from their works. However two men, Andrew Adam and Ambrose Tibbets were said by the Orsels to have heard of them and came to find them in their premises in Paris. They claimed to be able to make buttons and other articles in English steel. As there were no French workers who knew how to use it, they would work in Antoine's Paris factory and provide the necessary information there. But they needed one further workman who knew how to cast the metal. They could get a man called George Penn from Birmingham, but they had not the money to go back to bring him. Orsel carefully kept Tibbets in Paris and gave Adam the money to go and get Penn, providing letters of credit to Calais and London correspondents. Orsel, even with Tibbets as hostage, was afraid that the other two would take the money and disappear, but they kept their word and Adam and Penn turned up in Paris. Orsel quickly contracted with them and built them a separate workshop in his Paris factory so that they could retain their craft secret. He claimed to have lodged them and fed them and provided them with tools and raw materials, which he claimed, probably excessively, had cost 6,000 *livres* – he had even provided the men with coats, stockings, shirts and shoes! Things were initially going well but then the Englishmen abruptly started to slack off and do little work. He was tipped off that someone was going to suborn them, and reproached them with it, but they disappeared from their accommodation in May 1785.

Orsel determined to have the law on them, and got another manufacturer, who made buttons for the army, to enter the Englishmen's workshop and inventory what they had left behind, while the guild officers sentenced the Englishmen to a fine of 4,000 *livres* to be paid to Orsel. He discovered that the workers had gone off to the Alcocks at Roanne, but his attempt to seize them was frustrated by their appeal (or one by the Alcocks on their behalf) to the Parlement of Paris. Orsel at least wanted all the advances he had made to the Englishmen repaid.

> If the kind of conduct of the Englishmen towards Orsel was tolerated all the manufactures and workshops of France would collapse, for thereby any entrepreneur who was jealous that another had artisans or workmen who would be useful to him would suborn them away from him one after the other.

Most of the workers would only concern themselves that someone was offering them more money, and firms would be ruined and crumble to nothing. Orsel's own agreement with the English workers was written in English, he had paid them what they wanted, and 7.5 per cent more than such workers in England were paid. 'It is certain that if any English workman is able to leave freely whatever his contract, neither Sr. Orsel de Lamecourt nor any one else would take the personal risk of going to look for workers in England'. Orsel labelled Alcock a suborner who had taken advantage of the expenses Orsel had laid out for the workers and the costs of their trial operations in France. The men should be kept in prison until they could be returned to him.[69]

This was not how Joseph Alcock or the English workmen saw it. Alcock said that four young Englishmen had come over to France to sell their skills. When they went to Orsel he profited from their inexperience of the French scene and got them to sign a contract in which they had everything to lose. When they discovered their mistake, they realized they could not possibly fulfil the terms of their contract as Orsel insisted they should. They had then gone to Roanne in the greatest distress to ask work of Alcock. Orsel had them condemned, unheard, by the Paris municipal officials to pay him 6,000 *livres*, and tried to carry off to prison the only one of the four who was well at the time, and had been tending his sick friends. Fortunately a French copy of the agreement between Orsel and the English workers survives.

Adam Tibbet and Payne (the same man whose name in the other document is given as Penn) agreed to make silvered metal buttons for Orsel on condition that he gave them 7.5 per cent more than they would have got in England. Even allowing for the difference in the cost of living and their board this increase would hardly justify men going to work abroad. The money he had advanced them would be progressively deducted from their wages from the beginning of the ensuing year in proportion to their output, they would 'whiten' buttons for 3 shillings a double gross and chains 'à la figaro' (no doubt a current fashion item) for 3s. 4d. a dozen, and other items as required. Their board and lodging would be provided at the rate of £20 a year each. They bound themselves not to work for anyone else in France except Orsel for three years. Orsel made the agreement on the basis that the advance he gave would not exceed £100 sterling (about 2,400 *livres*). This is clearly at variance with the 6,000 *livres* he was demanding from the workers. The Bureau of Commerce refused to intervene, so the workers must have stayed with Alcock.[70]

While their manufacturing activities may not have recovered, for no record of them has been found after the Revolution, the Orsels seem to have continued to be highly prosperous as merchants. One of them appears in two lists of the highest taxpayers in the Paris district (Seine) in 1806 when he was twenty-fifth in the ranking and in 1812 when he was nineteenth.[71]

Contemporary English hardware experts were not unanimous on the number of their workers who would have to be seduced in order to produce an efficient production team in France, and one capable of training a suitable corps of French workers capable of carrying on the trade without continuous English assistance. The 'toy' trade had of course many branches, and much would depend on how wide was the range of goods to be made; some of the extension of the product range was a matter of design, fashion and market widening rather than the acquisition of fundamental new skills. Joseph Alcock's visits to Birmingham in 1777–78 were apparently to acquire knowledge of new developments and products; while he made an additional range of goods in new works on his return there is no indication that he brought new workers. On the design side two of the most important Birmingham manufacturers testified to a Commons Committee that there were drawing schools set up in the town 'for the Instruction of Youth in Designing and Drawing, and 30 or 40 Frenchmen and Germans are constantly employed in Drawing and Designing'. Whether this means that the aesthetic ability of Birmingham masters and artisans was low, or whether they recognized that to penetrate continental markets they needed to fit in with tastes different from their own, would be an interesting subject to explore, but evidence is lacking. In the same Commons Committee the same principal witnesses, John Taylor and Samuel Garbett, emphasized the attempts by foreigners to seduce British workers, and mentioned (though without naming him specifically) Michael Alcock's defection. They believed that 'if Ten of our Workmen were to go to any one place abroad they might raise a Manufactory, from whence they might supply Britain with some of the same Sorts of Toys made by the Petitioners'.[72] The estimate of the number of English workers needed to establish a 'toy' enterprise is probably not much different from the numbers Alcock had as a maximum at La Charité; of course he tried unsuccessfully to get more, but they were seized before they could emigrate.

When the Commons were petitioned in 1760 to prevent the export of buckle chapes Matthew Boulton believed the trade was largely confined to England because of the peculiar qualities of British iron and because 'there are Secrets in the Buckle Trade, which foreigners are Strangers to, which induces him to think that Buckles cannot be made so well abroad as in England', and he was against export. However, with typical inconsistency when his own interest was involved, he later exported chapes to Joseph Alcock at Roanne. Other witnesses to the same petitions said that 'if Foreigners could attain the Knowledge of those Arts, it would destroy their Trade and the Toy Trade in general; and that if Half a Dozen Buckle makers were seduced abroad, they would easily communicate that knowledge'. But John Baskerville, one of the most famous Birmingham men of the time, thought that 'a few Foreigners may be taught to do it, but in general have not the ingenuity'. One chape-maker, Joseph Green, thought that he could 'teach (foreigners) by a letter', but this probably applied to a method he had invented using charcoal as the fuel, and is at complete variance with all the other evidence about the transfer of craft technologies.[73] A French commentator on the La Charité partners' objections to the suborning of English steel toy-makers in the late 1760s,[74] who pointed to the several Birmingham workers needed to make a single article, was nearer to the mark. But if the workers were well chosen, and included men capable of making the machines and machine tools used in many of the 'toy' manufactures, and someone accustomed to supervise a varied group of trades, then a useful collection of articles in the Birmingham repertoire could be manufactured abroad, as Alcock's example shows. Here however, as has just been pointed out, it must be doubted if he had the full team of English workers he ideally required.

There are many instances of firms professedly producing hardware of the Birmingham 'toy' variety in France by the end of the century. In two cases, those of Gerentel and of Terry in Paris[75] we know the former had spent nine years in Birmingham, and that the latter was English, but in many other cases a direct Birmingham link cannot be proved. Daumy set up two successive companies in the 1770s and 1780s in Paris, received a substantial government subvention, and had a fly-press and powered rolls made by the famous engineers, the Périer brothers.[76] Dauffe attracted much favourable attention in the 1780s, being one of those manufacturers given premises by the Government in the old Quinze-Vingts hospital, where he constructed several machine tools, particularly a drop-stamp, which were thought very good. He concentrated on imitations of English polished steel goods, but though supposedly flourishing in 1788, his works seem to have disappeared in the revolutionary period.[77] The Daudiron family claimed to be producing high-quality English hardware, also in Paris. The celebrated mechanician, Merklein, claimed in 1780 to be carrying on a successful works at Clermont in the Auvergne, making English toys and military buttons. Cheret de Montignon had ambitious works at Rouen and Bordeaux in which English type hardware was one product.[78]

The Eden treaty had a considerable adverse effect on some firms, those of the Alcock brothers and the Orsels for instance.[79] To some extent the influence may have been indirect, in that once prohibition (however ineffective) was gone, smuggling, which could be done at an even lower cost than the moderate duty of the treaty, may have rather increased than diminished. While prohibition was renewed in the Year V, it was war rather than the evadable prohibition which protected the French hardware producer. Many of the new French firms were small, they multiplied as those trained at the older centres of the English-type button and other 'toy' trades left to found their own firms. By the Year III there were said to be around a hundred of them.[80] The trade was particularly flourishing in Paris, and by 1797 some of the firms were growing significantly, a few employing over 200 people. Even in the depression of 1810 the trade was active, but despite over half a century of development since English methods were introduced, buttons were falsely stamped to indicate that they came from London dealers, suggesting that there was still some conscious inferiority in quality.[81]

There was no dispute that the large-scale production of cheap decorative metal toys, particularly buttons, whether silver plated, gilded or of polished steel, made by the use of machines and particularly machine tools, had been first introduced to France by Alcock in the 1750s. By the end of the century it was clearly widespread, and the distribution of the technique from the firm he had founded at La Charité, largely through internal disruptions and subsequent defections, and then by imitation and a more natural diffusion, seems clear enough. None of his rivals ever claimed technical priority, which would have been a particularly good argument when seeking privilege or subsidy. There were some other attempts to spy in Birmingham or to take Birmingham workers to France, but one of the most ambitious, that of de Saudray, entirely failed. That of the Orsels flourished in the early 1780s, but their largest works had closed by 1788, and some of their English workers had joined the Alcocks. The main influence in the transfer of the relevant technologies thus was clearly Alcock's. While he was evidently an extraordinarily difficult man to do business with, and almost certain to quarrel with any associates, there can be no doubt that he had real genius in the design and working of machines, and in training other people, even adults with no industrial background, and youngsters. Even those who quarrelled with him later claimed expertise as having been his trainees.

The hardware trade was one where there was a successful transfer of British technology to France, if at a qualitatively lower level than that of the country of origin. While the first transferrer of techniques, Alcock, apparently went to France for his own reasons, and without enticement or inducement, there was subsequently a considerable effort by his own and later firms and entrepreneurs to seduce workers of the Birmingham hardware district to France, sometimes bringing their own tools. The success of these suborning ventures varied greatly, as we have seen, some had elements of the disastrous, others of the ludicrous. When there was a failure to secure all the different workers sought, this almost certainly had an effect on the quality of production, but there were other factors which probably influenced quality. France was very deficient in non-ferrous metals, particularly tin and copper. She was very much behind in the making of large iron castings, which must have given problems in the making of iron rolls, and in their turning. She was equally defective as a steel producer, and did not make cementation steel properly; she produced no cast steel. This would mean that steel for ornamental steel toys would have to be brought in. Cementation steel could be got from England or Germany, cast steel only from England. This would cause additional costs in tools, and often poorer, slower, and more expensive work. Coal was not always available and where there was a supply it was not as cheap (or supplied in the varieties) as that of the Birmingham hardware district. Given all these difficulties, France is to be congratulated on doing so well in adverse circumstances rather than criticized for not fully reaching the excellence of the output of the Birmingham hardware district.

9   Steel

Over most of the eighteenth century France regarded with a jealous eye the superior technology and production of steel in England. However greatly she coveted this technology, and despite considerable efforts to acquire it, the results were nearly negligible until well into the nineteenth century. An account of the rather unsuccessful attempts at technology transfer, including some industrial espionage, has already appeared and will be summarized here.[1]

France herself produced a certain amount of so-called 'natural' steel, well known in continental Europe but only briefly of importance in England, particularly in the late sixteenth century. This process depended on the smelting of certain qualities of high-grade iron ore, in which some manganese was often present. The resulting iron was then heated in a steel forge so as to lose sufficient carbon to become steel, and was finally consolidated and forged under a water-powered hammer. While of varying quality some kinds were regarded as much better than others, particularly that which came from Styria and Carinthia. The English in the early seventeenth century acquired a new method, almost certainly from Germany, that of producing cementation steel. Patented in 1613, the patentees quickly changed from using wood to using coal as fuel, and steel was incorporated into the wide coal-fuel technology which was continually being extended through national industry. Abandoning the original use of a reverberatory furnace, a specialized furnace was substituted in which refractory chests were put in furnaces with conical chimneys, a growing feature of several British coal-using industries. The refractory chests were filled with alternate layers of charcoal and bars of high grade wrought iron. In the early stages haematite iron from the Forest of Dean was used, later the industry came to depend entirely on certain high-quality Swedish wrought iron from the Dannemora region. Tyneside became important by the early eighteenth century, and Birmingham was also a significant centre of production. Sheffield certainly had steel furnaces in the first decade of the eighteenth century, and gradually became the leading centre from mid-century. Cementation or 'blister' steel was much more reliable in quality than natural steel, but its fuel requirements were large, as the firing of one or two chests took many days. By selecting the best of the resulting bars of 'blister' or cementation steel and binding them into faggots, reheating the faggots in a reverberatory or 'air' furnace and then repeatedly hammering and reheating the metal in a forge, 'shear' steel and other higher grades of steel were produced.

While this technology had basically been continental, but altered to the use of coal as the exclusive fuel, the next advance was entirely English. This was the production of the so-called crucible cast steel, invented in the 1740s by the Quaker, Benjamin Huntsman, and being employed by him and others from about 1750. This took cementation steel as the raw material and remelted it with a little bar iron in an elongated clay crucible and in a special furnace. The crucible was placed in a 'hole' furnace deriving its air supply from a cellar below. It was surrounded by hot coke and raised to a very high temperature; the steel remained entirely molten for four to five hours. This gave a steel of very high homogeneity and of a much superior hardness to those previously available, its quality making it excellent for watch and clock-springs, for razors, for edge tools for hand or machine working of metals, and for files. Files were of crucial importance in general metal-working, but particularly in the early development of mechanical engineering.

Though there were small amounts of steel produced in the Nièvre and as one product of the Catalan forges of the Pyrenees, most French steel came from the 'natural' steel forges of the area around Rives in the Dauphiné, which were dependent on the pig iron produced from a few furnaces of the neighbouring Allevard district, which alone was of sufficient quality. Though the main steel-producing area of eighteenth-century France, the Rives area was troubled by varying standards of product and by the incapacity to satisfy the demand of the national market, even for low-quality steel. A great deal of attention was given to it by important government technologists, as has been shown in a pioneering work by the late Pierre Léon.[2] Because it was there, and well established, French efforts tended to be concentrated on its improvement and extension, taking as a model the famed product of the

Austrian industry, and this may account for the limited initial attention given to the cementation method. The effort applied to the 'natural' process was largely futile, and only a 'fer aciéreux' (steely iron) resulted.

But the interest of the French in acquiring a good quality steel production, however it was thwarted, was intense and continuous. As the eighteenth century wore on, interest in the cementation and cast steel process as practised in England tended to increase. Curiously steel for arms is little emphasized before the Revolutionary period, steel for files is heavily concentrated on. The need for tool steel was such that its entry into France from Germany and to a lesser extent from England was not resisted, indeed a good deal of steel must have entered as tools, especially files, and at moderate duties.

A large number of attempts were made by French technologists to try to produce a good native steel. Only a few names are recorded but there is a statement from the great scientist Réaumur in a famous work of 1722:

> Particularly for the last three or four years ... Frenchmen and foreigners of every nation ... presented themselves [to the Court] claiming to have the true secret of changing iron into steel. But as we have seen no fruits of their operations ... one has virtually come to regard as searchers after the philosophers' stone those who undertake to change the irons of the kingdom to excellent steel.

Yet production in Germany, England and Italy showed that good steel could be made in quantity. If need be, he thought, the French, like the English, could use Swedish iron as the raw material. His own trials, beginning in 1715 and soon heavily subsidized, were in fact a failure, though much of his experimental work was good by contemporary standards and there were some notable gains in expertise. The large works he organized at Cosne were a disastrous venture, one problem being the use of French iron. But it was difficult for Réaumur in this works under the Regent's patronage (La Manufacture Royale d'Orléans pour Convertiree Le Fer en Acier) to reject a plentiful French raw material for a foreign import, especially when some of it was regarded as being iron of high quality when used for conventional purposes, and when contemporary chemistry could not isolate the critical differences.[3]

After Réaumur there was a steady procession of French and foreigners who claimed to have available techniques which would transform iron into steel; by the 1760s there was an increasing emphasis on emulating English steel, and crucible cast steel was now mentioned along with cementation. For some years Alcock's attempts at steel-making aroused much interest. He claimed to have had a share in one of the Birmingham steel making works, and to be able to bring over workers. In some of his early bids for support he also claimed to be able to make edge tools. Closely associated with this was his possession of an invention of a file-cutting machine, files being one of the most desirable steel products and France being notoriously defective here.

In the early 1760s, as we have seen, Alcock was trying to get away from investors he detested at his La Charité hardware works, and he emphasized his schemes for making steel as a main reason for his being allowed to go off and start a separate firm. When he moved to Roanne the hardware side of this new works was put in his sons' names, and they subsequently took over the direction. However, Alcock carried on steel experiments there, which continued some he had been carrying on in the La Charité neighbourhood as far back as 1759. Even in the first trials a problem surfaced which was to be a long-term one in attempts to develop English-type steel-making in France, the difficulty in getting fireclay good enough for the cementation chests. Alcock's talk of fluxes of sulphur, salt etc. at this time was probably an attempt to mislead the associates he mistrusted at La Charité, for he must have known that they were not used in England, though frequently employed by experimenters in France. If he could produce good steel then his file-making scheme could be revived, for he had early recognized that this was the main lack at Saint Etienne 'where coals are cheap as can be wished and very good workmen as there is in England [unlike at La Charité] who stand in need of nothing but Good Steel, and the English manner of finishing their work'. He thought he could quickly instruct them so 'France will never have occasion to Draw a single file, Either from England, Germany or Elsewhere in twelve months at furthest from when I begin it.'

While looking for the site of his new steelworks Alcock tried to explain to Trudaine the problems with the existing French product.

> It is true that among the quantity made one can choose some pieces which are passable and proper to make razors, cutlery etc., but the goodness of steel consists of it being of one even quality throughout the bar and having a body equally resistant throughout to other hard bodies; this one cannot find in the steels made in this country, and this not astonishing, for even if you break up bars of Berry iron, where the iron is held to be the best, or as good as there is in the kingdom, it is hard to find a [bar] which is the same quality throughout; quite on the contrary, one will very often find, even in the same fracture, two or

three different kinds of iron; how then is it possible to make good steel out of it?

There was, he said, nothing easier than to make steel, but nothing more difficult than to make good steel 'and there is none at present made in the kingdom at least among all I have seen or heard of'.[4]

While the final outcome is clear enough, some of the detail of Alcock's steel operation is confusing. He demanded wide privileges in 1767, and with his customary division of effort he was trying to develop a manufacture of heat-resisting earthenware at the same time as making steel. The steelworks was at Guegnon, not far from Roanne. The furnace went out of control on one occasion and some buildings were burnt down. He had to work unprotected in bad weather and fell ill, remaining so for almost a year. But late in 1769 he did produce some cementation steel, enough to have it tested at Saint Etienne by skilled workers who reported on it enthusiastically, and then more was tested at Paris with equal approval. All seemed well, and Alcock was urged by the Government to move on to imitate English cast steel 'which is suitable for fine goods'. Alcock described the cementation steel as having been made by his sons, possibly because he had initially been required to found the Roanne works under their names rather than his own. Some of the steel sent to Saint Etienne was to be made into files 'according to the pattern and cut of those of England', and into German-type saws. While he had earlier cautiously written 'You may naturally imagine that in the first days I cannot make the goods as perfect as I will do later', things for the moment seemed to be going well, and Alcock wrote to Trudaine de Montigny that his letter of congratulation 'has given me more satisfaction than I ever received because I see there that I have fulfilled his aims as well as the Council's for blister steel made from French pig iron'.[5]

But Alcock was in the same trap as others, able to make some small batches or selections of good steel, but not able to make it in quantity or with regularity. As the technical problems persisted he fell out with his financial supporters. The problems were just too great. There were once more difficulties in getting good refractory clay for cementation chests. He was trying to use French bar iron for conversion to steel when only Swedish would have given him the best, consistent results. He was using wood instead of coal as fuel, perhaps because the forge site owned by his associates was valuable only in terms of a superabundance of otherwise unmarketable wood. While he clung to the favourable reports which experts had made on his steel specimens his associates dismissed the workers and closed the plant. There was a further flurry in 1770 when there were plans for a steelworks at Dijoing on the Loire on the lands of the Marquis d'Equilly, but Trudaine corresponded with the marquis in discouraging terms, doubting if any product would be able to compete with the English article, and nothing seems to have been effectively launched. About Michael Alcock senior there is nothing known until his death in Paris was reported in the Birmingham press fifteen years later.[6] Perhaps he was running a warehouse in the capital for his sons, or just living on the 2,000 *livres* he was paid as a pension from the Roanne business; he is not referred to in correspondence from Roanne. There is a tantalizing mention of a steelworks his sons were attempting to set up at Moulins in 1790, but the rest is silence, there is no mention of them among the host of men who launched steelworks with the encouragement of the Revolutionary government in the early and mid-1790s.[7]

In the 1760s an additional inducement to the French to produce steel of good quality was the current rage for a new Birmingham fashion, that of fancy goods (particularly buckles), made in highly polished, often facetted, steel. Trudaine approached the French ambassador in London, de Guerchy, about the possibility of acquiring this skill. De Guerchy asked for more detail about the kind of Birmingham workers who should be suborned. There was a possible short-term solution based on the purchase of English steel to be fashioned and polished in France. There was also much to be said for obtaining the skill of making the steel itself, and de Guerchy was assured that if good reliable workers could be procured they would have their travel expenses paid, be installed at La Charité or Saint Etienne so as to earn their living, and would be well recompensed if their work was successful. They could be given the examples of Holker and Badger who had given important services to the French state. The way they had been looked after was an assurance to others who considered emigrating to France. While the link cannot be clearly made in the archives, the subsequent attempts by de Saudray to obtain both the plan of a Birmingham mill in which mechanical polishing was done and the method of English cast steel-making seems to be a natural continuation or a result of this earlier proposal for suborning, and de Guerchy was a later supporter of de Saudray in his appeals for justice over a pension for his services.

In the short term, however, the directors of La Charité poured cold water over the usefulness of the Trudaine–de Guerchy operation when asked to comment on it. In some respects this was a rational view. They were right to suggest that there was no native iron in France suitable for steel-making, and that English steel was made not only solely from Swedish iron, but from that of a few specialist Swedish forges for the output of which English firms had forward contracts. We can also understand their argument that English workers had been a serious problem, 'mauvais sujets' (a bad lot) at La Charité with the exception of Adam Tinsley. 'It is always to be presumed that when a man expatriates himself, partly by being suborned, he is, or will soon become, a bad lot.' Sanche and Hyde, the current directors of La Charité, had been keen to drive out Alcock and all those loyal to him, in order to gain management of the enterprise. The irony of their depreciating the possibility of steel production in France lay in the fact that they were later to launch a vast concern to do just that, in conscious rivalry with the English.[8]

The La Charité view did not go unchallenged. A commentator said that since there were steelworks in different English regions it was to be doubted if there was a formal contract by all of them in concert to buy all suitable Swedish steel, and there were independent iron and steel merchants selling Swedish iron. The writer (just possibly the scientist Montigny) knew some of the trade marks on the Swedish irons appropriate for steel-making. He knew too that the manufacture of decorative steel toys in England was highly subdivided into different workshops, so that 'it is very rare to find in any of these workshops a worker who can make a complete article, even for example a [steel] watch chain'. It was perhaps better to get a manager or an entrepreneur, but only one who had failed in business, or one persecuted for religion would be likely to come. Alcock may have been the example in mind in the first case. Even when well informed in some respects, there were often misconceptions in the minds of contemporary Frenchmen about England, like the idea of continuing Catholic persecution, perhaps derived from the recruitment of the group of Lancashire Catholics by Holker in the 1750s. In the same letter there is one of the very common French overestimates of the industrial significance of the Society of Arts.[9]

The mid-1760s was a time of particular interest in the English steel industry by the French government. Clearly all the efforts were not completely synchronized and co-ordinated, for about the time of the Trudaine–de Guerchy correspondence an outstanding metallurgist, Gabriel Jars, was sent to England with investigation of the steel industry as part of his remit. The main account of his mission is given later

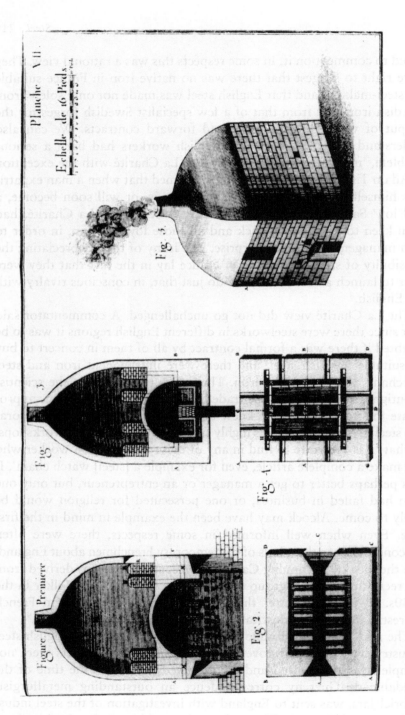

9.1 English cementation steel furnace drawn by Gabriel Jars, 1765

(Chapter 10). For present purposes it will suffice to say that polishing methods and file-making were to be looked into, and he was not merely to observe but to spy where necessary. He investigated cementation steel-making and file-making in the north-east and both cementation and cast steel-making in Sheffield. His report was detailed and illustrated by drawings. On his return to France he made small-scale trials of cementation steel production in Paris. He claimed that these were successful, but there was no full-scale follow up. Later he advised an arms-maker of Klingenthal on the possibilities of the cementation process and showed the firm his drawing of the English furnaces. He also tried melting steel in a crucible, though whether this was an attempt to make real crucible cast steel is unclear. He died young in 1769, and as a man with great practical experience of metallurgy and mining and a wide knowledge of European metal industries, was probably best placed to have improved the French steel industry.[10]

Between Jars's death and the Revolution there were continual attempts to improve French steel, and the methods employed were often said to be English, though we do not have much specific detail of them. The academicians Macquer and Montigny reported on steel made at a forge of the Comte de Broglie, by a process said to have been brought from England. The trials were supervised by Duhamel, the former colleague and travelling companion of Jars. In the 1770s a Franche-Comté experimenter asked for state help; he wanted to employ a foreigner of unspecified nationality, alluded to the great number of attempts to improve steel throughout France, and submitted a memoir on English steels. Duhamel reappeared at the Montbard ironworks of the great naturalist Buffon in 1774 (a works now splendidly restored as an industrial museum) and continued his endeavours to make steel, but despite his being given a healthy salary to spread steel-making methods, which was paid for several years, his methods had more promise than success. There are some important but eventually unsuccessful attempts at steel production which were at least inspired by the English example, but where there is no evidence of the recruitment of English technologists. The Chevalier Grignon, a former ironmaster and author of some treatises on the industry, was employed by the Government as a technical expert from 1773. In 1778 he petitioned the Government to set up an inspectorate (*des bouches à feu*) (for furnace industries) to look into fuel use and economy and particularly a shift to coal-using processes. A small inspectorate was established and had one or two distinguished members, for instance Faujas de Saint-Fond and de

Dietrich, as well as Grignon. Grignon conducted an enquiry into the iron industry in 1773–74 and in 1778 made a detailed enquiry into the steel industry in Dauphiné, heavily criticized for a decline in quality and quantity which particularly affected Saint Etienne. The Rives steel forgemasters in turn blamed the Allevard furnace owners and the quality of their pig. Grignon made a disastrous attempt to build a furnace of new design at Allevard. He experimented with steel-making, diversifying Dauphiné methods by Styrian ones. It might be possible, he concluded, to produce an English quality of steel by cementation methods, and at one point sent for coal for trials. The interest of his reports as an example of a knowledgeable technologist of the period giving opinions and devising experiments is great, the results negligible. He had been more successful earlier at a steel-making establishment he directed based at Néronville and Souppes, but these works only did well as long as Swedish iron was used. After his Dauphiné failure, he returned to experiment there, and also at the Buffon works.[11]

We have seen that de Saudray had plans to assist his Birmingham hardware production schemes by acquiring cast steel production also, that he eventually recognized the need for Swedish iron as a basis, and that he was concerned to bring in English steelworkers and even English coal for the purpose. It is not entirely clear whether he understood the relationship between the cementation and cast steel processes, or whether he thought cast steel was just cementation steel raised to melting point. Another steel projector who pressed his claims as long as de Saudray did was de la Place. His target was steel as good as English, claiming that 'hardware manufacturers, clock-makers, jewellers, cutlers, armourers only employ English steel, others are only used by the serruriers [literally locksmiths, but covers light metal-working generally] and for coarse work'. Once again we are told that his steel, like that of others, had been tried at Buffon's works, and that it was as good as English. He sacrificed time, energy and fortune to steel-making, 'one of the most important of secrets to the state'. Like other frustrated inventors at the end of the *ancien régime* he felt that the Academicians Vandermonde and Berthollet had reported unfairly on his steel, which practical artisans had said was as good as English. He had in Vandermonde and Berthollet two of the celebrated trio of scientists (the other being Monge) who announced to the world in 1786 that the difference between cast iron, wrought iron and steel was in carbon content. While his commission of inspection could hardly have been more eminent, de la Place, approaching paranoia, believed they were involved in a rival venture to produce steel. Though English steel was very much his target there is no indication of his trying to bring in English workmen.[12]

This seems also to be the case with Sanche and Hyde, who, after helping to get rid of Alcock at the La Charité hardware works, had supplanted him only to be sacked themselves in 1771, after which they had gone on to set up a similar works at Amboise during 1771–72. This seems to have performed disappointingly. There is no indication that steel production was a part of their original intentions at Amboise. What may have diverted the attention of Sanche and Hyde to steel was the efforts made by others at Amboise to make good files. The principal figure was Vaucher, who becomes prominent in the late 1770s in the exploitation of a file-making machine. He obtained a privilege and bounty in 1778. Another group, the Tricard brothers and Laa (the latter was German), were also involved. Vaucher lost his financial backer and sold out his business to Sanche and Hyde, very cheaply, in 1782. Over the next few years it is Sanche who seems to dominate the concern, and provides a stream of clever propaganda directed both regionally and nationally.

He emphasized that steel and files were products where government 'has had the mortification of spending great sums without achieving the goal of establishing manufacture', and recited the already long list of those whom it had fruitlessly supported. The large capital outlay on the Amboise hardware business initially limited their embarking on steel production, but in 1784 they got a fifteen-year privilege for a *manufacture royale d'aciers fins* to produce fine steel, files, coach-springs, cutting tools and steel hardware with an annual subsidy of 20,000 *livres*. Their steel was in the same year being tested locally and by a notable expert, Rosa, at the Hôtel de Mortagne in Paris. The concern built a large number of furnaces and forges, and eventually had a capital of 2 million *livres*. There were snags, however. While continually promising that English crucible cast steel would be soon in production, there is little evidence that it was ever produced except on a trial scale.

To some extent Calonne and his subordinates were captivated by Sanche's propaganda, to some extent they retained some scepticism, and this meant that they tried to test the entrepreneurs' claims by a series of powerful expert tests in which the conditions were specified with increasing vigour. Scientists as eminent as Berthollet and Vandermonde, technologists as eminent as de Dietrich (whose family were great ironmasters), trade experts as eminent as Tolozan, head of the Bureau of Commerce, went off to inspect Amboise. Dietrich was so favourable that the Government carefully advertised Sanche's product throughout the country. On the other hand the company had to admit that it was deferring cast steel production because of the lack of good crucibles; there were problems when it tried to get French wrought iron good enough to supplant Swedish as the raw material for cementation steel. Like Alcock in the Charolais nearly twenty years earlier they were trying to operate cementation furnaces with wood, not coal. There is no doubt that what Sanche and Co. were trying to do was to emulate the English; symbolically a money prize with an engraving of the king was offered 'to the worker who has most closely approached [the standard of] the English workers'. On the eve of the Revolution the reports on the Amboise steelworks began to show serious weaknesses, and Gille indicates that it was in a state of collapse in 1789, though Sanche still claimed to be producing some hardware (buttons) and some steel in the year II and once more dangled hopes of cast steel. The works was revived for file-making, but not steel-making, in the next decade. Sanche, it may be suspected, was one of those creators of bubble concerns who even deceive themselves. But the creation of this vast, highly capitalized, concern and the administrative, scientific and technological attention that was paid to it is testimony to the extent to which the French desired to have a native steel industry. Sanche, who had done so much to eliminate the English workers at La Charité, seems to have deluded himself that results of English quality in the steel industry could be gained without any significant transfusion of human skills from across the Channel, and without those materials – Swedish iron, good coal and excellent fireclay – that the English recognized as essential.[13]

While Amboise could be regarded as a typically overblown industrial scheme of the Calonne era, the interest in steel did not diminish with his fall from power. When a special meeting was held under de Brienne's chairmanship in 1788 to discuss industrial priorities it was stated that among existing industries those to make steel and those concerned with spinning were the ones which had been singled out for attention.

> With respect to steel, there was, and there still is, the received opinion that one cannot make it in France like they do in England, nor even in Germany, and in fact it has to be agreed that up to now we have not succeeded in making cast steel which is absolutely essential when highly polished products are required, no other steel will do for the

purpose, and we have always been dependent on the English for this material.[14]

Berthollet, who was making some of the last enquiries into Amboise, was commissioned to draw up a treatise to set out all the known processes for converting iron to steel and thus save the Government from all the bother which had arisen from those who falsely claimed to have new and secret processes.

Interest in steel-making was thus intense at government level at the last gasp of the *ancien régime*. It was stimulated after the Revolution when France found herself at war with the major European powers, one problem being that German steel supplies were cut off, and this by the closure of the same frontiers across which English steel had formerly clandestinely entered by a circuitous route. As usual with revolutionaries, those newly in power wrote and acted as if they were the first to make an attack on the steel problem. The desperate war situation of course gave urgency and intensity to their efforts but, in making an appeal to the scientists to answer the problem, they were often calling upon the same men who had given serious attention to the issue before the Revolution. Berthollet, Vandermonde and Monge, who had so successfully discovered the carbon content distinction in the ferrous metals, now produced an official handbook for ironworkers on how to produce steel. But whatever their scientific expertise, they had to fall back on Jar's reports of nearly thirty years before on English cementation and crucible steel-making at Newcastle and Sheffield.

The technical experts and manufacturers turned to, or offering their services, were largely the same who had been active under the *ancien régime*, and their results do not seem to have been much better, though enough steel of high price and often low quality was produced to see the military emergency over. Given the war, the number of English workers to be recruited was small, though some prisoners of war, English and German, were found, and when the Palatinate was occupied men were recruited there. The English industrialist, Edward Chamberlain, already involved in chemical manufacture in Normandy before the Revolution, claimed to have made some steel but needed more workmen and material to make a real contribution. Another works in Normandy, belonging to Lenormant, was among the more successful, and had English workers in charge of cementation steel production and file-making, though we have no knowledge of how they were recruited. Some cast steel had been made, but only enough for works purposes. Hassenfratz, a scientist and mines inspector who reported on their cast steel attempts, mistakenly suspected that a flux had been added to make cast steel. He reported that Lenormant's great problem was with making crucibles good enough to resist the molten steel. Of course the craft of crucible-making, with the use of high-quality fireclay (usually that of Stourbridge), and ground-down old crucible, with a long treading-out of wet clay before use, and a long and meticulous drying out of the finished crucible, was quite critical to English success. Even so, English crucibles rarely survived more than three firings. Hassenfratz was on the right lines in saying 'Crucibles are the soul of [cast] steelmaking, and it would seem that it is in this part of the business that we are behind hand. All the people concerned to produce cast steel have concentrated research on the flux ... and all have failed to concentrate on the crucibles'.[15]

The emergency ended once the Revolutionary armies had opened the way into Germany. Foreign, and particularly German, steel poured into France, and the Government, with total pragmatism and some cynicism abandoned its favour and financial support for those French works which had endeavoured to assist it by rising to the previous emergency. The civilian consumer, too, had a long-standing and justified preference for the foreign product. At the end of the Revolutionary and Napoleonic wars the French situation was still the same. In 1814 a short-lived Commission pour le Perfectionment des Aciers was set up testifying to the unsatisfied need for steels of English quality, but political changes prevented progress. In 1815 Pickford, who had been in France before and during the Revolution to introduce and develop textile machinery, returned and soon promised to send his wife back to Sheffield to recruit men from Huntsman's works, but though the authorities were favourable to the plan no result is recorded [below, p. 382]. It was only with the arrival of the Jacksons from Birmingham in the same year that the English cementation and crucible processes were finally acclimatized on French soil, though even then they had a long struggle before their operations were fully consolidated.

Why did the transfer of English steel methods to France take so long, despite the continuous and keen interest in them? There was the competitive attraction of natural steel production rather than that of cementation steel; it was already being made in Dauphiné and only an increase in quantity and some greater consistency in quality was apparently needed. It took a long time to appreciate that the critical supply of suitable iron ores for the iron needed for conversion to natural steel could not be expanded. The one change that may have carried some element of qualitative improvement, the Moiroud process, which claimed to save time and charcoal and aimed at achieving something like the Styrian quality, got government attention and technological and financial support. It became one of the hothouse projects of the Calonne era, and later was involved in the speculative schemes of the new Duc d'Orléans. Highly capitalized, it became mismanaged and largely collapsed, though Moiroud continued in business until his death in 1802. Ultimately then, the English solution was the real one.

Another disincentive to its adoption was its invariable use of Swedish wrought iron as its raw material. Even when French industrialists and technologists recognized its virtues, they did so in a provisional way, being prepared to use Swedish iron only in the short term until they could identify an equivalent French iron. Surely there must be an iron from one of the main French iron-making provinces which could be substituted for the foreign material? New steel ventures nearly always approached the State for privileges and commonly for subsidy. It was hard to ask for favours on the one hand and to make it plain that a foreign raw material would be imported on the other, especially when there was no reason explicable in terms of contemporary science to justify the unique properties of the foreign product. The cost of the import would also diminish the arguments for saving foreign exchange by producing enough steel in France.

There may have been penalties for France in the very heavy reliance that was put on scientists, or technologists with scientific pretensions like Grignon. This ran through the eighteenth century, from the efforts of Réaumur after about 1715 to the summoning of the savants to the aid of the Revolution and the State in the 1790s. As Gille says, 'of all the production processes which the scientists of the eighteenth century attempted to improve, that of steel was certainly the most widely studied'.[16] Perhaps the great reputation of Réaumur, despite his practical failure, established a powerful precedent. What may have appeared to contemporaries a matter of the transmutation of metals could have seemed a problem best solved in a laboratory.

There may be some truth in a later view that the limited scientific knowledge of the period meant that the testing by scientists of steel produced by French technologists was very erroneous and misleading, and led to grossly optimistic assessments of the product and the giving of wasteful rewards and subsidies to the undeserving.[17] The real scientific breakthrough of Monge, Vandermonde and Berthollet in 1786 may itself have been a misleading incentive to make industrial progress depend on more scientific investigation, for it had no useful technological spin-off. When appealed to in the 1790s they could only produce the 'Avis aux ouvriers en fer sur la fabrication de l'acier' (Notice to iron workers on the production of steel) (AN II). As a contemporary complained it was incomprehensible except to those who already knew how to make steel, while lacking in essential technological detail. The authors admitted they could not advise on how to manage the furnaces or where to go for crucible-making skills.

The apparently powerful array of scientific skills addressed to the steel-making conundrum may have diminished French interest in gaining the relevant technology by the suborning of workers. While Jars discovered a good deal in his British visit of 1765, he would not on an extended trip have wished to put the whole enterprise at risk by being arrested, or forced to flee, for suborning. Spying was part of his brief, suborning was not. Moreover, while in the end the solution was to take skilled workers to France, the need to take a full team, and exactly whom the team should consist of, were problems. It was only by the long experience of failure that the French were convinced of the critical importance of crucible manufacture in cast steel. Many of the difficulties stemmed from the lack of a wide coal-fuel technology in France. There was a need to select coal of the required quality, and, for cast steel production, the need to produce a good coke, a skill Jars saw the importance of, but which was still being wrestled with long after his death. Indeed France was not well endowed with good coking coals.

In the case of steel, furnace building was a very important skill, requiring good quality fireclay for firebrick. A very high quality fireclay for crucibles was essential. The material of the refractory chests for the cementation process was important, and for both processes furnaces had been designed which did not have existing parallels in France. Important as craft skill was in many British industries, it was absolutely essential in steel-making; as late as the 1840s a famous French observer said that in the Sheffield steel industry the skilled workers were still the true metallurgists of Yorkshire.[18] It would have been difficult to suborn well-paid workers whose skills were in high demand; they would also know perfectly well that unless the suborner recruited a full team of interdependent craftsmen he would have no chance of success, and it would be pointless to contract themselves to work abroad otherwise. It was only when the Jacksons took a full team to France in 1815 that a breakthrough began to be made. There was a disadvantage in the French failure to acquire a good steel technology which has not been often enough stressed. Poor quality steel meant poorer and expensive, slower working in all trades which needed good edge tools and good files. Before the extensive use of machine tools, hand tool quality was of great importance, but the humble hand tool has not received enough attention even from historians of technology and, with some mainly agricultural exceptions, has been overlooked by economic historians.[19]

10   The Metallurgical Traveller

Gabriel Jars, whom we have already met in relation to French interest in English steel processes, was a devoted servant of the French state, and one held in the highest regard by his compatriots, whether ministers, scientists, industrialists, or fellow inspectors. He acquired an extremely wide knowledge of European mining, smelting and metal manufactures, and his expertise was certainly unrivalled in France and was perhaps only approached by some of the leading experts who carried out international surveys for the Swedish mining administration. There is no doubt that he understood the nature and significance of the changes which had taken place in mining and metallurgy in Britain, and that he made important steps in encouraging and supervising trials of British methods, and in identifying raw material deposits and sites which were to be critical in pioneering those methods in France. His sudden and early death, however, means that we are left unsure whether he himself could have master-minded the key changes in the metal industries, particularly iron. In steel there is evidence that his own attempts to copy English procedures did not succeed, in iron he worked with several men who carried on the momentum of innovation on a large scale after his death, though their success was not perfect. All this has to be related to his extensive travels in Britain, and the question of how far they constituted industrial espionage.

Jars was born in 1732, his father being involved in some of France's few copper mines and smelters at Chessy [Cheissy] and Saint-Bel in the Lyonnais.[1] Educated at the Grand Collège de Lyon, Jars, like his two elder brothers, was trained in his father's mines. Once involved with the mines young Jars became a fanatic, spending very long periods underground, risking safety and health. His intelligence and hard work were brought to the attention of the Marquis de Vallière who recommended him strongly to Trudaine. The minister gave him a place in his new Ecole des Ponts et Chaussées, then perhaps the best centre of technical education not merely in France, but in Europe. While Jars arrived in Paris in 1751, aged nineteen, to pursue his studies at the Ecole a good deal of his training was not in an academy, but in the field. Within months according to Gillispie,[2] he was sent off to examine and report on Brittany lead mines and shortly after to mines in Alsace. In 1753 he was sent to the German engineer and mine inspector Konig at the Poulaouen lead mines in Brittany, Konig being one of the few experts on underground surveying in France, where this 'géometrie souterraine' was much desired, and the expertise of British and German mine experts much envied. Trudaine had arranged an annual fee for Konig for teaching the pupils sent to him. Konig's account of the instruction he gave covered many aspects of mining as well as smelting, casting and refining metals 'which we can undertake here using both the English and the German systems'.[3] He told Trudaine that he hoped all those who were sent to him would have 'just as much interest and teachableness as Sr. Jars has shown up to now', clearly the star pupil.[4] He was, as his brother recounted (largely repeating the Eloge of the Academy of Sciences after his early death) 'a kind of Pupil of the State', a member of a new technological species. After his training he returned to home territory and installed for the mines of Saint Bel and Chessy a large copper-refining furnace which saved the entrepreneurs much money, and other furnaces which were still working successfully after his death. He later installed a water-powered hammer there. Jars thus proved himself not just a savant and a theorist, but a man capable of practical success.

He was not left to concentrate his energies on the family copper concerns. He was next based in Paris, but soon sent on a tour of mines in the Forez, the Pyrenees and the Vosges, with another young Ponts-et-Chausées trained engineer, Duhamel.[5] Very quickly they were dispatched on another expedition, this time outside France, to Saxony, Austria, Bohemia, Hungary, Tyrol, Carinthia and Styria. The importance of travels to survey the progress of mining abroad was very much the concept of Trudaine, who had been in charge of mining policy since the early 1740s and had introduced the important mining legislation of 1744. The detail of the surveys to be made was worked out with the Academician Jean Hellot, whom we have already met with[6] who had a particular commission from the Government for investigation of coal-mines (as well as being inspector-general of dye stuffs) and had translated (with amendments) the famous German work on furnaces by Schlutter.[7]

While Trudaine was keen to train mining and metallurgical experts, giving them a good knowledge of chemistry and the relevant parts of physics, he was 'convinced that theory is only a fruitless operation without knowledge of practice, he cast his eye further; the same spirit which drove him to make scientists [philosophers] travel abroad to determine the external shape of the world', convinced him that only experience of foreign practice could train men to extract and work metals. The draft for the basic instructions to Jars and Duhamel survives.[8] They were first to go to Dresden where the Elector (also King of Poland) was friendly and to whom they would carry letters of recommendation. At the mining school of Freiburg they would first study German, as they would not learn anything until at least they understood 'the German idiom of the miners'. Hellot understandably not only wanted copper, copper/sulpher, and lead mines investigated, but the various materials and minerals which would give dyestuffs. They would keep a daily journal of places visited and submit a substantial monthly report. Even though they were visiting a friendly power there were some cases where secret agreements could be made – with suitable caution and explicit approval from their superiors. While tips or bribes would need to be given to the superintendants of workshops and chief workers 'to make sure that they would hide nothing', they were to keep these expenses down. Both in food and transport they were to exercise the greatest economy.[9] The later instructions for travel in Britain were already clearly anticipated here.

After these travels Jars, like so many scientific contempories, launched a campaign to attract the attention of the Academy of Sciences. He read several papers which led to him being received as a Correspondent in 1761, and also as an Associate of the Academy of Lyon. Such steps were essential to a career in the top levels of government scientific and technological service. After some time on home territory inspecting the Saint Bel and Chessy mines he was sent for a year to Franche-Comté to prospect for coal, a search which inevitably brought little return. Hardly had he completed the mission before he was given new orders for abroad by Trudaine.

This time he was to go to Britain, and Duhamel was supposed to accompany him, but in the event he backed out and Jars went alone. Now, as was again to be the case after the American War of Independence, there was a particular importance in seeing how far English industry had advanced during the war years. His instructions[10] are again very important: they convey an impression of existing knowledge in France of English technical advances, of the areas of ignorance, and the subjects on which the French government felt that information would be crucial. The main instructions, though supplemented by advice from other consultants, were once again from Hellot, now at the end of a long life in government service. It will be recalled that Ticquet's observations on the coal-based technology of England had been addressed to him in 1738.[11]

Jars's expedition was to appear scientific and educational, and his status as Correspondent of the Academy was to be emphasized.[12] He would get his main instructions after presenting himself to de Guerchy, the ambassador in London. Once there, as in the German expedition, he would take lodgings for three months in a house where no French was spoken. Eventually he seems to have made this preparatory stay near Newcastle, before his painstaking examination of that coalfield. One wonders whether he later hampered his conversations with the people of other regions of Britain by a 'Geordie' accent! The importance of effective verbal communication was emphasized by his brother when editing his papers: 'all the more necessary because he mainly had to deal with people with a defective understanding of their own language, and particularly with their kind of jargon more difficult to comprehend than the language itself'.[13]

His first target then, was to be the mines of Newcastle and lowland Scotland. He was to see what regulations existed for these mines. The French, given their own regulated system and their vague awareness of surviving regulations for British areas like the Derbyshire lead-mining district and the Forest of Dean, and of the existence of Cornish Stannary law, found it hard to comprehend the almost total freedom in other areas of Britain, especially the complete freedom of coal-mining, once royalties were satisfied. Were British mines run by entrepreneurs, and were royalty and other disputes settled by arbitration or by some court? Jars was to determine how the coal raised was used, noting the different uses of the different kinds of coal, and their price. Was it true, as reported in France, that the English smelted iron with raw coal?[14] Was it used to smelt copper? Was it necessary to purify it of sulphur for either purpose and change it 'to what the English call "coucke"'? In visiting the coalfields he was to take and carefully label coal specimens and note what the coal was used for.[15]

There was clearly a primary emphasis on coal and its employment, but if Jars passed near enough to lead or copper mines he was to visit them.

He was to look at some of the significant lead-silver mines in Britain, and see how their management differed from those of Germany. Eventually he was to work his way down to the Cornish tin mines; it was anticipated that the Godolphin family would be helpful to him. He should explore the smelting as well as the mining, and he was to give an account of Stannary law. Wherever he went he was to report back just as he and Duhamel had done in Germany, which had been found highly satisfactory. He was to get drawings and dimensions of the machines used in England which operated horizontal and vertical brushes to give a high polish to steel and copper hardware; this was (as we have seen) one of the preoccupations of de Saudray in the late 1760s and 1770s. English steel-making was to get particular attention. Was Swedish iron alone used for cementation steel? How did the English cut and temper their files so as to make them so much harder than German ones? How did the English manufacture sulphuric acid, did they use sulphur itself or pyrites as the material? Jars was also to make for the villages where the earthenware or pottery industry was carried on, particularly the white salt-glazed pottery which they had not been able to copy in France, but which the English exported in quantity. 'Throughout his journey he will keep down expenses as much as possible' and particularly not insist on having 'meals served in the French style'.[16]

To Hellot's draft of June 1764 various other persons added riders and amendments. Some were amplifications, like those giving the furnace and coal types to be observed in the potteries; porcelain was to be looked at as well as ordinary pottery. Jars was to discover where the good English fuller's earth was found and how it was used. How were red and white lead prepared? On a wholly different front he was to enquire into the means by which the English cared for and maintained the breed of their sheep and whether any could be exported. He was to look into paper-making processes.

> M. Jars will especially examine why industry is pushed ahead very much further in England than in France, and whether this difference arises, as there is every reason to think, because the English are not hindered by regulations nor by inspections, and that they have few means of enriching themselves save by trade and manufacture.

As of 1 July 1764 Jars was to receive 8,000 *livres* for all expenses of his tour, including the tips he would have to give the chief workmen at all the works he visited.[17]

Holker was involved, however, in a different way. Before Jars set off for England he got in touch with Holker while the inspector-general was in Paris so that Holker could recommend to him 'a person to be trusted', that is, one of his English agents, to give him detailed instructions on the itinerary he should follow. This seemed important to Jars because 'the English have the reputation of being very secretive'. On arrival in London he immediately made contact with the Marquis de Blosset, who seems to have been the intelligence adviser, perhaps virtually the spymaster, at the embassy, and he followed that by meeting Holker's friend who offered Jars his services. 'I will profit by them without abusing them.'[18] Next month he wrote to Trudaine that he would only be able to send him a full account of his expenditure of time and effort once he could find a secure route by which to do it, otherwise he would have to wait until he got back to London, which might be only after many months. 'This precaution is necessary because I shall be suspect from the moment when any of my letters have been opened, this happens very often in this country, in order to find out what the purpose of a foreigner's journey is.' He would however keep Trudaine informed of his movements by writing to Blosset, 'and I will write to him as a naturalist who wants to learn the language and satisfy his curiosity'. A letter reached Blosset in September from Newcastle. There Jars had accidentally met the Comte d'Ayen who would convey it personally 'because of the inconvenience there is in writing to you by the post'. Blosset handled Jars's expenses according to various letters of 1765.

By May of that year Jars was again in London and able to write to Trudaine by the diplomatic bag, enclosing his first large memoir of observations, though this had been done without time to clarify everything. He would revise the manuscript on his return. The style of the report might be excused in that 'I have been eight months without using my own language'. He complained of having large expenses and asked for 3,600 *livres* as an advance of pay due in September. The ambassador had offered to provide it, but the dutiful Jars wanted Trudaine to clear it first – which he did. There are various other indications of secrecy, for instance Jars's reluctance to count on information on industry gained from a single observation 'Above all in a country where the people are very secretive, and where often the simplest question can make a traveller suspect'.[19]

Again in July Jars wrote to Trudaine from London that he had not written him during his recent travels 'in the fear that my letters might be opened, but M. Bruyard will tell you of my route'. He told Trudaine that he had learned of clandestine British enquiries to be made in

France so as to learn the secrets of the famous plate glass manufacture of Saint Gobain. This would be made by a company of men 'who are amongst the greatest entrepreneurs in England with the purpose of setting up a similar works in Scotland'. This was very interesting intelligence, for such a company was set up by 1773, with Scottish East India merchants and other Scots very prominent, and with a manager and some workers formerly at Saint Gobain.[20] While in London Jars was also able to send Trudaine one of the brushes the English used for polishing hardware, and a bottle of the varnish used in Birmingham to give copper a good colour, with some of the ingredients.[21]

There can therefore be no doubt that Jars was in effect required to conduct industrial espionage when necessary, but given the multiplicity of things he was directed to enquire into, and the long time he was expected to spend in England, he clearly did not engage in the potentially dangerous game of suborning workers. On the other hand, where it might be advantageous, he was happy to be in the open as a travelling savant of the Enlightenment, and so was even able to seek enrolment as a corresponding member of the Society of Arts.

Jars's reports are most accessible in the three substantial posthumously published volumes, dedicated to the Academy, and published after his death with some editing by his brother (Lyon, 1774–81). There are some, however, in the main file in the Archives Nationales which covers his activities and there are others in the contemporary French Foreign Office files.

The published volumes contain reports roughly arranged by theme, and therefore not an unbroken account of the English travels. One of his earliest English reports covers the Newcastle mines. He emphasized the large capital required for the deep mining of the coalfield, £4,000 would be a small amount to open a new pit, it might be as much as £20,000 and there was thus an enormous responsibility on the boring expert. There followed a detailed account of Hartley colliery with its huge reserves and its large Newcomen engine with a 60 inch cylinder. The engine had been given the ancillary task of operating an early coal winding machine, but unfortunately an unsuccessful one because of its frequent breakdowns. He went on to describe the use of local coal for glasshouses at both Newcastle and Shields. He went into detail about coke-making in furnaces close to the Tyne, and the importance of a skilled workman in controlling air supply. The English practice of reheating pig iron for casting, rather than casting straight from the furnace was noted, and the use of such cast iron for pump barrels, engine cylinders and for wheels, presumably for use on railed ways. He made it clear that the English used for this purpose the 'air' or reverberatory furnace, whose widespread use was so distinctive of English practice 'that we in France call it the "English furnace"'. It was the same as was used by the English in copper smelting, and rather like that which had recently been introduced for lead smelting in Brittany. He saw a pump barrel 15 feet long being cast and admired the quality of the product. He visited the ironworks of the famous Crowley family at Swalwell with more reverberatory furnaces for casting and a large iron forge for making wrought iron. But it still used charcoal and was no different from continental forges, with the wrought iron not as good as Swedish. The forge however had an immense nose-helve hammer of 600 lbs. At Newcastle, as we saw earlier, he also examined the cementation (blister) steel process and the further working to improve some of the 'blister' steel to 'shear' steel quality. Commonly called 'German steel' this shear steel had removed the need for German imports. He was made aware of the critical importance of the quality of wrought iron used as the material for cementation steel.

At the Crowley's Winlaton works Jars noticed the great quantities of files made from cementation steel, and learned of local English attempts, parallel to contemporary ones in France, to cut files by machine, which had similarly failed. He also visited another works making small files and there were some differences in production. The importance of files as a product of steel and as an essential tool in the making-up of nearly all metal goods had meant that they had featured prominently in Jars's instructions. He took great care in describing the craft processes, indicating how cementation steel was forged under a water-powered hammer until it became what was called common steel. For watch files the steel was given the further specialized forging to turn it into 'German' steel. After the blanks were shaped according to the size and type of file wanted, they were exposed to an annealing heat and then had their surfaces cleaned up on a grinding-wheel. He described how the file cutters worked, as all observers have recounted them from the eighteenth century to the twentieth. The file was held in a channel by leather straps, the bottom of the channel being covered by what Jars describes as a lead plate [probably pewter] so that once the file was cut on one side it could be turned over and cut on the other without the cut side being damaged by the softer metal, even though the file was in the annealed state. He describes the special hammer which gave the hand-held chisel the repeated blows which produced the required cut. He realized that the skill was in the angle at which the chisel was held in making the cut, and that it should be kept constant. On the skill required for hand-cutting files, however, Jars was seriously adrift. He noticed that there were workers who specialized in cutting different kinds of file, and because he saw some boys of ten or twelve doing some cutting this led him to believe that the technique in general did not present any difficulty.[22]

The coal used for the heating of the files before tempering was roasted to a kind of coke-like cinder in the forge. Before the tempering process was carried out the file was coated with 'barm bottoms', the dregs of beer barrels, and then plunged into a mixture of burnt and crushed cowhorn and sea salt. This was to preserve the cut surface and give additional harding.[23]

He was rather puzzled by the tempering of the files. He had difficulty in accepting that the files were tempered by plunging them hot into salt-water. Particularly when looking at the manufacture of watchmakers' files, which were made of better grade steel, he would not believe the workers when they said tempering was done by plunging the heated files in water which had beer lees and salt in it. Even when he tasted the water and found it salty he disbelieved his own senses and thought that the taste was probably a metallic one from the immersion of the files – even though the workers insisted that it was 'sel marin' (sea salt) which gave the critical hardness. It is interesting to see that such a careful observer found it hard to accept something contrary to his own experience, even when verbal and physical evidence combined to establish the situation. One wonders if he would have accepted that the angle at which the files were immersed was also important; he simply describes the files as being plunged into the water 'perpendicularly'. As well as the observations on file-making near Newcastle, Jars also visited Sheffield file-makers, but added only a few supplementary observations, for instance on the use of swages ('moules') by which the file forger gave the required form to the blanks of files in the many different profiles in which those tools were made.

Jars's examination of English file-making was thus careful and largely correct. He was right to emphasize the quality of steel, and he knew the dependence of English steel-makers on Swedish wrought iron. He arrived before the general move from cementation steel to cast steel for quality files. But he was not appreciative enough of the skill of hand-cutting, and sceptical on the use of salt-water in tempering, showing the problems of assessing industrial processes in which craft skill was of the essence.

Naturally Jars was well prepared to assess copper mines and copper smelting and refining. However, the planning of his route was less than ideal from the point of view of the modern historian, who would have been better pleased if he had given more attention to the Cornish mines, and rather less to those of Middleton Tyas in Yorkshire and Ecton in Staffordshire,[24] whose importance was relatively brief, though Ecton made a significant contribution to national production for a time. He was too early to have assessed the Anglesey mines, which had hardly been discovered. The large smelting and manufacturing units which subsequently depended on them were visited in the 1780s by the de Wendel, de Givry and Périer group.[25] He did not visit the Swansea smelting district, already very important, and to become dominant; indeed the industries of Wales and parts of the West Midlands would ideally have repaid greater attention, but we have rather to marvel at how much Jars saw in the period of under a year he spent in England. He noted the repeated roastings and smeltings carried out in reverberatory furnaces in copper smelters near Derby, near Bristol and at Hayle in Cornwall, and the very tricky process of refining. But he was critical about what he was told or allowed to see. At the Derby smelter he was concerned about 'the mystery which the English make of all their processes' and was doubtful of the accuracy of his account. He checked it with a man in London who was an expert on smelters, establishing that there were ten or twelve smeltings in a reverberatory furnace before black copper was produced. He noted correctly that the smelters liked to have a mixture of ores from different mines to work with, but he was probably mistaken in thinking more roasting of ores before smelting would have been an advantage. Given the cheapness of coal the English would hardly have economized on roasting if they thought more would be helpful. Nor did the British smelters ever adopt the use of bellows in refining furnaces which he thought would be an improvement.[26] Jars did not get all the information he wanted from the major brass-making works at Cheadle in Staffordshire, a highly regarded supplier of good quality brass to Birmingham, 'the mystery which the English make of their proceedings allowed me only a few limited observations'.[27]

Understandably, given the time he had, and the wide diversity of industrial operations he was asked to observe, different industries were unequally described. Lead mining and smelting had detailed treatment, and Leadhills in Scotland, the mines of Alston Moor, other Northumberland and Cumberland mines in northern England and the

Derbyshire lead workings were well covered. Jars was always interested in comparative technology, noting that a water-column engine was being suggested for drainage at an English lead-mine, like the ones adopted at the mines of Schemnitz. While he was interested in (and included a plate illustrating) the Newcomen engine, he was a little dubious about the way the English turned so readily to steam-powered pumping, and thought that they neglected the possibilities of water-powered pumping and the long-term solution of the *stangenkunst* for drainage.[28]

Two commissions which were part of Jars's instructions for his English voyage must be discussed. One was the enquiry into English methods of producing sulphuric acid, and Jars's report may well have had an influence on the Holkers' plans for vitriol manufacture. When we know his instructions we can be sure that his statement that 'on the road from London to [Wandsworth] chance made me enter a large industrial building enclosed by walls on every side' is a clear economy with the truth. The excuse he gives for his limited information, that it derived from 'the four or five minutes I remained in the laboratory' again indirectly emphasizes the espionage element. The owners, prepared for espionage, had resorted to a remarkable tactic to defeat it. 'I only met there women from the Principality of Wales, of whom only a few knew more than a few words of English (this precaution is taken no doubt so that no one may divulge anything which happens in that laboratory).' He seems first to have found himself in a large building used for distilling and concentrating the acid. Deciding to look for the acid-producing process itself he 'traversed [the first building] without anyone opposing me' and entered an even bigger one with over 100 glass globes, each of at least 2 feet 6 inches diameter, running in ranks down the shop, and resting on a sand bed. He was not able to see exactly how the globes were being heated, but was able to see some with the little cast iron platform inside on which the sulphur was burnt in the presence of nitre. It seemed to Jars that the cost of the great number of glass globes was likely to make the enterprise unprofitable.[29]

Of all the branches of British industry which Jars looked at, and in which metals of course predominated, it was perhaps the iron industry in which his observations can be seen to have most effect after his return, and where his efforts continued to bear fruit after his death. However, we shall see[30] that several others were subsequently involved in coke-iron making, and that, even so, real technical success evaded the French until after the Napoleonic wars. High in importance in the instructions for his travels was to learn the prices and uses of coal, and to discover if copper and iron were smelted with raw coal, and if it were necessary to make the coal into what the English called 'coucke' first; the very use of the English term implying that coke was unused in France. As we have seen, Jars spent time and care in looking at the coking of coal in heaps near Newcastle, and at coke ovens, and in one of his reports he sketched a coke oven. Coke-iron making he saw at two places. One was at Clifton between Cockermouth and Whitehaven,[31] which he was able to compare with his notes on the Carron ironworks in southern Scotland. Jars's opportunities of seeing the operations were probably restricted. He noted that the company, apparently operating coke furnaces only, did no refining of the resulting coke-pig to wrought iron 'not being able to make a good wrought iron out of it, though refined with charcoal'. He exaggerated the importance of the import of North American charcoal pig iron, and the reliance on it in Britain for wrought iron production. At another new works near Workington there was the interesting phenomenon of coke- and charcoal-fired furnaces being built together.[32] The charcoal furnace was already in blast, using local 'kidney' ore and some from Lancashire, no doubt high-quality haematite. Charcoal, very unusually, came from a distance, in fact from Scotland, and one presumes that here sea transport allowed the usual problems of overcoming the friability of charcoal when carried by land to be avoided. The coke furnace, still in building, would make only pig for casting.

Jars's best and fullest account is of the famous Carron ironworks in Scotland, founded in 1760. He learnt correctly that they were founded by Birmingham entrepreneurs, though he does not give the names of Roebuck and Garbett. He emphasizes that the viability of the works was based upon the excellent local coal supply, the mines owned by the entrepreneurs, and the integration of ironworks and mines by railed ways. The mining itself was advanced in technique; Longwall working is indicated, wooden railed ways operated above and below ground and horses were employed below ground. There were two pits, each with its 50-inch Newcomen engine.[33] He was of course just too early to learn of Watt's improvements to the steam engine and his engine experiments at Roebuck's Kinneil colliery. He did know of a steam engine proposed to be built there, but if Watt and Roebuck only became acquainted in the summer of 1765, as Dickinson and Jenkins say, this cannot be Watt's separate condenser engine.[34] The existing collieries provided several grades of coal, one being a clod coal suitable for coking.

Jars described the coke-making, which took up to forty hours, and the advantages of the clod coal which did not stick together when burning. While there were soon to be four furnaces at Carron two were operating when Jars was there, and he pointed out that there was effectively no difference from charcoal furnaces in construction, though at 30 feet high they were on the large side.[35] The operation was much as at charcoal furnaces, and production was 4 tons a day. It is now becoming clear that single blast furnaces have alternated between charcoal and coke fuel, so that Jars was quite correct.[36] The iron produced impressed him, it filed well and could be cut, and he was surprised that there was no way that it could be converted into good wrought iron. However, the whole purpose of the firm was to produce cast iron products in quantity. The production of the great cylinders for Newcomen engines for the English as well as the Scottish market was a principal object. He described how a 50-inch cylinder was cast while he was there, which required the simultaneous tapping of both furnaces, as well as pig remelted in several reverberatory furnaces, which were also fed with scrap. Jars was told the cylinder production at Carron was done on the pattern of a large Welsh ironworks. Presumably it was based on the Wilkinsons' Bersham methods rather than the Darbys' at Coalbrookdale. The range of cast iron products was wide, and was beginning to include many items previously only made in wrought iron; one means used to make such goods more saleable was the polishing of them on water-powered grindstones, similar to those used in France at Saint Etienne.

Jars was impressed by the length of the campaigns at the furnaces, the first furnace built had been in continuous production for four years, the second for three, while the remelting furnaces operated for a year or more. The proprietors wanted the strongest possible blast and were dissatisfied with their original bellows. They had now built huge single bellows 24 feet long and costing £300. Jars believed that they would have done better to build double bellows on the French pattern. While the Wilkinsons were currently struggling to make Isaac Wilkinson's blowing patent practicable, the perfecting of the steam-powered cylinder-blowing engine by his elder son John was still about a decade away, so this development, important in enabling furnace size to be increased, was not yet available for Jars to see at British ironworks. For wrought iron production the Carron Company added imported American and Russian pig to their own, and Jars disbelieved their claims that they refined their iron with coal, observing that the finery used charcoal just like all those in Europe, but that the reheating or chafery hearth was fuelled with coal alone. Carron impressed Jars greatly, especially with the large coal-mining, iron-mining, coking and iron-smelting operations going on close to each other employing 800 workers.[37]

However, Jars does not seem to have been clear that it was East Shropshire, the West Midlands and a limited area of North Wales in which the dynamic developments were taking place, though he was informed that Carron cylinder making derived from Welsh practices. Had he diverted his journey into those areas he would have seen the successful conversion of coke pig to wrought iron using charcoal in the finery (without the addition of high grade American and Russian pig) and the first conversion of coke pig to wrought iron entirely with coal-fuel by the early versions of the stamping and potting process. Perhaps after nearly thirty years Hellot had forgotten Ticquet's enthusiastic report on Coalbrookdale and omitted to ensure that it was on Jars's route. Another remarkable omission is the Prestonpans vitriol works, which had originally taken Roebuck and Garbett to Scotland. We do know that the precautions against unauthorized entry there were strong, that the site was firmly enclosed, and that Garbett was perhaps the most industrial espionage-conscious and security-minded industrialist of the time. But a report on this great centre of the lead chamber process would have put in focus the other report on the obsolescent glass globe process.

For present purposes there has to be a concentration on those British industries viewed by Jars where there was a really significant element of take-up, or attempted take-up, in France, whether by open or covert means, before the end of the eighteenth century. But it must be emphasized that there are detailed and well observed accounts of other industries not mentioned here, for instance salt production, particularly a fine description of the famous Liverpool salthouse and the Northwich salt mines, of earthenware manufacture both in the North East and at the Staffordshire potteries, the Whitby alum mines and alum-making, Liverpool porcelain and the invention of printing on pottery there.[38]

Once returned to France after an absence of fifteen months Jars was again burdened with additional tours and commitments, but also received government and academic advancement. In the following year, 1766, he was sent on another major metallurgical expedition, with his brother as his companion, to view the mines of the Hartz, Saxony, Mansfeld, Hanover, Liège, Sweden and Norway, also reporting on manufacturing developments in Holland, and in Hamburg and Copenhagen. At the end of it he was given a permanent official status ('a department which M. de Trudaine will prevail upon the Controller-General to assign to him') as his brother cryptically states, which seems to mean a special inspectorate for metallurgy. In 1768, after being a Correspondent of the Academy of Science since 1761, he was a candidate for a vacancy in the Academy itself. He was a very close second to Lavoisier, but the ministry favoured Jars. Quite exceptionally the king agreed to a supplementary place for Lavoisier.[39]

Jars's last tours were again arduous, but in France. He made a circuit through the ironworks of Northern and Eastern France, also taking in Burgundy, in 1768 and was dispatched to Berry, the Bourbonnais, Forez and the Auvergne in 1769. On 20 August of that year he died from sunstroke which killed him as he went through the mountains of the Auvérgne.[40] For decades afterwards there was the strong feeling that had Jars lived he would have been able to bring to France the best techniques from abroad, especially from Britain. There is of course no way in which a confident view can now be given on this. On the one hand, as we have seen, his reports on British steel-making methods, with his accompanying drawings, were the best available to the savants and industrialists who organized the famous drive for war production of steel in the 1790s, but there was virtually no production of crucible steel in that great effort, and the cementation steel methods were not long persisted with.

Jars's own efforts to produce crucible steel soon after his return from Britain were not successful. Le Play, the finest commentator on English steel-making in the mid-nineteenth century, believed that Jars had been very important in criticizing Réaumur on the supposed furnaces needed to convert wrought iron to cementation steel, and in stressing that nothing was added to the charcoal dust in the cementation chests. However, Le Play thought that Jars had not been emphatic enough about that or about the sole employment of Swedish iron in English steel-making: 'Jars did not believe it was his duty to insist upon the differences which existed between the methods of the English workshops and Réaumur's precepts'. So despite his clear indication that the English only used Swedish iron, once he got back to France Jars was not sufficiently determined to stand against 'the continual preoccupation with native irons' and Le Play says that on the evidence of his writings Jars did not think he could contest the view on the appropriateness of French irons 'strongly rooted in France among both savants and state officials'. In the pilot steel production trials he conducted in the Faubourg Saint Antoine in Paris there was never any question of his using Swedish Dannemora iron, only native iron. Jars claimed success in these trials.[41] So Le Play's statement that he said nothing in his writings about the results of his experiments is not exact, but he certainly did not leave any detailed account of the experiments. Had it seemed likely that good results could have been obtained from a scaled-up plant Jars would certainly have strongly memorialized the Government, and asked for a reward of some kind, given the great interest in the steel question. Le Play states that documents in the mining administration archives indicated that Jars was in fact no more successful than Réaumur and that there was a loss of 200,000 *livres* on the experiments. He regarded Jars, however, as a 'learned metallurgist' and said that his criticisms of Réaumur's views on fluxes in steel-making meant that later French attempts at steel-making were nearer the mark.[42]

11 Attacks on the Problem of Coke-Iron: Jars to Wilkinson

If Jars seems to have got nowhere in his attempts to copy English steel-making, what about iron? This was perhaps his main preoccupation, and though he had not thoroughly sorted out his memoirs for publication before his sudden death, those for the first volume were already partly arranged, giving prominence to the relationship which the exploitation of coal-mines had with iron mines and particularly iron-works. He fastened quite sensibly on the need for coke of the right quality as a *sine qua non* for the successful imitation of the British use of coal in iron production. His approach to coke-iron making seems to have been a generalist one, and not dominated by military, and essentially naval, needs. This allows us to separate his attempts to answer demand in terms of technology from the subsequent ones of de la Houlière, De Wendel, William Wilkinson and their associates. One of his first visits in his 1768 tour was to the ironworks of the nobleman and scientist, Buffon, at Montbard, a centre of many experiments in the making of iron and steel. However, Montbard was as deficient in real results from the many serious experimenters who worked there, as it was notable for their celebrity and virtuosity. Jars does not appear to have discussed the making of iron with coal while at Montbard.

But Montbard was only a day's journey from Montcenis. Jars went there to look at coal-mines now being seriously developed by two entrepreneurs, La Chaize and Jullien, though there had been feeble and desultory operations over centuries. Before doing more the entrepreneurs were awaiting the necessary privilege from the commerce administration. Jars believed they should be given every assistance, the mines 'merit serious attention and every protection of which this sort of enterprise is susceptible', as there was coal there in great abundance and good quality. Hitherto the mines had been worked by inexperienced and undercapitalized men – the very problems Trudaine had tried to tackle in the mining edict of 1744. The entrepreneurs deserved encouragement, but they also needed a good mining engineer, and the miners were digging the coal so unskilfully as almost to reduce it to dust. Jars had made a pick like those used at Liège and showed the workers how to use it. There were various steps to be taken; the chief miner should be sent to the Belgian coalfields to gather experience, the road should be improved to give access to water transport and, most interesting, manufactures of iron and steel should be established on the spot, for which Jars believed Montcenis was better situated than Saint Etienne. The way to do this was for the entrepreneurs to set up a furnace to smelt iron ore with coal.

The main point however was Jars's opinion of the suitability of the Montcenis coal for smelting iron, that is to say for producing a good coke 'this method of smelting would be all the more essential to establish since it would be the first in France and thus it could serve as an example in a kingdom where wood is becoming scarce and where the consumption of iron and steel increases daily'. But it would be necessary to have the coal 'turned into what the English call "coaks", which they use for this purpose'. In fact one name in the immediate locality soon came to predominate over that of Montcenis, that of Le Creusot, though that internationally famous ironworks was of course founded on the availability of Montcenis coal. Jars immediately made a quantity of coke at Montcenis, was very pleased with the result and left instructions with the entrepreneurs how to produce it on a large scale. He also arranged to send some barrels of coke to be tried out at his family's copper furnaces at Chessy in the Lyonnais.[1] Though in Britain a portion of coke had been used together with raw coal as the fuel of copper furnaces in the early days of smelting copper with mineral fuel, by this time coal alone was used in Britain, so here Jars was not adopting British technology. He could hardly have known of this limited early use of coke in British copper smelting, and he believed that he was trying something not previously attempted in any country.[2] The long-term consequences of Jars's perceptive analysis of the possibilities of Montcenis can hardly be exaggerated, and if he had little else to his credit this would give him an honoured place in the history of French technology.

Jars continued his propaganda on the importance of coke, and particularly in iron manufacture. In 1768 he seems to have used it in casting iron in Alès, possibly for the reheating of coke pig. Early in the following year he was in Alsace. Here he visited the very large ironworks of a great family of ironmasters, the De Wendels of Hayange. The son of the family, Ignace de Wendel, was present. He had been commissioned as an artillery officer as part of his technical training. Ignace persuaded his father, Charles de Wendel, to allow Jars to experiment. He made some coke from local coal and a furnace was charged and the first coke-pig in France run off. The amount of coke-iron made was small and there does not seem to have been any follow-up at the Hayange works, though the story of the achievement spread quickly. But the most important thing was the capturing of the interest of Ignace de Wendel, who was to play a great part in the bringing of British methods to France, who was to lead the team of experts who investigated the British arms industry in 1784, and who is inseparably associated with the great Le Creusot project. Wendel was essential in directing the development of the iron industry to answering military demand.

Jars had thus made great efforts to fulfil the instructions he received for his British journey which required that he enquire into the use of coal in iron-making. The importance of, and the processes for, coke-making seem to have been his major preoccupation on his return, though the emphasis might have been different had his cementation steel experiments really succeeded. Even so, if he had thoroughly established that process, he might have subsequently moved to trials for making crucible steel, in which coke would have been needed, but he never got that far. His great interest in coke-iron manufacture was flawed in one respect; he firmly believed that it was impossible to convert coke-iron to wrought: 'the English smelt most of their iron ore with coaks from which they obtain an excellent pig iron, which can be cast very well, but they never succeed in making a good wrought iron from it'. This statement is a posthumous one in a pamphlet published by his brother from his surviving papers a few months after his death.[3]

The nature and efficacy of Jars's British investigations, and their relation to industrial espionage, we have examined.[4] For the present we will simply pursue the way in which his information on British iron-making was taken up, and how far it was found helpful or deficient. Just a year after Jars's death, Bertin, formerly controller-general and still a powerful minister, wrote to the Intendant of Languedoc on the importance of switching from wood to coal-fuel, both domestically and metallurgically, and cited Jars's attempts to develop coking in France as a means to that end 'when death overtook him and deprived us of this valuable expert', and enclosing a pamphlet of Jars's which discussed coal use not only for metalworks, but in the home 'without any bad smell' – presumably coked.[5] But Jars's example was not neglected, though the next significant step was taken just over the French border, not far from Hayange, when the Prince of Nassau-Saarbruck tried to copy the English methods on his estates. At Sulzbach he set up coke-iron furnaces, and with some initial success, though the furnaces were abandoned after two years.

After Jars's death the link with later attempts to obtain technical knowledge and expert technologists from Britain is provided by De Gensanne, a French metallurgist who visited Sulzbach. He was most enthusiastic about the trials, which he wrote up in his *Traité de la fonte de mines par le feu de charbon de terre* of 1770. He involved himself with a group whose speculative fervour may have outrun their expertise – William, Count Stuart, a former army officer, Charles Kessling, another former officer, and two others, one of whom was a financier. Their scheme was to set up a large company to make coke which was then to be directed to iron-making. They turned for help to Gensanne and an architect, Ling. Their technological grasp was unsure; on Gensanne's persuasion they tried coke-smelting in a reverberatory furnace at Hayange in 1773, reminding one of the disastrous trials of William Wood in England in the early eighteenth century. Stuart and Ling rightly favoured the blast furnace, and broke with Gensanne.[6] They revived operations in Nassau-Saarbruck in 1774, initially mixing charcoal and coke in the furnace charge in different proportions, claiming to have produced good pig. Some of this they said had been converted to wrought iron with a mixed charcoal and coke fuel. While Stuart and Kessling sought an exclusive privilege, and experimented with improved coking, Ling was forced out of the association and contested their claims with the Government. Back at Montcenis the coalmasters la Chaize and Jullien also experimented with coke-iron production, claimed success, and got an *arrêt* for privileged manufacture. This included, very interestingly in view of future developments, the making of 'iron cannon cast in the English manner.' There was now a successful take-over bid by Stuart and Kessling for their Montcenis rival.

A period of confusion and irreconcilable claims followed. There were experiments at the ironworks of Buffon and in the Montbard neighbourhood with charcoal-coke mixtures. By 1777 the Chevalier Grignon, a government technologist, entered the lists. He was formerly an ironmaster, it was he who proposed the furnace-industry inspectorate to encourage coal use.[7] He was experimenting with coke and iron at Lyon.

The Stuart company contested an exclusive privilege for coke-iron making with a company led by Ling; eventually they settled for separate privileges, each company being given a monopoly period in several provinces. Finally Stuart seems to have sold out to others, but there is no real evidence of long-term success from any of these concerns. Ballot, who gives the best account of this period, considers that no one made any money out of the trials; the consumers of iron were apathetic, the dirty smoke of coal put many ironmasters off, the quarrels between those claiming new processes made for confusion. The use of existing charcoal furnaces for coke-smelting, however, was probably not as serious a disadvantage as he thought.[8]

Iron and Armaments

The next development was very important, it led to massive state intervention in the iron industry, and to a celebrated technological collaboration between an English ironmaster family and the French government.

A brigadier in the French army, Marchant de la Houlière, became fascinated by the possibilities of making coke-iron after reading Gensanne's publication on the subject, and began an enthusiastic collaboration with him. De la Houlière searched for a good site for coke-iron production and was attracted to Languedoc, where the Estates, with a more progressive economic policy than most similar provincial institutions, were pressing the use of coal because of a real and serious wood shortage, and the partners were invited to the coal-mines of Alès by the local bishop. In 1773 they made pig iron with a coke-charcoal mixture, but mainly coke. However, they used a Catalan forge, not a blast furnace. Though they received a small subsidy from Languedoc, de la Houlière decided after two years that his resources were insufficient, and Gensanne's knowledge incomplete. He concluded that it was essential to go to England, and supplement the information which Jars had brought back, and he appealed to the Government and the Estates of Languedoc for financial assistance. Together they provided the 4,000 *livres* he asked for.[9]

Fortunately de la Houlière's report survives, a document of the first importance.[10] De la Houlière's aims were seemingly in the first place to investigate English coal and iron ores, to see if there were any reasons in raw material quality or preparation why English progress was so marked, and to look at iron-smelting equipment, especially furnaces and bellows. But he in fact went further. He looked into the methods of converting coke-pig iron to wrought iron with coal. A key element was added, that of the 'casting (of) excellent naval guns as practised in England'. How far this was in de la Houlière's mind before arriving in England is unclear. He states that he got great help from the Comte de Guines, the French ambassador in England, who had been briefed about de la Houlière's visit both by the Archbishop of Narbonne on behalf of the Estates of Languedoc, and by Vergennes, the great French foreign minister. The ambassador (very remarkably) provided de la Houlière with letters of introduction to those ironworks where there were foundries casting guns for the royal Navy 'as it was principally in these establishments that there was a ... hope of securing the most essential information'. Does this simply mean that some of the best of the relatively few British coke-smelting iron works were prominent in cannon casting because of the qualities of their iron, and that these ironworks were the ones where best practice could be observed? This would eliminate the most famous coke-iron producer of all, Coalbrookdale, which no longer made cannon. There were two further pieces of assistance which were provided by de Guines. One was the loan of his chaplain, MacDermott, as a translator and travelling companion to de la Houlière. Another was a letter of introduction from the Birmingham industrialist Matthew Boulton to his acquaintance the ironmaster John Wilkinson, at a time when their famous technological collaboration in the successful realization of the Watt steam-engine was in its early stages. The first cylinder cast and bored by Wilkinson had just been delivered to Boulton in April 1775.[11] Boulton's recommendation of de la Houlière to Wilkinson is one important incident in Boulton's highly inconsistent pattern of behaviour in relation to the encouragement or prevention of the transfer of British technology abroad.[12]

De la Houlière's report was a most penetrating and perceptive one. He was not always completely right of course; it was fine to indicate that coking coal was not confined to a small number of coalfields, but it was wrong to imply that it was only coal which contained stone and shale which would not coke properly. Nor were there coke furnaces in all parts of England; many of the places he mentioned were correct, but

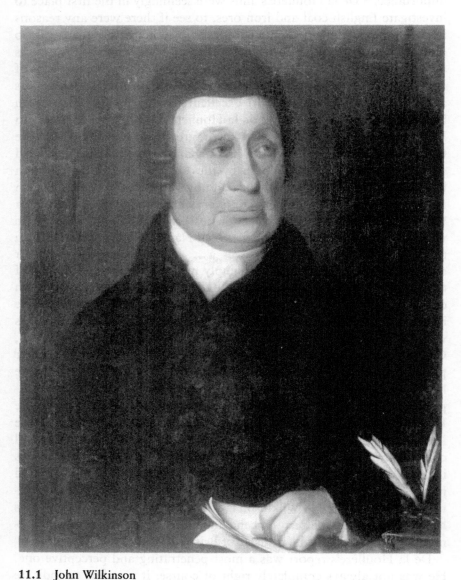

11.1   John Wilkinson

it would have been interesting to know where the seven or eight he referred to as being in London were sited! He confirmed Jars's information on coke-making, that it was usually made in the open air in coke-heaps, but sometimes in specialized but simple ovens of more than one type. He gave a few details about the common practices of mixing iron ores for the blast furnace and about rather rough and ready methods of giving ore a preliminary roasting before charging the furnace, but he probably exaggerated the proportion of limestone sometimes used in the charge.

De la Houlière noted that coke-iron as it came directly from the furnace was fit to cast large cooking pots for common use, or bars for the grates of coal furnaces in other industries, but that it made rough-looking castings, anything but smooth, and with coke and cinder stuck in it – as one can see today by looking at the famous Iron Bridge in Shropshire. For more exacting uses he realized coke-iron was run off into pigs and later remelted in reverberatory furnaces. The iron resulting from remelting in such furnaces was very fluid, it produced castings of very high quality, the process 'consolidates and unites it at the same time, so that it forms a compact mass, without interstices, capable of resisting the strongest action of gunpowder'.[13] It had the further quality of being able to be filed and chiselled.[14] De la Houlière describes a visit to the famous Bersham works of the Wilkinsons where he saw two large reverberatory furnaces which when charged with coke pig and cast iron scrap brought their contents into complete fusion in two and a half hours, and they were then tapped, producing enough iron to cast a 32 pounder cannon. Similarly the worn-out cylinders of Newcomen engines could be broken up and recast in reverberatory furnaces, facilitating new monster engines of 76-inch cylinders. The range of goods made in cast iron was increasing fast and included pump barrels, water pipes, and gear wheels. He made it clear that the reverberatory furnaces were fuelled with raw coal, and unlike Jars, does not seem to have been diverted into ideas of using coke in them.

De la Houlière had been well advised on the works to visit. He went to West Bromwich near Birmingham and visited the premises of Wright and Jesson who were pursuing their patent process[15] for converting coke-pig to wrought iron, the so-called stamping and potting process, which historians now recognize as being of great importance. It was the main method of conversion with coal before Cort's puddling and rolling process overcame its difficult teething period and took on generally in the mid-1790s. 'The owners were away', he wrote, 'but I got on good terms with the workmen in the way which usually succeeds', by which he meant giving them drink money. He gives a very careful and exact description of the process, which had originally been developed by the Wood family of Wednesbury, very close by, but significantly improved by Wright and Jesson. It was the first process to undercut the prices of the charcoal forgemasters for the conversion of coke-pig to wrought, and thus achieved a wholly coal-based production of iron. De la Houlière's observations were excellent, but they unfortunately did not lead to any take-up of the process in France, and even the successor process of Cort did not make any progress there before 1815.

Though De la Houlière does not seem to have known that the Wright and Jesson process he had just seen was founded on methods developed by the Wood family, he did make the short journey to Wednesbury to see the Woods' works and also their coal-mines with their steam engines, one with a 76-inch cylinder. He described Wood's own stamping and potting process which he was using to convert wrought iron scrap. This he was obtaining from much of Europe as well as from Britain, and turning it into iron equal to the best Swedish, which was extensively used locally for musket barrels.

De la Houlière listed the main points he had established; that iron ore was being smelted without charcoal, that not only pig but wrought iron could now be made in districts where woods were few, and that the iron ore and coal mines in those districts could be profitably exploited and not remain unused. Scrap could be recycled into high quality iron. The reheating of coke-pig in reverberatory furnaces made it much superior for casting, and it was now possible to produce elegant shapes for architectural iron like balconies, balustrades, railings, and gates. But to him the remarkable finding was that about armaments made from iron. It was now possible to have mortars, gun carriages, cannon balls and bombs made from coke-pig iron, without any charcoal iron, and have the work done 'with extraordinary speed'. More significant still, cannon could be made from this iron which could be made lighter in weight and yet proof against bursting. He had believed, like many others involved in the iron industry, that any iron made with coal-fuel would be brittle and coldshort. This was not so; 'we must acknowledge the facts and bow to the nation which pays most attention to everything making for economy in man-power'. The English put great emphasis on the remelting of coke-iron pig in coal-fired reverberatory furnaces.

Since that technique had been employed (for twenty years according to de la Houlière) the English had never had a case of a burst cannon among those so manufactured. Such appalling accidents did occur on French ships 'so that our sailors fear the guns they are serving more than those of the enemy'. Sailors were killed or maimed, there were liable to be secondary explosions in gunpowder and cartridges, and the vessel itself could blow up. In a naval engagement in 1765 guns on two ships had exploded, causing seventy to eighty men to be wounded and some killed.

According to de la Houlière his sole reason for making his English tour was to explore the possibilities of coal use in iron-making in order to save on charcoal, which the scarcity of wood was making dear in France. As well as some civilian demand, he had anticipated that coke iron could be used in cannon-balls and bombs but now a much more important military use had been made evident, and 'he realized, with the greatest satisfaction that a good citizen can enjoy, that his journey could serve a more useful purpose than he had hoped'. As 'a zealous military man and having the interests of the King's service at heart' he had the idea of bringing a man with the right experience to France. He therefore tentatively approached 'an eminent ironmaster who owns four foundries and has brought the casting of iron to the highest pitch of perfection', saying that anyone fully possessed of the necessary skill who came over to France 'could make a large fortune'. The man spoken to, of course, was the man to whom he had been introduced by Boulton, John Wilkinson. It was he who had in the previous year (1774) taken out a patent for cast iron cannon bored out from the solid, a patent he did not long enjoy because the British government was unwilling to have him in a monopoly situation.[16]

Wilkinson had no scruples about discussing the possibilities of such an emigration. However an Englishman would not trust an arbitrary government or its ministries who could get rid of him at any time, 'but if it were a question of a private arrangement between individuals, then he saw a tidy profit was to be made, with all the benefits accruing from an assured market on a long-term basis'. John Wilkinson said that he could send over his younger brother, unmarried and without family responsibilities, who was currently managing the Bersham works in North Wales, where cannon founding was a main activity. At this point a Wilkinson–de la Houlière partnership was the idea, with Wilkinson insisting on a guaranteed market for twelve years in France and prompt payment (he was only too aware of the fluctuations between wartime and peacetime demand for armaments) and free export from France for all cannon, cannon-balls and bombs surplus to French government requirements, 'for these Englishmen never set a limit on their field of trade'. De la Houlière did not find this unreasonable, but pointed out that the Government would control exports in wartime and make sure that they only went to allies or neutrals. Next day he was with William Wilkinson at Bersham, who liked what he heard of his discussions with his brother, and 'had a great desire to see France'.

De la Houlière urged the French government to follow up this possibility with all speed. It could ensure better cannon at no greater cost, they could be proved very rigorously indeed, which would reassure French sailors, with the cannon being made in the French style and tested at French ports. The transfer of the technology would be a permanent asset to France. Export of munitions above French requirements would produce foreign exchange for France. Given that the French government allowed the immigrant ironmaster a good profit, and stuck faithfully to its agreements with him this 'would attract all those arts and trades into France which it may be thought desirable to transplant'. In other words a successful deal with William Wilkinson might have more general implications for the transfer of technology; he might have an impact on metallurgy like that of Holker on textiles. De la Houlière went on to suggest possible outlines of a contract, in which his estimate of the amount of time needed to set up a cannon foundry in France seems highly optimistic. William Wilkinson's proposed removal expenses at 2 to 300 guineas appear generous but not unreasonable. Wilkinson was familiar with coal-mines and could give valuable advice on them, and particularly on steam pumping, as he frequently made steam engines 'which are used in almost every coal mine in England' at Bersham. De la Houlière thought he could go it alone, but he modestly suggested that it would be better to recruit Wilkinson. For himself he would be willing to set up coal-fired reverberatory furnaces at or near Paris so that ministers and members of the Academy of Sciences could see solid cannon, water pipes and other things cast from coke-pig. He understood only too well the difficulties of getting the French establishment, ministerial, financial or scientific, to take with full seriousness industrial experiments carried out in the distant provinces or reported on by a provincial Academy.

De la Houlière was also aware that there was something of a cultural credibility problem about the Wilkinsons for French ministers and administrators. Their industrial capital was very large, £80,000 he believed, they sold naval cannon not only to their own government but to the Dutch and the Turks, they were limitless in their ideas of trade expansion, they were businessmen first and patriots second. While their type might be unfamiliar in France, de la Houlière assured his government that 'they are no mere upstarts, but persons of good breeding, actuated solely by that spirit of gain which is all too common in their nation'. The French government should be quick and decisive if it wanted to secure William Wilkinson, and not give him too much time to change his mind, or wait until Anglo-French relations deteriorated and the countries were again at war. For him to help arm the French in wartime might be held treasonable, 'whereas if he had taken this step in time of peace, he would be allowed, by virtue of his rights as an Englishman, to follow up a business on which his fortune depended'.[17]

The report is a remarkable one in the accurate way in which it fastened on to relevant technologies and then explained them well, and in the fewness of misconceptions; there was an absence of inflexible received ideas and nothing was set down which was superfluous or of low significance. It raises interesting questions. De la Houlière, despite his military background, had come over to explore the commercial manufacture of iron with coal-fuel, not armaments, and there is no need to discount the genuineness of his statement that the importance of coke-iron for cannon and the new technique for their manufacture were new and unexpected to him. But his advisers at the French embassy had directed him to ironworks supplying the British navy as the best source of information on coke-iron production – had they done so hoping that he would come back with military as well as civilian industrial intelligence? That he was directed so firmly to John Wilkinson probably simply depends on the embassy using Matthew Boulton as an intermediary. Boulton and Watt had found that they were greatly dependent on Wilkinson because of his ability to bore accurate cylinders which satisfied the closer tolerances demanded by the Watt engine, which the Carron works could not. This achievement was eventually based on Wilkinson's cylinder-boring machine, a separate invention from his cannon-boring one.

John Wilkinson was the more likeable brother, and had long friendly associations with some of the most powerful and successful businessmen of his time – for instance with the copper tycoon Thomas Williams and the iron merchant and ironmaster Richard Crawshay – and he seems to have retained the loyalty and trust of his workers. But both Wilkinsons had a high opinion of themselves, and a strong distrust of restrictions, whether deriving from government and taxation, or from associations with other ironmasters. They believed they knew their business better than anyone else, and were impatient of deals and diplomacy, and simply wanted to get on with making iron. William took his arbitrary and imperious manner to France, and while the French found themselves very dependent on him technologically he was not as attentive to their needs or to their commands as they would have wished. It may be speculated that if William Wilkinson had given the close care and attention to detail that Holker did to textile matters the French might have had a securely founded coke-iron industry thirty years or more before they did. It was the elder brother from whom the inventive ideas came, William simply transmitted some of them to France.

William Wilkinson made a preliminary visit to France within weeks. One of the first requirements of the French was that eight cannon made by John Wilkinson should be imported and examined. This was done in an entirely overt and aboveboard fashion and the permission of the Privy Council obtained, apparently on the basis that another country had been allowed to give a much larger order to the Wilkinsons.[18] William Wilkinson seems to have remained in France for some months, and it was with MacDermott (the guide and translator for de la Houlière's English visit) and with de la Houlière himself that Wilkinson visited the cannon foundry of Ruelle on 26 January 1776, meeting there Secval, a marine officer who was inspector of artillery production, and it was probably at this early point that he examined the site at the isle of Indret on the Loire, not far from Nantes and a naval arsenal since 1691.[19] Wilkinson travelled extensively, visiting de la Houlière's ironworks at Alais, and examining a reverberatory furnace near Marly, possibly one which de la Houlière had undertaken to build on the Wilkinson pattern so that the Academy of Sciences could pronounce on its production. Wilkinson said that the firebrick was deficient and that cast iron parts were needed for its construction. He promised to get the necessary materials from Britain, but we hear no more of the furnace.[20] After his tour Wilkinson believed, according to de la Houlière, that it would be quite possible to make coke-iron in France.[21]

Wilkinson returned to Britain for a time, and remained at Bersham until the winter of 1776, but was back in France early in the next year, probably travelling in the company of J. C. Périer, whom we will encounter later in his relations with the Boulton and Watt engine and with Le Creusot. Navy experts, concerned at the superiority of English cannon and the deficiency in the supply of French ones, urged the Navy Minister, de Sartine, to agree with Wilkinson, and a contract was signed in May 1777, perhaps a revision or confirmation of one of 1775. Indret was agreed as the site, and indeed work may have already begun there. Wilkinson was named as director of operations; his initial salary was 12,000 *livres* raised two years later to 50,000 *livres*.[22] Wilkinson was to supply all the plans; the construction and the assembly of the machinery was to be done under Secval and another French officer. Indret was to melt down old cannon in coal-fired reverberatory furnaces, and to cast iron cannon solid in sand, a practice new to the French, and then bore them out from the solid with machinery like that the Wilkinsons used in England. Secval was in regular correspondence with Sartine; he showed himself to be critical about the supposed overwhelming superiority of the English processes, and to be resentful of Wilkinson's domineering manner, saying he always met 'le despotisme Anglais' when with him at Nantes. Sartine tried to get Secval to reconcile himself with Wilkinson and hoped that 'by continuing to flatter his amour propre you will regain his confidence',[23] but in the end Secval was partly replaced by another and celebrated naval engineer, Toufaire, who continued the association with Wilkinson beyond the Indret project.[24] The naval director of the Brittany ports wrote to the Minister in October 1778, hoping that Wilkinson would not exceed a ten- or twelve-day absence that had been agreed, though admitting that his zeal had been unremitting so far. He was trying to keep the peace between Wilkinson and Toufaire on the one side and Secval on the other.[25]

There were considerable difficulties in building a tide-mill and the related hydraulic works to power a battery of water-powered boring mills. But the mills were at work by August 1778 and there were important ancillary features new to France, like an iron railed way. However, the works had cost 2 million *livres*, only a few cannon of small calibre had been turned out, and Wilkinson was talking about going back home. With a war now on it might be impossible to recruit anyone else to replace him. It became urgent to have an appraisal of the essential problems at Indret. Sartine turned to the great artillery expert Gribeauval, perhaps the most famous name in the history of artillery. He in turn recommended an artillery officer we have already met, Ignace de Wendel, of the important ironmaster family at Hayange, where as we have seen he had already been involved in coke-iron experiments.[26] Wendel had the delicate job of basing himself at Nantes and visiting Indret, where he gave out that he was just an interested industrial expert and artilleryman, without declaring his mission of inspection,[27] but by the time Wendel had completed his findings, Wilkinson was suspicious that he was about to be replaced by a Frenchman. This was exactly what Sartine wanted Wendel to do.

Wendel reported to Sartine at Versailles. He was clear that there were management weaknesses which were affecting Indret. However, the serious problem was the source of iron for it to work on. The supply of old cannon for remelting in the reverberatory furnaces was drying up, and not all of this material made good metal for the Wilkinson process. Berry pig, thought the best in France, and fairly close to hand, had been tried and failed; clearly charcoal pig would not do. With war with England now under way, and England the only source of coke-pig, there was now no hope of importing it, though some may have been previously brought in. The only thing to do was to tackle the whole problem at the roots, and find a centre where large quantities of coke-iron could be made in France. Indret, though few cannon had been made after a vast capital expenditure, was not necessarily a failure, there were five water-powered boring mills and one horse-powered, the four reverberatory furnaces should be raised to seven to match potential. With a proper material supply well over 1,000 guns could be made there in a year.

Wendel moved in several directions at once, he intensified the search for old French cannon and bought Dutch ones. He also obtained Spanish ones, but with a requirement to return some of them to Spain when refabricated. He took over Indret on lease from the Crown and had it made a *manufacture royale*, while the great cannon foundry at Ruelle was associated with it, so as to take for boring some of the cannon to be cast at Indret. Another foundry at Forgeneuve joined the other two as a *manufacture royale* under Wendel. Though Wendel undertook to produce guns at the same price at which they were currently made in the old way at Ruelle, he failed to do so, and had to endeavour to justify his higher costs to the new Navy Minister, de Castries.[28] In 1781 Wendel delivered good cannon to Brest and other ports 'without any fault interior or exterior', but during the following year production fell off. Rambourg, the superintendent, and later a famous ironmaster, said that the remaining iron at Indret was not of a type suitable for a second melting in the reverberatory furnaces, leading to a pitted casting if employed, and by October operations were halted 'for lack of good quality material'.[29] Nevertheless the Wendel administration soon had the foundry expanding its production and improving its equipment. In 1783 he added two water-wheels capable of boring four cannon at once. In his later Le Creusot project he became involved with the famous engineer Périer and with him explored the possibilities of steam-power at Indret, Périer putting in an estimate in June 1785, and pointing out that a steam-engine was unaffected by frost or drought.[30] Large boring machines were installed powered by the engine. It is interesting that after the end of the American war some sizeable orders for coke-pig iron were sent to England and that John Wilkinson offered a contract of this kind in 1783. In 1785 the navy minister authorized Wendel to buy from England the quantity of coke pig he needed to keep the Indret cannon production going, but the cost of the purchase was being looked into.[31]

But if the radical solution to the problem was to be the setting up of an English coke-fired ironworks, that put the French back, at any rate during the course of the war, into the hands of William Wilkinson. Wendel admitted that he himself could not reliably build coke furnaces. 'There is only in France a single man who has the idea and he (Wendel) was forced to turn to Sr. Wilkinson, the English expert who built the Indret works.'[32] 'It is a compliment to British industry, in this branch of the Arts, that it is essential to France to acquire it.'[33]

During 1781 Wendel worked with Wilkinson, with whom he had managed to form a good relationship, to find a site for coke-smelting.[34] Wendel was attracted to Saint Etienne, but eventually they settled on Le Creusot, adjacent to Montcenis in Burgundy, thus confirming the choice indicated by Jars just before his death. Wendel, Wilkinson and Toufaire went to Montcenis to view the ground and plan operations. There seems to have been a stepping-up of the proposed scale of operations from two coke-furnaces looking to Indret to consume their pig, to a larger complex of four or five furnaces, all cylinder blown by steam-power, with associated forges to convert some of the pig to wrought iron by English methods. This would need steam-powered hammers, for little water power was available at Le Creusot. This larger works would look to have a wide civilian market, as well as a naval one.

Even before leaving for Le Creusot William Wilkinson insisted that he should have a personal contract with the new Navy Minister, de Castries, 'as contractor for the Crown'. He agreed to prepare all the plans and sketches for the blast furnaces and forges to be operated by steam-power. A draughtsman was to be appointed, who would be paid by the king, providing Wendel with copies of plans signed by Wilkinson, of which he would retain a copy. The plans were to be approved by de Castries.[35] Wilkinson undertook to provide the steam-engines at an agreed price and set them up,

> These steam engines could then only be obtained in England. The Wilkinson family being the owners of the chief works where these kinds of machine were made, once again we turned to him to obtain them and also to obtain the precise dimensions of the workshops that it was intended to build.[36]

Wendel was briefly worried that Wilkinson might be tempted to join up with another French firm proposing to make iron with coal,[37] so he was to teach the necessary workers and not to leave the enterprise until 'The English method shall be perfectly understood'. He thought the concern could be got going in three years.[38] At a point when Wilkinson had thought the project might be finished in two years 120,000 *livres* was suggested as his payment. He would now be paid 72,000 *livres* a year, 216,000 altogether, one-third of the salary would be at the king's expense, the rest at that of Wendel, who (with business associates) would pay the other two-thirds and the costs of machines, furnaces etc. On de Castries's orders, Wendel would have 'the effective position of King's commissioner'.[39] It was recognized that building English-type furnaces would be costly. 'English blast furnaces have much larger dimensions than those they work in France, and thus the building is much more expensive.'[40]

It is interesting that William Wilkinson declared that the contract he made with the French government was not only on his behalf but on his brother's ('equally for him and for his brother Mr. Wilkinson'), indicating that his elder brother and partner was keeping a close eye on his activities. He contracted for two years at least, but to stay longer if need be. He might take absence for his own business affairs; he also made it clear that he would need to return home for technical consultations with his brother.[41] In either case he would arrange for his replacement by an English expert. He interestingly indicated that the English voyage was essential so that 'he could see once again all the operations which he will be practising in France and become informed of all the progress made in the Art since he left England', a good indication of the rate of technical change in the English iron industry at this period. He also needed English cast iron pipes for the blowing mechanism and a special English vehicle, apparently for the carriage of the engine cylinders from a seaport to Le Creusot. He contracted to answer all questions put to him by Wendel frankly and truthfully so as to enlighten him fully on his operations. On top of his salary he had living expenses of 1,000 *livres* a month and full travel expenses. However, he could leave if either of two things happened; if his brother died and he had to take over the British business, or if he was recalled by the English government. The latter shows that Wilkinson did believe it a possibility that he might be summoned home on due notice under the terms of the 1719 Act.[42] It was clearly indicated that Wilkinson might bring over workmen from England; they would be under him and any special pay and conditions should be respected, and Wendel was to pay as agreed 'with the greatest exactitude'. For a steam-engine to blow two furnaces Wilkinson was not only to provide the steam-engine itself on terms and timetable to be agreed, but to 'bring over from England a workman to operate it', and this workman was to teach a French worker how to manage it, and not leave until the Frenchman was perfectly *au fait* with the engine. The English worker's salary was to be fixed by Wilkinson but paid by the King. In the matter of coking, Wilkinson was to make trials of coal and teach workers how to do it, leaving at least two trained workers when he left. He was also to survey the district for suitable iron ores. Among other stipulations, once the furnaces were at work Wilkinson was to stay long enough to instruct two foundrymen and also two forgemen who refined pig iron to wrought.

The story of Le Creusot has been deeply investigated, particularly by Ballot, Gille, Woronoff and Ozanam. Of central significance are the great financial problems which were involved and the measures taken to solve them, and the fortunes of the great capitalists who were brought in, but then found their finances fatally threatened by the pre-Revolutionary economic fluctuations. While the State was involved, the attitudes of administrations differed. Necker needed much convincing, 'he thought that the public interest ought not to get itself involved with private industry except to share in the results when they have been achieved'. This early Thatcherism was not appreciated by Wendel, who emphasized that this kind of industry could be got off the ground much more readily in England where the whole atmosphere was highly commercial and a large amount of capital was always in circulation, whereas in France great capitals were centred on Paris and the public finances.[43]

Under Calonne, however, there was a different atmosphere. That minister had a vision of Le Creusot as a point of concentration of the new English industrial technology, with the extensive employment of steam-power and the use of coal in industry on a great scale – all the more marked when the queen's glassworks for the production of

English crystal (flint glass) was added to the Le Creusot establishment, and Indret too was brought into the same financial and entrepreneurial complex. Taken together all this should be an example to French industrialists of how things were done better in England, all the more pointed because there were grave and exaggerated worries about the potential exhaustion of wood-fuel supplies in much of France, and a national survey of fuel use, with a desire to shift to coal, was about to be undertaken.[44] Under Calonne the French monarchy made large advances to the Le Creusot firm and effectively also took a share in the enterprise; eventually it became a company with a large shareholding. Périer, even though deeply involved with the great Paris waterworks scheme of the time, also became an investor in Le Creusot, and a major influence in the entrepreneurial team, and his approach was always risk-taking and expansionist.[45]

However, from 1782 the works at Le Creusot went ahead rapidly, despite canals on which hopes had been founded being unfinished, a great labour shortage having to be overcome in an underpopulated region, a huge and expensive cartage operation mounted, and grave problems of discipline among the large new labour force being encountered. Four blast furnaces were erected, twice the height of normal French ones, an unparalleled blast of 3,000 cubic feet of air a minute supplied by a steam-engine making 15 strokes a minute, while two more similar blowing engines supplied other furnaces. There were four large reverberatory furnaces for remelting pig for casting. Then there was a forge for converting some of the pig to wrought iron, with large steam-powered hammers, while the small source of water-power available was also used by employing steam power for water-returning. There was a large area used for coking coal in heaps. To French eyes a remarkable feature was six leagues of railway, with iron rails and trucks with cast iron wheels, partly horse-drawn, but with some downhill runs by gravity. The first smelting of coke-iron took place in December 1785.

But there are two aspects to be noted which somewhat reduce the importance of Wilkinson at Le Creusot and of Le Creusot itself. First, while Wilkinson certainly prepared the plans, and thus introduced the basic technology, the actual construction of the vast complex was carried out by Toufaire. There were initial problems over the linings of the first furnaces which were due to a mistaken choice of stone by Wilkinson or an English supervisor. French authorities then and since carefully pointed out that in the critical period between 1781 and 1784

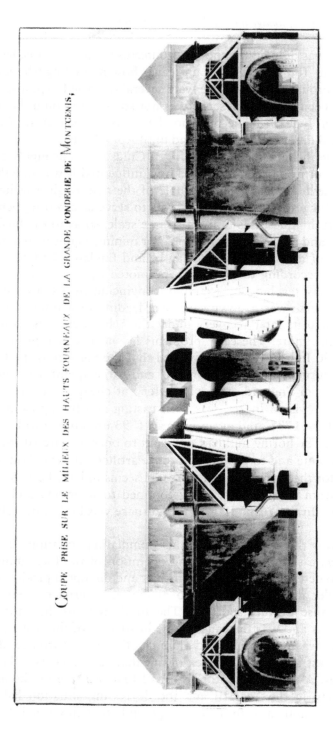

COUPE PRISE SUR LE MILIEUX DES HAUTS FOURNEAUX DE LA GRANDE FONDERIE DE MONTCENIS;

11.2 Section through the Wilkinson furnace, Le Creusot

Wilkinson was only on the spot at Montcenis for ten months, leaving a great deal to Toufaire. What is unclear is how many English workmen he in fact brought over; if there were several of varied expertise it may well have been that his presence was not so essential on a day-to-day basis. After June 1784 he may not have been much at Le Creusot, though he did not return to England until April 1786.

More significant is how successful Le Creusot was as highly capital-ized centre of iron production, and how influential it was in either the short or medium term as an example of the new English technology. 'This, the biggest works in France, was to serve as a testing bench for new iron techniques, this time on a large scale, so as to establish their solid basis and then advance further.' For mining engineers it was to be the means of making good their lag behind England. Le Creusot was also to be, according to those who promoted it, 'a school for others, that is to say teaching by example, convincing by its own success'. Sadly its course was a downward one, leading to a total collapse in 1814, though its later recovery under the Schneiders was to make it famous once more. The early problems lay in defective products. As late as 1790 Indret was not convinced that the pig iron of Le Creusot could be turned into good cannon, and large quantities were still imported from England, not only better but cheaper. Le Creusot, in-tended to provision Indret, was itself casting and boring cannon, but some made in 1788, and again in early 1793 are known to have been too brittle. The boring mill had to be put to boring charcoal-iron from Franche-Comté and to producing bronze artillery. It turned out ballast and shot for the Navy, but by the Year II seems to have been getting its pig iron from other works, being confined to remelting and cannon production. In the Year VIII a further furnace was built, but a charcoal one.

What was the explanation of this humiliating situation? The coal supply was a serious problem. The operation of the local mines was allowed to deteriorate, and the inefficient and disrupted production got worse under the Revolution. Two of the coke furnaces were closed down because of fuel shortage. The local iron ore had too much phosphorous and was the cause of the brittleness of the cast iron. The coke made was full of lime and alumina. The limited iron production from the vast industrial complex meant that capital costs inflated the iron prices. A technical visitor who had first seen the works in 1787 visited them in the Year III and the depressing situation led to his despairing comment 'Can it then be possible that those high hopes of

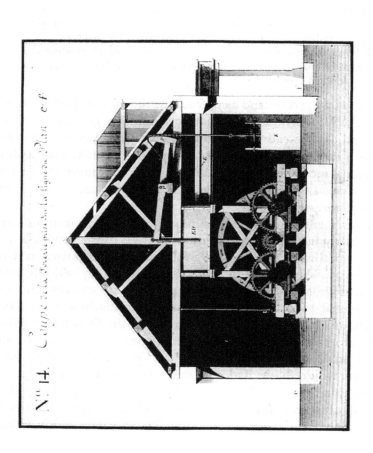

11.3 Wilkinson boring mill at Le Creusot

fortune and success were only in fact an illusion?' While good technical judges realized that the processes themselves were perfectly viable, they saw that fuel, ore, coking, were all adrift, and that the great works was sited in what was, for contemporary communication systems, a very inappropriate spot – whatever changes the future might bring.

Naturally, ironmasters in the rest of France were not the least inclined to try to copy so disastrous a venture. Conservative in general, possessing in charcoal iron-making under the 'indirect' method a system which had worked since the fifteenth century, nothing but a critical raw material shortage, or a flood of cheap foreign imports, or decisively demonstrated savings from a new production method would influence them, and then only with great reluctance. Rambourg the prominent ironmaster who had at one time supervised Indret, wrote as late as 1814:

> the people who so readily propose the use of mineral coal in place of charcoal don't seem to stop and consider that this implies changing almost everything in the furnace, the refineries, the machinery, the workshops, that ore has to be situated near mines which produce the right kind of coal, to have the ores near the fuel and train workers in the new kind of process.[46]

While seen on the one hand as potentially 'the most important works in Europe', Woronoff shows that 'cette usine grandiose parait monstrueuse'. At the end of the empire Le Creusot was insolvent and apparently a failure. For the past twenty years it had been difficult to urge a national movement towards British technology given the adverse publicity which Le Creusot inspired. Le Creusot was, in his telling verdict 'un contre-example'.[47]

The involvement of William Wilkinson in the French iron industry, and particularly in units of the industry directed to the production of armaments specifically intended to rival British naval power, is a remarkable story. The Wilkinson brothers took a totally self-interested business attitude to demands for their products or services, and this was exemplified by John Wilkinson's supplying machinery for naval copper production as well as his contribution to the French iron industry.[48] The brothers were as willing to offer their technical advice and services to Austria or Prussia as to France.[49] It is doubtful if all other ironmasters would have had the same uninhibited attitude; the Wilkinsons were strongly confident in their ability to lead the field, to dominate the British industry technically, and even more to maintain their lead over any continental competitors. The ease with which William

Wilkinson was able to pass between England and France, the absence of secrecy or cover-up in his contracts with the French government, shows the impotence of the British government when it came to dealing with significant businessmen as compared with mere managers or skilled workers who involved themselves in suborning, or were themselves suborned to go abroad. William Wilkinson probably took few workmen to France (it is a matter where evidence is incomplete) and as these may well already have been in the employ of the Wilkinsons in Britain it would be difficult to bring the 1719 Act to bear, for they could have travelled as domestic servants of some kind. Why the British government did not summon William Wilkinson home is not easy to understand, and he clearly thought it was a possibility. Over the war years communication would perhaps have been impossible, but there were periods before and after the war when he could readily have been recalled. Was it simply that in practice there was one law for workmen and another for entrepreneurs? De la Houlière's appraisal when first recruiting Wilkinson may have been a remarkably accurate one in this respect.

12 A Tale of Two Navies: Copper Sheathing

There was a second type of metal technology, and in this case an entirely naval one, in which the French quickly recognized an important British advance, and wished to secure the advantage for themselves. While the practice of coppering had other merits, its fundamental purpose was to defeat a grave problem, long recognized in both naval and mercantile shipping. This was the serious damage to the hulls of ships by the teredo or ship worm, and this pest was particularly prevalent in tropical and sub-tropical waters. These were increasingly penetrated both by European merchant ships, and – given the territorial disputes and quarrels over trade in these waters by the European powers – by naval vessels as well. This serious problem was the object of some ingenuity and experimentation by the maritime nations.

One solution was to put a temporary layer of wood planking over the underwater part of the hull. This did not eventually prevent the action of the worm on the hull itself, but it reduced and delayed it, and enabled ships to remain longer at sea without needing to be docked. An increased sea-life between repairs materially improved the economics of ship operation; in the case of naval shipping it was an effective increase in naval power if ships could spend longer at sea and less time in dockyards. But wooden sheathing was a useful palliative, not a real cure. Not only would the worm soon penetrate the sheathing, but the sheathing itself had to be replaced, and the ship had to return to a shipyard, have the old sheathing ripped off, have any hull damage which the sheathing had not prevented repaired, and new wooden sheathing put on. There was naturally a considerable cost in time, labour, and materials, and the ship's role, whether commercial or warlike, was interrupted, though of course the removal of the sheathing would be combined with other repairs and refitting. The earlier practice of sheathing with wood has sometimes led historians to confuse this with copper sheathing and predates that practice.[1]

The possibilities of the metal sheathing of ships were explored over the centuries. It appears to have been tried by the Romans, then by Spain and Portugal in the sixteenth century and subsequently in England. A major period of experimentation followed the development of rolled lead sheet in England towards the end of the seventeenth century. Here it was soon recognized that some deleterious process (much later identified as a galvanic action) took place between the lead sheathing and the iron fastenings of the ship, including the large bolts. This meant that the latter were eaten away until the whole security of the vessel was put at risk by its defective fastenings.

The failure of lead shifted attention to copper, and in 1708 the navy was offered a sheathing of copper and in 1740 of a brass-like alloy. It was also understood that if the process succeeded not only the worm but barnacles would be adversely affected, and that this would give improved sailing qualities.

It was in 1761 that the Royal Navy first seriously tried copper sheathing, on the *Alarm* frigate for the West India station. There ships were sometimes so worm-eaten and leaky as to be nearly unserviceable after two years, and resheathing with wood presented great difficulties. The gains in time at sea with coppered ships because of virtually complete protection from the worm, and the gains of speed and manoeuvrability because of the clean bottoms, were so appreciated that the results of galvanic action between copper sheathing and iron fastenings, though quickly perceived, were accepted, and the replacement of eroded iron bolts at refits became normal. High as were the costs of coppering, they could be reduced by recycling copper when it became worn, or when the ship was broken up. We cannot here go into the various devices which were turned to with limited effect to reduce galvanic action, the alternative to coppering with sheet by 'filling' with copper nails, the painting of the inner sides of the copper sheets, the placing of tarred paper and various compositions between copper and hull.

The practice of coppering had hardly taken hold in the navy much before the end of the Seven Years War, but the pace of sheathing with copper was greatly increased at the outset of French involvement in the American War of Independence. Its effects on ships' performance, as well as on time at sea, were enthusiastically marked by naval commanders. During the extreme difficulties of the British navy in that war the proportion of the fleet that could be kept at sea was highly important. Over a two-year period virtually the whole of the navy was coppered. However, the galvanic problem took its toll. Towards the end of the war there were some terrible losses of ships by sinking at sea, and as the larger ships carried huge crews of 600 to 850, the shock was all the greater, and it became irrefutable that many of the losses were due to the failure of iron fastenings by galvanic action. By the end of the war the Admiralty and Navy Board were coming round to the view that coppering was too dangerous, its installation was slowed down and complete abandonment contemplated.

Naturally this was a matter of serious worry to the copper industry, which had just found itself a lucrative market; the larger vessels could take around £700 of sheathing each, and coppering had been spreading to East Indiamen, West Indiamen, and slave-traders. The problem clearly could only be answered by a technical solution. Galvanic action, though imperfectly understood, obviously depended on the use of dissimilar metals in proximity. If copper could replace iron where both had been exposed to sea water, the difficulty might disappear. The central problem was that copper was so much softer than iron, not only for sheathing nails, but particularly for bolts. These had to be driven tightly into holes of smaller diameter bored in the timbers, so as to make the fastening watertight, and ones made of ordinary copper would bend hopelessly if so driven. Consequently, some of the best technical minds of the time concentrated on this question, but this effort will simply be summarized here, for it was only the successful solution which concerned the French, and led to their attempts to acquire it.

There were three sets of experiments. One was that of the West Midland industrialists Matthew Boulton and James Keir. This had begun at least as early as 1779, for at the end of that year Keir patented a copper-zinc-iron alloy bolt, and such bolts were already being tried at a navy yard. But by 1783 the bolts were abandoned as a failure. Two other powerful figures in the copper trade backed experiments which had important similarities. One was William Forbes, the existing copper contractor to the navy, who had made a fortune in the trade, and clearly did not want to lose a main element in his navy business. He took up the idea of Henry Cort of rolling metal through graduated rollers with incisions of decreasing size, which Cort had originally devised for recycling iron (for which he was a navy contractor) but which he later combined with the puddling process to produce the classic method of refining coke-pig to wrought iron. The speed of take-up of Cort's rolling process in the copper industry is astonishing. Cort's patent of January 1783 was followed up by one of July of that year taken out by Forbes for rolling copper in grooved rollers, either hot or cold. The third person to intervene in this technological race was Thomas Williams, the man who dominated the British copper industry in the late eighteenth century, and was to be its monopolist between 1787 and 1792.[2] Williams worked with Westwood and Collins, 'two ingenious artists of Birmingham'. William Collins developed a system by which copper bars were turned into bolts by being gripped between the grooved rollers of a rolling-mill and then pulled through steel drawplates until they were of much greater length. Westwood patented a system whereby copper was to be passed through graduated rollers with incisions of decreasing size. But his system has important advances on Forbes's. He made the rollers adjustable, so that they could be brought closer together or further apart at will, increasing the potential number of passes at different apertures. Secondly, he made the process one of undisputed *cold* rolling. Copper bars were to be passed between the rollers while under a cold water jet so that the friction of rolling did not heat the copper. It was probably Westwood's patent which predominated, but both were being employed by Williams's Parys Mine Company by January 1784.

For naval orders a comfortable agreement was arrived at between Forbes, Westwood and Collins at the end of 1783 which must have had the blessing of Thomas Williams, for he was clearly the patron of the Birmingham men. While the situation on the naval copper contracts is not easy to unravel, in 1784 the navy ordered all new ships to be fitted with the patent bolts. The Williams organization also supplied copper for many merchantmen, assisted by its control of the Liverpool market under the 1785 agreements which created the Cornish Metal Company, intended to divide up the national copper market. In that same year the Parys Company were said by Matthew Boulton (at that time deeply involved in the politics and organization of the copper trade)

> to have created many new uses for copper, particularly Forged Bolts and Nails which are used in all the Dockyards and their Rolled Bolts are sold to all the naval powers in Europe as well as their Sheathing: they have travelling agents abroad negotiating with France, Spain and Holland and workmen to show these states Experiments with the Bolts etc.[3]

Thus an apparently insuperable technical problem which was about to cause the abandonment of copper sheathing by the navies of Europe, and would certainly have prevented the extension of coppering to merchant fleets, had been resolved. How far had the French navy been an active rival or an imitator in these developments? How did it attempt to get this British technology for itself?

Hardly had the British naval trials begun to produce results than they were known of in France and a matter of keen interest to the French government. On 30 September 1764 Choiseul wrote to the Marquis de Blosset, who seems to have been in charge of intelligence at their London embassy, citing correspondence which had already passed between them, and mentioning information which Choiseul had already asked for about the attempts of the British navy to sheathe in copper ships of different types which were destined for colonial service. Blosset had obtained from a British peer some information indicating that the trial had not been too satisfactory. But Choiseul continued to urge Blosset to pass on to him everything he could possibly learn 'on the details of the putting on of this new sheathing'.[4]

The French navy certainly took up the practice, as did the Spanish, for a Spanish prize taken by the British in 1781 was coppered, and a special study was made by the Admiralty in 1782 of the *Pégase*, a French coppered ship taken by Barrington.[5]

In coppering the French had some serious handicaps as compared with the British. Their own copper mines were of small importance and the mining and manufacturing of indigenous copper made little impact on national demand. Britain in contrast had replaced Sweden as the leading mining and smelting country for copper, had pioneered the coal smelting of the metal, and was using rolling-mills to produce it in sheet form. The French had to import smelted copper, principally from Sweden, and their lack of a significant copper industry of their own also left them behindhand in the techniques of working the metal. However, by 1783 they were in a position to make their own rolled copper for sheathing. Before examining the very important and successful works in which this was done, it is worth noting the great and continuing interest which the French navy took in the subject of coppering and their close concern with what was happening across the Channel. A series of proposals was made to the Marine, particularly in the early 1780s.[6] The copper shortage inspired proposals to sheathe in lead and in tin (no doubt in ignorance of the unfortunate experience of the British with lead a century earlier); there was even a proposal to use tin plate.

Just as in Britain, in France the early 1780s was a time when the whole future of coppering was in doubt because of the loss of ships at sea from the failure of large iron bolts, critical in their basic construction and fastening. The French were also disturbed because of the excessive requirement to pump the ships, due to the leakage of sea water through the crevices left by bolts which shrank in diameter as galvanic action ate them away. There were therefore very naturally doubters in France: some officers stressed that it would be very sensible to see whether the British judged their early experience with copper sheathing a success before committing their own navy to what would be a highly costly process. The costs themselves were debated. If it would be possible to have a coppered ship at sea for four or five years without major attention to sheathing or hull, this would make the apparent relative cheapness of wood sheathing much less significant. Some commentators believed that the problems were even worse for French warships than British; the French used iron nails more freely, while the British used more trenails and wooden fastenings, which were of course unaffected by coppering. The French seem to have had problems with the quality of their copper nails, which was probably the reason why a considerable number of copper sheathing plates were lost during voyages. It was even proposed to secure copper sheathing with iron nails. Before copper was successfully rolled in France in 1783 the hammered plates previously used were not as smooth as the British rolled ones, and not so useful in preventing the adhesion of barnacles.

There was a seemingly excessive worry about the patina of verdigris on sheathing and various preparations were devised to coat the copper to avoid its formation. As in England there were several methods used to try to delay galvanic action, by painting the copper with various compositions, daubing with tallow, and by using a layer of tough paper between sheathing and hull, sometimes applied after heavy tarring with the best Baltic tar. Anything which might provide an acceptable alternative to copper was reported immediately to the Marine. Le Turc, the important industrial spy in Britain whom we will meet in other contexts, hurriedly reported on a British ship sent to the East Indies with a sheathing of sheets of compressed paper!

Even when the key copper-rolling processes were brought over from Britain, an operation which we will describe in the next section, there is evidence that the dominant French firm at Romilly was not prepared to make sheets, or bars for bolts, except to certain regular thicknesses for which there were large orders, which suggests that there was still a lack of technical flexibility. As in England there was experiment to find alloys which might be, in ease of working or durability, an improvement on pure copper; two cases reported in 1792 of trials with such alloys had proved disappointing.[7] High remelting costs, particularly when coal was not cheaply available, caused the French navy in 1786–87 to try to use again the old copper sheets from ships being resheathed or broken up. They apparently employed convict labour with iron-tipped mallets to reshape the sheets and close up the old nail holes. Convict labour was no doubt used because the verdigris dust caused much sickness and even deaths among their workers. Even so, many sheets were wasted. It was proposed in 1792 to set up a machine with cast iron screw presses and cylinders to do the job.[8]

All this indicates that the French fully appreciated the importance of the English invention of copper sheathing ships, and having quickly put it into practice themselves they equally understood its advantages and its problems. A great deal of ingenuity was exercised on their side to try to eliminate the difficulties, as we have seen. But the French did not arrive at any solutions to the main galvanic action problem equal to the British one which Westwood and Collins had found, and in the beginning they did not even have any ordinary rolling-mills which were suitable to make good copper sheathing plates.

The initiative in producing rolled plates was taken by Le Camus de Limare, a Louviers industrialist who was also one of the entrepreneurs in a very early machine spinning factory in that town. Born in 1736, son of a prominent tanner and leather merchant, he had three uncles who were major woollen manufacturers. He himself progressed towards banking and finance and became also a tax collector.

In one of the most remarkable pieces of military-industrial espionage of the eighteenth century Le Camus was in England in 1781 at the height of the war examining the production of copper sheets for sheathing and engaging English workers to make them. We can be sure of the date because Le Camus wrote to the Marine on 10 March 1782 referring to a memoir he had written to them on the technicalities of copper sheathing on 1 December 1781 'on my return from England'.[9] A much later memoir from the proprietors of the works he founded[10] stated that 'this branch of industry (copper sheathing) was in large degree confined to England. The founder of the Romilly works had managed by 1782 to obtain for himself at great expense, and even greater risk, workmen of that nation, who, backing up his inventive genius' had set up at Romilly melting, refining, rolling and other plant.[11] Le Camus, his successors stated, had at least enabled France to share 'avec son ennemi capital' a branch of industry of which Britain previously had the exclusive operation, and in which it had made the French its dependents. Sadly, there are no details of this outstanding piece of espionage. A surviving letter from Le Camus to Matthew Boulton,[12] would indicate that his English was excellent, which would have been an important advantage. How many workmen he originally secured is not known.

The Marine archives give some further background. In March 1782 the Comte de Hector at the Brest naval base wrote to the Minister enclosing a memoir from Le Camus on the way in which the English coppered their warships and merchant vessels. As he had travelled in England, and had observed English production methods, Hector thought his observations would be very valuable to the French navy.[13] He believed the English dimensions for the sheathing sheets were more suitable and the thickness of rolled plates was more regular than those of hammered ones. The long, uneven, French hammered plates became holed within a few months. The English nails were better shaped and the sheathing was more surely attached to the hulls, while they varied the thickness of the sheathing which covered different parts of the hull. Though having doubts about some of Le Camus's proposals, including those about copper fastenings for rudders, Hector wanted to keep in touch with him and have him over to Brest for an extended visit. It is clear from the correspondence that Le Camus was not simply passing on his English experience, but that he had already embarked on English-pattern manufacture. He had in fact proposed such a manufacture to the navy as early as 1780, promising to provide them with all the cast, hammered and rolled copper they needed.[14] Even so he would be basing his production on the original technology of copper sheathing over iron fastenings, but this would not yet be a relative disadvantage, for the great British breakthrough to copper fastenings, made possible by the Westwood and Collins inventions, only occurred after the war ended.

Le Camus picked on the site at Romilly in the valley of the Andelle, where there was a cluster of old fulling-mills, for water power was of the greatest priority for operating rolling-mills and powered hammers. This was shown by Thomas Williams's great British works both at Hollywell in Flintshire and on the Thames at Marlow and Wraysbury. Already, when the Comte de Hector was writing to the Marine, Le Camus had started building his works. At this point, as we have shown, rolling sheet copper by water-power, not the cold rolling or drawing of copper bolts was involved. While Le Camus's works would, when it came into production in 1783, have potentially solved the problem of coppering the French navy, it would not have been in a position to solve the problem of galvanic action. The French navy would, like the British, soon have been brought to the point of abandoning coppering unless it could have cracked that problem. The long-term success of Romilly is recognized, but this could not have been achieved unless it had been able produce hardened bolts. How was this technology gained?

Once the war was ended a highly qualified team of French experts, largely military men, quickly went to England. They concentrated heavily on two industries which were essential for armaments, where British leadership was indisputable, and they wanted to check up on the wartime advances made in Britain. The party included Wendel, already deeply involved with William Wilkinson at the Indret cannon works, and currently replacing him in its operation. He was the leading light as we have seen in the creation of Le Creusot, with William Wilkinson as the technical adviser. There were two other artillery officers in the team, with whom he was closely associated, de Givry and Dulubre. These three were accompanied on part of their trip by the brilliant engineer J. C. Périer, and his younger brother, Augustin. J. C. Périer was the main intermediary, as we shall see, in the importation of Watt engines into France in most remarkable circumstances. The cylinders of the engines had of course been supplied by John Wilkinson.

John Wilkinson indulged in a certain amount of play-acting, as on other occasions. Périer had naturally come on steam-engine business, with a visit to Boulton and Watt at Soho which included engine payments.[15] Watt wrote to Wilkinson that the party were on the way to see him at his Broseley and perhaps his Bradley works too. The French visitors he said, apart from the Périers, consisted of three 'ironmasters and not ignorant ones' de Wendel not being the only one to combine industrial and military functions. Boulton and Watt advised the Coalbrookdale Company and their neighbours, William Reynolds and Co., that the Frenchmen were about, and very inquisitive concerning 'the new processes for making barr Iron. I learnt what they know already and took all the care I could to give them no fresh knowledge'. He said they had complained about the difficulties experienced in getting into works in England and the refusal of the owners to show them off – all the more interesting in that they reported on this matter to their own government in a very contradictory way.[16] In writing a warning to Reynolds, Watt did indicate that some of the Frenchmen already knew Wilkinson.[17] However, giving a warning to Josiah Wedgwood[18] a day or so later, Watt deluded himself that 'Mr. Wilkinson to whom they are gone will not be very communicative'. He was not certain that they would go spying in the Potteries, but forewarned Wedgwood that 'they are clever people'. Wilkinson told Boulton and Watt that the party consisted of a Champagne ironmaster, two artillery inspectors and a small arms works director, besides the Périers. Here he was being much less than candid, he knew perfectly well that Wendel was not only an artillery expert, but a major ironmaster, and his brother's collaborator in both Indret and Le Creusot. And Périer was not merely involved with the engines of the Paris water company, he too was now deeply involved with Le Creusot. William Wilkinson at this point took over the party and guided them to the Cheshire saltfield, Manchester, Liverpool and Ravenhead.

It is the last name, Ravenhead, which leads us from the maze of steam-engine and iron business with which the French party was concerned and concentrates on the third major target of the Frenchmen – copper sheathing. Ravenhead was the newest and largest copperworks in Britain, having been recently built by the Parys Mine Company, a dynamic mining, smelting and manufacturing concern, based on the Anglesey mines, and led by the outstanding lawyer-entrepreneur, Thomas Williams of Llanidan. The Parys Company had sited their great smelter on the Sankey (or St Helens) Canal, and on the rich coal-mines of John Mackay, a daring Scottish industrialist who had bought the adjacent Ravenhead estate. He developed the policy of inducing very large industrial enterprises to site themselves on his lands and consume great quantities of his coal, where other local coalmasters had merely thought to export local coal to Liverpool or the Cheshire saltfield by the canal. In 1773 he had attracted to his lands the huge glassworks which first exploited French plate glass technology in Britain.[19] In the late 1770s, once in control of the cheap copper ores of the Parys Mine in Anglesey, Thomas Williams as their manager had contracted with Mackay to build the great Ravenhead smelter.

Williams and Wilkinson were soon closely linked in business deals. Already by 1780 Wilkinson was sending iron to Williams for the equipment of his works. Wilkinson also supplied Williams with an illegal or 'pirate' Watt engine for Ravenhead. In 1781 they made a journey to Scotland together. Williams was in 1785 to take over the half of the Anglesey mines he had not previously controlled, forming the Mona Mine Company. John Wilkinson was from the outset a partner in one of its two subsidiaries. The year 1785 was to see profound revolutions in the British copper industry, overthrowing the long monopoly of the Associated Smelters, and in this John Wilkinson lent Williams powerful and decisive support. The Ravenhead works was the principal supplier of the works near Holywell in Flintshire of which the main output was naval copper.[20]

The report of the Wendel party is one of a handful of descriptions of British copper smelting available for this period and one of the best. The French experts described Ravenhead as 'a famous copper smelter'. There was clearly no restriction or inhibition on their examination of the works, and the manager, Joseph Harris[21] must have been given instructions by Thomas Williams to allow them every facility. As we will see, the Parys Mine Company was in negotiation for huge contracts with the French navy in the same year. Williams had the same policy of openness to foreign visitors as his friend John Wilkinson, and he must have known through Wilkinson exactly how closely his visitors were integrated into the French armaments programme. There was, of course, little likelihood that the French would be able to set up a great coal-fired copper smelter, they lacked the copper ore in the first place, but we will see that Williams's policy of openness went beyond his Ravenhead operations. The French party gathered condensed but accurate information on Ravenhead, its forty-eight reverberatory furnaces, the yield of Anglesey ore smelted, the degree of preparation of the ore by washing and roasting (which had been done at the mine) and the extent to which some ore needed preliminary treatment at the smelter. They learnt about the charges of the reverberatory furnaces for preliminary roasting, and of the repeated smeltings, up to six for fine copper. The final refining process they did not remark on, possibly it was not being carried out on the day of their visit. But they learned of the coal/ore ratio, the price of coal (under 5 shillings a ton) and its consumption by the works, which was 30,000 tons a year. This great smelter could produce about 1,300 tons of fine copper a year, probably nearly one-fifth of national production. They were given a price at which standard grade copper could be shipped to Dunkirk by the Parys Company.[22]

So far the de Wendel party had gained much information on the efficiency of the British copper industry without obtaining much military-technological intelligence which they could directly employ on their return. But they now moved to the Holywell works of the Parys Company, equally under the control of Thomas Williams and built with astonishing speed on the powerful Holywell stream as it ran down to the Dee estuary. They were new works, completed in 1780. There smelted copper, largely from Ravenhead, was turned into manufactures. By the time of the de Wendel party's visit naval copper seems to have predominated over the original primary purpose of the works which was said to be producing copper goods for the slave trade, and their report called it 'manufactory of copper plates for ships'. They entirely concentrated their report on naval copper.

They described the rolls for manufacture of sheet copper which were made of cast iron, each being 18 inches in diameter and four feet 6 inches long. They were powered by the fast-flowing Holywell stream, as were other rolls for the production of copper bolts of different diameters 'which are to be substituted for those of iron in vessels which are copper sheathed because experience has shown that the iron was very quickly destroyed'. The new rolling-mills with graduated channels were discussed and drawn, though the drawings do not seem to have survived. The use of rolls with incisions of decreasing size, and the ability to further vary the size of the apertures by altering the distance between the rolls by means of adjusting screws on the roller frames, are clearly described. The French observers seem to have missed the water cooling of the rolled bolts, but were aware that the final shaping was given by cold working under a water-powered hammer to remove the rough edges and give perfect roundness. The use of powered shears to trim off the bolt lengths was also noted. The strength and elasticity of the bolts was shown by a test where 1.5 inch bolts were weighted so as to bend an inch out of true, and then returned to perfect straightness when the weights were removed. The importance of these works for naval demand was shown by their contract to supply the navy with 20 tons of bolts a week.

Givry and Dulubre had been given special permission as artillery officers by the Maréchal de Ségur and the king himself to accompany Wendel and report on mine working, smelting of minerals, refining of metals and other English manufactures. Wendel was clearly regarded as the most expert, by whom the others were to be guided. Their report of 27 March 1784 is remarkable not only for their good account of copper smelting and the making of sheathing and bolts, but for a great deal of detail on Woolwich Arsenal, which they seem to have got into with little difficulty. There they obtained details of the strength of the artillery units, the proving of guns, and the making of bronze guns. They were able to converse with the famous Dutch master cannon-founder Pieter Verbruggen, apparently without constraint.[23] Givry and Dulubre seem to have obtained much information about both land and sea artillery, and reported on the first, adverse, reaction to the new carronades by British naval officers. They also reported on the number of muskets held in stock nationally and the British reliance on the commercial market, including that of Birmingham, for muskets and side-arms.

Their conclusion was that the comparison with Britain indicated that France had little to fear on the supply of arms. This of course took into consideration the expertise already brought by Wilkinson to Indret and the expectations for Le Creusot. But they were seriously wrong in thinking that Jars had obtained all the needful expertise on cementation steel. They also believed that all the hardware manufacturing skills were now as perfect in France as in England, and mentioned the works of the Orsels. They stressed the extensive use of coal in England, particularly in the iron industry, and at another point admitted that French ironworks were not commercially competitive with the British. Their trip was just too early to enable them to appreciate the developments by Cort, but like de la Houlière in 1775 they gave a short account of the stamping and potting process for refining iron. They believed that the combination of coal and the new canal network was of the greatest importance, given the low canal tolls and the absence of internal customs dues. They remark on the ease of manufacture of cast iron, and its adoption for larger engineering parts, particularly gears, and for railed ways.

Their favourable conclusion on the general question of arms was perhaps influenced by a desire not to decry too much the efforts of their own government and their military superiors. But the considerable part of their report given to the copper sheathing issue runs counter to that overall optimistic view, as does the urgent need felt by the French government for their early and energetic post-war enquiry into the industry of a nation which the French had just defeated. They admitted that the time they had had in England, only two months, had been a problem, referring to 'the great difficulty one experiences in being able to see the different premises, and the rapidity with which we had to hasten through them'. Here there is once again a contradiction about the ease of admission to industrial sites to which we will return.[24]

At the beginning of 1784 Le Camus was announcing that his works at Romilly was fully operational as far as rolling sheet copper for naval vessels was concerned, and he was also able to supply copper parts for the fastenings of ships' rudders, but there was no mention of bolts. Romilly was the sole French provider of sheathing to their navy, and Le Camus claimed that this had removed a need to get expensive sheathing from England. He demanded *manufacture royale* status for his firm. Once the war was over it became important for Romilly to open up a civilian market as the naval one declined, and outlets were looked for in making blanks for copper coinage, and goods for the slave and East India trades.[25]

Obviously if Romilly could make copper bolts as well as sheathing the copper naval market would be increased, and the French navy would no longer need to import bolts from England if it was to avoid the problems of galvanic action. How did the French set about getting the bolt-making process? Again we are back to John Wilkinson. On 22 May 1784, only a few months after the visit of the Wendel–Givry party to the Parys Company's works at Greenfield near Holywell, John Westwood, who with William Collins had patented the processes used by the Parys Company, wrote to the Navy Board. While at the mills to advise on an aspect of bolt-making for an order which Collins was fulfilling for the Navy, he had learned something very startling. 'I have received such information concerning Tools which have been made by Mr. Wilkinson of Bersham Foundry and I have every reason to expect there are Grooved Rolers [*sic*] on a ship which is now at Cnars Quay in Chester River' [Connah's Quay on the Dee]. He had no legal proof because he had not been able to find any customs officer to search the ship, but his own staff and the clerks of the Parys Company were quite sure that the equipment was made at Bersham and was now on the vessel, which had also taken on material for engineers, cast iron pigs[26] and lead. Wilkinson of course had a large interest in lead mines.

The Navy Board should organize a search of the vessel, thought Westwood. There was no doubt of her destination, which was France. Westwood realized that powerful people might be involved – 'I hope this information may not be made publick' – and he suggested that the Board get in touch with Collins who might be in London or with John Dawes, the important East India Company Director and banker, who was Williams's partner in the Parys Mine Company. In fact it is certain that the export of tools and machinery was legal at this date, apart from that of the textile industries, and it would have been impossible for the authorities to do anything about Wilkinson's exports before the Tool Act of 1785. Though Westwood does not specifically say so, it seems probable that Wilkinson could readily fulfil the French order for bolt-making rolls because he had already supplied Williams with those at the Holywell works; not only was he the leading founder and turner, but his Bersham works (near Wrexham) could hardly have been handier. No one could have better understood than Westwood the importance of this particular export for French naval power.[27]

This seems to solve the mystery as to how the new British bolt-making technology got to Le Camus's works at Romilly. It does not mean that Romilly immediately replaced British suppliers, particularly the Parys Mine Company. In June 1785 the Navy Minister, de Castries, was following the example of the British Navy Board and forming a project to replace iron fastenings by copper ones under the waterline of French ships. He regarded this as the preferred technique, but he was carefully costing the price of iron as compared with copper fastenings, taking the example of a seventy-four-gun ship. He was examining favourably estimates prepared by Pascoe Grenfell, a business associate of Thomas Williams, for sheathing and for fastenings: 'These prices seemed all the more moderate to me in that his samples of every kind of item have now been recognized at Brest as being of superior quality'.[28] In December at the naval base of Rochefort the Comte de Vaudreuil (the commander), de la Grandville (the intendant), 'all the Members of the Marine Council' and two technical experts carried out trials on a range of materials produced by Pascoe Grenfell. We can be sure that the materials were from the Parys Company because the relevant translated document comes from the archives of the Anglesey Mines.[29] The British copper products were tested against French iron ones, and the tensile strength and elasticity of the British copper bolts found much superior. A bolt of Grenfell's copper well over 6 feet long was driven into the stem of a French battleship through a hole of smaller diameter. It took over an hour to drive it in and was so tight that it took four hours to pull it out! Copper spikes supplied by Grenfell were satisfactory but not always as hard as iron ones.

There were no French copper bolts tried in comparison with English, clearly because Le Camus de Limare was not yet producing them at Romilly. His copper nails, however, were compared with Grenfell's. Rather more of Le Camus's nails broke, but not disastrously (fifteen out of 207). The outstanding differences were in the heads of the nails; the English ones were able to form a surface flush with the sheathing, the French ones, clumsy and uneven, would have affected the fouling of the ships. The heads were not well attached, and flew off when the sheathing was stripped off again, which probably indicated that they did not secure the sheathing so well. The metal of the British and French nails was examined when broken, and the French copper was found badly melted and full of air holes. Large copper screws provided by Grenfell were excellent and capable of being reused. His sheathing was remarked on as being 'perfectly well rolled and of an equal thickness throughout', implying that Le Camus's, which was also tested, was not. Some of the heavier copper work, for rudders for instance, supplied by Grenfell was highly approved, and much harder than any formerly cast and used at Rochefort, while there was a noticeable saving in weight. At the end of 1785, therefore, the French production of naval copper was still qualitatively behind the British, and they were not yet producing bolts, while their prices were much higher; in nails the English produced more good nails per pound of copper, and overall their nail contract price bore a 13:30 ratio to Le Camus's, 'which is immense'.

There can be no doubt how Le Camus got over his technical difficulties; he did it by recruiting English workers in large numbers, but exactly how is not clear. If Le Camus was able to examine English works in 1781 he may have recruited some English workers then, despite the difficulties of wartime, but these would have only been skilled in reheating furnaces and in plain rolling. It would only be after the English advances of 1783–84 that he could have recruited English workers able to manage the graduated rollers obtained from Wilkinson. Some of the plain rolls at Romilly were very poor by British standards, being heavy wooden rolls covered with iron plate. According to John Vivian, Le Camus had to import some large English plain rolls for making copper sheathing, which he got from a London founder, and as 'the French do very little in the Copper trade without English implements', when one broke he had to send it to London to be recast. But the passing of the Tools Act in 1785 prevented it being returned to him, and according to Vivian, had a very adverse effect on his production. The anticipation that the Tools Act might be repealed in 1786 had, he said, been an important reason why Le Camus had been able to find additional financial backing with the aim of increasing production, because that depended on his being able to get more English rolling machinery, which would be possible if the Act was repealed. In fact rolling-mills were specifically included in the new 1786 Act.[30]

A fairly detailed description of the works was published in 1787[31] with information supplied by Le Camus. Romilly did not smelt, but remelted old copper, melted down copper cakes or ingots from various sources, and mixed different coppers and refined them. There were some rolling-mills for square bars, which the reporter had not seen, but Romilly claimed that the relevant machine was now 'more perfect and quicker than those they use in England'. Reverberatory furnaces were used not only for melting and refining, but for reheating at the various stages of manufacture. Romilly was producing the copper bolts and fastenings which were now replacing iron on copper sheathed ships. Cold rolling by rollers with graduated incisions is described, and then the final shaping on channelled anvils under heavy powered hammers, with hammers of different weights for different thicknesses of bolts. Of the six water-wheels which drove the plant with great economy of water, four were over 20 feet in diameter.

A knowledgeable account of about the same date forms part of the report of the local inspector, Goy, on the industries of the town and Generality of Rouen. He had apparently recently prepared a prospectus on the manufacture at Romilly. The concern was particularly interesting 'because it has withstood for several years the efforts of the English companies which operate in the copper trade.' While capable of producing manufactures for the civilian market 'at this present moment this works is solely occupied in the King's service' that is, for naval copper.[32] However, as late as 1787, while supply of the French navy was supposed to be entirely from the 'works in its infancy' at Romilly, the great Norman and Paris banking house of Lecouteulx was in fact importing naval copper from England.[33]

Many of the reports and observations on Romilly do not bring out the importance, or even the existence, of an English workforce. But a report on the manufactures of Alençon, Caen and Rouen, possibly for the information of Louis XVI on his visit to the great harbour works at Cherbourg, mentions the Romilly plant, though not under that name. It says critically that 'it has not yet arrived at the extent and perfection of which it is capable', but adds encouragingly,

> one can forecast from what is already there that this concern will become one of the finest and most useful in the kingdom. The greater part of the workers are English, and have brought with them their wives and children in such a way that it constitutes a kind of colony that deserves particular protection. At this very moment they are

asking for letters of naturalization for them, and they propose to put the request before the Controller-General in the next few days.[34]

This statement is fortunate, because it backs that of Arthur Young in 1788 on 'a manufacture of copper-plates, for the bottoms of the King's ships; a colony of Englishmen'.[35] It is unlikely that all the workers were English, however; it would have been a prime object of the proprietors to see that French workers participated and thus domesticated all the skills in France.

One reason for the fall in the total number of workers from between 200 and 250 before 1789 to 120 in 1805 may have been the departure of English workers under the pressures of revolution and war. Certainly in 1805 there were only four Englishmen listed. They were all foremen, probably even what would now be called 'department managers', or would contemporaneously have been termed 'agents' in British copper works. These were 'Grist' (Griffith?) Powell, the master of the foundry [given as 'Griffey Poley' in another return], John Harris, the master roller, and William Harris the master hammerman. Two years earlier there had also been listed Daniel Grimpret [sic] the foundry inspector.[36]

The whole question of the recruitment of the once large English team at Romilly, of whom these four were the remnant, is unanswered. We may perhaps guess that Powell, with his Welsh name, could be of Swansea origin, as of course that was a great smelting centre, where remelting, refining and alloying skills would have been fairly plentiful. The two Harrises make one wonder if there was a connection with Joseph Harris, the manager of Thomas Williams's Ravenhead works, and if he recommended them. While the names of their places of origin are garbled in French, one, William, was domiciled at Wraysbury, Buckinghamshire, and John, his brother, was also recorded as being of Buckinghamshire origin. At Wraysbury and Bisham Thomas Williams had two mills which were mainly devoted to the production of naval copper, but were his own possession, and not part of the Anglesey Mines organization. As he seems only to have acquired Wraysbury in 1788, the Harrises may have left for France before then, but rolling-mills had been operated there by the previous owners, Pengree and Company. A First Empire list of English civilians, officially 'hostages', but men not confined to prison camps after the resumption of war in 1803, lists a John Daniel Grimpret, inspector at the Romilly works, John Harris, 'master hammerman in copper', a William Harris and a Victor Harris. The last was born in France, presumably the son of one of the other Harrises, and was certainly a metalworker.[37]

In 1785 Le Camus increased the capital of the firm by taking in several partners. One was the Spanish scientist, diplomat and businessman Yzquierdo. Though officially 'vice-directeur du Cabinet du Roi D'Espagne' his activities went far beyond the cultural, and he normally lived in Paris. It was through his intervention that Romilly was turned into a joint-stock company with a capital of 800,000 *livres*. The Rouen and Paris banking houses of Lefebvre and Lecouteulx and a Paris notary were brought in. The capital was doubled again in 1787. As Belhoste and Peyre rightly insist, Romilly became 'a perfect example of very large scale enterprise', like Le Creusot or the Paris water company, which were created at the very end of the *ancien régime* with massive backing from financiers and bankers. Yzquierdo at about the same time was also participating with Le Camus in one of the first great cotton-mills in France at Louviers, and then the two, with the Lecouteulx and the Duc de Rochefoucauld, set up a large stocking-frame factory at La Roche-Guyon, using the latest English machines. In all three cases Yzquierdo was clearly trying to get a hold on the latest English technology entering France, with the intention of transmitting it to Spain.[38]

With the reorganizations of the Romilly concern in 1792 and 1795 we need not concern ourselves,[39] as there is not so much an infusion of new British technology as an extension of that already acquired. It is an interesting sidelight on the necessary auxiliary parts of British coal-fuel technologies, that in 1787 Romilly had to set up a special brickworks to free itself from the need to import English firebrick for its furnaces. But while Romilly displayed a combination of technologies quite new in France at the end of the eighteenth century 'the technological level of the equipment however still remained poor as compared with the English plant' and this was particularly noticeable in the water-wheel arrangements and the wooden transmission drives, deficiencies which Belhoste and Peyre think were due to leaving these aspects to French technicians.[40]

Before Romilly there had been only small rolling-mills for non-ferrous metals, for instance one erected by d'Haristoy at Deville near Rouen in 1764, and even this was a foreign machine; given his keenness to import English processes it was probably an English one. Lead seems to have been the metal rolled. Another mill was built at Saint Sever in Rouen in 1776, and in this suburb dominated by the Holkers it would be surprising if it were not English. One mounted for the de Dietrichs in Alsace was built for them in England, but on a German pattern, and since they were famous ironmasters it was probably used in that industry.

Once Romilly was operative there were imitators. A substantial works was built nearby at Maromme in 1789, but was turned to bronze cannon-founding and was integrated with Romilly in 1797.

An interesting works, which seems to have been largely overlooked, is reported on by the American industrial traveller Joshua Gilpin. This was in the neighbourhood of Avignon, and was run by an Englishman called Richardson. A brass founder on the Thames near London, he had been nearly ruined when his works burned down uninsured. He worked for a Mr Elliot in Normandy from 1787 until 1796 – Gilpin unfortunately forgot the name of the works – but Richardson then came to work for Elliot at the Avignon works. Like so many in the Revolutionary period it was sited in a great monastery and its church, coal was piled high in the cloisters, the refectory had become a rolling-mill, the smoke of the furnaces hung in the roof of the splendid church, it all made 'an odd and striking contrast'. The works with its five melting furnaces, two pairs of rolls and two tilt hammers were 'employed wholly in making copper sheets and compound [alloy] bolts and nails for the Navy'. The coal came down the Rhône from Montcenis, and Gilpin knew of Wilkinson's Le Creusot works there. The workmen were all French, and Richardson said 'he never found persons who were more apt to learn and better disposed to work. Some difficulties occur in first training them but since then he has them busy and attentive without trouble.' These works were no doubt directed to supplying the Mediterranean ports with naval copper, as Romilly was to the Channel and Atlantic ones. But Gilpin after talking with Richardson about this and other industrial plant found that it 'still seemed to conform to my idea of the infancy of most manufactures in France ... these works of which every little stream affords an example in England [were] here boasted of as capital manufactories'. But, as with Romilly, there had been 'numerous English families which came here before the war, there now remain only two'. A member of one family had become a French army officer, and the other family in fact came from America.[41]

The French naval copper manufacturers were much concerned that the Eden Treaty of 1786 allowed British manufactured copper to enter at reduced rates, and the Romilly Company was supported in its complaints by the public representations of their Norman neighbours, pointing to the importance of the industry at all times and 'have become of such great importance in time of war'. If the treaty could not be overthrown, at least Romilly should be helped by having import duties on the raw copper it imported abolished.[42] However, the terms of the Eden Treaty, limiting the duty on imported manufactured copper to 10 per cent *ad valorem*, were not allowed to operate. They were not observed by the customs officers on the basis that the bars and sheets coming in were not fully manufactured and as semi-manufactures should pay the old higher duty on raw materials. While the avidity of the farmers-general was blamed by the British, one may suppose that the Romilly firm gave them every encouragement.[43]

Romilly was at a peak just before the Revolution; for a time after the outbreak of war it was threatened by a shortage of imported copper, but this was overcome by the famous device of the Revolutionary government in ordering the melting-down of all church bells, which normally had a one-third yield of copper. The Peace of Amiens briefly reduced naval demand and endangered Romilly's prosperity, but the renewal of the war led to a lengthy period of prosperity and good trading. Prosperity had a kind of problem of its own, new French firms wanting to go into naval copper production sought to entice workers away, while the proprietors complained loudly in the Year XIII that 'The Englishmen who are the heads of the workshops and have been at the manufacture since its foundation have had their loyalty unsettled' by 'a scandalous practice, which had as its object to engage them for a similar works, set up at Ferrol'.[44] The entrepreneurs had to divert this plot of their Spanish allies by getting these chief workmen to renew their contracts at some financial cost to the firm in higher pay.

The French attempt to obtain by industrial espionage and the seduction of workers the vital technology of coppering ships is a remarkable episode in the history of the transfer of technology in the eighteenth century, and like the cannon-founding at Indret and Le Creusot, was driven by military needs. It is however a complex story. It shows that it was possible to recruit and remove to France large numbers of skilled English workmen, but not possible to retain most of them for long. While through the intermediacy of the Wilkinsons it was possible for French military men and engineers to inspect British copper smelting and sheet and bolt-making plant, their testimony about the ease of viewing manufactures in general is varied, even contradictory. The role of the Wilkinsons is again critical in the securing of the incised and adjustable rolls which had been developed for copper bolt manufacture in England – it is interesting that the use of such rollers in the Cort iron process (for which they were first devised) did not happen in France until Dobson introduced them *c*.1800, and even then they did not immediately catch on.[45] Again, though the Romilly plant achieved its basic purpose, it was not for some time thought of as being as technically efficient, or as economical, as its British rivals. In 1819, when Romilly received a gold medal for its copper sheathing sheets, it was said of the firm 'the name alone is praise enough'. But the left-handed compliment that its huge works enabled it to arrive at perfection 'which it is on the point of achieving' seems to imply some reservations even at that date.[46]

Two Other Industries: Steam-Power and Glass

PART FOUR

Two Other Industries:
Steam-Power and Glass

13 The Steam-Engine in France: Newcomen and Watt

Newcomen

The steam-engine was the single most famous technological development in Britain in the eighteenth century. Its transfer abroad began at an early stage both in the case of the Newcomen and that of the Watt engine. Given the degree of foreign interest and the potential importance of the inventions it would naturally be expected that they would be a focus of industrial espionage, but while some clear cases of espionage can be found, it does not play a great part in their diffusion abroad. On the one hand there was no resistance by the authorities in Britain to the export of the mechanical parts of the engine, or to the journeys abroad of expert artisans who would erect it.

In France, with which this study is particularly concerned, both the Newcomen proprietors and the Boulton and Watt partners took formal and official steps to obtain a privileged and protected status for their engines in France, and it was not their fault that such privileges, though obtained, were of no real value to them. During the eighteenth century, the period of this study, the impact of the steam-engine in France was very limited. This seems not to be due to any obstacles which the British put in the way of the French acquiring engines – indeed there is a remarkable episode in which the British government assisted their export in wartime – but to the limited extent to which France had been able to follow Britain down the path of creating a coal-fuel economy. With only a small number of large coal-mines, and an extreme paucity of metalli-

ferous ores, a major potential employment for the steam-engine in draining mines and (late in the century) winding coal and ores, hardly existed
in France. When towards the end of the century it became possible to
follow the British example in erecting large spinning factories, French
industrialists preferred water-power to steam except in a few instances.[1]
There is thus a kind of paradox, by which the flow of a leading-edge
technology abroad was not inhibited, yet resulted only in a trickle of
transfers. In this section this situation will be looked at and commented
on, but there will be no attempt at a detailed account of every instance of
transfer, as espionage was not the normal means by which it was achieved.

Knowledge of the existence of the Newcomen engine on the Continent was very rapid. This has to be seen against a change in the
historical view of the early years of the Newcomen engine in Britain.
Once thought of as an instance of slow diffusion, the spread of the
Newcomen engine (even during the years when it was affected by the
costs of patenting under the extended patent originally granted for the
very different Savery engine) is now known to be very rapid. Over
ninety engines, despite a cost of around £1,500 a time, were erected
between 1712 (when the first Tipton engine was built) and the expiry
of the patent in 1733. Similarly, the view that the Newcomen engine
was the creation of mere mechanics, quite outside the purview of the
scientific world, is now exploded.[2] The interest of the Royal Society in
the successive experiments with the vacuum, steam pressure and condensation is well established, and if Newcomen, unlike Papin and
Savery, was not a Fellow of the Royal Society, this was possibly for
social and religious reasons relating to his extreme non-conformity, not
to any intellectual inferiority. He, after all, produced a classic solution
to a problem that fascinated contemporary minds, and from 1712
onwards his had to be regarded as 'a phenomenally successful machine'.[3] Alan Smith has pointed out that contributions to the evolution
of the first steam-engines were made by the following Fellows (or
foreign members) of the Royal Society: Huygens, Leibnitz, Papin, Boyle,
Hooke, Sloane, Desaguliers (of Huguenot descent but an Englishman)
and Newton, as well as lesser known Fellows like Savery, Thomas
Ayres, Henry Beighton, John Meres and James Lowther. Ayres, Lowther
and Meres were all members of the Fire Engine Proprietors, the company which exploited the Newcomen engine after 1716, and of which
Newcomen himself was for a time a member.[4]

Given the contacts and correspondence between leading European
scientists the Newcomen engine could hardly escape being quickly

known internationally. We know that the first successful engine at Tipton was very soon visited by the Spanish ambassador 'with a large suite of foreigners, to see the new engine, (he) was not even allowed to enter the engine house however large a reward he offered, and had to return very dissatisfied without having seen anything but the wonderful results that this ... engine was able to produce'.[5] However, some foreigners soon had an intimate knowledge of the engine.

Marten Triewald, the young Swede just quoted, who was studying science and mechanics in London under the influence of Desaguliers, was recruited to accompany Samuel Calley, the sixteen-year-old son of Newcomen's partner, who had been given the responsibility of building an engine near Newcastle for the important Ridley family of coalowners. Triewald worked for them for several years and was involved in the erection of four engines near Newcastle. Like Desaguliers he was involved in the 1720s in giving public lectures (in his case in both Edinburgh and Newcastle, together with John Thorold) devoted to 'Natural and Experimental Philosophy'. These lectures may have assisted in spreading the knowledge of the Newcomen engine in Britain. In 1722 he astonishingly patented the Newcomen engine in England, apparently on the basis that the Newcomen engine as an atmospheric engine was being sold under the Savery patent for a quite different engine. This was an argument which others, including the Parrot family of early erectors, had advanced with some justification.[6] His partnership with Nicholas Ridley and Samuel Calley probably indicates a scheme to break away from the Fire Engine Proprietors, as it was for the erection and maintenance of engines.[7] Triewald was to be much involved in attempts to transfer Newcomen technology to Sweden, but he was not the first in the field, though there was early Swedish interest.

Foreign knowledge of the engine, as we have pointed out, came rapidly, and as Hollister-Short has shown, the secrets of the engine were not well guarded. The German, Johann Keysler, pointed out in 1729 that he had been present in 1718 when a scale model had been demonstrated at the Royal Society, another indication of how the British scientific interest in the early steam-engine made for international scientific intelligence of it.[8] By July of the same year the Imperial authorities in Vienna knew of the engine and instructed Joseph Fischer von Erlach, then on a study tour of England, to learn something about the engine's operation. Here apparently enters an element of industrial espionage, for von Erlach 'had to disguise himself in labourer's clothing and work as a day-labourer during his time in England in order to come at the secrets of atmospheric steam engine work'.[9]

This may suggest a significant difference between scientific intelligence about the engine and the technical, or craftsman's, knowledge of how to make it. It may also explain Triewald's later statement that 'I am the first and only foreigner to have obtained *free access* in England to this magnificent invention',[10] implying perhaps that others had to obtain the technology, as opposed to the scientific knowledge, by spying or suborning. For the science von Erlach could have turned to Desaguliers, whom he knew. But he did not rely solely on the fruits of his own espionage to secure the technology for the Hapsburg Empire, for during late 1718 or 1719 he approached Isaac Potter, a member of a notable family of early engine builders, and persuaded him to emigrate, and he arrived in Vienna by the early summer of 1720. For reasons which Hollister-Short explores[11] building the first engine did not begin until 1721, at the Konigsberg mine in Hungary, and it was operative in 1723. By that time von Erlach had built an engine for ornamental garden waterworks at the mansion of Prince Schwartzemberg just outside Vienna, and possibly another engine at Cassel. Potter built two further engines in the Schemnitz area, and two more were in hand at the time of his death in 1735.[12]

The plot continued to thicken internationally. A Lieutenant-Colonel de Goumoens, who had joint ownership of a mine near Liège, had been in English military service in Scotland. He was in Newcastle in late 1719 and saw a Newcomen engine at work, obtained one of the early prints of it and sent it to his partner, who got the English Jesuits at Liège to make a model of it in order to obtain a patent. However, it was another Liège group who brought over a Colonel John O'Kelly, an Irishman who had served in the British army in England, who built an engine between 1720 and 1721. The cylinder and valve gear were brought over from England, but problems at the mine meant that it was not at work until 1723, and was moved to another site in 1725. O'Kelly's subsequent success was small, he had to leave the Liège mine partnership, and was involved in negotiations to build engines in Spain and Sweden, where one of his assistants was simultaneously being persuaded to join a different group of venturers. O'Kelly's schemes seem to have got nowhere, but the adoption of the engine in what is now Belgium was more successful than elsewhere on the Continent. Saunders, formerly an assistant to O'Kelly, built four engines at a lead-silver mine at Vedrin during the period 1730–40, and by 1732–35 he was also building steam-engines at coal-mines on either side of the border with France in the Hainault region. Native engineers were building engines in the Borinage from the late 1730s, and considerable numbers of engines continued to be built in what is now Belgium. But there 'the craft of engine building ... remained throughout the eighteenth century and well into the nineteenth at much the level that George Saunders had left it about 1740'.[13]

The knowledge of the early steam-engine in Sweden did not depend initially or solely on Triewald. Emmanuel Swedenborg was in England, mainly London and Oxford, *c*.1710–13, principally studying mathematics and astronomy, but resided with London craftsmen (a watchmaker, a cabinet-maker and an instrument-maker) to learn something of their skills. After leaving England, and on his way back to Sweden, he wrote to a correspondent at Uppsala about the value of what was clearly the Savery engine for water returning to operate mills.[14]

Swedish industrial observers had visited England with some regularity from the late seventeenth century, generally with the support of the Swedish Board of Mines, and they were very conscious of the new British developments in metal-mining and coal-fuel technology. Erik Odhelius had made such a visit in 1691–92, Anders Swab in 1712. By 1718 the Board was concerned that those with foreign experience had been absorbed into its own domestic hierarchy, and that a six-year information gap had now arisen. Another very well-trained young expert, Henrik Kahlmeter, was selected and sent to Britain in 1718, and stayed four years. At an early stage of his visit, while in Scotland, he learned about the Newcomen engine, and he visited at least three engines erected or building in the Newcastle area. He sent several letters and reports back about this 'exceedingly beautiful invention', one of which came to Swedenborg. His report was enthusiastic. Kahlmeter had met Triewald in Newcastle, and was getting him to send drawings[15] and a detailed description, to Sweden. Thus, as Lindquist put it, 'the first detailed knowledge of steam power technology was brought to Sweden, not as a result of a random diffusion or a bold private initiative, but as a matter of routine by a Swedish civil servant on official duty'. Kahlmeter was quickly followed by an unofficial observer, Alstromer, a Swedish merchant of scientific ability who resided long in England as a commercial and government agent, acquiring dual citizenship. His great preoccupation was bringing advanced industrial processing methods from abroad, overwhelmingly from Britain, in order to advance Sweden's industrial base from that of a mere primary producer, particularly of unmanufactured metals. He visited Wolverhampton, saw the Tipton or 'Dudley Castle' engine of 1712, met Thomas Barney and obtained his recent (1719) print of the engine.[16]

The story of the attempted domestication of the Newcomen engine in Sweden has been excellently told by Lindquist, and to follow it in detail would divert us from our main purpose. It need only be said that two propositions were before the Swedish government as early as 1723, one by a Frenchman, Colonel de Valair. He appeared in Sweden claiming some unspecified invitation to display his knowledge of several techniques, which boiled down to two, a water-raising engine of great power and an iron-steel conversion process, for which he wanted exclusive privileges. One of his business associates is known to have been in England during 1715–16, and it became clear that de Valair's engine was a Newcomen one. Though the group got a patent they seem to have been clueless as to how to build the engine; they briefly brought over an Englishman, probably Saunders, but he soon left. Then in 1725 O'Kelly put in a proposal to the Swedish ambassador at The Hague, dismissing Saunders as an able workman but without a knowledge of the scientific principles of the engine, and eventually himself sending a drawing and description of it. The administration decided not to proceed with either entrepreneur, one consideration being the issue of wood consumption in a country without coal.

Given that the Newcomen engine was only successfully established in England in 1712, it is astonishing that it was actually being proposed, or even in the early stages of contract, in several European countries about the end of the decade. As Lindquist puts it this shows 'the potential *mobility of technical information in terms of speed and distance*'.[17] Its introduction into France was closely parallel to the earlier introductions into Belgium and the Hapsburg Empire, it followed very quickly, and within the lifetime of Newcomen. However, in the French case the evidence seems to suggest that the impetus of its introduction came on balance more from British initiative than from insistent demand in the technologically recipient country – but the picture is a complex one.

John Meres, FRS, Clerk of the Apothecaries Company, and instigator of joint-stock ventures, including the Fire Engine Proprietors (of which he was Treasurer) went to France in the summer of 1725 with the approval of the Committee of Proprietors. He had already memorialized the controller-general, Dodun, before the middle of March of that year, and he had discussed the matter with the Regent, Orléans, who was ready to give Meres an exclusive privilege for the engine in France, once it had been approved by the Academy of Sciences. Dodun wrote, 'it is also an Engine of a new invention, so that there is no similar one up to now in France'. The site and purpose of the engine in that country seem to have been already determined. It was to be a water-supply engine for Paris, like the York Buildings one in London, and was to be sited by the Seine in the garden of the Marquis de Bully at Passy. That these things had already been determined implies that there must have been preliminary discussions well before March 1725, and that the planning of the introduction of the Newcomen engine into France may have been fairly close in time to that in the countries we have already discussed.[18] As Meres was accompanied by John May, whom we have already met in another context (as a naval architect and engineer endeavouring to introduce the steam-bending of timber during and after the Law scheme), he was obviously concerned to install a full-size engine and to operate it where it could have hardly been more prominent. However, others were aware of the invention and the potential of the engine. Particularly dangerous was the royal architect, Germain Boffrand. He had engaged a Lorraine craftsman who had studied under Desaguliers in London to make a full-scale copy of a Savery engine and a one-twelfth-scale model of a Newcomen one. He claimed that he had done this a year before the Passy project was launched, and the models are known to have been in Paris before July 1725.

However, in the autumn of 1725 the building of the Meres engine went ahead, though with a number of bureaucratic difficulties, particularly from the city authorities of Paris. The Prévôt des Marchands after receiving representations that the engine would be so powerful as to dangerously lower the level of the Seine, stopped the operations and fined Meres. The controller-general sternly intervened and demanded that the matter be settled, and, after the Prévôt had solemnly visited the site with the city engineer building was eventually allowed to proceed, emphasis rather amusingly being placed more on the fact that the water raised would inevitably find its way back to the river (its state of pollution not being specified) than the inability of the Newcomen engine to make a significant difference to the Seine's level.

While formal permission to proceed was only granted to John May in late November, by the following month Boffrand was renewing his campaign. He gave demonstrations of both his Savery and his small

Newcomen engine, obtained witnesses and encouragement from the architectural profession in the capital and publicity in French and foreign journals. But in May 1726 the Passy engine was operative and was visited by commissioners of the Academy of Sciences, very distinguished ones, Réaumur and d'Onsembray. As it happens we have not only their observations, but the witness of some young English aristocrats and gentry who were in Paris at the time as part of the usual Grand Tour of the Continent. The engine made 14 strokes a minute, a good rate, and was burning a cord and a half of wood per day. The Academicians considered it 'a machine which does great credit to the genius of its inventors', but made criticisms based on the possibility of the more efficient use of wood-fuel and the better condensation of steam in the cylinder. However, the Academy gave its official approval and recorded the successful report in its official publication.

At this point, however, Meres died in Paris. As the business leader of the Fire Engine Proprietors this was a blow in itself, and the social standing of May in the Paris governmental and bureaucratic milieu, as a working engineer, would have been less than that of Meres with his obvious gentility. We do not know if May preserved effective links with the Fire Engine Proprietors back in England. While the details do not concern us here, there was now a revived attempt by Boffrand to advance his own scheme, and an additional French contender appeared. The plot was further thickened by the appointment of a new controller-general, favourable to Boffrand for nationalist reasons. There were lengthy intrigues, and examinations of Boffrand's machines – he seems to have been shy in confessing that his engines were simply filched copies of English ones – but the Academicians were remarkably objective and faithful to their original assessment of the Passy engine. There is some suggestion that May was less diligent and effective in his advocacy and lobbying of the Academy and government than Meres had been. Nevertheless on 6 July 1727 May received a privilege for twenty years, much more realistic and conformable to custom than the fifty years he had at one time asked for.

Thereafter there is virtual silence. We have no information about any application to May for licences, and no later mention of him has been found. There is no account of the dismantling or sale of the Passy engine or its removal elsewhere. Oddly the only commemoration of the engine seems to be in the street name Rue de la Pompe and that of the Métro station which echoes it. Alan Smith is strictly correct in saying that the Passy engine itself resulted in no transfer of technology.[19]

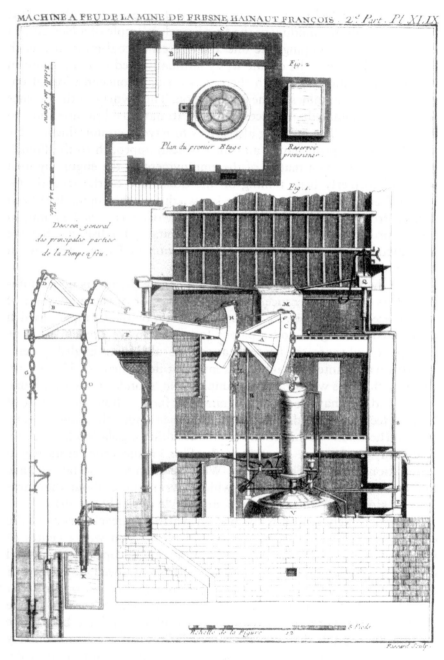

MACHINE A FEU DE LA MINE DE FRESNE HAINAUT FRANÇOIS. *2.ᵉ Part. Pl. XLIX.*

Échelle des Figures.

Fig. 2

Plan du premier Etage.

Reservoir provisoire.

Fig. 1.

Dessein général
des principales parties
de la Pompe à feu.

Echelle de la Figure.

13.1 Newcomen engine at Fresnes, 1732

A transfer of technology nevertheless did take place within about four years with the building of the first French example of a Newcomen engine for mine pumping, the one at the Fresnes coal-mine in French Hainault. Thereafter the engine was continually used in France, but in very limited numbers, though there was a small concentration of engines at the Anzin mines in the same region. The owners of the Fresnes engine and its immediate successors seem to have paid no attention to the May patent. The building also seems to have been uninfluenced by the Meres–May propaganda and their official approach to the French government. It was a matter of the employment of the engine by men who had formerly been mining on the other side of the recently redrawn French frontier, and whose knowledge of the engine had been derived from its early adoption at mines in what is now Belgium; in other words while the technology was indubitably English, its effective introduction, as opposed to its *demonstration* at Passy, came by an indirect route.[20]

From the first appearance of the steam-engine there was no prohibition of its export, to France or anywhere else, or of the movement of men to erect it. There was a direct application by the Company which distributed the engine under patent for an exclusive French privilege for a period of years, the nearest national parallel to an English patent, and this was granted though apparently not implemented. There is no evidence that this was attacked as unpatriotic or undesirable by anyone in England. We have to set this against the furore about the export of English technology and technicians to France under the Law scheme; the reverberations of this affair and the resulting legislation had hardly died away at the time Meres and the Fire Engine Proprietors began negotiations with the French state. Why the difference? So far we have found no contemporary sources which say anything about the paradox, let alone offer an explanation, and so we can only speculate.

The most likely reason is the way in which the development of the early steam-engine of Papin, Savery and Newcomen was a centre of intense interest in the scientific community of Europe. International intelligence about the engine diffused with great speed, the speed of correspondence between the scientific luminaries of Europe of that period, which is one of the chief cultural phenomena of the age. While the pioneering work of Newcomen and Calley may have been done outside the capital, the constellation of Fellows of the Royal Society involved in some way with the discussions, demonstrations and actual promotion of Newcomen engines shows that the invention was deeply involved in, not extraneous to, this milieu. If the scientific appreciation of the engine quickly became international, was it really morally possible to prohibit the export of a machine (in effect its key parts together with an erecting staff) which seemed part of the scientific enlightenment? If the Newcomen engine had rapidly contributed to industrial development in the recipient countries in a way which made them dangerous rivals to Britain, some means of restraining the export of parts and the (usually temporary) emigration of expert builders might have been resorted to. But there were constraints on its spread. There was the high cost (commonly around £1,500 all told even in Britain) in its early decades.

The use of fuel was critical. In those cases, as in Hungary, Sweden and Paris, where wood-fuel was used, the consumption and cost must have been great. Of the Konigsberg engine it was recorded that it would need over 13 cubic metres of wood a day, and 5 square miles of forest would have been needed to keep it going for a year. No wonder that when the imperial mining authorities were able to develop water pressure engines for draining purposes Newcomen engines were relegated to a subsidiary role and no more new ones were installed. Only in the Belgian coalfields and at some French mines did the Newcomen engine find a permanent home, and there were probably only about seventy to a hundred engines in Belgium at the end of the eighteenth century. Hollister-Short hits the nail accurately on the head when he writes 'a steam engine during the 18th century and for much of the nineteenth was so symbiotically linked to the mining of coal ... that it could not in any significant or lasting way break through the technological matrix in which it had come to maturity'. As Britain was the only nation to have achieved a largely coal-fuel technology by the end of the eighteenth century, the export of the steam-engine did not become a threat which prompted any countervailing measures from the initiating country.[21]

Watt

The introduction of the Watt engine into France was a remarkable affair, but not initially one of industrial espionage. Indeed the first engines were exported to France after that country had joined in the American War of Independence, and by an astonishing arrangement which depended on the availability of passports and safe conducts issued by the French, American and British authorities. However, there were two earlier attempts to obtain the engine for France without regard to the British patent rights of Boulton and Watt. Though they quickly obtained a privilege to protect their engine in France, it was never fully implemented and was successfully infringed. The important infringer, Périer, was the very man who had been the principal benefi-ciary of the wartime exports. We will see that he subsequently obtained the secret of Watt's double-acting engine from a Spanish engineer who had gained it by blatant industrial espionage, and went on to manufac-ture such engines himself.

How did the French learn of the Watt engine? Three men are known to have been in touch with one or other of the engine partners and to have then informed the French government about it. However, it is now clear that yet another person offered to act as the agent of Boulton and Watt in taking the engine to France. To those already recorded – D'Hérouville, Joseph Alcock and J.-C. Périer – must now be added the business magnate Le Camus de Limare, whom we have already met as the prime actor in introducing copper sheathing manufacture for the French navy. Count D'Hérouville, a lieutenant-general in the French army, had a long interest in steam-engines, going back to the late 1750s. He seems to have had two purposes in mind, one being the installation of a Newcomen engine at coal-mines in Anjou. There he was apparently associated with the Duc de Chaulnes, but there was a fire that damaged the engine at Montjean in which he was interested, and though steam-engines continued to be used on that coalfield it is not clear if he was involved with them. But very early he developed a project for draining the marshes round Dunkirk by steam-power.[22]

Unfortunately some very interesting correspondence which has survived is largely undated.[23] It shows D'Hérouville in active correspond-ence about the cylinder and 'working barrels' of a pump, which were being made in England. The calculations necessary were being made in England by Steven Glover, but there were other calculations made by the great watchmaker, Le Roy fils, who in turn consulted the famous English watchmaker Graham, 'perhaps the most precise man in Eur-ope', apparently on the amount of water that could be raised. The watchmakers came in because of their mathematical rather than their engineering ability. The calculations about the performance of the Newcomen engine made in 1717 by Henry Beighton were still being relied on. This project was probably going on in wartime, for there are discussions about bringing coal in vessels from Newcastle with both

French and English government passes, an interesting precedent for the later intergovernmental co-operation about obtaining the Watt steam-engine in wartime. D'Hérouville certainly also explored the possibility of importing Newcomen engines from Liège, though this idea seems to have been abandoned.

There is a series of letters of a Thomas Stephens of London in 1758, who had received an order for two engines from D'Hérouville, but passed on the cylinder part to 'my founder in Shropshire', probably the Coalbrookdale Company. The building of an engine house was in active preparation, and Stephens had been over to France to see D'Hérouville on the spot where it was to be erected. But some of D'Hérouville's associates were confused about the nature of the engine. 'They mistake mine', said Stephens, 'for another Fire Engine called Savery's Engine, which raises the water without Pumps' but Stephens had thought he had made it clear that it would not raise enough water. He had achieved 'almost 40 Years Practice in Most sorts of Engines', and knew what he was talking about as he had made one of the largest Savery engines ever built to raise ornamental waters in the gardens of the Earl of Burlington. Stephens also had problems in convincing D'Hérouville that British pumps were better than a wooden pumping system that had been suggested; his system had the authority of Desaguliers. 'Dr. Desaguliers, who was my Master, was the best Engineer we ever had and has left the best Instructions of any I ever read'.[24] There was a problem about finding an engine erector who could speak French, but Stephens proposed to get over this by employing at Dunkirk an English boiler-maker, now resident at Bruges, 'who speaks French indifferently' who could interpret for the erector. The erector would have the high wages of 6 guineas a month, but Stephens himself would come over to put the engine to work. The engine seems to have been erected and employed, but wind-mills were also used to help drain the Dunkirk marshes.

D'Hérouville now became an advocate of steam-engines to supply Paris with water, and advanced a seven-engine scheme in 1759. He went over to England, perhaps while the Seven Years War was still raging, and brought back the plan of a steam-engine. He produced further schemes in 1765 and 1766, which did not come to anything. However, from now on plans for a steam-powered Paris water supply were in continuous agitation; for a time the running was taken up by Joseph Auxiron, more celebrated for his steamboat project, but his efforts were soon superseded by those of J.-C. Périer.[25]

Périer's ideas seem to have been conceived about 1775, and received powerful and decisive backing from his close association with, and patronage by, the house of Orléans. Naturally it was Newcomen engines which were originally thought of. Watt had only joined Boulton in Birmingham in 1774, the vital connection with John Wilkinson for the supply of accurate cylinders had only recently been made, and the first successful engines were only operative at Wilkinson's Broseley ironworks and at Bloomfield colliery in the early summer of 1776.

The city of Paris approved Périer's scheme in October 1776, though he did not receive his royal privilege for the waterworks until early in 1777. He went over to England late in 1776 or early in 1777 to deal with the ironmaster John Wilkinson for the great quantity of iron pipes which would be needed.[26] Périer, once in touch with Wilkinson, of course learned of the existence and superior efficiency of the Watt engine. The trickiness of Périer was at once apparent, he tried to persuade Wilkinson to make him such an engine without dealings with, or payment to, Boulton and Watt, on the basis that the Watt patent was not legally enforceable in France. Though later on Wilkinson made a number of 'pirate' copies of Watt engines for sale to customers, he was not prepared to do so on this occasion, and Périer had to deal with Boulton and Watt direct. But it was only in October 1778 that Périer was finally authorized by the waterworks company to order two engines from the Birmingham firm, and in December he was back in England to contract with both Wilkinson and Boulton and Watt.[27]

Meanwhile others had taken a more open and honourable part in introducing the Watt engine into France. Joseph Alcock, the hardware industrialist whose father, as we have seen, first took Birmingham methods to France, had come over to Birmingham in June 1777, partly on private affairs, partly commissioned by Trudaine de Montigny to look into new hardware methods and new machines. During the visit he had got to know Boulton, who told him that he had 'perfected' the steam-engine a few years before – Boulton was not above claiming the chief part in the invention.

Alcock stressed the importance of the engine in mine drainage, rather over-emphasizing its significance for coal-mines. He thought that it was important to acquire one of the machines as soon as possible, even if a high price had to be paid for it by the Government. It could be used to replace the very old hydraulic machine of Marly for pumping water from the Seine to Versailles, for a major mine, or for the water supply of a great town. Once one was acquired French craftsmen could try to

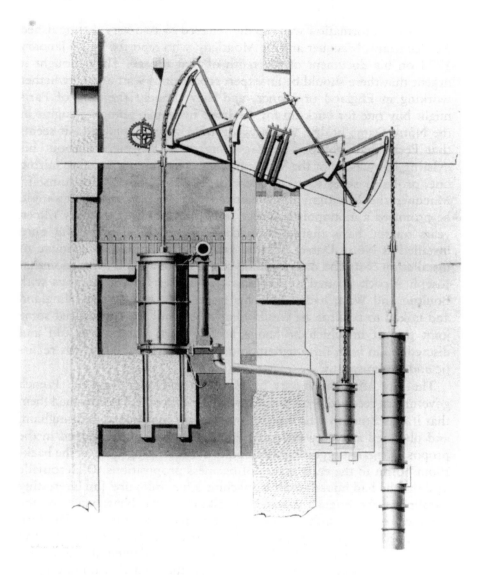

13.2 Boulton and Watt original drawing of a Périer engine for the Paris waterworks, 1779

reproduce it at leisure for 'working from a model even under our immediate direction the most capable workers would take several years to imitate it'.

Alcock's information was rapidly referred to two very distinguished Academicians, Macquer and De Montigny, who reported by 14 January 1778 on his document of the tenth of that month. They thought it urgent that there should be an expert report on a Watt engine whether working in England or France, and they thought the City of Paris might buy one for back-up for the large hydraulic pumping engine at the Nôtre Dame bridge, which was getting very dilapidated. (It seems that Périer had not put the Government in the picture about his existing knowledge of the Watt engine and his intentions of acquiring one, probably so as to retain some degree of monopoly for himself.) Macquer and Montigny recommended that Boulton and Watt should be promised a monopoly privilege in France for the customary fifteen years on the basis that their machine proved itself successful once installed at Nôtre Dame, Boulton and Watt providing an estimate of installation costs and daily running costs. There was no suggestion that Joseph Alcock wanted any commercial interest in the dealings with Boulton and Watt; had it been his father who had revisited England and talked to Boulton he would almost certainly have advanced some joint project in which he had a leading part, but he was old and discredited in both Birmingham and Paris, whereas the son was realistic and circumspect.[28]

The day after the report of Macquer and Montigny the French government received propositions from D'Hérouville. He informed them that it was Boulton who had set up the new machine at Birmingham, and obtained a twenty-five year patent. Watt is not mentioned in the proposals, again suggesting that Boulton was treating Watt as the backroom boffin in the early stages of business propositions. D'Hérouville said that he had himself built a 'machine à feu ordinaire' [an interesting parallel of the English practice in talking of the Newcomen as 'the common engine' once Watt's had appeared] to drain the Dunkirk marshes sixteen years ago, but he had learned from 'scavans' [*sic*] and 'connoisseurs' that the Boulton engine was fundamentally different, mechanically more efficient, and used less fuel 'but that no one up to now has yet been able to get to know exactly the true construction' of the engine. D'Hérouville had proposed to Boulton that he should alter his existing machine to the new type and provide him with another new one. But Boulton not wanting to 'reveal the detail of his steam engine to any curious observers in France' was demanding that he should get for his engine a similar kind of protection in France that his patent provided in England, but once given that protection, he would come over, supervise the building of the Dunkirk marsh engine, and then build as many more in France as were ordered from him.[29]

D'Hérouville's propositions received rapid attention. They reached Tolozan, the most influential intendant at the Bureau of Commerce and, through him, Necker, who wrote to the Count in the following month. Necker found only one objection, the twenty-five year term of the privilege requested, when a firm edict had previously been issued from the royal council that exclusive privileges should never exceed fifteen years. In effect Boulton could have almost the same monopoly period as an ordinary English patent would have given (fourteen years), rather than one paralleling the special extension by Act of Parliament that he and Watt very exceptionally enjoyed. By mid-April a draft *arrêt* had been prepared for Boulton and Watt, Watt's name now being equally prominent with Boulton's, and setting out the importance of the separate condenser, but not getting this very clearly distinct from Watt's favourite project of the 'steam wheel', a rotary engine which he of course never fully implemented.[30] The Watt engine was advanced as valuable not only for its great fuel economy over the Newcomen engine, but for employment in working forge hammers, in blowing furnaces, in rolling copper and other metals, and in all the uses that water-mills were put to (probably based on the use of the reciprocating engine for water-returning rather than presuming on the success of the steam wheel) and in draining marshes. Boulton and Watt offered to come over to France to set up their machines and demonstrate their superiority to the older type, at either the Dunkirk marshes or any other places indicated, under the inspection of commissioners appointed for the purpose. They wanted exclusive rights to make, sell and distribute their engines in France. In fact even at the draft stage it was stipulated that the privilege should only be for fifteen years, that the comparative test should be at either Dunkirk or Paris, that any privilege would only begin after a successful trial, and that those making or using Newcomen engines could continue to do so untroubled by the privilege. The *arrêt* was granted by 14 April.[31]

The liaison between Boulton and Watt and D'Hérouville did not work out successfully, though D'Hérouville had done a great deal for them. An undated paper, probably of April 1778, shows Boulton and Watt offering to supply all necessary parts both in cast and wrought iron, and in copper and brass, for the Count's engine, and to send over an engineer to erect it. D'Hérouville, probably for health reasons which prevented him travelling, relied on intermediaries to visit London and Birmingham on his behalf and negotiate with the engine partners. One had been the Marquis de Puysegur; at this point the intermediary was J. A. de Magellan, a Portuguese savant who seems to have been equally at home in France and in England, where he became an FRS.[32]

Some of the correspondence suggests that while the engine partners were grateful to D'Hérouville they were backing off from total commitment to him. Boulton did not himself come over as D'Hérouville hoped. On 17 April Magellan wrote that he had not been able to get a date from him for his visit to Dunkirk, and if the imminent war broke out a passport would have to be obtained for him. Magellan wrote again a week later that the engine partners were indeed in London, but said they were overwhelmed by steam-engine orders for mines. It is not entirely clear, but it seems that there was also a scheme afoot in which Boulton would be willing to be indirectly involved with a French hardware manufacture to which he would send out semi-finished parts, even 'completely finished except for the last touches'.[33] If some other person would undertake the hardware project, 'he would not fail to undertake all that part which would be consistent with the Law, for in effect an Englishman cannot go and set up himself a manufacture in another country, without denaturalizing himself and submit to enormous fines'. This was quite specious; closely acquainted with the Wilkinson brothers, Boulton must have known that William Wilkinson was doing that very thing in the most blatant way, and that the law was directed at artisans and suborners, not entrepreneurs. Reverting to the steam-engine business, Magellan reported that Boulton and Watt would prefer to have French workers employed in the building of the Dunkirk engine, 'for in effect it is not permitted to send workers from here to another country; and it is only an Engineer or director to erect this machine according to the ideas and designs of the gentlemen [Boulton and Watt] whom they are obliged to send from here which is permitted'.[34]

D'Hérouville pointed out that the *arrêt* he had obtained was not the final stage of the administrative procedures. There would have to be a confirmatory *arrêt* when a successful comparative trial had been made, while the inclusion of the steam wheel in the first *arrêt* added a complication, which might mean other trials. Nor was he able to take on the job of registering the final *arrêt* in all the Parlements of France, necessary if it was to be effective. Boulton and Watt were saying that they could not produce the reciprocating engine and make the trials in less than a year, yet the French government usually wanted projectors to implement their schemes within a year in order to confirm a privilege. This might allow someone else (perhaps someone who had obtained knowledge of the engine by espionage) to come in and anticipate them. However, there were now suggestions of a trial of the engine at Paris as an alternative to the Dunkirk marshes.[35]

Early in June Boulton wrote once again, putting off a visit to D'Hérouville in Paris. He claimed that his hardware trade partner, Fothergill, was objecting to his going to France at a time of year when accounts were to be settled – though in many years they never did so! He assured D'Hérouville that these were not 'mere Excuses, there are matters of fact and of the greatest moment to my general concerns'. Through Magellan Boulton insisted that he would not go back on any of the terms that had been agreed in the negotiations that had been conducted on his behalf by the Portuguese intermediary. However, he had an English military plan of the Dunkirk marshes and saw no need to go there himself. His customary penchant for secrecy was prominent. 'The less said about this business until it is concluded the better and therefore I hope Mr. Magellan will put a seal upon his Mouth.' Boulton's second refusal to go to France, and his demand for secrecy for a project already covered by a French *arrêt*, are suspicious. One wonders how far he already knew that once Périer had full financial backing he would immediately be ordering Watt engines for the Paris waterworks.[36]

D'Hérouville's position now weakened significantly. He had to inform the Government that the effectiveness of the draining of the Dunkirk marshes had been made more difficult by demolitions by the British at the end of the Seven Years War. His company was selling out to a Dutch company with Necker's agreement.[37] He now suggested that Boulton and Watt carry out their trials at Paris, but in such a way as to make this part of a viable project which could cover some of their costs in erecting an engine there. One possibility was that it could be erected in a place where it could provide water for the gardens and buildings of the king. An engine at the Samaritain could produce ten or twelve times as much water as the hydraulic pump now there. While D'Hérouville sought means to keep his project alive, Magellan reported to him that Boulton was still willing to fulfil his part, but he was under a daily increasing pressure of business, which might hold him up; the

Prussian government was now sending officials to investigate the purchase of engines for that country.[38] In August Boulton wrote to Magellan asking him to tell D'Hérouville that they knew that he had done everything possible to accelerate the project, and 'that he has fulfilled with honour the part he undertook'. But they needed to show the superiority of their engine by comparison with a Newcomen one, but there was no such engine at Paris to compare theirs with.

But now a new engine purchaser entered the picture. This was Joseph Jary, who had a coal-mine near Nantes. He was already using a Newcomen engine and wanted to replace it with a Watt engine; this could provide the ideal opportunity to test the two engines side by side. But Boulton and Watt had carefully refrained from putting Jary in the picture about the terms of the *arrêt* they had been granted, and were going slow on his order until they had learned whether the required trial could be shifted to Brittany. Their only suggestion to D'Hérouville at Paris was to send a scale working model of one of their engines for test, with a three- or four-inch cylinder, though they knew well, as many modern model builders have come to appreciate, that 'it is so much more difficult to make Models work than large Engines, that no man hath ever been able to make a Model of the Common Fire Engine work with half the Vigour or with double the Quantity of Fuel [in proportion to the work done] of those on a larger Scale'. Their proposal seems to have been a bad joke, and not a worthwhile return for D'Hérouville's long efforts on their behalf. They also informed him that the steam wheel had not come to fruition, and indeed had now been abandoned, so that that would have to be struck out of the *arrêt* before it could be confirmed. They still believed in the principle, and that it could eventually be feasible. Boulton, possibly as some compensation to D'Hérouville, was proposing to send him prices and samples of some higher-quality Birmingham toys which were going to be manufactured, presumably so as to allow him some agency in the French import trade.[39]

By October Jary had been brought into the negotiation by Boulton and Watt, and they wrote rather shamefacedly to D'Hérouville to explain why they had not followed up the engine business with him. They asked for 'another effort of the same generous spirit which you have all along shown in the affair'. They had come clean with Jary and explained the terms of the *arrêt* to him, an *arrêt* which would now have to be altered. He had come to England and 'taken great pains to inform himself of the effect of our machines' and made extensive journeys in order to thoroughly investigate the properties of the Watt engine. There survives a list of Watt engines erected so far which they had provided for him, and a certificate given by the officials of the great Cornish Chacewater mine to show the superior performance of the engine they used.[40]

Jary's conduct had not been honourable initially. Just like Périer (though Boulton did not mention Périer to D'Hérouville) he had 'endeavoured to obtain an engine without our permission'. This suggests another attempt to seduce John Wilkinson, for his co-operation was essential for a suitable cylinder. But having failed in his underhand scheme, Jary had now come openly to Boulton and Watt and joined them in an approach to the French government to arrange the comparative trial of a Watt engine against his Newcomen engine at his Brittany mine. They wanted this, they told D'Hérouville, to be 'agreeable to your sentiments'. However, they again seem to have been trying to soothe D'Hérouville with trifles, sending him examples of the mechanically copied paintings they were experimenting with; whether just as a present, or with a view to his being an agent for their sale, is unclear.[41] Magellan wrote to him a few weeks later,[42] trying to act as a persuasive intermediary in getting D'Hérouville to agree to the Brittany trials. After Boulton and Watt had given Jary a letter of introduction to D'Hérouville there was some correspondence between the two about progress with the Brittany engine, and in December Tolozan at the Bureau of Commerce agreed to the comparative trials being held in Brittany. But the suggestion made by Jary to D'Hérouville that they should join to advance a Paris waterworks scheme in opposition to Périer was in fact an idle hope.[43] Périer had scooped the waterworks deal, and with the effective co-operation of Boulton and Watt.[44]

By 27 August 1778 Périer had been able to set up the powerful organization of the Compagnie des Eaux with the backing of the Orléans interest, and by late October the company had empowered him to contract with Boulton for his new steam-engine. It was specified that all parts would be imported which could not be made in France, and that Wilkinson should be contracted with for pipes. It is very unlikely that Périer advanced the proposal to contract with Boulton and Watt without first sounding them out. But that wily and shifty character preserved a fall-back position by which he would see what Liège ironmasters could provide in equipment and in price, to make sure that he was not overcharged by the English, while if Boulton and Watt proved too expensive he had the saving option of going to English Newcomen engine builders.[45] By 29 October Périer was already in

London and writing to Boulton in Cornwall that he was anxious to contract with him for two engines; he would be going to Wilkinson to contract for iron pipes, but wanted to see Boulton before he went north. Successive proposals were made to Soho by Périer, particularly plans to pay for the two engines by shares in the Paris waterworks. These Boulton and Watt resisted in favour of a direct payment. However as late as January 1779, Watt was still trying to arrange payment from Périer on the basis of coal savings over a comparable notional Newcomen engine, for a given weight of water raised.

Boulton and Watt told D'Hérouville that Périer was playing tough, he insisted he would order Newcomen engines if Boulton and Watt did not supply theirs. Even if they were more expensive to run he nevertheless had an effective monopoly, a captive market, in the water users of Paris, and all he need do was raise the price a little to compensate. He claimed his own *arrêt* excluded anyone else from building water-supply engines for Paris, so that Boulton and Watt would not be able to deal with anyone else for that purpose. Thus, unable to build and demonstrate their engine in Paris, they would lose their own *arrêt* for a French engine monopoly. 'You Sir, can be better judge of the weight of these arguments than we can', they wrote plaintively to D'Hérouville.[46] Périer's hectoring was really pointless. There was no way in which by supplying engines to him Boulton and Watt were going to be able to carry out in Paris the comparative trials with a Newcomen engine that their *arrêt* demanded. They persisted with the plan to carry out such a test at Jary's mine.

At this point D'Hérouville really ceases to be of significance, though as late as January 1779 Boulton and Watt were making a show of seeking his advice and consent in their negotiations with Périer.[47] There are references to his ill health in Magellan's correspondence, and in one of his own letters,[48] but until the selling of his Dunkirk lands he had certainly done everything possible to advance the claims of Boulton and Watt in France. Even the considerable delays faced in France by the most enterprising inventors and projectors in obtaining privileges from the Government had not deterred him, he had acted with speed and efficiency on behalf of his English associates, and without much attempt to advance his own personal interest.[49]

Before Boulton and Watt finally argued out the terms of their agreement with Périer, yet another entrepreneur appeared on the scene, offering to take over and guide the fortunes of their engine in France. It is perhaps a pity that his overtures came late, in effect a day after the fair, for his standing as a businessman could have provided an effective opposition to Périer, in a way which D'Hérouville's perhaps could not. This potential intermediary was Le Camus de Limare, whose successful founding and direction of the great copper sheathing works at Romilly we have already examined. He wrote to Boulton at the end of December 1778. He knew Magellan and D'Hérouville, and had gone with them to Dunkirk the previous May, hoping to confer with Boulton there, but, as we have seen, Boulton embarrassingly failed to turn up. His acquaintance with Boulton went back to a visit he had paid to Birmingham as early as September 1773, when Boulton had told him and his companions, 'about the discoveries you had made for bringing fire engines into perfection'. This is another instance of Boulton taking credit for Watt's work. He had finally taken over Roebuck's interest in the Watt engine only in the previous month, and Watt was not to arrive in Birmingham until May 1774!

Le Camus had heard of the later progress of the Watt engine from a very enterprising character whom we have already met and of whom we shall hear more in another context, 'Mr. Izquierdo, Director of the Cabinet of Natural History of the King of Spain', who had been to Cornwall, where he had 'seen and admired' the Watt engines already built. Le Camus believed that the best thing for Boulton would be 'to have them known in France, in order that the privilege granted to you by the King's Council for that purpose may be as beneficial to you as possible'. Had Boulton come to Dunkirk, Le Camus would have come back to England with him to unfold his ideas on the exercise of the privilege in France. He knew from D'Hérouville of the transfer of the test of a Watt engine against a Newcomen one to Jary's mine in Brittany, and intended to be present when it took place. It was important that Boulton should find means to diffuse his engines through France; they would sell well once

> their great effect and their economy is experimentally [i.e. by trial] known here. ... It would, without doubt, be a very troublesome thing to you to correspond from London [*sic*] with all the provinces of France; besides the difference of language must be an obstacle and a delay. If it was agreeable to you, Sir, I would treat with you about the exercise of your privilege in France; and as I know you to be an honourable and reasonable man, I make no doubt but we should easily agree about the conditions. Mr. Magellan and Monsr D'Hérouville could testify to you how careful and diligent I'm in business.[50]

The implication seems to be that Le Camus was intending to come in as a major businessman to take over the D'Hérouville operation now that Périer seemed to be at the head of a much more powerful business interest than the Count could command. What reply the engine partners made to Le Camus we do not know: had he made his bid six months earlier, before the Compagnie des Eaux was formally launched, the story might have been very different. As Boulton and Watt were hammering out their contract with Périer in January 1779, while still making protestations that they would do nothing without D'Hérouville's consent, Magellan, still acting as the Count's agent, correctly saw that 'it seems, from several pieces of evidence, that M. Périer won't fail to do all he can to invalidate their [Boulton and Watt's] privilege'.[51]

Périer set up an engineering works alongside the Paris water company's steam-engine site at Chaillot. One early function was to produce those parts for the two Watt engines which were not being made in Britain. The works went on to be the first great engineering works in France capable of producing machines of large size and was of an efficiency comparable to the first generation of large engineering works in Britain.[52] The quality of the work was very favourably commented on by Watt when he visited the plant in 1786. However, there is little doubt that from the outset Périer intended to copy the Watt engine and sell it in France without any compunction about the intellectual property of Boulton and Watt, and that he had no real intention of helping them to get their French patent amended and finally implemented.

Boulton and Watt had now agreed to provide the two engines, one to Périer and one to Jary. But they seem to have lost interest in the possibility of a trial of their engine against a Newcomen one at Jary's mine in Brittany. They made no effort to expedite his engine before Périer's, though after the original difficulty caused by Jary asking Wilkinson to make one of their engines without their permission or participation, they found him a good man to deal with.

Of course Boulton and Watt now had orders for three engines in the middle of a war. That throughout the century there was never any concern in Britain about the export of steam-engines is remarkable enough. That these engines were sent to France in the course of a desperate war, fought by Britain over vast distances, and on frequently unfavourable terms, is astonishing to modern minds. It is hardly less so that Jary and the Périer brothers turned up in England in wartime with no apparent difficulty to negotiate with Wilkinson and with Boulton and Watt about their engines. Jacques-Constantin Périer was in England in November 1778, and was at Soho in January and February 1779; his younger brother Augustin was in England in 1782, and being shown places of interest around Birmingham.[53]

Boulton and Watt coolly wrote to the Privy Council, stating that they were in business to make the new kind of steam-engine for which a twenty-five year extended patent had been granted to Watt in 1775. They had orders to send 'several of the said Engines to France together with a very large quantity of cast iron pumps and pipes for the purpose of conducting water through the City of Paris (all being the manufactured goods of this kingdom)' but were prevented by war. How to justify breaking the wartime prohibition on trade?

> Your Majesty's memorialists apprehend that if the said goods cannot be transported safely to France, the French will be obliged to establish Manufactories capable of furnishing them not only with Fire Engines but also with many other kinds of Cast Iron goods of a larger size than can now be made in France with which they are at present supplied from the British Manufactories: by which means your Majesty's subjects may lose a beneficial branch of Commerce.

It is interesting that Boulton and Watt emphasized the French inability to make good large iron castings as a way of giving an additional justification for the engine's export – an inability that their friend William Wilkinson was soon to help the French to overcome by building the great coke-iron works at Le Creusot, though the effects were disappointing.[54] The great irony was that by exporting engines to Périer, Boulton and Watt were providing models to copy to perhaps the only engineer in France then able to set up his own works and produce engines with the higher tolerances required if Watt engines were to be successfully built. In fact Boulton and Watt's application to the king in Council was approved without difficulty, possibly because of Watt's good standing with William, Earl of Dartmouth, Lord Privy Seal, whose seat at Sandwell Hall, West Bromwich, was close to Boulton's works. When approached he saw 'no reason to discourage your application' and agreed to use his influence with influential members of the Privy Council.[55]

Their approval was essential but, once given, arranging the actual export of the engines was a different matter. There had to be British, French and American passports,[56] engine parts and pipes had to come from John Wilkinson's Bersham, Willey, and Bilston works, while some specialized items had to come from Soho, so that shipments were made from both Chester and Chepstow. With deliveries for both Jary in

Brittany and Périer in Paris there were problems about the French ports to be used; war conditions meant high insurance and the pressganging of sailors; the right passports had to be at hand, and shipmasters of some courage were needed to take a ship into enemy waters, however well provided with proper documents. In Captain John Williams of the *Mary of Chester* John Wilkinson found a man of considerable resource, who made two voyages, though only after many delays and difficulties for which he was not responsible. Among the problems was ill feeling between Périer and Jary. Périer did not want his goods to go on the same vessel as Jary's, and he seems to have intervened with the French authorities to delay passports for Jary's shipments. But it was a later cargo of Périer's water pipes which was long delayed and remained very prominently on the wharf at Chepstow. This caused information being laid with the Customs that John Wilkinson was exporting not only cylinders but cannon to France. There was an understandable confusion between his activities and those of his brother, known to have been in French government service since before the war. Only a little exaggeration was required to turn the iron pipes into cannon and create the long-lived legend that John was supplying the French with artillery; this could easily be confused with the fact that his brother was currently making cannon for the French at Indret.[57]

Both Périer and Jary raised the risks by demanding that supplies of metals be shipped with the steam-engines. Both wanted to ship both copper and pig iron, Jary wanted lead, and Périer was particularly concerned to have steel. It made the whole enterprise more risky, for there were wartime proclamations against metal exports, and there was an Act of Parliament to enable Orders in Council or proclamations to prevent not merely the export, but even the coastal shipment, of copper sheet or bar 'lest the same should come to the use of an enemy by capture', so important was the practice of copper sheathing of warships.[58] As early as May 1779 Périer sent Boulton and Watt a note of various materials he wanted, 'you have promised to obtain steel for me, I would consequently be very obliged if you would load it with our machines and pipes'. He wanted 2,000 lbs of steel, of the different kinds which Boulton and Watt had explained to him – an interesting indication of how far the expertise of an outstanding French engineer fell short of the English practice – 'and particularly of the sort which is most successful for turning metals'.[59] His need for a large quantity of tool steel was no doubt dictated by his intention of disregarding Boulton and Watt's privilege in France and building engines himself. At one point it was suggested by Watt that pig iron for Périer should be cast into plates, grate bars or some other readily convertible form in order to evade Customs vigilance for pig iron. The Jary shipment of December 1780 apparently included a clandestine loading of pig iron, so that despite 5 guineas to the Customs officer at Chepstow Watt was 'surprised she was let go with such a cargo'.[60]

The first Chaillot engine was finished by 1781 and tried out on 8 August when it operated successfully, though not immediately at full power. There were delays in payment to Boulton and Watt for which the real reason was the finances of the water company, though various excuses were given. Eventually they received a belated double payment, because this was specified by their contract if the company made a second share issue, which it did. During the attempts of the company to delay payment, they raised some queries about the evidence for the Boulton and Watt *arrêt* for a privilege, though, as Payen makes clear, they knew about it perfectly well, and could hardly have expected the Birmingham firm to obtain confirmation of the *arrêt* from the French government in the middle of a war, or certainly not quickly. The Périers conducted the delaying correspondence 'sur [un] ton d'amiabilité hypocrite'.[61]

Already in 1780 John Wilkinson had suspicions of Périer's conduct when an engine erector, Vickers, who was sent out to him on one of the special government-approved voyages, returned having been refused landing permission in France: 'this is a plain proof that he [Périer] does not choose to have even an English workman employ'd in putting the Engine together ... such a jealous Temper is a bane to undertakings of this nature – and a weed of luxurious growth in France'. Neither he nor Boulton and Watt yet saw the real problem, that Vickers, had he gone to Chaillot, would have learned of Périer's plans to build Watt engines himself. The Périers, however, both visited England early in 1782 with the intention of seeing Boulton and Watt, but we know nothing about discussions or negotiations on either side. A letter from the Périers in July 1782 refers to the patent rights of Boulton and Watt in England, and to the agreement of Wilkinson not to make parts for the engine without their consent, but significantly says nothing about the French privilege as part of the basis of the contract with the water company and Périer for the Paris engines. Thereafter little correspondence is known of until the Périers finally settled the water company account in August 1786.[62]

In the meantime the Chaillot works had begun to make steam-engines, and there is no question that some of them were Watt engines.

There is however some doubt about numbers and types. There were some 'garden' engines for the waterworks in the parks of the nobility, and a number of these were Savery engines. Engines supplied to the Anzin coal-mines may have been Newcomen, and the cylinders were certainly British. While contemporaries said that Périer had built forty engines before the Revolution, and a hundred before he ceased business in the second decade of the nineteenth century, it has not proved easy to trace them. Of the forty, Payen was only able to find a quarter.[63] Périer himself in his important pamphlet, *Sur la machine à vapeur*, of 1810 wrote 'We hardly have two hundred in France, whether on the old principle [Newcomen's] or on the new one' (Watt's). We may assume that he is talking of France under its contemporary boundaries, which would include perhaps a hundred Newcomen engines on the Belgian coalfields, which casts more than a little doubt over whether Périer himself made a hundred. There is no doubt that he built some splendid engines, a number of which had long working lives. Particularly important engines were those at Gros Caillou in Paris to increase the water supply, and at the Ile des Cygnes, also in Paris, for flour-milling, one at Indret to power cannon boring machines on Wilkinson principles, and cotton-mill engines, including some for firms in which the Périers themselves had an interest. Watt visited Chaillot during his industrial consultancy visit to France with Boulton in 1786–87,[64] of which more later, and had no doubts about the quality of the work done there. 'He has succeeded ... in having erected a most magnificent and commodious manufactory for steam engines, where he executes all the parts uncommonly well.'[65]

Watt's observations are generous considering what his feelings must have been. Périer had totally ignored Watt's original *arrêt* for a privilege. Watt had approached the French government again in 1783 or 1784, at a point where the water company was refusing to pay up for the engines supplied, and when he was without a scrap of support from Périer. In his memoir to the French government he said that this and wartime problems had prevented his asking for confirmation of his *arrêt*, but once the war was over he and Boulton renewed 'the offer of our service to the Kingdom of France', provided the authorities confirmed the 1778 *arrêt*, including the latest developments of the engine (principally rotative motion and the ability to work large forge hammers and corn-mills), and provided the engine partners were granted letters patent. The operation of the Watt pumping engine at Paris was sufficient proof of the superiority of their engine over the old type. If it

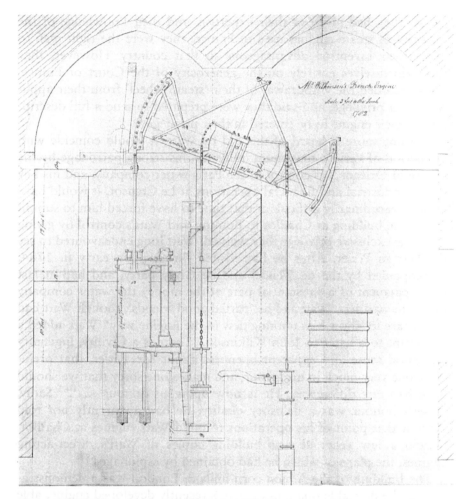

13.3 'Mr Wilkinson's French Engine', 1782: Boulton and Watt engine drawing supplied to Wilkinson for Le Creusot

were argued that it would be wrong to give them an exclusive privilege 'en qualité de sujets d'une nation rivale' [given their situation as citizens of a rival country] they could point out that their engine had been introduced into France far better by their assistance than it could have been without it. As well as their co-operation in building the engines at Paris and Nantes, they had provided William Wilkinson with plans and instructions to set up an engine to blow the furnaces at Le Creusot and they were making the drawings for a small one for Rochefort. From the proofs they had given of their expertise, and their knowledge of the majority of steam-engines used in France, they were the right men to make their invention advantageous to that country. However, they threw themselves entirely on the generosity of the Court of France. They recorded the withdrawal of their 'steam wheel' from their application for privilege, and said they were prepared to send a full description of their engine to be entered in their privilege.[66]

Nothing more is heard of this bid by Watt, it would coincide with the period of Périer's maximum influence, his strong patronage by the House of Orléans, his control of the Paris water company, and his key role in industrial and financial operations at Le Creusot. It would have been extraordinarily difficult at that time to have forced him to submit his engine building at Chaillot to Boulton and Watt's control by giving them the exclusive privilege they wanted. Watt long endeavoured to see the best in Périer. After he had visited Birmingham early in 1784, accompanied by the de Wendel and de Givry party, and had at last made payment of a substantial part of the money the water company owed the partners, Watt and he 'parted good friends', though Watt had taken care to 'show him nothing new in the Engine way'. Watt added a postscript to a letter to John Wilkinson. 'There is a Civility, Ingenuity and good sense and apparent openness about Mr. Périer, that prejudices one very much in his favour, and makes one sorry that we should have had any differences. He is now upon his honour ... '.[67] Sadly, Périer's honour was a delusory quality; he had apparently not told Watt at that point of his operations to build Watt engines at Chaillot. Within a few years he was building copies of Watt's direct-acting engines, the plans of which he had obtained by espionage.[68]

The building of the Albion corn-mills in London was a demonstration of the desirable qualities of Watt's recently developed engine, able to deliver rotative motion with the smoothness conferred by the direct action of steam on either side of the piston. But while Albion Mills provided a showcase from the point of view of the British consumer, it was also an attraction to foreign visitors, for whom London was more readily accessible than Birmingham. While Boulton and Watt and their engineer John Rennie tried to keep a careful control over visitors, this was not always easy. Boulton wanted to be thought a leading member of the European scientific enlightenment, and found it difficult to refuse access to his works to eminent scientists.

In June 1787 there was a visit to Albion Mills by two eminent French Academicians, together with a French marquis. The marquis was 'a good draughtsman', and while Boulton was showing the others the granaries of the mills, the Academician Coulomb and the marquis 'stole away and could not be found'. After Boulton and the others, including Barthélemy of the French embassy, had seen over the granaries they found themselves waiting for a long time for the others to rejoin them. Then one of his employees came to tell Boulton that

> he had seen them concealed in the dark hole where the rotative wheels are and that one of them had his handkerchief in his hand with a book or paper in it in which the Marquis or Coulomb was sketching, and when he came up to them the sketch was concealed [*sic*] in the handkerchief as if practised in Dexterous Arts [i.e. conjuring] finding themselves thus disturbed they came and joined their Company. I had great difficulty to suppress my indignation but I thought it would then do no good to show it. ... They set out this morning to Birmingham. Pray show them Hospitals but I must object to such thieves going into Soho Mill. They might have obtained more Knowledge if they had behaved like philosophers and gentlemen, but they are thieves and should be treated as such.

The interest of the Academicians in British hospitals was sincere, but the incident shows how the most innocent-seeming visit of investigation could be diverted to espionage.[69] Coulomb had been one of four commissioners appointed by the Academy to inspect and evaluate Périer's Chaillot engines in the early months of 1783, and so was no stranger to the Watt engine; it was he who reported in detail to the Academy on 19 March, though all the commissioners signed the report.[70]

Perhaps the interruption of the observations of Coulomb and his aristocratic draughtsman colleague occurred at a critical moment, for we know of no result of their examination of the Albion Mill engines, and it seems unlikely that anything so important would not have been passed on to Périer. But another knowledgeable visitor carried out a highly successful piece of industrial espionage in 1788. This was Augustin de Betancourt y Molina. Betancourt, though of French ancestry, was a Spaniard from the Canaries. Betancourt was given a commission from the Spanish Crown in 1788 to put together a collection of models relating to hydraulics. He wanted in this connection to see the latest version of the steam-engine, and came over to England. At first he approached those expert in mechanics and physics in London, but they could only tell him about the Newcomen engine, well enough known in France.

He then made his way to Birmingham, having learned that Boulton and Watt were ahead of the field. He was kindly received, but only shown the hardware and silver-plating side of Boulton's business, not the steam-engine. He learned that engine speed could now be regulated (by the centrifugal governor) but he was not told how, or how new economies in fuel consumption had recently been achieved. He returned frustrated to London, but did not give up. Through an unknown London friend he got permission to see over Albion Mills. He immediately fastened on the importance of Watt's parallel motion linkage, he noted the different arrangement of steam pipes and valves, and that an engine of a smaller size of cylinder than he would have expected was delivering considerable power. He correctly deduced that here was a double-acting engine with steam applied successively to each side of the piston. Perhaps, as Payen suggests, these conclusions would have been arrived at by anyone who, like Betancourt, was a good mechanical engineer but he must at any rate be congratulated on knowing his business. Some features, like the centrifugal governor, he seems not to have been able to observe. Interestingly, he did not hang about, but set off back to France the next day. Once back in France he set about making a model of the engine, which he did successfully.

He then prepared a paper for the Académie des Sciences, delivered in December 1789, in which he coolly reported on the new technology developed by Watt, and the fact that he had obtained it by espionage! Having not seen the centrifugal governor he advocated the cruder 'cataract' method of controlling engine speed. He described the sun-and-planet motion and emphasized the importance of the latest Boulton and Watt engines for producing rotative motion and driving machinery. He was able to say that Périer was convinced by his report and model and was going to build double-acting engines. This Périer did rapidly, employing them to drive the large government-subsidized flour mills built at the Ile des Cygnes at Paris. Needless to say, the resentment of Boulton and Watt against Périer and Betancourt now ran deep. When visiting the great French engineer Prony in 1802 Watt was ready to forgive him for publishing an account of the engines – including a claim by Périer that he had really thought of the key ideas before Betancourt showed him his model, but his resentment against Périer and Betancourt had only increased with time. In 1788 the Périers were removed from the Paris water company; they involved themselves in many other ventures, particularly in several cotton-mills which did not have a long-term success, but their Chaillot engineering works had passed its peak: 'from the beginning of the Revolution, the story of the Chaillot foundry is one of a long, slow decline'.[71]

Taking the Newcomen and Watt engines together, the story of the transfer of British steam-engine technology to France is a curious one, with differences from, and contrasts with, that of the other transferred technologies. Industrial espionage played a part, particularly in the case of the Watt engine, but a subordinate one. The main inventions were introduced into France by the inventors or their appointed representatives, and in the cases of both engines this was done by seeking a royal privilege in France, conferring a monopoly for fifteen or twenty years; in other words they applied for the nearest equivalent to an English patent. In the instance of the Watt engine the interest of D'Hérouville in acquiring one of their engines provided an initial stimulus to obtaining a privilege; as far as we know in the case of John Meres and John May the initiative came directly from the English side, from the Fire Engine Proprietors, the company promoting the Newcomen engine. Intelligence about the invention of the engines in both cases passed rapidly to France. It was aided by the existence of a wide and much travelled European community of enquiring and curious men, many of whom had good contacts with their home governments, were full members or corresponding members of national scientific societies, had close contacts with industry or business, or were indeed industrialists themselves. Both the Newcomen and Watt engines were excellent examples of the speed of international transmission of industrial and technological intelligence in the eighteenth century. The information stage in the process of transfer, often emphasized as a serious problem in modern formal analyses of that process, is here seen as very rapidly achieved and with little difficulty. Le Camus de Limare learning from Boulton's lips of the important new engine that was under development, even before Watt joined him at Birmingham, is a remarkable instance.

In the case of the Newcomen engine in France we do not know why the privilege granted to May was not effective. He may not have had the resources to obtain the necessary letters patent from the Paris and provincial Parlements. We do not know how far he had the support of the Fire Engine Proprietors back in England, particularly after Meres's death. In any case their organization ran down after 1733, when the Savery patent, under which the Newcomen engine had been sold, expired. We do not even know when May died.

That Boulton and Watt also sought an exclusive patent in France is interesting, demonstrating that British entrepreneurs believed in the controlling power of the French state over French industry. How far they, or Meres and May before them, made a simplistic analogy between an English patent and a French privilege is uncertain. Their relationship with Périer was founded to a large degree on a misjudgement of his character; charm and apparent candour were vitiated by a fundamental untrustworthiness and trickery. It may be that Boulton's fascination with power, political and business power on the one hand balancing the physical power of the steam-engine on the other, helped to influence him to favour Périer. For Périer with the finances of the great water company behind him possessed power in a way that D'Hérouville and Jary did not. 'Périer was more strongly situated to win the contest. With his privilège in his pocket [for the Paris water supply] and backed by all the excellent connections which his close association with the house of Orléans provided', as Payen puts it, the cards were stacked in his favour in France, and Boulton, with his fascination with power, would have been strongly influenced by that.[72]

Boulton and Watt basked in the interest in their engine of cultivated and informed society throughout Europe, and not merely that part of society which had scientific achievements or pretensions. On the one hand they wanted to display the engine to advantage, on the other they sought to keep the details of much of the technology, especially newly invented features, and the methods of manufacture, from foreign observers. They relied considerably on the fact that Wilkinson's excellently bored cylinders were available only to them. Here Périer proved to be a better engineer than they had anticipated, and soon had no need of Wilkinson cylinders. John Wilkinson was visited by Périer even before Périer was in touch with Boulton and Watt, and several other trips were made by the Frenchman to Wilkinson's various works. With his general contempt for secrecy Wilkinson may have allowed Périer to see everything he wished, including his cylinder-boring machine.[73]

In the case of France then, the Watt engine was originally exported without industrial espionage, and after Boulton and Watt had been granted a provisional exclusive privilege, though it was not eventually validated. Of course, as we have seen, both Périer and Jary had at first endeavoured to obtain their intellectual property by improper means by getting Wilkinson to build them an engine without the permission of, or payment to, the engine partners. But if industrial espionage was not immediately involved, there is no doubt that once he possessed the Boulton and Watt engine, and had the equipment to copy it, Périer intended to make it in France, without further payment to them, whether in consideration of their English patent or their French privilege.

It was only with the development of the double-acting engine that Frenchmen turned to straightforward industrial espionage, without success in the case of the Coulomb party, with remarkable efficiency in that of Betancourt. His paper to the Academy, and the open building of direct-acting engines by Périer for the French government, indicate that official France regarded the espionage with equanimity, even with favour. However, though French scientists may have paid him the dubious compliment of espionage, in 1808 they elected Watt as a corresponding member of the mechanical section in the first class of the Institut – a section of which Périer had been appointed a member in the Year IV.[74] Finally it should be pointed out that, despite the engineering brilliance of Périer, and the keen interest of many of the scientific community, the Watt steam-engine, though copied in France, was not significantly developed. Payen puts it clearly: 'The machines built under the Empire were exactly the same as those which Watt made in 1785.'[75] Isolation, as he says, engendered stagnation, but the interesting question is why, in so many cases where the French imported English industrial methods, they were dependent for further development on fresh infusions of men and machines from across the Channel, why the vitality and originality of one industrial culture was so much greater than the other.

The spread of the steam-engine abroad, whether Newcomen or Watt, attracted little concern or anxiety in Britain. Had the spread been numerically significant the reaction might have been different. But as we have seen in the case of the Newcomen engine, the steam-engine was tied to the 'coal-fuel matrix', and while coal-mining took place in a few other European countries, in none, except in what is now Belgium, was it considerable enough to have wide implications for the economy. There it was built at a much lower technical level, and without the critical innovations which gave greatly improved performance at the hands of Smeaton, and a revolutionary improvement at those of Watt. Where the Watt engine was used abroad for supplying water to cities, draining docks, or operating mints, these were not cases where the competitive industrial strength of foreign countries was being dangerously advanced at the expense of Britain, and these exports could be viewed with a friendly eye. In the case of France not only was the endowment of coalfields vastly poorer than in Britain, but the possibilities of marketing were also much poorer, for the problems of terrain made the extension of river improvements and of canals less attractive. Even in the post-Restoration years there was the greatest difficulty in bringing in private investment to join with the State in their development.[76]

There were no non-ferrous mines of significance – there was no French Cornwall to provide a great first market for the early Watt reciprocating engine. Once cotton began to be manufactured by powered machinery at the end of the century, it was overwhelmingly water-power that was turned to. While the French interest in the Watt engine as a scientific and mechanical masterpiece was high, it did not translate to any large number of orders; there were twenty-eight enquiries made to Boulton and Watt: only five orders resulted. Indeed there were only twenty-two export orders altogether for the Watt engine during the twenty-five years of the extended British patent down to 1800. This is virtually no advance on the foreign rate of take-up which the Newcomen engine had under the Savery patent between 1715 and 1733, thirteen engines in eighteen years. There was thus no reason why there should have been any lobby or any hostile legislation against the export of the steam-engine during the eighteenth century.[77]

14 Glass

The technological connections, and the relative mutual indebtedness of France and England in the eighteenth-century glass industry are not simple or straightforward. At its briefest it can be said that a great deal of French bottle-glass making, though by no means all, was imitative in product, fuel, and to a considerable extent in methods, of what was done in England, and that the introduction of English practice began with the century. In plate glass, mainly made for mirrors, the French were predominant. Their great achievement was in developing the processes which produced plate glass by casting, not blowing, though blowing long continued to be used in parallel with casting. The British did not make a lastingly successful attempt to copy the French cast-plate process before 1773 and, even so, were not firmly on their feet before the early 1790s. Their glass as a material was probably poorer in quality than that of the French monopoly, the Compagnie des Glaces, but the British made some important improvements in the preparation of their glass for market. A third variety, flint glass, was developed in England in the late seventeenth century and was outstanding in clarity, solidity and ability to take cutting, and led European technology in crystal glass throughout the eighteenth century. Most remarkable attempts were made to secure this technique for France in the last decades of the eighteenth century, but the results were more notable for the patronage and intervention of the aristocracy and the Crown than they were for serious qualitative rivalry with the English model.

The glass industry, therefore, is a remarkable example of technological flows in opposite directions between England and France in the eighteenth century. It should be remembered, however, that the English glass industry had, in the sixteenth and seventeenth centuries, been indebted to, and heavily dependent upon, inflows of continental technology.[1] In the 1560s Le Carré and Becku, both arriving from the Low Countries, but Le Carré a native of Arras, had been given a patent for window glass manufacture by both the main continental methods, the making of 'crown' glass by the Norman system (hence the common term of 'Normandy' glass) and the 'broad' glass made by Lorrainers. Through Le Carré Italian experts, formerly settled in Antwerp, particularly Jacob Verzelini, were brought to set up crystal-glass works in London. The persecution of Protestants in the Low Countries and in France made emigration more attractive and the English glass industry continued to receive skilled foreign immigrants into the late seventeenth century. One of them began the glass industry in St Helens in the 1680s, so inaugurating what was much later to become the world's most celebrated glass-making centre. By the beginning of the seventeenth century, however, England was making its own typical contribution to glass-making, by bringing it within the scope of the gradually growing coal-fuel technology.[2] This seems to stem from developments under the direction of Dr Thomas Percival at the Winchester House glasshouse in Southwark, probably c.1609–10. The coal-using system was soon made the basis of a patent and the use of wood-fuel was prohibited for all kinds of glass. Sir Robert Mansell gained control of the company operating the patent in 1615, and he obtained a renewal of patent in 1623, and a further one from Charles I in 1635, but it was cancelled by the Long Parliament in 1642. While the effects of the monopoly and the prohibition of wood-fuel have been much debated, it is probable that together they carried through the conversion to a coal-fuel technology with a rapidity which could have hardly been achieved otherwise, and gave to the English industry its distinctive character.[3]

One of the consequences of these changes was a continued interest in experimentation. An obvious problem in coal-use was the pollution of the glass from the soot and flying coal fragments of a coal furnace. In one branch of the industry it was discovered that the lower costs and higher temperatures attainable with coal were not seriously affected by this pollution; bottle glass had to be cheap and in the middle of the seventeenth century a new type of bottle began to be made, largely by a specialist branch of the industry attempting to produce in standard sizes. It probably derived from methods devised by the versatile Sir Kenelm Digby in the 1630s, but only widely taken up after the Civil War. The new bottles were thicker and stronger. The coal-using glassmakers had introduced underground tunnels beneath their furnaces to increase draught and heat, allowing the use of a batch with a higher silicon content and less potash and lime. The bottles made in such furnaces were very dark in colour, often virtually black, which meant that there was no problem from the soot and flying fragments of fuel of a coal furnace falling into the pots, which could be left uncovered, enabling them to be more readily heated.[4]

The other important British breakthrough was in the invention of a new type of fine crystal glass, the so-called flint glass, though it was the addition of a proportion of about one-third of lead oxide into the mix which was the critical departure. This heavy white, clear, lustrous glass proved capable of being cut, giving a beautiful range of attractive patterns, and it was eventually used to produce brilliant lustres for chandeliers. Its invention is ascribed to, or at least associated with, George Ravenscroft, a glass merchant who had imported Venetian glass, and, we now know, also negotiated an English monopoly for the importation of the plate glass of the French Compagnie des Glaces. While he brought in some Italian workers, the famous lead flint glass with which he is associated does not seem to have been made in Italy before or afterwards, though the Venetians were worried from the outset about its potential threat to their exports because of its 'extreme beauty'. There are many unresolved questions about Ravenscroft and his 1674 patent, which have been carefully explored by Dr McCleod.[5] One contemporary stated that a Signor Da Costa of Montferrat introduced the process and that Ravenscroft then 'carried it on' and patented it. But it is unlikely to have been carried out successfully in a wood rather than a coal-fired furnace, which suggests that if Da Costa was the real inventor, he invented it after settling in England. While Ravenscroft was basically a merchant, it cannot be entirely ruled out that he made some technical contribution. Some men of commercial background have been important inventors, Henry Cort being one. Though Ravenscroft seems to have given up the manufacture of flint glass, if not of plate glass, before his death in 1683, other English glassmakers moved in very smartly about that time and by 1696 there were nine flint glassworks in London, four in Bristol and five in Stourbridge, and several others elsewhere.

There were a number of changes in the technology of English glassmaking associated with coal-use and beginning in the seventeenth century, but their chronology and their state of diffusion is by no means thoroughly established and understood. Coal furnaces, unlike wood ones, had to use grates, and this encouraged a strong air current.

Existing wood furnaces, as Godfrey points out, in the French and particularly the Italian forms, had a reverberatory element, and this would have enabled some separation of fuel and crucibles. From the beginning of coal-use underground air access passages were introduced in England to increase the air flow through the furnace. Higher, bee-hive shaped, Italian-type furnaces probably gave an advantage to the early coal-using glass-makers in drawing the smoke off to the top of the furnace. But we know that the first important coal-using glass furnace in Southwark employed some kind of chimney, an important new departure. Other early coal glasshouses seem to have been in fairly tall buildings. By the late seventeenth century some English glasshouses were designed so that the glass-working took place within a large brick cone which enclosed both furnace and working places. This however was not universal, and it has recently been pointed out to the writer that illustrations of seventeenth-century London coal-burning glass-houses show high louvred roofs, not cones; but the cone seems to have been general in the provinces by the eighteenth century.

Similarly there is some doubt about when crucibles were caped or covered to avoid the problem of soot and coal particles falling into them. This practice may have been known before Ravenscroft's time, and it has generally been assumed that he must have used it in produc-ing his high-quality flint glass. Certainly when French glass-makers tried to make flint glass themselves they regarded caped pots as essen-tial to operating with coal. The caping, however, meant it was harder to raise the temperature of the melting batch sufficiently, for the flame of the furnace no longer played directly on the surface, so coal furnace design and stoking had to be of a high standard. However, in the case of English bottle glass with its dark colour there was no great need to cover the pots. One existing problem for glass-makers was the need to find good-quality fireclay for crucibles, and particularly where coal furnaces were operated at high temperatures (for instance with caped pots) the fireclay was critical. The need to renew crucibles was itself costly, but a burst crucible could also mean a very expensive loss of glass. Hence the success of Stourbridge with its superb fireclay, not only in attracting glasshouses to that district, but in supplying fireclay for crucibles, and for furnace bricks, to glasshouses in distant parts of the country.

Bottle Glass

The French glass industry, longer and more solidly established, naturally did not hasten to copy the changes in the English glass industry, which after all had been fairly recently dependent on the infusion of French technology. In 1700 English coal-fired furnaces were still unknown there, but by 1710 there was already one, in 1720 four. All these were bottle furnaces and 'thereafter, their popularity grew at a revolutionary rate'. Scoville believes there could have eventually been as many as forty-six. This increase was related to several factors.[6] There was the great extent of the French wine industry and its exports, and there was the additional element of brandy production where coal, often English, was already frequently used in coastal distilleries. There was the serious concern of the French authorities that an expansion of forest glass industries for bottle-making would put wood fuel supplies for domestic and general purposes under great strain in some districts and raise prices disastrously. Lastly, the relatively unsophisticated nature of coal-fired bottleworks made them relatively easy to copy.

The fuel situation was underlined by an *arrêt* of 1723 which insisted that new furnace owners had either to prove that their reserves of fuel were such as not to make them a threat to existing industries or to households, or alternatively to guarantee that they would use only coal, a rule which led to the virtual stagnation of the wood-burning bottle furnaces, while the coal ones grew rapidly in numbers and output. Many bottle furnaces were close to the ports, which enabled them not only to take advantage of the export trade but to obtain British coal when peace and the level of duties made it possible, as its quality was preferred. That English coal-fired bottle furnaces were readily adopted, and long in advance of the introduction of English methods in other branches of the industry, is certainly due to the simplicity of the technology, for open crucibles were used and there were no cones. Consequently it is unlikely that any serious espionage was needed to obtain the technology, as only the underground air passages and the grates would be very different from existing practice. However when, with great apprehension, the manager of the Tourlaville works of the Compagnie des Glaces decided on using coal for part of their production process in 1747 he turned to a certain Jean Mol who he said had built all the coal-using glass furnaces then operating in France, suggesting that even in this relatively simple area of coal-fuel technology in the glass industry the necessary construction skills did not diffuse with great rapidity.[7]

The first coal-fuelled dark-bottle factory was probably that of Thevenot in Picardy, set up in 1709, and already reported on as being very successful in 1712.[8] He was making bottles and carafes in the English fashion and perhaps emphasizing his independence of English assistance by claiming only to employ Catholic workers. Naturally those who were prominent in the French coal-mining industry tended from its early stages to move into coal-fired glass production. Desandrouin, a leading figure in the Hainault coal industry, had a works near the important mine of Fresnes in 1716 and had two others at Boulogne in the 1720s.[9] It is interesting that when setting up such works the entrepreneurs continued for decades to call them 'English-type', virtually until the Revolution. In setting up a works of this kind in southern France, on the Alès coalfield, Chatal emphasized in 1733 that he would use only coal. His venture was attacked by local master glass-makers, still clinging on to their claim to be gentlemen – 'gentilshommes verriers' – and as such to have a monopoly of produc-tion, and they boasted that as recently as 1715 they had enforced their pretensions to the point of going to law and closing a non-gentry glasshouse. Though the master glassworkers insisted that 'it was im-possible that gentlemen glass-makers could put up with the smoke of stone coal because it is so dense and is the reason why gentlemen glass-makers have always continued to use wood', the authorities did not consider their pleas for industrial gentility worth attention.

Another document stated that English-type bottles were already widely used, and a glassworks at Cette was also being authorized (though it may not have been completed) and allowed to employ workers whether they considered themselves gentlemen or commoners.[10] Already the important bottleworks at Sèvres near Paris was producing great quanti-ties of bottles, not far short of half a million a year between 1737 and 1739. Nevertheless, despite this assured success, it is remarkable that in the 1760s a string of applications to be allowed to build new dark-bottle furnaces that used coal continued to describe the product as 'façon de Angleterre' or 'a la manière d'Angleterre' in such widely dispersed sites as Normandy, Picardy and the Auvergne.[11] As late as 1786, when the brown-glass bottleworks of the important coal propri-etor Solages at Cramaux were favourably commented on in the famous report of de Dietrich on fuel use, they were still described as 'façon d'Angleterre'.[12]

The large bottleworks were extremely successful in the second half of the century. Sèvres produced about 1 million bottles in 1768 and 1.2

million in 1788 (nearly 1,000 tons) and this despite its position in the fuel-hungry Paris district, and the need to get some of its coal from a great distance, even from the Saint Etienne coalfield.[13] This would have been a source of astonishment to English glass-makers, many producing very close to coal-mines, or at least, like the Londoners, with coastal transport for their coal, and they would have quailed before the problems involved in river transport between Saint Etienne and Paris. Two Lyons works were at least as large as Sèvres.[14] While there may possibly have been some industrial espionage in the first acquisition by France of English bottle glass methods, and possibly some seduction of workers, it would have happened before the 1719 Act, and not at that time been liable to any penalty. Once the idea of underground access passages (*caves*) for air to the hearth had been mastered, together with the making of passages (*arcades*) for the entry and removal of pots, for fuelling with coal and for tending the fire, no further call was made on English technology. French bottle houses continued to have square furnaces in a rectangular building, often wooden, with a tile roof on a wooden frame, just like a domestic building. While contemporary experts were critical of the French glassworks, and compared them adversely with the English ones which melted the glass batch more rapidly and were more economical on fuel, the French bottle-makers preferred a second-best technology and less costly plant than the great English cones.[15]

Flint Glass

When we turn to flint glass the situation is very different. There was a great growth in the production of good white glass in France during the eighteenth century and some of the works where this was made (sometimes alongside the commoner kinds) became large and celebrated, like Saint Louis, Saint Quirin and Baccarat. Frequently there was a German or Bohemian transfusion of technology to such works for fine white glass, never, it would seem, an English one. The makers were eager to call their glass 'crystal'. But it was generally realized that it was of a lower order than the English flint glass, or 'cristal anglais', lacking the clearness and brilliance, the solidity, the ability to cut or engrave well, to produce the finest flashing lustres for chandeliers, or be the material for the best optical work. In the decades before the Revolution the claims for parity by French white glass-makers became louder, though never completely accepted by the Government, but at the same time desperate attempts were made to acquire English flint-glass making by intensive espionage and suborning.

While the main effort to gain flint-glass technology starts a decade later, there was already real interest in doing so in the late 1760s.[16] Not long before his death Gabriel Jars reported on the glassworks of Letebach near Saint Quirin 'perhaps the most important in the kingdom for white glass'. They told him, however, that no lead went into their glass. They complained of trouble with the breakage of too many pots, and he made several recommendations, based on what he had seen of English practice, on the fineness to which old pots and baked clay should be ground before being used in the composition of the pots. He also advised on the treading out of the clay, and the time the mixture for the crucibles should be left to stand before use, and on how to make a brick box in which to dry out the materials 'as the English do'. He 'advised them to make all sorts of white glass and that with lead, otherwise *flint-glass*, and send specimens to M. Trudaine de Montigny in order to get our opticians to try it out'. But they told him 'that they had already attempted the *flint-glass* but that it had not come out pure, and had marks in it and a lot of lead left at the bottom of the pot'. He thought that the potash they were using was possibly the problem. There was no mention of either covered pots or a cone furnace.[17]

About the same time an English glass-maker was memorializing the Government. Robert Scott Godefrey[18] said he had come to France late in 1767 'at the solicitation of the Count de Guerchy' – in other words he had been suborned through the French embassy. At first coming to France he had been commissioned by the Marquis de Marigny, the head of the royal buildings, to exercise his skill as a painter on glass, producing a window with a portrait of the king, who then appointed him his painter on glass, but without fixing a special pension. Though he had continually waited on de Marigny he had not been given an audience or any pension. He had 'spent all he had in the world to set up his Furnaces, purchase utensils, and support his wife and children'. His main aim was to produce the flint glass for which he had come over. 'He flatters himself that he may one day deserve [Marigny's patronage] by establishing in France a manufactory of Flint Glass, so well known and of such utility in England. He knows how to model it in all its forms, and to adapt it to all its known uses.' He needed a privilege to set up a flint-glass works in Paris or the environs, and to be paid for the work he had already done for the king.[19] Ill luck dogged

Godefrey. After ten years he got a privilege for a glasshouse for English crystal near Paris, saying he could produce it at half the price of the glass which was imported from England. But just as he was about to exercise his privilege Godefrey died 'without disclosing his secret, or training someone able to follow him in his enterprise'.

The next to claim the knowledge to make flint glass was Joseph Koenig. A Bohemian, he said he had worked for twenty-six years in one of the chief crystal glassworks in London in making 'le beau Cristal appellé *flint glass*'. He rather suspiciously claimed to have made it in all colours. He also claimed to have attempted to make it in Paris with 'the most satisfying success'. Godefrey had proposed making enamels, and so did Koenig, who also mentioned watch glasses, and glass for practitioners in medicine, mathematics and optics. In another paper Koenig insisted that English crystal was 'incomparably finer, more brilliant and purer than those made in the very best French glassworks, it is an article of trade which we do not have'. He wanted the Crown to provide a site, build the works and the necessary furnaces, and provide the tools and a 5,000 *livre* subsidy. Mignot de Montigny of the Academy to whom the proposals and specimens were referred was very suspicious of Koenig, of whom nothing was known, and who had no money or security to give to the proposed firm. If he could find a backer the king might give him an annual subsidy, a privilege for an area of ten or twelve leagues diameter (probably intended for the Paris area) and a title of royal manufacture. But it must be proved that he had himself made the flint glass samples he had submitted, and that he had the equipment and machinery needed to cut glass.

But when the inspector of manufacture for the Paris district went to see Koenig's works in September 1779 he found that he had a partner, whom Koenig had never mentioned in his petition for a privilege, and that the partner had just thrown him out because while he had fulfilled all the partnership arrangements Koenig had fulfilled none. The firm had thus collapsed and government support was pointless. But the inspector suggested that 'the secret which the Sieurs Lambert and Boyer claim to have of making cristal and enamels in the English fashion is that of Sieur Koenig, and that they have it from this foreigner who has made it known to them'. It is in this way that the two men enter the story who were, after many misadventures, to establish flint-glass making in France.[20]

The early years of the Lambert and Boyer enterprise were very tangled. Boyer was a senior official (intendant) in the household of the

Duc de Guines, which suggests some continuation of aristocratic patronage back to Godefrey's arrival, though the partners were to seek more powerful support still. Lambert, originally from Autun, was a chemist. The pair seem to have been partly reliant on German expertise originally but employed some senior French workers with whom they hoped to produce English crystal.

They set up a works in the park of Saint Cloud, then owned by the Duke of Orléans and under his powerful protection, and by 1782 they were attempting to produce crystal, but also enamel, which may help to confirm some continuity from the Godefrey venture. At this point they first submitted their products to government inspection, carried out by a celebrated scientist, Macquer, much employed as a commissioner. He approved the white enamel, which was particularly needed for clock and watch dials, and was much better than that on the market. If flint glass was important for watch glasses, dial enamel was clearly a useful complementary product. Macquer much approved the flint glass specimens they submitted which were clear and brilliant and the glass just as heavy as English flint glass and fit for chandelier lustres, decanters, drinking glasses and equipment for scientific laboratories. But there were stringy marks in the glass which seemed to rule it out for optical purposes, and he would get an expert on optics to check.[21] If rather more keen on their enamel than their glass, Macquer nevertheless recommended Lambert and Boyer for government support. This July report was followed by another by Macquer in December, by which time the entrepreneurs were making some glass on a production scale, while the specimens Macquer had seen had come from a pilot plant. Macquer had himself assisted at the first melting, where he thought the furnace had worked well, and now a glass-blower had turned the glass into articles 'on English patterns which he has imitated very well'. The blower had trouble in producing some of the more difficult forms, but Macquer was generally pleased with the glass. Some of the glass was later engraved and seemed comparable with English. Consequently he felt 'that the product of this manufacture will very soon be as perfect as could be desired, and in these matters we will not need to be at all envious of foreigners'.[22]

But as so often in these official reports, ordinary working of the glasshouse did not match the results of these special examinations, and English methods and standards had not been assimilated. Shortly afterwards Macquer reported that the partners had had to seek workers from England 'to be more sure of certain manual skills'. They were now crippled in extending their works by financial stringency; they wanted an exclusive privilege for their manufacture and an annual subsidy to cover their interest charges. The first they did not get, the second they did, not exceeding 5,000 *livres* a year, dependent on favourable reports by Macquer. The English technological infusion was emphasized in a document submitted by the Duke of Orléans, as the Saint Cloud works was on his land and under his auspices. In search of perfection, the entrepreneurs had

> taken themselves off to England to examine the glass furnaces of that country in order to be able to make similar ones so as to consume only coal [which shows that wood fuel had been used, at least in part, up to then] and further to find means to get hold of workers for blowing and cutting, those who work in French glasshouses not being able to work with this material which was absolutely new to them.

This indicates how little, outside bottleworks, coal had been assimilated by the French glass industry. The Duke's letter goes on to show how troublesome the English workers had been and how other French glass-makers had tried to entice them away, and asked the Government to enforce the extensive existing legislation against this practice.[23]

To the labour problems we will return. There exist fairly extensive accounts for the expenses of the Lambert and Boyer manufacture, both at Saint Cloud and later in Burgundy. The first one seems to date from 1783. Some of the costs are for the experimental plant, for what is probably the manager's residence, and for the first working hall, a furnace and an enamelling oven. It is interesting that brick and furnace clay had to come from a distance. The original furnaces were still being made by Germans 'Ficher [?Fischer] and his German friend and master-blower', and they were certainly given their first warming up by wood fuel.

But then there is an entry 'for the complete demolition of the said two furnaces which were found to be so badly built as to be unusable'. So the funds for building two new ones had to be found. For some of the building Lambert and Boyer turned to the mason from the *manufacture royale* of glass at nearby Sèvres thus drawing on the expertise of the expert from one of the oldest coal-using glassworks in France. Again wood was used to dry out the furnace. They then took on master blowers, a blowing-pipe maker, and stokers, all French. These men must have insisted on having uncovered crucibles, but these proved useless once real English furnaces were used and were discarded. In interesting contrast to Macquer's praises, it proved that when large scale manufacture was tried 'none of the pieces produced could be retained'. The glass itself was good but it was badly formed into vessels.

Then the working hall was found to be too small to contain both the furnace and the blowing teams which worked round it, wood which was still being used as fuel was too expensive for the high temperature needed and, even with wood, flame and sparks harmed the material in the uncovered pots. Taken together these considerations led Lambert and Boyer to knock down the furnaces once again and build new ones in a much bigger hall. Not only were these things constructed, but also new or altered buildings or plant, including a fritting furnace, underground access passages, a laboratory and a store, were put in. Of course all this rebuilding was expensive in skilled labour and materials. Again there was expense for wood to dry out and prepare the furnaces. A water-mill was built for grinding and sieving materials. For some of this work a brass-wire sieve was bought in England.

At this point it was once again seen as desirable to obtain expert English workers, a blower, a cutter and an engraver 'so as to get the necessary instructions to be able to make the furnace according to the dimension of English ones, and only consume coal, without doing damage to the crystal and also get the method of making pots suitable for the said furnaces'. The Company asked two partners, Lambert and Dusauchay, to pass secretly into England. The journey, which only secured a single worker, cost 2,700 *livres*. Now the firm set about building a new great working hall, and new access passages to the furnaces, 108 feet long, 8 feet deep and 8 feet high. Again special firebrick and furnace clay were bought. This time the furnaces were again dried out with a wood fire, very slowly, the process lasting a full month, but the final seasoning of the furnace was done with coal. Once again recourse was made to England for cast iron marvering tables, testifying (as in so many other cases) to the superiority of English iron casting. Iron furnace bars and some iron tools were bought in, and the moulds for all the glass vessels or parts which could be cast or blown in a mould.

Then came the critical piece of English technology, thirty-six pots covered with lids of special clay. The accounts go into the greatest detail about the large hall attached to the mill, the workers' housing, sheds, even the latrines, paving and other facilities. One gets the impression of the employment of the dignified and over-expensive industrial architecture common in prestige projects in France.

The chief French workers were now paid off and dismissed; they had been trying to work with coal, but had failed. A boatload of coal costing about 1,800 *livres* had been consumed 'being a complete loss for the entrepreneurs'. It was thought that there had been a comparable loss of materials for the batch, of over 1,200 *livres*. There now had to be an additional trip to England, for which a Sieur Gutter (possibly German?) was employed. He contracted two English glass-blowers with their assistants (*garçons*), a lustre cutter and three cutters for other decoration. Interestingly the French firm had to pay off the workers' debts in England, and then those who did the actual suborning of the individual workers had to be paid for their services, no doubt generously in view of the potential legal penalties. Then the expenses of the men, their wives and children, had to be paid on their travels from the port of London to Paris. Gutter had to be paid a good fee for organizing the whole operation.

The operation had been carried out before the Tools Act of 1786, for blowers' tools and cutters' tools were straightforwardly exported from England, paying duty in both countries, together with a collection of moulds and wheels for the men's work, not to mention their personal baggage. Then six glass cutters' lathes were made at Paris and Sèvres for the considerable sum of 1,800 *livres*, and three engraving lathes. Finally there were beds, chests, and wardrobes for the English workers – and interestingly chimney pieces and hearths, so that they could enjoy the coal fires they did in England. The costs of the enterprise down to 1783 were listed as 134,517 *livres*, but there seem to have been some other accounts not incorporated. An English visitor to France in 1785 said that the glass being made at the Queen's Glassworks was 'Parker's Cut-Glass ... two-three Renegade-Journeymen of that ingenious Artist, are making fortunes'.[24]

There is a quite comic picture of technological tangles as Lambert and Boyer sought to take up a specialized English industrial process on wholly inadequate information, the most important errors being related to their lack of understanding of the technologies related to coal. These included the necessity to use coal for the temperatures needed for flint glass – no instances of successful production with wood are known – the need for covered pots, the qualities of firebrick, the type of crucible clay and the making of crucibles. They got them all wrong, and the continual scrapping and reconstruction of plant must have made the site seem a sort of industrial madhouse.[25]

Once they had brought in a selection of English workers and their tools and looked at English glasshouses and their arrangements one might have expected smoother operation, but the entrepreneurs still had a rough ride. We find the Duke of Orléans writing on their behalf to say 'that after all these efforts and troubles ... Lambert and Boyer hoped to enjoy their enterprise without further trouble. They were deceived. On the one hand the workmen left their employ and absented themselves without permission, to the great prejudice of the firm', while there was the enticement away of workers by French firms which we have already mentioned.

In August 1785 the entrepreneurs informed Calonne that 'the English workers, when they had hardly arrived, did everything they could to ruin the manufacture. There was bad production, time wasting, and often complete stoppage of work. Lambert and Boyer then decided to train French workers'. They claimed to have succeeded in both the quality of product and speed of work, and could now do without the Englishmen, but they had sacrificed much to reach this position: 'it has been a very expensive school for the petitioners'. Up to now they had been working more for the good of the State than their own benefit.[26] The troubles at the works were extensive and a nuisance to the civil authorities. The head of the local *maréchaussée* wrote that 'there are difficulties every day between the entrepreneurs of this glasswork and the workers' and he was frequently called on to arrest them. His most recent case had been an Englishman who was paid weekly piece-work rates, and having made his quota he wanted to stop work, even though the furnaces were still alight. In this case the official had been able to settle the dispute. The proprietors would not have had trouble with this worker if it had not been for another Englishman, George, who was the more skilful of the two but 'the worst scamp in the world'. They believed themselves irreplaceable, and that they could come and go at will.[27]

Much later in 1808, Lambert, now apparently no longer connected with the glassworks, and making enamel at Sèvres, recounted the problems with England and English workers. On one of the English trips their interpreter had been arrested (apparently a relation of Boyer) and had committed suicide in an English prison. Once the Saint Cloud works seemed likely to succeed with its English workers, the British embassy in Paris intervened. The secretary of the ambassador gave the workers money for drink to keep them from working properly, after which the British government made continual requests that the workers be handed over to the ambassador and 'the French government of the time was weak enough to give into the demands'. The workers who 'had cost us such sacrifices' were handed over. Lambert said that he and Boyer were allowed a three months' delay, but in fact it was for six months as, under the 1719 Act, emigrant English workers summoned home had the right to six months' notice and the French authorities insisted on their remaining for that time.

In a letter to the minister in April 1785 the entrepreneurs said that there had been an unofficial approach to the workers by 'London merchants', presumably on behalf of their former English employers. They had got into the works, presumably warning the operatives that they were going to invoke the legislation against the emigration of skilled workers. This clearly disturbed the men, who became undisciplined. They only worked when they wanted and tried to avoid working in front of French workers. Overall the Lambert and Boyer episode is a remarkable example of what could happen when the British government got its act together both in catching those who were suborning workers, and in demanding their repatriation.[28]

During these troubles the ownership of the Parc de Saint Cloud changed hands, passing from the Duke of Orléans (the father of Phillipe Egalité) to Marie Antoinette. The Duke had provided the land for the works and on several occasions the partners recorded their gratitude to him, 'the enlightened protector of useful firms', as Lambert described him in his article of 1808. He claimed that it was the keenness of the English diplomats to get back the English workers which fixed French government attention on the firm. But Marie Antoinette clearly took a personal interest in the works, perhaps because of her reputed fascination for chandelier lustres; the works was immediately called the Queen's Glassworks, and retained the name when the site was changed. This happened in 1786–87, the specific *arrêt* for the change being made in February 1787. An explanatory document stated that while the glass produced at Saint Cloud was getting so close in quality to the English that it was hoped that it would soon equal it, the Saint Cloud works was still of too small a scale, and other local problems prevented it being completely successful. The quality of the glass often varied because the coal available near Paris was not always equally good and the fuel problem meant that there was no regularity in the production process nor a constant output of glass. With too low a heat the alkali was not properly incorporated, the fluxing effect diminished and the melting was imperfect, so that the glass had a gelatinized appearance and looked stringy, and it had air bubbles. But product quality problems deriving from the quality of the coal itself were compounded by the high price of coal at Paris, the high cost of labour near the capital, and the somewhat cramped site.

The very drastic step was taken of removing the whole operation to Montcenis in Burgundy, and installing it alongside the ironworks of Le Creusot. The machinations which led to this step are not explicit, but a manufacture which was not merely a *manufacture royale*, but also named for the queen, had to have some degree of grandeur or even magnificence. From the point of view of Calonne, by integrating iron-works and glassworks he was able, according to Dietrich, to gather on one great site examples of the latest British technology, showing both what could be accomplished with coal fuel, and how well the French could master the technology. As another account puts it, it was an attempt to 'obtain for the industry of the nation, the advantage of not having any longer to resort to foreigners for goods of common and even daily necessity', and to gain two industrial processes 'possessed exclusively up to now by the English'.[29]

The *arrêt* for the removal of the enterprise to Le Creusot is brief and stresses only the better supply situation there, but makes it clear that the firm would be absorbed into the business complex to which Le Creusot and Indret already belonged, so that Lambert and Boyer were to concert with Wendel, Périer, and the powerful financial group supporting them, in which there was already a royal investment. This was paralleled by a similar investment of 150,000 *livres* in the Queen's Glassworks.

Fortunately the building of the Queen's Glassworks survives, illustrating the quite sumptuous standards to which the most prestigious royal manufactures were built. Now it is a part of the Ecomusée of Le Creusot and serves to facilitate the historical understanding of this famous industrial region, now with only its past to celebrate. It survives because its elegance and quality of construction caused it to become the mansion of the Schnieder family when they took over the great ironworks in the next century. The mansion had an English glass cone at the end of either wing! One is said to have contained a private theatre.

By the time the move to Le Creusot was approved the number of English workmen remaining was small. There seems to have been a third attempt at recruiting more workmen around the time of the move in 1786. A German approached Lambert and Boyer in February 1786 proposing to obtain English workers 'of all kinds and all this with the utmost secrecy. The singular advantage presented by engaging English workers led Messrs Lambert and Boyer to begin negotiations'. Apparently an instant decision had to be made 'in the fear that the matter

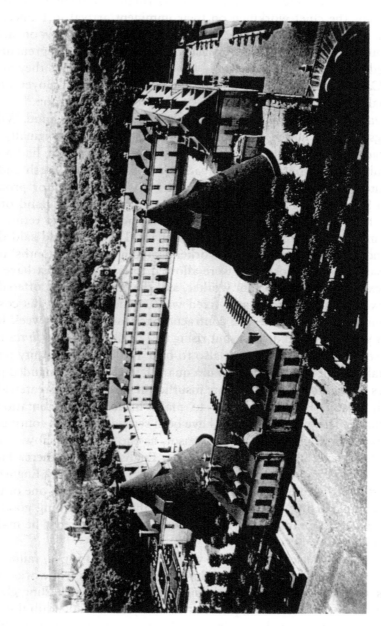

14.1 'Verrerie de la Reine', Le Creusot: modern view of the eighteenth-century glassworks. Photograph, 1916

should be discovered in London'. The German then demanded 50 *louis d'or* for the chief workmen on their imminent arrival in France; time was not to be lost for the men would have no money on arrival. Though they thought the sum asked too great, the entrepreneurs decided to accede. Someone would have to meet the men as they arrived at Calais and take them directly to Burgundy, which Boyer did on behalf of the new enlarged Indret-Le Creusot-Verrerie group.[30]

One of the original group of English workers at Saint Cloud, William Biggs, a lustre cutter, went on to Le Creusot. He had originally been attracted by the promise of higher wages in France, as he had a large family. But he considered his treatment at Saint Cloud harsh and had wanted to go home. Not only had the British ambassador promised him his travelling expenses, but his old employer in England offered him his job back. It is to be noted that he had arranged to return after six months, the statutory period under the 1719 Act, and said that a French *arrêt* insisted that the workers complete the six months' notice at Saint Cloud before they were allowed to leave. He must have been an exceptionally important worker, and the entrepreneurs offered him a six months' contract, at a fixed wage, which included his costs of training an apprentice. The contract wage was 9 *livres* a week in the first year, hardly luxurious, but rising to 12, 18, 20 and 24 *livres* in the subsequent years. There was also to be a 1,000 *livres* gratuity paid in instalments. However, there was a quarrel when Biggs demanded piece-rates after finding the fixed rate insufficient, and Boyer threatened him with prison. Biggs demanded to make his own representations to Calonne. The quarrel seems to have been settled, for Biggs continued to be paid for some years at Le Creusot, as the accounts show.[31] There were, however briefly, one or two other English workers there. 'Here is also a pretty considerable crystal glass work, in which two Englishmen are still left' wrote Arthur Young in 1789. He talked with one of them: 'he complained of the country, and said there was nothing good in it but wine and brandy; of which things I question not that he makes a sufficient use'.[32]

The Le Creusot glassworks was not as depressing a failure and counter-example for English technology as the great ironworks which was its neighbour; as the sole significant producer of flint glass in France it received various prizes at the early industrial exhibitions and laudatory testimonials; during the long war period it was able to export to the parts of Europe under French occupation or influence, but it did not survive beyond the early decades of the nineteenth century. There were other attempts to set up flint-glass manufacture in France; the total number of such attempts was probably, as Scoville says, about seven. Their importance was not always as great as the archival mentions would indicate. Meyer Oppenheim, originally from Pressburg, had settled in England where he worked for many years, particularly in Birmingham, in making flint glass and coloured glass. He appears in Rouen in 1783, working with a pilot production plant. He obtained a privilege for making flint glass with coal in the following year, but quickly fell out with his partner. They employed briefly eighteen blowers, three being English and three German. Oppenheim wanted to produce English coloured glass as well as crystal. Coloured glass was important in Birmingham where it appeared in various of the ornamental or 'toy' products of the town. While living there Oppenheim had taken out a patent for red glass in 1770; as early as 1755 he had taken out a similar one when living in London.[33] By 1786 Oppenheim had fallen out with his French associate and the glass he produced was said to be poor and tasteless in design, and he seems to have been prevented from creating further works at Rouen and Le Havre.[34]

Once war caused trade with England to be again broken off there was a grave shortage of optical glass and in the Year II the Committee of Public Safety backed a works at Boulogne-sur-Seine where the glass was said (as in the cases of so many other works) to equal English crystal. It lasted at least to the Year VI when its glass was exhibited with the Le Creusot product and said to be as good. There were two brief attempts at English crystal in the Bordeaux district in the late 1780s and another in Paris in 1797,[35] but they seem to have had little significance and we know of no English workers at any of them. At the very beginning of the Revolution a man called Belesaigne appeared. He had been chief workman and manager of a white-glass works at Cork in Ireland and had been in Britain for thirty years. He was born French, but had fled from France with his family because of 'persecution of non-catholics', and had worked in all the most celebrated works in England. He wanted to go and set up a glassworks at Castries in Languedoc to produce flint glass for optical purposes on the pattern of the English product. His project was referred to the opinion of several outstanding Academicians, Berthollet, Desmarets, Cassini and Abeille, before whom he was to demonstrate his abilities. But they had by now learned caution and wisdom in making assessment of new glass projects and of selected specimens from pilot plants. Belesaigne, they said, could only turn out flint glass once he had built his works: 'it will only be over time and with a continuous and thorough operation and in a furnace which has in the course of events been constructed with care that this artist will be able to produce samples of glass by which his intelligence and talent can be judged'. They simply gave him a permit to build a furnace using only coal in any place he considered suitable in Languedoc. His further activities are unknown.[36]

Plate Glass

The technological exchanges between England and France in the plate glass industry are complex, but quite fascinating. They will only be summarized here, and the concentration will be on those transfers of technology which were achieved by subterfuge, usually by the entice-ment of managers and the suborning of workers. While each country desired some of the processes developed in the other, in the case of this industry there is no doubt that the most important innovative process was French, and that British efforts to obtain it were remarkably parallel to the efforts the French made to obtain British technical advances in other industries.[37]

The French in the late seventeenth century were chiefly jealous of Venetian skills in the production of quality flat (plate) glass with a soda alkali. The glass was blown in a long cylinder, flattened, and then ground and polished with great care to make large and handsome mirrors and strong and clear glasses for coach windows. The Venetians made great efforts to prevent the emigration of workers. But Louis XIV, driven by his great projects of palace building, encouraged Colbert, already concerned to bring prestigious luxury industries to France, to secure the necessary skilled Venetians. The Royal Plate Glass Manufac-tory was set up by the king in 1665 and began operations in the following year. Manufacturing of the raw glass was soon moved to Tourlaville in Normandy, while the final preparation of mirror glass remained in Paris.

However, to condense the story radically, a rival company appeared in 1688 which was also privileged by the Crown. This was based upon an entirely new method of forming the glass, by casting it on a metal table instead of blowing it into a cylinder. While the actual invention is obscure, there is no doubt that it was French, and that it was made into a technically and commercially successful process by Louis Lucas de Nehou, formerly with the other company at Tourlaville. The new company eventually took over the site of the huge ruined castle of Saint Gobain in Picardy, partly using its materials for their buildings. The great advantage of their casting method was that much larger mirror glasses could be made. The rivalry of the companies became ruinous, and in a vain attempt to save them the king amalgamated them in 1695, but the united company was bankrupt by 1702. Royal prestige was too involved to let the concern founder, and a new firm was set up in the same year. Ironically for the catholic monarch the financial side of the concern was greatly strengthened by the introduction of Swiss investors, Genevan Protestants. There were subsequent periods of difficulty, both technical and organizational, but from 1710 de Nehou gave inspired management to the works at Saint Gobain and Tourlaville. For a long period the Saint Gobain works employed both blowing and casting, while casting was introduced at Tourlaville by David Oury, one of the best managers to emerge after de Nehou's death.[38]

Though the company was supposed to have a monopoly within France, there were several attempts to set up rival firms in France or its dependencies. There was an early works in the principality of Dombes under the patronage of the Duc de Maine, though under restriction on its sales. It only lasted a short time. But a large works at Rouelles in Burgundy was protected by the provincial Estates and existed for about twenty years before succumbing. Naturally the industry, and essentially the new casting process, was wanted beyond France. The former director of the defunct Dombes works took the manufacture to Spain under royal protection around 1720, while the difficulties and temporary closure of the Compagnie des Glaces around 1700 led to the creation of a German works in the Archbishopric of Mainz, though it did not permanently continue casting. In 1691 there was an attempt in England to set up a company to cast glass plates, a patent was taken out and parliamentary incorporation unsuccessfully petitioned for. Almost certainly, as Professor Barker has suggested, this was an attempt to safeguard the enormous capital which was needed for the casting process.[39] The problems of the French company *c*.1700 are said to have led to the emigration of workers to England too, for we hear of the casting of plates of large size at a Vauxhall glassworks in 1701. Plate continued to be made there, and it was reported on as we shall see by a French visitor in the 1760s,[40] but the works were not casting then, and had certainly long ceased to do so by the time the great effort to set up a British casting works was made in the 1770s. A works at Southwark was also both blowing and casting plates in the 1740s. The situation however was that the casting process had failed to become permanently established in Britain, and by the 1770s only blown plates of limited size were made in this country and the French company was exporting large cast plates to the value of £60,000 to £100,000 a year to Britain.[41]

At this point an influential group in Britain made strong efforts to obtain the casting process. Of great importance was Admiral Philip Affleck, and he was backed by a strong Scottish group, many of whom were important in the East India Company. There were a few men of French background involved in the early days, including the principals of a great French merchant house in London, Bourdieu and Chollet. But Affleck's other connection was with his brother-in-law, John Mackay, the Scot who took a decisive part in the development of the St Helens coalfield in Lancashire, where he had bought the coal-rich Ravenhead estate and had also invested in the nearby Thatto Heath colliery and the adjacent glasshouse. As already mentioned in connection with the copper industry, Mackay's policy was not simply to export coal from the coalfield but to attract industries which were large users of coal to his mines. A few years before his agreement with the Parys Mine Company of Anglesey to site their great copper smelter at Ravenhead, he had already brought the British Cast Plate Glass Company to that estate, no doubt through his family connection with Affleck, and he was himself an original investor.

How did the British company obtain the necessary expertise? As the French would have done if the situation had been reversed they sought technical skill from their rivals in the originating country. They did so at the highest level, approaching Delaunay Deslandes, the director of Saint Gobain, and one of the most brilliant managers in eighteenth-century Europe, who controlled the vast works both technically and organizationally. After a period of weak management and technical disasters Deslandes led the company to prosperity, discipline, technical efficiency and larger markets at home and abroad in a long period as Director lasting from 1758 to the eve of the revolution. Deslandes said that he was approached by Lord Mansfield to join the new British concern, but refused. It would have been an astounding coup if he could have been recruited, and the wealthy Compagnie des Glaces and the French state itself would have left no stone unturned to prevent his leaving. His memoirs have the cryptic comment on the incident 'I always have had a French heart and I always held to the principle that while one must eat bread it did not have to be gall' – presumably his

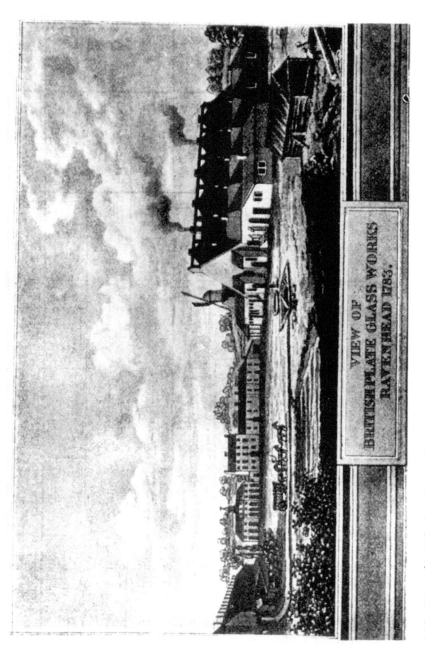

The text within the image reads:

VIEW OF
BRITISH PLATE GLASS WORKS
RAVENHEAD 1783.

14.2   View of British plate glassworks, Ravenhead, 1783

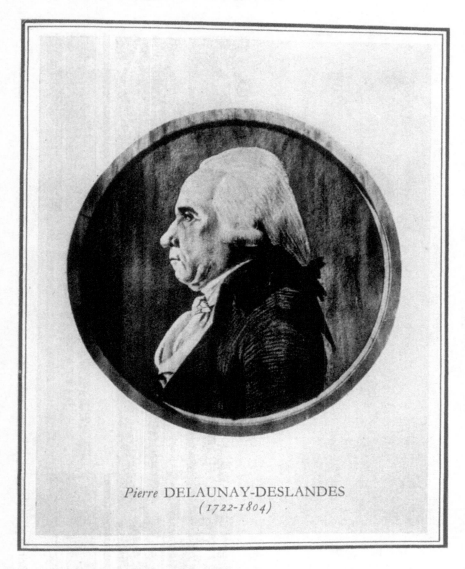

Pierre DELAUNAY-DESLANDES
(1722-1804)

14.3   Pierre Delaunay Deslandes (1722–1804), director of Saint Gobain from 1758 to 1789

view on English cooking. But when Mansfield and another British peer visited him at Saint Gobain soon after, they told him that, given his unwillingness to move to England, they had recruited Philip Besnard, formerly a manager at Saint Gobain, but dismissed by Deslandes. He had then gone to manage the rival works at Rouelles in Burgundy, from which he had later also been dismissed.

Besnard was in Britain by 1771 and carried out the first stages of obtaining a patent for cast plate, but did not persist, perhaps because his British partners preferred secrecy to patenting. While there is much highly complicated detail, the upshot would seem to be that Besnard did not agree with the embryonic British Cast Plate Glass Company which intended to set up at Ravenhead, and began to make overtures to a second group headed by the Duke of Northumberland and to be based in the North East. Negotiations were conducted through the diplomat and writer, Louis Dutens, whom we have already met with when giving the remarkable account of Holker's escape from Newgate, which Dutens had heard while he and Holker were being entertained by the Duc de Choiseul. Dutens had been attached to the Duke of Northumberland's household as a chaplain and tutor. In these discussions another foreign technologist was involved, Pierre Théodore de Bruges, presumably from the Austrian Netherlands, though little is known of him. He claimed to have various chemical processes including ones for improved soda, and soda would be sold on the market as well as being made for plate glass manufacture. However this scheme, though being discussed as late as 1777, never got off the ground. The Lancashire scheme had been launched under parliamentary incorporation (giving it effectively limited liability) which would hardly have been repeated very soon for a second company. There was little likelihood that the market could have supported the output of two companies, and Besnard's terms for his services were unrealistic and greedy.[42]

Besnard was replaced at Ravenhead by Jean-Baptiste François Graux, another defector from Saint Gobain, perhaps disillusioned by his brother's imprisonment for defecting from Saint Gobain to another French glasshouse. Deslandes regarded him a 'Mauvais sujet' in the same class as Besnard, 'but absolutely without any kind of knowledge and talent', which seems perhaps too harsh a judgement. Graux brought over two skilled workmen, Couturier and Poirier, who were soon disenchanted with Ravenhead, and considered Graux did not pay them well enough and so sought employment at the Cookson glassworks at Newcastle. Couturier told the Cooksons that Ravenhead would soon collapse as 'the person who manages the same [Graux] knows nothing of the nature of working the Glass to Perfection'. However, he and Poirier soon applied to the French ambassador to return to France, and though doubts about their readmission were raised by both the foreign minister and Deslandes, they eventually were allowed back to Saint Gobain. About this time some of the Ravenhead proprietors, but not Affleck, who did not believe additional French expertise was needed, toyed with bringing over Paul Bosc D'Antic. He was a savant as well as an industrialist. He was for two years at Saint Gobain, where his scientific talents, particularly for soda manufacture, were greatly over-estimated by some of the Company, and he had eventually been thrown out and went to law with the firm. He had then helped to found the rival firm at Rouelles, but had been dismissed after two years to be replaced by Besnard. Bosc seems to have been very concerned to be elected to the Royal Society, and when he was narrowly rejected his interest in Ravenhead seems to have ended.

Graux, who now added 'de la Bruyère' to his name, presumably to suggest his gentility, was persisted with at Ravenhead until his death in 1787. On a personal level he was well regarded, but he did not succeed in making the company either technically or commercially viable. He seems to have operated the basic casting operation well once he had obtained large copper casting tables to a high enough specification. His main technical problem was a general one; having been trained in a wood-fuel system he found great difficulty in changing to a coal sys-tem. There was a saving in fuel costs by using coal, but much of the glass was bad, and a high proportion was mere waste because he did not use covered pots and glass suffered from coal smoke and coal fragments which discoloured and spotted it. Possibly he was unable to use covered pots because he did not know how to get sufficient heat from his furnaces, though such pots were tried.

It was only when Robert Sherbourne who had been with the Com-pany from the early days, but not on the manufacturing side, took over at Ravenhead in 1792, that a great turn-round took place. In effect Ravenhead fully exploited British coal-fuel technologies, the caped pots were used successfully and permanently, the cuvettes, in which the final stages of heating took place before the glass was poured over the tables, were given a separate furnace. Waste was cut down to a fraction of its former extent so that what was left over was able to be absorbed as the cullet element in a later batch. It was found possible to take advantage of the coke-iron revolution by using large glass-casting tables made of cast iron. Sherbourne was a lucky general; excise regulations were not so onerous as they had been in Graux's time; instead of facing an invasion of Saint Gobain glass in one of the few French triumphs under the Eden trade treaty, and one where they could

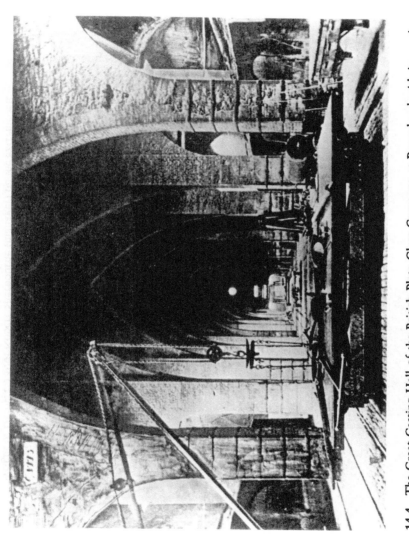

14.4 The Great Casting Hall of the British Plate Glass Company at Ravenhead with its casting tables, date unknown

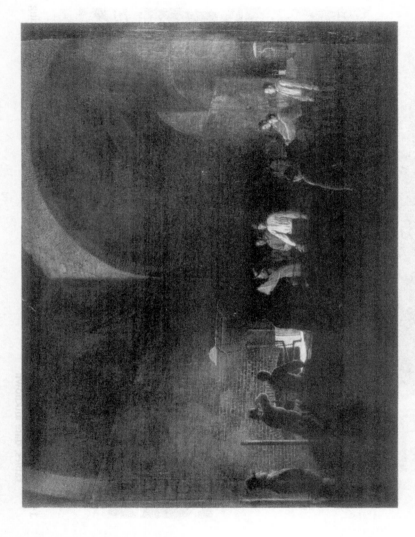

14.5 Casting plate glass at Ravenhead. Photograph of painting believed to be after Joseph Wright of Derby, c.1800: Robert Sherbourne (manager) on the extreme left

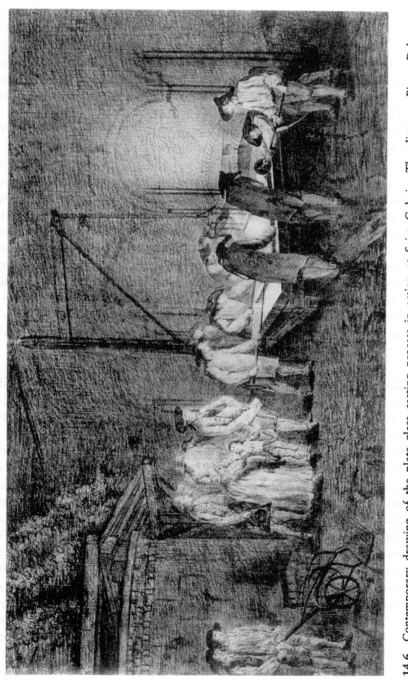

14.6 Contemporary drawing of the plate glass casting process in action at Saint Gobain. The director, Pierre Delaunay Deslandes, attends the moment of casting wearing his sword and the cordon of the order of St Michel

be confident of superiority, he had only to face a Saint Gobain distracted by the Revolution, and then from 1793 enjoy a home market
secured by war. In these conditions the Company was able to obtain a
renewed Act of incorporation in 1794 with reorganized finances. By
1806 Sherbourne was making £48,000 worth of glass a year 'and that
of such glasses as had never been made in England'.[43]

While Ravenhead was dependent on a basic French technology for
casting, it had developed a new technology for the grinding and polishing of glass, and it was only there that it had a superiority to French
production. Here again there was a recourse to coal-based technology,
natural for a company sited on excellent and plentiful coal, but upon
the Lancashire plain, where hydraulic power was limited. The idea was
to turn to the newly available rotative power of the steam engine.
Previously Ravenhead had sent its glass out unpolished, which meant a
considerable loss of profits. Like Saint Gobain they preferred to face
the lesser breakage losses on raw as compared with polished glass, but
they did not have, as Saint Gobain did, finishing facilities in the met-
ropolis. An important factor in their change of policy, and decision to
export finished glass from Ravenhead, may have been the rapid spread
of the canal network, improving the transport of a fragile product.

In 1786 they approached James Watt, not only to supply an engine,
but also to devise the machinery which would be needed to grind and
polish. This he did by designing grinding and polishing tables in which
pairs of glasses were moved over each other in a circular motion with
the abrasive materials between. The tables were installed on two working floors, each with a set of ten, and in such a way that the movement
of any single pair of glasses could be stopped separately. This was a
brilliant but now almost forgotten invention of Watt's; it was the basis
for finishing plate glass until the twentieth century. While Saint Gobain
devised a hydraulically powered polishing system at a subsidiary works
of Saint Gobain c.1800, the French recognized the superiority of Watt's
system as soon as they knew of it and in the 1820s they obtained the
equipment from the celebrated iron founders and engineers, Halls of
Deptford. Neither Saint Gobain nor Ravenhead was now in a
monopoly position in their home country and, unable to penetrate
Ravenhead, Hall suborned a foreman and workers from another plate
glass company in order to be able to make the Watt system, first for
Saint Gobain and subsequently for the Saint Quirin company. Incidentally the laws still in force on the export of machinery were possibly
broken.[44]

There were other important instances where the French tried to copy in the plate glass industry the coal-fuel technologies that were well established in English glass-making. But these particular efforts were not, on existing evidence, based on industrial espionage. The motives of the French managers were in each case a need to save wood-fuel, or to allow an expansion of production without driving up the price of fuel, and so making the expansion unprofitable. In the 1740s David Oury, manager of the Tourlaville works of the Compagnie des Glaces in Normandy, was pressed by the company to investigate the possibilities of using coal-fuel, the main incentive being the growing shortage of local wood supplies. He started from the expertise in furnace building and operation already gained in bottle-glass production and he left a splendid account of his enquiries, experiments and problems which has been described in detail elsewhere.[45] There was a limited expertise in building coal furnaces, and he had to use the services of the one man, Jean Mol, who had built most of the existing coal furnaces in France. The difficulties lay not only in furnace construction, but in the whole business of managing and stoking a coal furnace, which though a matter of general knowledge in England, was virtually unknown in France. Mol should be retained to train stokers and furnace hands, those who could use coal were rare, dear and obstreperous. Nevertheless, despite great anxiety, Oury did manage a partial conversion of the furnaces at Tourlaville to coal, but a full conversion was never achieved. There is no mention of covered pots, and how the pollution of the product was controlled is unknown, or whether Tourlaville's concentration on blown plate made any difference. The conversion to coal was not only partial but imperfect, and in 1758 an Englishman, Egleton, was at Tourlaville teaching French workers to use coal, but we do not know how he came there, or whether or not he was suborned.

Saint Gobain was surrounded by much greater forest reserves than Tourlaville, but these were mainly in the hands of powerful aristocratic proprietors, though the company subsequently sought to buy its own forests. Wood remained the main fuel until 1829 and was not dispensed with until 1850. But in 1762, soon after Deslandes assumed control, he began to plan new casting halls where coal could be used as well as wood, one motive being to keep the wood suppliers in some anxiety about their market, and moderate their price demands. His use of coal was not timid or tentative, and one or two of the four great furnaces used coal for extended periods between 1768 and 1784. The interest here is that Saint Gobain and Ravenhead were both trying to use coal in cast plate production over much the same span of years and both having great problems. Finally in 1784 Deslandes gave up:

> I have not been able to succeed except very imperfectly. The English have tried likewise, and they have spared no expense. They have devoted to it the genius which no one will deny them, and the persistence they give to all they undertake. They have succeeded even less well than I have.

At that time his view of the failure of the British attempts was quite justified, and shows that he was obtaining good intelligence about Ravenhead.

The main reason Deslandes failed was his inability to use caped pots. He knew all about them, and drawings of them survive in his papers, but he seems to have lacked confidence that he could raise the temperature of the melt to a sufficient level in such pots. He made the most careful attempts to ensure that the standard of stoking in his furnaces was of the highest and the actions of the stokers were controlled to the last degree. But he was not always able to get British coal, and some of the French coal he obtained was not of equal quality or had high transport costs. The draught control for the upper part of his furnaces may have been defective. However, he admitted that though 'I have put the effort into this that I have given to everything I have done ... we have not been able to succeed'. The situation is full of irony. Deslandes produced a most remarkable essay for the Académie des Sciences on 'the means of making glassworks coal-fired' of which a copy is attached to his splendid 'Mémoire' or 'Historique'. The greatest irony is that his work in operating with coal was made a principal justification for his being ennobled and honoured with the cordon of Saint Michel, and that this was received just as he was throwing his hand in and giving up the use of coal. In the case of Deslandes's experiments with, and employment of, coal there is no way he could have profited by industrial espionage in England. There was no successful British coal-fired plate glass industry to imitate, and there was not much he could have learned of direct relevance from other branches of the glass industry. In fact the boot may have been on the other foot; Deslandes's preparations for a move to coal-fuel began in the late 1760s, some use was made in 1768 and extensive use in 1770 and 1771, so that Graux may have had experience of it before he came to Ravenhead.[46]

The British attempts to gain the technology of the French plate glass industry show that there was as little scruple on the British side in suborning key managers and workers from France, as there was in the instances of the many other industries where France endeavoured, and often succeeded, in suborning British ones. The difference was simply that there was a British technological lead in far more industries, and the value of obtaining French workers was generally less significant to the British. The problems of acquiring the process of casting presented some initial problems at Ravenhead, but with persistence they were overcome. What proved the great headache was the problem of connecting the glass-making to coal-fuel. The eventual breakthrough at Ravenhead gains all the more interest from the parallel attempts to use coal by Deslandes at Saint Gobain, while the brilliance as managers of both Deslandes and Sherbourne, and the strong support both received from their companies, means that we do not have to ascribe the eventual French failure and British success in coal-use to non-technical factors. Had Deslandes been operating in an industrial environment where the large-scale employment of coal in furnace industries had long been common, and all the related know-how and skills were in place, and if he had assured supplies of excellent coal a few hundred yards away, as was the case with Ravenhead, the short distance he remained from success might have been crossed.

Two examples of French reports on English glassworks in the eighteenth century should be noted. Both were connected with Saint Gobain. De Roux, a chemist employed at various times by the Compagnie des Glaces, apparently on a consultative basis, was sent in 1769 to visit English glasshouses. He seems to have discovered only two plate glass works then operating, and both blowing and not casting. Both sold their glass raw and not polished, leaving that to the mirror-makers. One was at Newcastle, one at Vauxhall near London. The Newcastle works sold through a warehouse in London's Fleet Street. Roux seems only to have visited the Vauxhall works. Though it had three halls only one operated at a time, probably reflecting the abandonment of casting, which had been carried on earlier in the century, and Roux regarded the works as insignificant compared with the 'grandeur' of Saint Gobain.

Coal was the main fuel, but the pots were heated with wood during the working period, which suggests that they were not then covered. The furnace was vaulted in a kind of refractory sandstone, the pots made of Stourbridge fireclay. The furnaces could last four years, but had to be put out occasionally for repair to the 'sièges' of the furnaces on which the pots stood.[47] Though the life of the pots varied, he was told, from a week to four months, he thought that from the large number in store an average life would be a fortnight. He thought that because the old glass (cullet) which was put into the batch was partly the flint glass only found in England, that there would be some small lead content in the glass. Blowing only took place on three days a week, and Sunday was not a work day. The works claimed to be able to blow glasses of great size, but one of these took a whole night to produce and the general run of glasses made was much smaller. Roux considered the glass had been well refined, but was of a very bad colour, though it had melted well, which he believed was due to added arsenic and lead glass cullet. He had not visited the Newcastle works, but the glass of theirs which he had seen had string-like markings and a green colour. He did see some mirror-polishing, and learnt about the making of beaten tin leaf for backing mirrors, watching the leaf being cast in a cast iron mould at a critical temperature. The great shortage of tin in France led him to enquire about prices and freight to France. Considering the limited working time and the single, if large, furnace Roux's statement that Vauxhall produced £50,000 worth of glass a year is surprising and perhaps mistaken.

Deslandes's reaction to the report was strange. At one point he gave the report considerable attention, as can be told from his surviving notes on it, later he claimed that Roux had never seen the Vauxhall works, which seems incredible. The detail of Roux's report seems unlikely to have come from an intermediary or agent, and it gives every indication of being his own work. It may not have been exactly what Deslandes looked for, and he does seem to have a poor opinion of scientists, particularly chemists, though himself proud to be a corresponding fellow of the Academy of Sciences. Roux was apparently readily admitted to Vauxhall works and to the mirror-makers and tin workshops. He probably enjoyed the special indulgence from which savants commonly profited, and one would not have expected him to advertise his connection with the Compagnie des Glaces.[48]

The Ravenhead works very carefully hid its operations from the British public behind high walls, and it generally maintained considerable security. After a slacker period, however, things were considerably tightened up in 1790. The British Plate Glass Company then announced in the press that:

> having experienced many inconveniences, by the admission of stran-
> gers to view the works at this place [Ravenhead], they are much
> concerned to be under the necessity of enforcing the order on the gate
> of the Works, and that the public may not be offended at this appar-

ent rigour, they are informed that the proprietors themselves are
deprived of the pleasure of seeing the Works, without an order of
admission from the Committee in London.[49]

As late as 1816 proprietors who did not come on official inspection
had to give ten days' notice. But occasional persons, 'strangers ... who
go recommended by the Committee', were then allowed to see parts of
the works, and by that means Henry Saladin, a young member of a
Swiss family who were major investors in Saint Gobain, got to see
some of the works in that year, including the Watt engine and the
attached polishing and grinding machines. He proposed making a model
of the machinery for Saint Gobain. The Committee member who recommended him was probably ignorant of the family interest of the
young Swiss in Saint Gobain, or of his practical gifts.[50]

Security had certainly not been forgotten at Ravenhead. Sherbourne
retained information on the ingredients of his glass, the proportions of
materials that went into the batch, as a personal secret. It was only
once he had reached an advanced age that an anxious company was
able to prevail on him to part with it, and that only in the strictest
confidence. 'Mr. Sherbourne has ... forwarded to him [the Governor of
the Company] a list which is now sealed up (to be lodged in the
Company's strong box) not to be opened but in the event of Mr.
Sherbourne's death, or his resignation of his charge at Ravenhead.' It is
likely, however, that this degree of security was inspired more by worry
about British rivals than continental ones.[51]

The experience of the glass industry as a whole in terms of technological transfer between the two countries was not a uniform one, but
differed much between the main branches of the industry. In the
instance of bottle glass the product was unsophisticated and the
tolerances in the techniques of manufacture fairly slack. Enough of the
essentials of English methods of production were readily acquired to
produce a perfectly viable industry in France by the early eighteenth
century, which soon moved to production on a very large scale. It is
interesting, however, that the French continued to call bottle glass
made with coal-fuel 'English-style' glass virtually down to the Revolution. Flint glass presented much greater problems; few French attempts
to acquire it from Britain met with much success, the one that was
fairly successful required a remarkable effort in industrial espionage,
but exhibited many of the difficulties of obtaining a novel coal-based
technology, sometimes to a ludicrous extent. Whether this effort would
have survived without the successive patronage of the Duke of Orléans

and the queen, and the ministerial support of Calonne, which allowed its assimilation into the Le Creusot complex, is most unlikely. In plate glass a basic French technology was transferred to Britain by the usual method of suborning, but the British had to work out painfully for themselves how to assimilate it to the coal-fuel on which British glass production had been based since the previous century. Their long difficulties meant that there was nothing worthwhile to be transferred from England to France before Deslandes gave up his attempts to use coal at Saint Gobain in 1784. British success only came after his retirement; the Revolution and war put cumulative impediments in the way of any transfer of coal-use from Britain to France, and there was no attempt to leap the barrier.

PART FIVE

The Transfer of British Textile Technology in the Late Eighteenth Century

15 The Arrival of the Water Frame and the Mule

This study has shown that the transfer of technology from England to France in the eighteenth century embraced a wide range of industry, and that it was already important in the early decades of the century. However, there is no question that the great series of English mechanical inventions in textiles in roughly the last third of that century attracted an unprecedentedly strong interest among French businessmen, manufacturers and administrators. To some extent this was due to the obviousness of the results of the employment of machines. For instance, textile machines seemed much more straightforwardly intelligible than many of the processes of the metal industries, where the qualities of raw materials in primary production (as yet inexplicable by contemporary science), and hardly acquired craft skills (both in primary production and in much of the manufacture of metal goods) were less readily reduced to clear principles than the mechanics of textile machines. These seemed intelligible to anyone with some simple mathematical knowledge. The French fastened perhaps too firmly on to the idea that the one great principle driving British textile invention was the saving of labour.[1] They learned with some disappointment and over time that it was possible to obtain British machines and endeavour faithfully to copy them, while still leaving some technological gap attributable to the quality of materials and to the skills of construction and operation, so that, even though a great technical advance might be achieved, it did not deliver complete technical equality with the English product, or equal or lower costs.

It is evident that for English textile skills and machines to reach France the law must have been broken. Any suborning of workmen to take their skills abroad was illegal on a broad interpretation of the Act of 1719. Moreover, in 1750 a further Act specified that artisans in cotton, wool mohair and silk were prohibited from emigrating. The same Act tackled for the first time the export of tools and utensils, which included machines; but here the wool and silk industries alone were covered by its terms. While the 1750 Act came too early to have been aimed at the great succession of cotton spinning inventions, and was probably mainly directed at equipment in the finishing trades, the statutory response to the dangers of the export of the new cotton machinery came quite early, in an Act of 1774. This was directed against the export of tools and utensils for cotton and linen manufacture. It was obviously intended to protect the jenny and the water frame; the successful theft of the jenny by John Holker junior in 1771 would already have been known in England. Exporting these items was subject to a fine of £200, and there were similar fines against those who collected machinery for export, or against shipmasters knowingly carrying it. Not only machinery itself was forbidden to be exported, but from 1781 models or plans for woollen, silk, cotton and linen manufacture were included. The definition was 'machine, engine, tool, press [this would include the calender] paper [probably directed to the glazed cardboard used in pressing which the Holkers had tried to imitate in France] utensil or implement, or any model or plan' of such. In 1782 the export of equipment for calico-printing was prohibited.[2]

We will now look at the known instances of British citizens who appeared in France and engaged in the transfer of textile technology, roughly in the last third of the eighteenth century. We will trace, wherever possible, how far they were suborned by the French state or by French businessmen, and how far that recruitment involved the clandestine export of machines; in other words how far deliberate industrial espionage was involved. If expert workers turned up in France without being enticed, in other words, they simply went of their own free will to a land of seeming opportunity, where their technological knowledge would be at a premium, knowing well that they were breaking the law; that distinction will be made. The way in which the immigrants contributed to French technology will be examined, and how far their efforts succeeded in the spread of the new textile machines and in the quality of their product. However, no attempt will be made to follow these issues into the nineteenth century, nor into the countries outside France that were conquered by the Revolutionary armies, or brought under the aegis of the First Empire. Nor is there an attempt to give a general account of the cotton industry of late eighteenth-century France, which has recently been excellently and exhaustively covered.[3]

We know that the number of Britons involved in France as managers or mechanics in textiles after the end of the peace of Amiens was surprisingly large, but for the last decade of *ancien régime* and the Revolutionary period the notable immigrants are only about a score, though in some cases they may have fronted small dependent groups of assistant artisans of whom no record has survived. Perhaps the most celebrated of these immigrants, and the earliest, were the Milne family.

The Milnes were particularly associated with the Stockport district. Early in the 1770s John Milne, previously a wire manufacturer in Manchester, had moved to Sharston, close to Stockport, where he had developed an ambitious patent machine for dressing flour. Entering into a partnership which included men already involved in the cotton industry, John Milne was next operating Castle Mill, an Arkwright-type cotton factory at Stockport which was in production in 1778. The factory was built by, and on the land of, Sir George Warren, an MP who had been prominent in securing the 1774 Act against the export of tools and machinery in linen and cotton. Milne seems to have devoted himself to improving roving machinery, for which he was given a premium of £200 by the Manchester Committee of Trade in 1782. The factory seems to have been commercially unsuccessful, and Milne had left it and it was to let by the end of 1782.[4]

However, the family had already made a connection with the French cotton industry. According to one account they were approached by a French government agent within a few months of their occupation of Castle Mill and one of John's sons, James, was put in touch with John Holker, with the particular purpose of going to France to build the latest carding machinery. He was offered 2,400 *livres* to go over and build such a machine.[5] John Holker, however, wrote to the French government in September 1779 that Milne had been sent to him three months previously by friends of his.[6] To test his ability, Holker had got James Milne to make a cotton carding machine, which he had done with complete satisfaction. By it a single man could card 23 lbs of cotton a day and better and more cleanly than by any other method. Holker promised Milne 2,400 *livres* for the machine, confident that it would fully cover its purchase price in a year by the reduction in labour costs it would achieve. Normandy alone could keep 200 such machines busy, without considering the other provinces in which cotton goods were made. Holker enclosed a list of other machines Milne said he could produce, but which he would not make public without reward. Milne was learning French, would soon be able to make himself understood, and would be ready to meet Necker himself, or the Intendants of Commerce if they so desired. Apart from the carding engine Milne offered a cotton-cleaning machine suitable for Indian or West Indian cotton, a machine for spinning wool, for which he wanted 120,000 *livres*, a machine for coarse-spinning cotton – no doubt his father's roving machine – for 70,000 *livres*, a silk-doubling and twisting engine for 48,000 *livres* and a flour-dressing machine, which was certainly that developed by his father.[7] Twenty-four thousand *livres* was asked for it. It is interesting that at this point there is no mention of the main Arkwright roller-spinning machinery; possibly James Milne had been mainly involved with the carding equipment of the Stockport factory.[8]

A much later document advancing the claims of the Milne family speaks of Holker in flattering terms, 'as commendable for his patriotism as for his great diligence and the extent of his insights' and says he was impressed by the continuity between carding and spinning processes which Milne proposed, which suggests that some of the Arkwright system was disclosed to him. Milne did go to Paris in the same year and made there a model of the carding machine for Tolozan, the Intendant of Commerce. He said that it was approved by members of the Academy of Sciences. While his expenses were paid, his total demand for 440,000 *livres* for his bundle of technical advances was understandably thought excessive and he was instead offered an annual pension of 15,000 *livres*, and a premium on machines made. James Milne's brother, John Milne II, had come over for a time, but returned when the family's full demands were not met.[9] Early in 1780 James Milne wrote to Necker listing various 'mechanicks' he had on offer for flax, worsted and wool spinning, and a cotton-spinning machine of inestimable value, very likely the Arkwright one. He made it clear that 'the property and secret of the aforesaid Mechanicks are only belonging to Mr. John Milne of England', the father of the James Milne now in Paris, who had vested his rights in James for purposes of negotiation. James had 'spared no pains in prevailing on his Father to furnish him with these commissions on the most reasonable terms'.[10]

Perhaps because of the failure of the Stockport mill the Milne family soon joined (or rejoined) James in France. They first vainly asked the Government for 500,000 *livres* for the introduction of their inventions – they long resisted the truth that they were basically the same as

Arkwright's.[11] They then joined a highly adventurous entrepreneur, Francois Perret, in a scheme to set up a cotton-spinning and cotton velvet manufacture. This, after some successful trials, was sited at Neuville in the Lyonnais, on the lands of the Maréchal de Luxembourg. Perret seems to have originally dealt with James Milne, whose Paris machine he had bought. He had a remarkable facility for raising capital. Early in 1782 he had obtained for his firm the title of 'Royal manufacture for the spinning of cotton by English machines'. By July, for reasons which are not specified, John Milne the father had replaced his son James in the enterprise. James for the time being returned to Manchester, one of the younger sons now stayed with the father. The complications of funding the Neuville enterprise have been thoroughly examined by Chassagne and need not concern us.[12] The cotton velvet weaving resulted in large unsold stocks. The upshot was that the Milnes departed on the grounds that new partnership arrangements reduced their influence. They clearly realized that the firm faced disaster. They left in November 1783 and their shares were forfeited early in 1784. That the departure of the Milnes was timely is shown by the fact that Perret died in the same month, hugely insolvent.

While attempts to reorganize and refinance the venture continued there were visits to the pioneering spinning-machinery by several interested persons. One of these was the engineer J.-C. Périer, whom we have already encountered in the context of the Boulton and Watt engine. He was accompanied by the important Academician Vandermonde, who was much used by the Government as a commissioner to examine inventions, and was also closely connected with the House of Orléans. They were 'attracted by their wish to see machines which they did not as yet know and to estimate their performance'. They decided that 'nothing more ingenious or useful has been thought of than these machines which have been seized from England'. Périer was part of a new group which sought to take over the concern in 1785; he was convinced that the machines could be run much faster and produce more and better yarn. After much difficulty the firm was restarted and ran until 1804.[13] The Milnes subsequently claimed that, after their departure from Neuville, Martin (of the firm of Martin and Flesselles) also came to examine their machines, but in his case surreptitiously.

The Milnes, back in Paris, now cast about for partners and government favour so as to relaunch their spinning-machinery. At this point they found themselves with rivals in the construction of Arkwright's machines. In May 1783 Holker wrote to the administration that the previous day two Englishmen had turned up on his doorstep with an interesting proposition – an indication of his reputation as the key to recognition and favour by the French government. The men were Lancastrians like himself, and their home was only 6 miles from his own birthplace at Stretford. They were skilled workers in iron and copper, and machine-makers and millwrights. They had been employed in one of the biggest cotton manufactures in England, apparently the Peels' factory at Radcliffe Bridge near Bury, at which all the processes were carried out from beating and carding to fine spinning, and all the machinery was operated from a single water-wheel. The labour force of this highly mechanized unit was almost entirely composed of children and young girls. Apparently John Holker junior had tried to get into this works on an English visit, but had not been allowed to enter. The two men described to Holker the mill's powerful water-wheel, and the great size of the main building, 110 feet long with five floors. There were up to forty spinning-machines, each of forty-eight spindles, and 250 young people were employed. Holker's visitors could not only carry out the necessary millwright's work and erect such a building, but make all the various machines, and produce a yarn in which the amount of twist could be varied according to the type of cloth it was intended to make.

Holker forwarded a specimen of warp yarn the men had brought, and he waxed ecstatic about it; it could allow the French to imitate some cloths which were now imported from India in huge quantities and which they had been unable to copy successfully. The spinning-machines were different from any Holker had previously seen and he succinctly described the grooved and the leather-covered small cylinder rollers of Arkwright's water frame. But these were not the only important features; there was a carding engine which he believed was superior to those already introduced by Milne and Hall[14] which had a tendency to 'tear' the carding. If they could get hold of good workmen, both metalworkers and copper and iron founders, the Englishmen could make the mechanical part of a factory such as they described for an estimated 100,000 *livres*, leaving the water-wheel and mill building out of the reckoning. The mill itself would have to be built with very strong floors 'for the slightest irregular movement would derange the working of these machines'. The gear-work could be made by men used to making large clockwork. The drive shaft from the water-wheel should be fitted with an 8-foot iron drive-wheel made in four sections keyed together, and this should engage with another toothed iron wheel of 3 foot 6 inches or 3 foot 8 inches diameter. Holker doubted if any French foundries could make such iron castings, and they might have to be got from England. This was all the more vexing because such iron gears not only lasted longer, but moved much more smoothly, and drove the machinery infinitely better than wooden ones.

Holker suggested that the men be provided with a water-mill and building to set up a couple of spinning-machines (and one each of the other machines) for demonstration purposes, before the State or private investors were turned to for substantial support. The two men wanted wages of 24 *livres* a week during the trials. If expert commissioners appointed by the Government regarded the trial as a success, then the men wanted a single payment of 500 *livres* each and an annual pension of 1,200 *livres*, so that they could move from the service of one enterprise and help to set up others in different provinces if they so chose. Despite their very unusual requirements Holker believed the men should be welcomed, as he thought the yarn their machines could produce could be used in the making of cloths for calico-printing, which could substitute for the East Indies cloths which had to be bought on the Lorient, London or Amsterdam markets. Some of the larger calico-printing firms, like those at Bourges or Beauvais, or particularly Oberkampf[15] and Holker's associates, could well provide finance. The two Englishmen wanted to know quickly if they would be supported; if not, they would go on to America.[16]

While Chassagne believes that Holker's two visitors were Theakston and Flint (alias Wood and Hill), to whom we will return,[17] they are not named in the document just quoted. The visitors mention only their Lancashire connections, while in other documents Theakston and Flint emphasize only their connections with Arkwright's original Cromford works in Derbyshire, making no mention of Bury.[18] It is most likely, as Chassagne states, that the works at Bury which Holker's visitors came from was that of the Peels, and correspondence with Charles Aspin, the expert on textile-machinery history, confirms this view. Rémond, who quotes the document in full, says that it was not possible to tell with certainty who the two Englishmen were, but that they were 'doubtless' Wood and Hill.

The letter certainly has some interesting implications. First, it shows that, despite his advancing years, Holker was able to grasp the critical importance of the Arkwright system, especially the roller-spinning, and its particular significance in producing excellent warp thread, which could be the basis for improved all-cotton cloths, suitable for printing. At the same time he saw some of the engineering problems in installing powered cotton machinery in the inferior mechanical engineering environment of France. It reinforces the case that James Milne had not fully communicated to him the mechanical detail of the Arkwright system beyond the carding stage, either because he himself was not fully *au fait* with it in 1779, or because he wished to preserve some degree of secrecy. Holker was evidently not aware that the Milnes had installed a parallel system to the one his visitors described at Neuville in 1782; it is perhaps worth speculating that the replacement of James Milne there by his father and brother may have been because of their superior knowledge of the spinning-machinery.

Whether or not the two men who visited Holker were Theakston and Flint, and whether he can thus be allowed a very important intermediary role in the introduction of the Arkwright system to France,[19] he certainly took an active interest in obtaining new textile machinery. In 1779, the year that James Milne had been sent to him, he brought over from England William Hall, brother of one of the managers of the Sens manufacture with which he had himself been closely involved. Hall was to provide carding engines and the improved English jennies which carried more spindles and were easier to operate, because they were worked by a vertical rather than a horizontal (in fact inclined) hand wheel. While his cotton-carding machines were tried not only at Sens, but at the Holker works at Oissel and also at Amiens, they were not persisted with in these other places. On the other hand Hall continued to make machines for carding and spinning both cotton and wool at Sens between 1780 and 1786, and as he made 104 machines, eighty-one for wool and twenty-three for cotton, they must have been of value.[20] Hall was paid 1,800 *livres* for his expenses in coming over to France and received a pension for some years. The early types of jenny had been employed at Sens since the younger Holker had introduced them from England in 1772. Hall petitioned the Government from Sens as early as May 1783, claiming that some of his carding machines there worked perfectly and that he had installed jennies with double the number of spindles of the earlier ones. He particularly stressed the satisfaction that his wool-spinning jennies gave at Elbeuf, where he had repeat orders. He had been urged to make a wool-carding engine, which he had done. Interestingly the manufacturers' motive had been that 'the carders held the whip hand and often would not do the work they were supposed to and carded badly'. He was ready to go and install the engine at Elbeuf, 'but as it is quite usual that when one invents something people are to be found who are very ready to copy it', he wanted some safeguarding agreements before making his invention known. He also wanted some further reward from the Government. They would see 'that I do not at all resemble many others who demand recompenses and encouragements before executing their projects'.

In 1786 Hall was complaining that the Government was giving the Milnes much more help than they gave him, and recounting his sad state as a widower with nine children, ill for a year himself and with illness among the children. But in 1787 Brown, the very judicious inspector of industry, reviewed Hall's case and believed that the Sens manufacture had been more than generous to him and that the Government should not feel it necessary to give him further assistance.[21]

The interest now shifts to other English innovators. Once returned to Paris, the Milnes began to look for fresh support. They issued a document about the potential profits on spinning particular counts of yarn on their machinery. They wanted the backing of a company to establish carding machines, and to carry out coarse and fine spinning and winding, one which would provide a capital of 400,000 *livres*. They would operate for nine years as Milne and Company, with the elder Milne having half the shares and a salary of 6,000 *livres* as long as he directed the business. Their inability to conduct commercial transactions in France is indicated by the award of a one-twentieth interest to a merchant, Reboul, who would look after the external affairs of the firm for the nine years. Milne sought to protect his technological contribution by putting under seal with a senior magistrate in Paris 'the geometric drawings of his machines, explaining the movements of each individual part and the detailed description of the means employed to govern these movements so as to produce the different degrees of fineness and evenness which it gives the yarn'. This advantage could only be known to the inventor and would be wanting in those who stole or imitated the machines. Clearly the Milnes already scented rivals. In another memoir Milne claimed that Arkwright's machines were only an imitation of his and that his inventions were superior. But the French administrators quickly pointed out that Arkwright's patent and the advantages he was known to have secured for his country showed how ill founded Milne's claims were.[22]

Two groups of rivals had now appeared. There was, first, a group of Louviers industrialists who were exploiting the talents of the two previously mentioned English workers named Theakston and Flint, now calling themselves Wood and Hill. Secondly there was the firm of Flesselles and Martin, cotton velvet manufacturers of Amiens, who were already using the skills of Price, an English cloth finisher, and were now making great efforts to procure the Arkwright system. Jean-Francois Martin had gone to Manchester in the summer of 1783. On his return the firm petitioned for government help to set up a machine 'exactly like that invented in England by Arkwright, and of which the English are so protective, as the spinning done by this machine is so perfect that it allows them to produce work if not superior, at least equal to that of India'.

Martin had visited both England and Ireland. He had initially gone over to England to pick up information useful to the cotton velvet business, but had then heard of the Arkwright machinery. He next abandoned his Amiens works for a time 'to give himself over completely to the means of getting to know this machine; for this he spared neither trouble nor money'. He took various precautions in England and Ireland so as to get into the manufactures more easily and avoid suspicion. He had, he claimed, run the greatest dangers, and without these measures he might have lost his liberty and perhaps his life. But these risks and expenses resulted in his having a perfect knowledge of the workings of this machine, of which he had a full set of plans.[23] According to one of the associated documents (a report of March 1784) Martin spent no less than three years in England to collect all the information needed to set up an Arkwright-type mill in France. On his return the partners had a model of the Arkwright machinery built and sought government help; the machine enabled the scientist Vandermonde, on behalf of the Government, to go and verify their claims. In a letter to Vandermonde an official suggested that it would 'doubtless have a connection with the machine built by the Mills [sic] of Manchester in the manufacture of Sr. Perret near Lyon of which I have heard much discussion'.

Martin and Flesselles, however, wanted an exclusive privilege, which would have been harmful to the Milnes, and the Louviers group were making similar requests. Martin and Flesselles had the backing of the Duc de Noailles and of the Amiens Inspector of Industry, Roland de la Platière, now emerging from his virtual disgrace over the Holker quarrel.[24] The justification of an exclusive privilege (now become distinctly unfashionable) was that a single firm could quickly acquire the size and regularity to push through this new technology to the point of supplying demand.[25] But the administration wanted to know that the technology possessed by the firm was unique within France, and whether other innovators had been at work with the same equipment before the proposed privilege was asked for. Roland, a close friend of Flesselles, was probably being economical with the truth in his backing of the priority of Martin and Flesselles. He had written in 1783 to Montaran, giving him what was supposed to be the first intelligence of a set of English textile machinery which is obviously Arkwright's, saying 'that this machinery is a secret even in England'. Perhaps he was deriving his information from Martin while he was still pursuing his English espionage. But Montaran had consulted with another Flesselles (Jacques Flesselles, the Intendant of Lyon, not Martin's partner, Pierre Flesselles) who told him that his remarkable machinery was exactly the same as that which had just been set up at Neuville by Milne 'who has come from Manchester'.[26]

The Louviers group was dependent on the expertise of the two Englishmen who for some time continued to insist on aliases, John Theakston ('dit Wood') and John Flint ('dit Hill'). They had apparently arrived in France in May 1783, being brought over, according to Ballot, by one of their associates at Louviers, Alexandre, a member of the Fontenay family.[27] The firm included two of the greatest business houses at Louviers, J.-B. Decretot and the brothers Pétou. They were concerned with wool rather than cotton, and seem to have believed that the Arkwright machinery could be readily adapted to wool. In fact Arkwright, though he had envisaged it as early as 1772, was only preparing a plan to spin wool on his machinery in 1785, and then under a scheme by which he sought a national statutory monopoly for some years. Though Robert and Thomas Barber of Derby had been using Arkwright's machinery for coarse-wool spinning before his patent was overthrown, and there were a few other experiments, the real beginnings of water frame use for worsted in the north of England are regarded as being at Dolphinholme, near Lancaster, in 1784, and Addingham in the West Riding in 1787. The machinery only reached the West Country in the 1790s.[28]

Thus Theakston and Flint seem to have been recruited to take on a project which would have been innovative by English, let alone French, standards. In a request for an *arrêt* for a privilege from the Government they said their original operation had been that of building a wool-carding machine at Louviers. While there were some machines for this purpose in England which had given them the basic idea for theirs, they claimed that their machine was equipped with a kind of very positive chain drive and sixteen cylinders, and would only deliver the slivers of wool when they were properly prepared. It 'has seemed very ingenious and daily excites the admiration of all the best manufacturers and the most eminent mechanics'. But as far as spinning wool was concerned Wood and Hill (as we will subsequently call them) said they had not had an opportunity to do it – they presumably meant back in England. They could not propose it as a certainty, but they thought that by playing about with modifications to the cotton machines, which they were well acquainted with, they were 'morally certain' to succeed equally with wool. They pointed proudly to the three wool-carding machines they had now built at Louviers; without having detail of every French carding establishment, they were sure the differences between their machines and any existing ones were such that no single piece of mechanism which could be employed in their own machine was in existence elsewhere. The carded wool of the French works, even those at Rouen and Sens, went on to be spun on 'spinning wheels' where the spindles were turned by cords – probably their dismissive way of referring to the jennies there – and were not a part of a connected set of centrally driven machines like the Arkwright system, 'with an even and controlled movement like that of a clock'. On that system it was possible for a single water-wheel to turn 6,000 spindles.

The petition had opened with a classic account of the machinery of the Arkwright system. Unlike the Milnes, who claimed that they had devised the original machinery and Arkwright was their imitator, Wood and Hill took the opposite tack, and stressed their association with Arkwright's most famous works. Their 'machine for carding and spinning cotton is entirely similar to the famous machine invented and built in England by the Sieur Arkwright now at Cromford in Derbyshire, in which [place] the said Wood and Hill have been managers, the one for seven years and the other for ten'. Ballot says that Wood had been a builder and Hill a mechanic, and that Hill was only twenty-one years old about this time. If this is correct he had presumably just completed his apprenticeship at Cromford when he left; he could hardly have had significant experience at a Bury mill as well, which further indicates that the two visitors reported on by Holker in 1783 were not Wood and Hill.[29]

The two Englishmen went to Paris to discuss their claims with Tolozan who had a particular responsibility for Normandy. He got the Inspector of Manufactures, Lazowski, to examine their plans and models at

Louviers, and he then conferred with Holker, the investors, and the local inspector, Goy. The upshot was that it was decided that, as competition forced the French to imitate England, Wood and Hill ought to be encouraged to establish in France a technology found useful in that 'knowledgeable and industrious' nation. Holker was for giving them a privilege only for an area of a few leagues round Louviers, Lazowski would have been willing to extend it to one or two provinces. The term envisaged was for twelve years rather than the fifteen generally granted in privileges. But Wood and Hill dug their heels in: they wanted a national privilege for fifteen years. If they did not get it they would take their technology to Switzerland. The Government gave in, and they got their fifteen year national exclusive privilege together with the status of *manufacture royale* and the usual bunch of tax and other concessions that accompanied it.[30]

They were to make at government expense, and distribute to five named towns, models of their machinery. There were some changes in the entrepreneurial group in the early stages. Le Camus de Limare was early involved, then withdrew, but briefly reappeared when a company was set up to exploit the privilege, at this point being associated with Eugene Yzquierdo de Rivera, a tricky Spaniard, a director of the 'cabinet' of the King of Spain. As Ballot put it he 'sought to purloin the secret of new machines so as to introduce them into Spain'.[31] One argument for an exclusive privilege seems to have been that it would be a means of more gradually introducing a technology which would otherwise be too disruptive in reducing the price of labour, though this reduction was seen to be necessary to meet English competition![32]

Wood later described the difficulties which faced him in setting up such complicated machinery 'in a country where everything had to be created [for it] cannot be expressed, you will only appreciate [the difficulties] very imperfectly ... when you learn that (Wood) had to make with his own hands the tools and instruments needed to fashion the different parts of the machines, of which he himself built the first examples'. He later claimed that men he trained had gone on to build the machinery in many other works of the same kind.[33] In 1786 Wood and Hill brought a group of English workers to Louviers to help in machine-building, though some of the machines were hand operated, possibly jennies to complement the water frames by providing weft. The Louviers entrepreneurs were highly pleased with their skill and dedication: '[our] Englishmen work without respite and with an intelligence which daily strengthens our hopes'.[34] The Louviers partners were badly hit by the effects of the Eden Treaty in 1787, and vainly requested government financial help. Interestingly, the partners admitted 'we are nowhere near the perfection which the English have attained'. Nevertheless their machinery was set up and 200 workers, many of them children, were employed. The firm survived and the works were part of a very large factory complex of 600 workers in 1810.[35]

While the Louviers company started business with a monopoly privilege, it does not seem to have insisted too strongly on it. There was more argument and difficulty with Martin and Flesselles and their claims. Even as early as June 1784 they wanted their original ten-year privilege extended. In July Vandermonde was being turned to to arbitrate as to the respective claims of Martin and Milne. They both wanted him to go to see the machines at Neuville to judge if they were the same as those cited in the privilege given to Martin. Vandermonde was willing to do this, but claimed to have doubts as to what the Government wanted: 'all the motives which can govern the Administration's decision'. But his letter was not immediately acted on.[36] In the following year an official of the Council of Commerce sent the controller-general the report of a group of Academicians on Milne's machines. Milne wanted the same commissioners to examine the machines of Martin and Flesselles; there was some doubt about their willingness, but it was thought their reluctance could be overcome. The official, D'Angervilliers, a secretary of state, said that not only he but Vergennes, the foreign minister, wanted the matter settled as it was holding up a projected scheme for a manufacture at Rambouillet in which the minister was involved. If there were further problems the Milnes might take off for foreign countries, especially America. There was some move through the Duc de Mouchy, on whose lands they were established, to have different commissioners and Academicians inspect the Neuville machines from those inspecting the works at Epine (Arpajon). In fact there was an independent inspection of the Epine works by an able inspector, Brown, in June 1785. He was very cautious about the yarn quality achieved so far, but enthusiastic about the spinning-machines which could only be appreciated by those who had seen them – they did the greatest honour to their inventor. Flesselles and Martin deserved the support they had received so far.[37]

The key inspection and report was that of the Academicians, Desmarets, Coulomb and the Abbé Rochon, which had been made a month before. They had looked at Flesselles's and Martin's machines and then compared them with those of the Milnes. They were clear that it was a Milne (James) who had first brought the cylindrical carding engine to France, and they knew of the involvement of Tolozan. But they had, when recently examining this machine (while very keen on its operation and the carding produced), been very disturbed by the amount of repair and upkeep it required. The complicated mechanism and gearing resulted in heavy friction and thus led to repairs 'by craftsmen more skilful than are generally to be found in the provinces'. The 'Manchester machine' as they called it, that is the unmodified version of Arkwright's, was in contrast a well recognized success. The mechanism was simpler and needed less maintenance, and Martin and Flesselles had single-mindedly applied themselves to 'copy faithfully the Manchester machines'. They recognized that Arkwright's crank and comb device as used by Martin was a superior method to Milne's horizontal comb. But Milne's machine was better finished, though when Martin and Flesselles's machine was more carefully mounted they would equal the quality of Milne's carding, and by means which were better for large-scale manufacture. The drawing operation of Flesselles and Martin was done in several stages, the Milnes in a single one, though the principle was the same. Martin and Flesselles's spinning-machines gave quite a good yarn, even though they were rather crudely made and the water-wheel which drove them worked jerkily and irregularly. Oddly, however, there was little breakage of thread in spinning. Milne's machine only differed in that it used gearing where Martin and Flesselles's machine used pulleys and (presumably) a cord drive. The principle was exactly the same but the Milne's yarn was better because more even. Output was similar, even though Flesselles and Martin's machines were water powered and the Milne's driven by hand with a crank.

While the Milne's machines were much more carefully made and gave a better product, the commissioners, as seems often to have happened at this period, tended to prefer machines which were simpler, which needed only operatives of lower skill to work them, and less highly trained mechanics to repair them. But the final conclusion was that the machines of the two disputants were the same in principle and were in fact Arkwright's, 'the sole inventor of this kind of spinning'. The only difference was in the pulley drive of Martin and the gearing of the Milne's, and they preferred the former.

They had been asked to find out who first brought such machines to France and the papers they had seen favoured the Milnes. Though the Milnes had installed five machines at Neuville, on which they were also reporting, the commissioners pointed out that they had not demanded any privilege on that account 'which is always fatal to the nation that grants it, since it discourages ingenuity, harms the progress of the industry and finally causes a loss to the state which is infinitely greater than the profit which results to the individual who possesses it'. It would be best to give every citizen complete liberty to copy and to improve this kind of spinning so the French might come to contest superiority with England and even take it away from her. The commissioners thought Arkwright's patent ('privilège exclusif')[38] would harm British trade by restraining the spread of the machines in England, during which time they could be carried abroad by industrial espionage to foreign countries.[39] The commissioners concluded by hoping that the firm of Flesselles, Martin and Lami should have some unspecified encouragement and protection, the Milnes should be suitably rewarded for first introducing the Arkwright system, and they all should be encouraged to spread and perfect their spinning-machines but without the least right to prevent anyone else taking up the business.[40]

In fact the Milnes came out of the period of dispute and rivalry rather well. In October 1785 they became part of Calonne's drive for industrial growth. James Milne on behalf of himself, his father and one of his brothers signed a contract with the controller-general. The Government would provide them with a site and give them 24,000 *livres* for introducing their machines, they would get an annual fee of 6,000 *livres* starting in the same month, and a premium of 1,200 *livres* for each set of Arkwright machines made, sets which were henceforth commonly called the 'assortiment Milne'. They undertook to provide one set of machines for the Government to be made available for demonstration purposes; to stay in France; to supervise their machine-building plant themselves; to supply the machines to all who required them, and to allow disputes on price to be resolved by intendants of commerce. The Milnes could also involve themselves directly in spinning enterprises unhindered by those who claimed privileges – this clearly told the Louviers and Epine manufacturers to forget their monopoly claims.

The machine-building site the Milnes were given was in the kitchens of the Chateau de la Muette at Passy. The products of this oddly placed works in fact were well regarded. John Milne, the father, worked to simplify their version of the Arkwright system, and to reduce complication and cost for both manufacture and repairs, so that there were finally only three types of machine, for carding, for coarse spinning and for final spinning. The first sets of machines only came off the culinary production line in 1787, they seem to have been operable by hand-power, and though an early delivery to Lecler at Brive proved faulty, they generally succeeded well.[41]

The fortunes of the Milnes were further improved by their gaining the patronage of the Duke of Orléans. Their agreement with him was full of contradictions with that made with Calonne; perhaps they could get away with this because of the way in which Calonne's projects were generally regarded as under an anathema after his fall. In 1789 the Duke contracted to have sole right to the Milne machines from the following June; every two months they were to supply him with a complete 'assortiment' until twenty-four had been delivered. The Duke's mills were at Orléans and Montargis.[42] The first was managed by Thomas Foxlow, who had married Sarah, the daughter of John Milne I. He had been a fairly successful fustian and calico manufacturer in Manchester, a member of the prestigious Literary and Philosophical Society there from 1782, and also prominent in the first of the Manchester commercial societies, the Committee for the Protection and Encouragement of Trade. However, he failed in business, and arrived in France in June 1785 to join the Milnes. He was soon building machines with them.[43] The family were soon actively disposed in various cotton ventures. Foxlow was developing the Orléans works, one of the very few French works to be steam-powered. This he was to take over in the Year III, when his former patron, Phillipe Egalité, succumbed to the Revolution he had once encouraged. The Duke's other factory at Montargis was supervised by Thomas Milne, though he installed machines for other purchasers as well. Thomas also directed a works at Foulonval near Dreux, set up in 1790, Robert one at Montivilliers near Le Havre, while another son-in-law, Newton, later set up as a spinner at Dreux. La Muette turned out eighty-four 'assortiments' between 1786 and 1797, which would each typically consist of a carding engine, a roving machine, one for coarse spinning and four for fine spinning.[44] Thanks largely (but not entirely) to the Milnes the technology of the water frame had been added to that of the jenny in the French cotton industry by the early years of the Revolution.

The introduction of the mule into France is attributable to Philemon Pickford, though he was closely rivalled. It is said that it was on Calonne's authority that he was brought over to France. The first connection seems to have been with Brown, the French inspector of

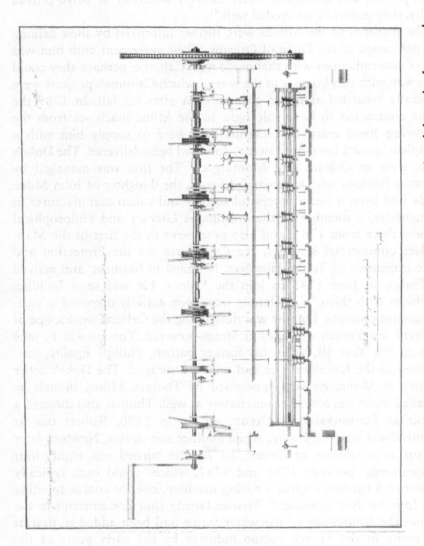

15.1 An Arkwright-type machine built by the Milnes at Passy, viewed from the front and (facing) from the side next to the wheel

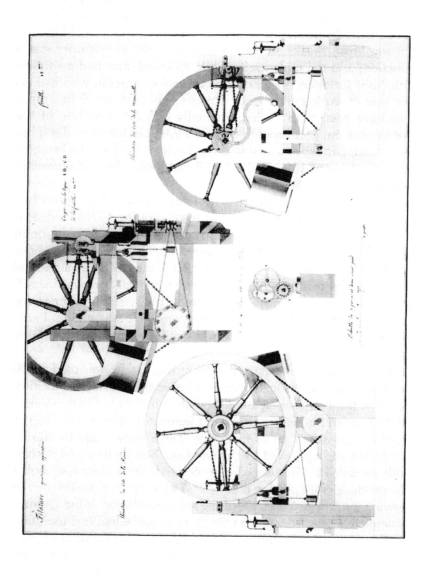

Filature, première opération.

industry of English origin. The son of a gardener of the King of France, he had been inspector at Caen, and then was made 'inspector ambulant' in 1787.[45] On a visit to England Brown seems to have had careful discussions with Pickford, a machine-maker of Ashton, near Manchester, who was able to make all the machinery for the preparatory stages of production, and the mule itself. While Pickford later had a connection with Abbé Calonne, brother to the controller-general, who had (as we have seen)[46] strong industrial interests, his first work in France seems to have been with Lecler, originally called Clark, one of the group of English émigrés brought over by Holker in his early days, but by now operating independently at Brive. Lecler organized the bringing to France of a mule of 109 spindles[47] and Pickford, who had arrived in France in 1788, erected it for him.[48]

This was a fairly rapid transfer of technology, since Crompton had only brought his invention to fruition at the end of the 1770s, and, as it was not patented, it could not have been drawn to French attention in that way. It was only modified for powered operation in Britain about 1790, so that its operation in France by Lecler and others as a manual machine did not at this point constitute any technical backwardness.[49] By early May 1790 Pickford had completed his new machines for Lecler, and repaired and improved existing ones. He was now in Paris, where he was prepared to stay to build similar machines for 2 *louis* a week.

The Bureau of Commerce agreed to his terms, and he was paid 3,000 *livres* at once.[50] There was a first agreement between Tolozan and Pickford, by which he was given housing and a workshop in the old Quinze-Vingts hospital (like several other inventors and innovators about this time) in order to complete a first set of machines. These were ready by March 1791, inspected and approved by the Academicians Le Roy and Béchet, and highly regarded by Tolozan who pronounced them 'the most perfect of all the machines for spinning cotton'.[51] A new contract was signed in the following month, giving Pickford the accommodation in the Quinze-Vingts completely rent free, and for the three years he had free use of all the tools the administration provided for him. On each set of machines, those for the preparatory stages plus the mules themselves, he was to get a 300 *livres* bounty, up to a quota of twenty sets, which he had completed by January 1792. There was a further substantial grant in three-monthly instalments if he established a workshop which was able to satisfy the demand for machines by entrepreneurs, and he could charge them 7,400 *livres* per set; this could be reviewed if demand exceeded expectations. He was to mount a sample set of the machinery at the Quinze-Vingts to be kept for purposes of comparison with the machines of others. The mules in the contract were only able to spin relatively low counts, but he was going to produce a new specimen mule, able to spin finer, for which materials had already been delivered to him. He was also to make an improved jenny. For this he would have a salary of 48 *livres* a week in addition to his bounties and free materials, but these new machines when built would belong to the administration. Pickford's machines would be examined by Le Roy and another commissioner to be named by the Academy of Sciences.[52]

From this time we have only rather disjointed evidence on Pickford's activities. In Year I of the Republic he was involved in a cotton manufacture at Rochefort near Dourdan (Seine et Oise) which was said by the municipal authorities to be in full activity, with complete sets of cotton carding and spinning machinery, including the mule, specifically said to be like Lecler's at Brive. The Dourdan works was directed by Brown, the former inspector of manufactures under the old regime[53] and was supported by the Duc de Rohan. Pickford had been granted a 'brevet d'invention' in 1792.[54] He is said to have left the Quinze-Vingts in 1793; as we shall see when we look at the case of another occupant, Le Turc, things were very disturbed there at that time.[55] Pickford founded a second spinning venture at Dourdan, but in the Year V he had problems for which he blamed the assignats and removed his manufacture to Paris. There he sought to take over the space from which Le Turc had been ejected in the Quinze-Vingts, to which his own works could be removed as a going concern.

We know he returned to England in 1799. But he is said to have been setting up a water-powered spinning-mill near Dourdan for C.-F. Lebrun in autumn 1805. This makes his later statement 'I was a victim of the Revolution and was obliged to leave France until 1814' more than suspect; but it was no doubt a good thing to say to the Restoration government. He claimed to have been reviled in England because of his work for France, and so left and spent some time in Spain, but was driven out by the war of 1808. He certainly came back to France in 1814 and, apparently successfully, asked for his old quarters in the Quinze-Vingts back with a government loan, his justification being newly improved spinning techniques he had acquired in his absence. He received a loan of 15,000 francs. His stock in France thereafter tended to decline though he built looms of 192 spindles. A memoir of the Comité Consultatif des Arts et Métiers in 1824, while agreeing that he had introduced the mule into France, claimed that he had trained very few apprentices before his wartime departure from France, not the 300 he claimed. His tenancy at the Quinze-Vingts was ended in 1825 and his machines were regarded as government property and were to be removed to the Conservatoire des Arts et Métiers. But he was recommended for some support in recognition of his early services, his situation as a foreigner, and his poverty (*détresse*): 'it would be honourable for the Government to treat him with some indulgence and a mark of humanity to assist him a little'.[56]

Pickford soon after his return to France had made an interesting but apparently fruitless attempt to carry out some industrial espionage by seducing English workers. In this case they were in the steel industry. His wife, Sarah Charlton, was to be given 3,000 *livres* to go to England to bring back two workers from Huntsman's famous Sheffield steel works, one of them being a relation of hers. On their arrival in France the workers would be given 300 francs each month until they could build cementation and cast steel works, and the substantial award of 1,000 francs each if they succeeded. Nothing seems to have come of this, probably because of the short life of the Commission Pour le Perfectionnement des Aciers which was sponsoring Mrs Pickford's journey. The Jacksons of Birmingham, emigrating about the same time, proved to be the successful introducers of cast steel in France.[57]

Very close in time to Pickford's first making of mules in France, another venture was launched by men of British descent, but long resident in the country. Jean-Baptiste Morgan's forenames suggest he was born there. He was a large merchant at Amiens where he became president of the Chamber of Commerce. By 1765 he had set up a large cotton velvet manufacture, and he profited from Holker's help in obtaining the services of one of the spinning-mistresses the inspector-general sent to train spinsters in various provinces. He was also an early user of the jenny, which he obtained from Hall at Sens, where the early jennies based on the one brought over by John Holker junior were employed. A Hall carding engine was later obtained. The cotton velvet firm became a *manufacture royale* in 1766, carrying through all the processes from spinning to weaving, dyeing and finishing. There were 400 workers in 1781 when Morgan had his son and another merchant, Delahaye, as partners. Some English workmen were employed. Two of them, Spencer and Massey (later a partner), were sent back to England in 1788. The expenses of their trip were paid by the new Bureau d'Encouragement at Amiens, concerned by the depressed state of industry in that year, and believing that the acquisition of the improved English machine-spinning methods was the answer. The two men came back with not only an Arkwright machine, but a mule of 160 spindles, and Spencer soon set it up. Perhaps because a large part of the costs of the Spencer and Massey expedition were paid by the Bureau d'Encouragement, other manufacturers were freely allowed in to the works to examine and copy the mules.[58]

The works was quickly visited by savants and inspectors.[59] The firm seems to have been known as Morgan and Massey in 1790, when the important British weaving expert, McCloude, was installing new types of English looms there, possibly including those for Manchester-type small wares, and effectively reintroducing Kay's fly-shuttle.[60] In 1791, however, the acquisition of mule technology was not yet assured. Massey was then writing to Molard at the technological exhibition centre at the Hotel de Mortagne in Paris saying that his partner Morgan had obtained Spencer's tools to use in his operations – whether Spencer had died or left the firm is unclear – 'one would very much wish to have a machine like Spencer's, but one doubts very much whether the construction would be possible in France'. If Molard visited them they would be able to assure him that theirs was the first of the type known in France. They were presumably contesting Pickford's priority. They were bringing more English workers and mechanics over and requested that the Committee of Agriculture and Commerce pay up for the cost of bringing them, as had been promised. They were keen to equal the finish of English cotton velvets, and were trying to bring a Manchester finisher to their works for that purpose.[61]

While many of the English mechanics who first introduced the new English textile machines to France did not, as we will see, end in a state of prosperity or even modest comfort, one of them, George Garnett, seems to have been under an unpropitious star during most of his time in France. He outlined his earlier career in France in a letter of October 1787. He claimed that he had developed in England a number of machines for spinning not only cotton, but also all kinds of wool. While machines for the same purposes had been tried in France, he believed them to have been unsuccessful. He said he could not use the machines he had developed in England for legal reasons – they were presumably in some cases basically Arkwright patent machines, with some of his own variations.[62]

Unlike many other English artisans who went to France after having been suborned, Garnett specifically states that he came over 'without knowing the first principles of the French language, and even without knowing a single individual'. He reached Paris, saw there the machines imitating English ones (probably Milne's) but concluded that his own were better. Learning that a major manufacture at Sens was conducted by an Englishman, Hall, he wrote to him and was invited there. 'He is the only friend I have in France.' However, Hall was not able to persuade his partners to invest in a large establishment using Garnett's machinery. But he did persuade Maigret de Serilly, a major capitalist, and an important investor in Le Creusot, to fund the construction of Garnett's machine, with the eventual aim of setting up a 2,000-spindle cotton factory of the English type. Garnett claimed that his machines worked well, and having completed them he and Hall came to Paris to demonstrate them to Serilly. But here came Garnett's first misfortune: Serilly went bankrupt.

Hall knew Tolozan well, now the dominant figure among the intendants of commerce. Tolozan revealed that he was going to pur-chase an estate in the Barrois, nominally at any rate on behalf of his son, and there he would set up a series of complementary textile enterprises. Garnett said that if Serilly was unable to continue as his patron he would be delighted to come under Tolozan's wing, and this in preference to another patron who had proferred support, with whom Garnett now broke off negotiations. But Garnett was initially unwill-ing to move all his machines to Paris for assessment as Tolozan wished, but finally gave in and Tolozan inspected them in the Quinze-Vingts in November 1787. Back at Sens, Garnett worked at a machine for worsted spinning. Serilly having finally signalled his withdrawal, Garnett de-cided to get Hall to approach Tolozan again, no doubt in a meeker spirit, but not unnaturally the intendant kept him waiting for a couple of months. The situation now was that Garnett had several cotton machines on offer on which Hall had reported enthusiastically, praising Garnett as both a machine builder and operator, and saying that women and children alone could work the cotton-spinning machinery. Garnett claimed that he had quickly gained enough French to understand and be understood, and went to Paris to tell Tolozan about his completed wool-spinning machine, taking a specimen of yarn with him. He al-ready proposed to the Government in May 1787 that he should have a reward of 30,000 *livres* if the machine on inspection was able to produce yarn equal to the sample.[63]

Garnett said his prototype wool-spinning machine could be enlarged to take as many spindles as were required without any falling off in efficiency. Tolozan seems to have agreed with Garnett's terms, but on the condition that Garnett should also include his cotton machines, and would receive 20,000 *livres* for them. Tolozan would take them for his own use on his estate if they proved viable. Until inspected they should be mounted in accommodation at the old Quinze-Vingts hospital.[64] The machines at the Quinze-Vingts were examined by Tolozan in person and by four inspectors of industry, who all admired them, and Tolozan considered they were worth further investigation. He arranged a high-powered panel of inspectors, Desmarets the inspector and Academician, Le Turc a general engineer who was an expert on knitting machines and whose star was currently, but briefly, in the ascendant after some years of successful industrial espionage in Britain (see Chapter 17, p. 446), and Béchet, now in charge of the Quinze-Vingts. While there was a few weeks' delay before the inspection, and the cotton and wool machinery was examined separately and with an interval between the two visits, Garnett was dealt with relatively quickly.

But the reports of October 1787 were not very good. The three commissioners had submitted the machines to 'repeated trials'. Garnett's carding engine was a simple one, and French experts often had a penchant for simple rather than complicated machines. On the one hand a simple machine often readily illustrated the principle of the process, and French intellectuals liked to have the principles of an innovation clearly exemplified, for it supported that process of industrial demystification which was the main technological element in the French Enlightenment. Moreover, the simpler the machine the easier it was to maintain, repair and operate with labour of limited skill. Nevertheless Garnett's machine did not impress; the commissioners felt that like many workers who copied machines (in this case Arkwright's) he had made changes in the hopes of improvement, and 'unable to analyse and grasp the essence of each element of the whole' he had cut back on the most useful features, resulting in the tearing and stretching of the carded cotton, so that a dry, uneven and weak thread would result at the spinning stage. Similar criticisms were levelled at the later stages. For instance the final spinning machinery embodied changes introduced by Garnett 'which served to make it less good than the one already known in France', and the successive small pairs of rollers did not draw out the thread properly. The resulting thread could not be employed in any kind of textile. The worsted spinning equipment was also partly condemned, but much depended on the fact that the wool cardings used were of uneven length. The commissioners were not sure whether the process was much quicker than hand-spinning; here they felt that some further trials and comparisons were possible.

Garnett, not unnaturally, contested the results. The commissioners had not been hostile when with him; he had not had opportunity to sign the commissioners' report as was customary. No doubt they were trying to be tactful, but he was shocked when Tolozan told him his machines were worthless, and felt that the intendant had gone back on his word. But a letter of expostulation tended to weaken into a demand for expenses, for Garnett had not even enough money to travel back to Sens from Paris. The controller-general, presumably advised by Tolozan, rejected his bid for support, but allowed him 600 *livres*. Garnett not very realistically asked for another trial of his machines, and another audience with Tolozan: 'please forgive, Sir, the frankness of an Englishman who perhaps, consistently with his own character, has spoken his mind too freely'.

Hall reported Garnett's annoyance and disquietude in the following month, and maintained that there had been some doublespeak by the commissioners; while viewing the machines they had been full of praise on the quality of the moving parts and the beauty of the yarn, and then reported the machines as worthless. But Hall's regard for Tolozan would not have allowed him to recommend and praise Garnett's machinery to the intendant if he, as a textile manufacturer, had not thought it excellent; he thought a great mistake had been made, that Garnett's talents had not yet been fully exploited, and that this was unfortunate at a time when the Anglo-French commercial treaty 'has handed victory to the English'. French manufactures languished, and would stay deep in depression 'until we possess the same machines that they do'. He particularly regretted that Garnett's worsted-spinning machinery would not be available to the great manufacturing centres which could have used it, and could have been relatively quickly in competition with England where the machine-spinning of worsted was still not widely taken up. He believed that Garnett's cotton machinery was better than that of the Milnes or that at Louviers or Arpajon. The commissioners who had seen Garnett's machines should not have given the impression that they could have made similar ones: if they had been presented with the machines in parts without having them completely set up, they could not have made them work properly. Their report, Hall deeply regretted, must have greatly reduced Tolozan's reliance on his own opinions. He tried to salvage Garnett's position by offering Tolozan his cotton machines for nothing if he got the originally suggested 30,000 *livres* for his worsted-spinning machine. If Garnett was not supported by the Government Hall believed he would 'carry his talents into another kingdom', destroying the machines he knew he would not be allowed to take with him.[65]

Garnett now had an apparently hopeful break, but which was to end in a highly traumatic experience. One of the new Bureaux d'Encouragement which were trying to stimulate depressed industry in manufacturing centres, that of Rouen, invited him to come and set up a workshop after he had offered to build jennies and carding equipment in March 1788. The building of carding engines was to be concentrated on as a way of providing quicker and cheaper supplies of carded cotton for jennies, which the Bureau particularly wished to encourage. Garnett was to have 2,000 *livres* a year wages and a bounty of 8,000 *livres*. However, his arrival in Rouen coincided with the problems caused by both the Eden Treaty and the disastrous harvest of 1788, and severe unemployment resulted which caused a natural reaction among the workers. Grain riots extended into riots against machines; while the higher reaches of local society represented in the Bureau d'Encouragement saw machines as the salvation of the local textile industries, the lower social ranks regarded them as their own ruin. This was reflected in the *cahiers de doléances* of the region: 'Let us forget the very name of these spinning machines which have stolen the bread from innumerable poor citizens who have nothing but cotton spinning as their sole resource'. So on 13 July 1789 what seems to have begun as a grain riot diverted itself to Garnett's workshop. The rioters, many of them women, stoned the works and, despite the appearance of Garnett and three workmen – one probably his brother – with guns, advanced on the shop. One of the defenders fired and the crowd fled, one man being fatally wounded. The following day the rioters were back. 'A lawless mob arrived at his premises' and Garnett saw them break down the doors with axes, run through the workshops, smash all the machines and tools, scatter the metal debris and burn the wooden parts nearby.

Garnett appealed to the members of the Bureau d'Encouragement and local merchants for compensation, but understandably they did not respond rapidly; in any case there is some evidence that his carding engines were not as economical as had been hoped. Later, having moved from the Saint Sever district of Rouen to set up a spinning-works on another site (Lillebonne) in the same department, he appealed to the Government 'to help a foreigner who has brought to France the machines without which it will be impossible for French manufacturers to enter into competition with those of England'. Not only the local inspector of manufactures, Goy, but the inspector ambulant, Brown, had been in Rouen at the time of the riot, and would be able to support Garnett's demand for 9,700 *livres* damages, including the loss of five carding and five spinning-machines.[66]

One might have thought that at this point Garnett would have carried out his earlier threats to leave France. But despite the national Revolution which coincided with his private revolutionary experience of 14 July 1789, he continued to memorialize the Government. In April 1791 he claimed to have further improved his wool-spinning machines which were displayed in the Quinze-Vingts, and in June they were highly approved by Le Roy of the Academy of Sciences. But Le Roy thought that it would be better to enable Garnett to set up his own manufacture with them than to pay him the large bounty he demanded – perhaps he was still asking for 30,000 *livres*. Nevertheless, he should be paid the purchase price of the machines and given assistance to get one of the new *brevets d'invention*. Garnett was given 300 *livres* to tide him over while Tolozan asked for a full report by Le Roy and Béchet. There were three machines made by Garnett and his brother, one probably for the final stages of carding, one for coarse spinning and one for finer spinning, all for worsted. They were still in principle like those Garnett had first made, and based upon Arkwright's cotton-spinning machinery, but with some modifications for the adaption to wool. Some problems in the first machines seemed to have been overcome in the new ones, but their output was not particularly fast as yet, as only four spindles were being used, while when fully mounted there would be two sets of twenty-four spindles in each of the water frames. The speed was not very constant, but this too would be easily remedied when fully operational. Mechanically the machines were good: 'Their action, of the kind in Vaucanson's machines, is well thought out'. A full production set of machinery, culminating in four 48-spindle spinning-machines, could be had for 12,000 *livres*. The brothers were still in search of their bounty and a production site.

However, in late 1792 George Garnett was still arguing with the local authority, now the administrators of the Department of Seine Inférieure, as to whether he had properly submitted his claim for the damage done in 1789, saying that the Bureau d'Encouragement was in his debt, not the other way round, and that the 2,700 *livres* the Department offered was ridiculous against his just demand for 9,700.[67] In 1806 his widow was fighting her late husband's battles. She pointed out that he had never received any of the 30,000 *livres* once promised him for his worsted-spinning machine, and that though a Bureau de Consultation during the Revolution had allotted him 6,000 *livres* he had never received any of it. The specimen machine had been kept for a time in the Conservatoire des Arts et Métiers, but then returned to his widow. Remarkably, as late as 2 May 1806, the widow was granted a *brevet d'invention*, valid for ten years, for her husband's wool-spinning machinery.[68]

Garnett prompts some interesting reflexions. Though many years in France and continually putting his technical abilities for sale to national or local authorities, he seems in the end to have achieved very little. In all likelihood his machines were not particularly good, but the great sense of urgency in France about the need to close the technological gap with the British in spinning made it possible for him to appeal to successive administrations and receive some temporary encouragement, if sometimes more moral than pecuniary. He seems to have come to France without being recruited by any individual businessman or by government. He may have genuinely been trying to push some variations of his own on Arkwright's machinery and before 1785 had felt hampered in England by the existing patents. But he clearly arrived in France without funds, and it could be that he came over to evade creditors. Like other English émigrés, a good example being the Milnes, he tried hard to avoid the charge that he was simply importing machine technology that others had invented. The French were fairly quick to realize that he was largely purveying the Arkwright system. They appreciated that it would have been better to have had immigrants who simply imported the latest state of the art as proved and tried in Britain, rather than the idiosyncratic versions of the English machinery thought up by men who were genuinely inventive, but of second-rate abilities, and often intensely committed to their own particular variants.

16 Further Textile Espionage and the Efforts of the Bureau of Commerce

There are a number of other British artisans of some importance in the transfer of English textile technology to France not associated with the first critical establishment of key inventions. John McCloude [the name is variously spelt in French archives and published sources, but the only signature seen is 'John McCloude'] had been a Manchester foreman and was a highly specialist weaver. His principal attachment seems to have been to the *manufacture royale* at Sens.[1] However, in September 1789 a letter to the inspectors at Abbeville, probably from Tolozan, shows that McCloude was in that town, and enquired about the difference between his muslin looms and existing ones. He was to make a loom for the Government – provided it did not cost more than 120 *livres* – which was to be sent to Paris where it was to be operated under McCloude's own eyes and with a thread of specimen fineness. This trial would decide if McCloude should get a government pension, or other allowance. He had asked for a payment 'for the time he lost in making himself intelligible to the (French) workers'.

In 1790–91 the Sens firm seems to have encouraged him to offer his services to the Government, saying that he had made there a whole variety of small stuffs, including types of muslin, as they were made in Manchester. He would be able to set up looms for this purpose and train French workers so that when he moved to a new district they could carry on independently. Once he had completed the work he was doing at Amiens and Abbeville, he wanted to be given another destination where he could repeat his activities. He asked for his own expenses and the maintenance of his wife and child, two *louis* a week regularly paid each Saturday. Work should also be provided for his wife, either in making bobbins or spinning, and a bounty should be paid at each place at which he operated, which should match the services he had given there. In May 1790 it was decided he should go on to Troyes, where he demanded 48 *livres* a week, double what he had had at the other two towns. But the Bureau of Commerce thought 30 *livres* a week plenty, for he needed an eye kept on him; he wanted his booze 'like all the English who like to drink'. He would be able to teach the weaving of seven or eight new English-style cloths in a period of four to five months. However, the municipal officers of Troyes rejected the project and he was sent back to Sens. A year later the new Ministry of the Interior headed by Roland de la Platière enquired about McCloude's activities at Sens, complaining that earlier requests for information by Brown, the inspector of manufactures, had not been answered. A main feature of McCloude's work was the reintroduction of Kay's fly-shuttle into areas where it had fallen into desuetude, though it had not been universally abandoned, for instance the Saint Sever works at Rouen had continued to employ it.[2] Though in 1789 McCloude with another British artisan, Lord, had offered to build not only looms of new types, but also a worsted-spinning machine, nothing seems to have been done about the second proposal.[3]

A file of material survives for 1791–92 showing that McCloude then wanted to return home to Manchester, but hoped for a reward for his services to France, and wished to leave at a convenient time, retaining the favour and good will of the authorities. Even if the earlier aspersions on his love of drink were true, they had not prevented him collecting high opinions from very good judges. Desmarets dug out an earlier enthusiastic report made while McCloude was with Morgan and Massey at Amiens in 1790 where 'This very clever manufacturer has shown the greatest intelligence in the way he set up looms'. He had also demonstrated at the Quinze-Vingts a loom capable of producing quilted cotton of the English type. With his looms there was nearly twice the output of the French weavers with an ordinary loom. Massey urged the Government to reward McCloude but to get all possible information from him before he returned to England. There was similar strong support from the directors of the Sens factory (where McCloude still had his main home), from Pajot de Charmes, the former Abbeville inspector, from the industrial scientist Hassenfratz of the Bureau de Consultation (who recommended a reward of 1,500 *livres*) and from Molard, the future head of the Conservatoire des Arts et Métiers.

McCloude had his proposed gratuity, but seems not to have left France immediately, for having received it in 1792 he went to set up twenty-three fly-shuttle looms for a works belonging to Périer near Nonancourt, then fifty others at Evreux. At a place four miles away he and another Englishman had set up a small enterprise with a dozen looms, but this was about to be sold in the Year III. He is next heard of in 1795 at Chantilly where he was involved in training workers in English cotton spinning processes, then at Mello where he had completed a contract for Alexandre de la Rochefoucauld-Liancourt in the Year VII. In 1807 he asked for government help to set himself up at Tarare and between 1819 and 1822, now in his seventies, he received two small sums to help him in financial difficulties.[4]

The list of British immigrants coming to France can be further extended. John Collier had been brought to France by Périer in 1784 for one of his textile ventures. His brother James Collier, whom we will mention again in connection with the activities of the Toulouse industrialist, Boyer-Fonfrède, came to France in December 1792 and first set up the Toulouse spinning works and then one at Saint Foy in the Dordogne. With Charles Albert (with whom we will deal shortly) he later set up works spinning cotton, linen, hemp and wool at Coye at the beginning of the Year VII. Like many other English residents the Colliers were seized as hostages at the end of the Peace of Amiens and dispatched to prison camp, but quickly released. James developed water-powered machinery for spinning hemp for sailcloth which was capable of making vast quantities with a labour force almost entirely of women and children; he claimed a large factory could go a long way to providing the needs of the French navy and would reduce labour costs by five-sixths. In 1806 he and his associate Berthonneaux invited the minister of the interior to send a commission of 'enlightened, honest, discreet and patriotic technicians' to examine their machinery, so that the minister could provide them with all possible help, protection, privileges, and encouragements which the law permitted. A few days earlier, as part of the same campaign for subsidy, a representative of the Gironde wrote in to support Collier because of his successful work in mounting cotton machines and organizing baize production locally on the English pattern – in his two and a half years in the department he had comported himself 'in a manner to merit the esteem of true Republicans'.[5]

The brothers had jointly operated a cotton spinning venture in Paris in 1805 and 1806, employing thirty workers, and there was a joint patent taken out for carding cylinders in 1806, in addition to the hemp-spinning innovations of that year. In 1811 they said they had spinning-machines available which were of interest to manufacturers in various parts of the French Empire; the prospective purchasers however insisted on an inspection of the machines by Molard and one of the Milnes. By 1814 John Collier was working with a merchant and cotton and woollens manufacturer of English origin, Valentine Rawle. Rawle, whose enterprises were for some years large and important, had been a merchant at Rouen since 1787. Initially he had employed another English mechanic, John Newton Ford. Ford had previously migrated to the United States, but had been suborned thence to France by the French minister at Philadelphia. He submitted details of eight textile machines in the Year IV, before joining up with Rawle. He later asked for large sums in grants and a loan in order to introduce and put to work a new English wool-carding machine and wanted buildings which the State had confiscated ('batiments nationaux') to use as premises. For this scheme a considerable number of 'extremely clever workers' had been obtained, who included John Hulse (of whom more later) and William Lowry. But the Government was going through a period of disillusionment with English mechanics: 'these English skilled workers who perhaps have no other purpose than to sow corruption and discord among us'.[6]

While there are other British names which could be followed up, there are few that can be connected with major transfers of technique in spinning and weaving textiles before 1800, when our study ends. We will look at calico-printing briefly and separately. It is, however, important that we should examine some notable cases of French industrial espionage in England which were carried out by men who were already, or were to become, important industrialists. A certain Lecomte, while travelling in Italy in 1788 as tutor to a young Bordeaux man, made the acquaintance of Charles Albert, a Strasbourg citizen who had taken an early interest in mechanics. Albert, then aged twenty-four, had spent a year in Manchester and was engaged on a business trip to Italy on behalf of an English industrialist. In 1790 Albert was offered a job in Manchester by the (unnamed) manufacturer he had been acting for, and he accepted it quickly, for it offered a chance to learn about the new English textile technology at first hand. On his way to Manchester Albert met Lecomte in Paris. Lecomte was planning a new career as a merchant in England, Albert proffered help and they arranged to keep in touch.

Soon Lecomte came to meet Albert in Manchester accompanied by Boyer-Fonfrède, the son of a wealthy Toulouse merchant and West India plantation owner. He was four years younger than Albert. Lecomte and Boyer-Fonfrède told him of their plan to open a large cotton factory near Toulouse. Albert could be very useful to them, he was not only in an excellent position to know about the latest machinery and get plans, models and tools, but very well placed to suborn workmen. In his account of the operation Albert calls it 'a delicate and perilous mission, given the keen look-out kept by the English, and the severity of the penalties imposed by the law'. Albert said he was encouraged to take part in the scheme because of the love of country and liberty which so closely affected many young men like him in the early revolutionary years. Soon his espionage had taken such a successful course that it was no longer safe for him to continue to work for his Manchester employer – presumably because discovery of his activities would soon become inevitable. So Boyer-Fonfrède wrote him to say that he would pay him a salary equal to his existing one until a point was reached where he could become a shareholder in the nascent enterprise.

By November 1791 the operation seemed close to completion. Models and tools had been collected, some others contracted for, and yet others were under negotiation. In all this Albert had used an intermediary, 'T' as he was called. Two principal workers engaged were Thomas Crookes, who would emigrate to France with all his family, and Thomas Holt. They were separately to rendezvous with Albert at a place outside Manchester to begin their journey, initially travelling to London. But Holt failed to turn up. Albert met Crookes and his family, supplied them with funds and with directions how to take ship for France, and then returned to Manchester to sort things out. The worker-agent 'T' had learnt that Holt was going to denounce him to the British authorities. As an English subject he had to flee to escape the penalties of the law, but said Albert should remain to help to steady the nerves of the other recruits, who had not yet left the town. Albert put all the tools and models in a trunk and sent them via London to Toulouse where they arrived safely. A group of workmen, including a spinner referred to as 'J.C.', the suborner himself, 'T', and several others were successfully dispatched to France. A Bolton weaver, Jeffrey Scholes, was urged to follow. But in December 1791 Albert was denounced by Holt. He was offered his freedom if he would say where 'T' and the other suborned workers were – they had not at this point crossed the Channel. As this would have wrecked the whole scheme Albert refused to give them away. The British newspapers carried the story of Albert's arrest, and in his view this prejudged his case – though his guilt was clear enough. To make matters worse, Scholes, who had not yet left, was intimidated by the campaign in the press, and turned King's Evidence. Crookes was arrested in London, just as his ship was about to sail for France, and had Albert's letters of recommendation to his French partners on him at the time. After another refusal to give information which would help arrest 'T' and other accomplices, Albert was put into Lancaster gaol at the end of December 1791.

Hearing of his arrest Boyer-Fonfrède and Lecomte wrote from Bordeaux to Albert's father that there was nothing dishonourable in the arrest, and that all good people and friends of France would esteem him the more, that he should lack for nothing, that even if it cost £1,000 to set him at liberty it would be raised, and that there was no obstacle that their friendship for their imprisoned colleague would not overcome. Shortly afterwards they said that the necessary bail had been raised and would be forwarded to England. They wrote similarly to Albert, saying that the bail was on its way and whatever the outcome 'we will never abandon you'. Though Albert said he had not received any earlier letters they insisted they had written to him six times. Albert appealed to be moved to London, where he thought the bail would be more quickly arranged, and was transferred to Newgate. No bail turned up from his partners, but the French embassy offered £500 for the purpose. But it was now pointed out that while the bail required for suborning one worker was £500 Albert was now charged with suborning three, and there was a similar bail needed for each case, so that £1,500 was needed. No one offered that, and Albert went back to Lancaster Castle. Now Crookes joined Holt and Scholes in testimony against Albert. In fact it seems that only Scholes's evidence was taken, perhaps because Albert had spent his last money in trying to influence potential witnesses not to present themselves at the trial.

Albert was convicted of 'having persuaded and suborned this worker to carry the cotton manufacture abroad'. He was imprisoned for a year and fined £500, but the imprisonment would continue so long as the fine was unpaid, even if the year had elapsed. Now Boyer-Fonfrède and Lecomte assured him that when the year was out he would have his fine paid, and could come and join their enterprise if he wished – he would never be left to his fate. But after some months Albert was told that the money would not be available at the year's end and that another year would have to be spent in prison, while it still remained possible for Holt and Crookes to bring forward their evidence and increase Albert's fine to £1,500. However, he was able to get his eight months in prison before trial taken towards his sentence, and the two other charges were dropped.

Boyer-Fonfrède and Lecomte were not short of money at this time. After creating a very large and celebrated works near Toulouse, Boyer-Fonfrède had begun to set up others in the Midi and had a luxurious mansion in Paris; Lecomte had set up a branch merchant house in Philadelphia which he directed from his Paris base. But while they cruelly abandoned their associate, well-to-do Englishmen took pity on him. A Manchester evangelical church mounted a campaign for his release on the grounds that he would remain a prisoner for ever if his fine was not paid, and a magistrate arranged that the High Sheriff of the County of Lancaster would order his release, and in December 1796 he was set at liberty. His English supporters provided bail, the condition being that Albert could not re-enter England without paying the original fine. The Governor of Lancaster Castle had himself petitioned for his release, and Albert had strong support from the Johnson family on Bolton-le-Sands whose daughter Elizabeth he married in the few weeks between his release from prison and his return to France.

Back in France he was received by Boyer-Fonfrède and Lecomte with hypocritical sympathy and condemnation for the cruelties of the English, and the insulting offer of 23 *louis* compensation, while they each put the blame for their lack of help on the other. He went to law demanding the costs he had had to pay in Britain, and damages. While both resorted to exploiting legal delays, Boyer-Fonfrède eventually had to pay 75,000 francs.

Albert went on to be an important cotton manufacturer at Coye, where (with James Collier) he was associated with the financier J.-F. de Rougemont. His Paris textile machinery works was valued at 120,000 francs in 1806, and he received a gold medal for a collection of cotton-spinning machinery at the national industrial exhibition of that year. In 1809 – with a partner – he was awarded 6,000 francs for a small steam-engine by the Société d'Encouragement pour l'Industrie Nationale. For some years he was an important industrial lobbyist for the cotton industry and was involved in attempts to grow cotton in Tuscany. Though his cotton business declined at the end of the Napoleonic regime he was later an associate of the Englishman Humphrey Edwards, who was important in the introduction of the economical Woolf steam-engines in France. According to Henderson[7] Albert, despite the generosity he had received in England, on his return directed in Paris an agency for the importation of smuggled English machines, and he resumed this activity in the 1820s and ended his business career as a major importer of English and American textile machinery.[8]

Boyer-Fonfrède had embarked on his great cotton venture near Toulouse, obtaining substantial concessions of lands and buildings from the authorities for little expenditure, and claiming that he would employ 30,000. Part of his scheme was a huge English-type water-powered spinning factory, in which Arkwright-type machinery was used, and for which a collection of splendid plans and drawings survives in the Conservatoire National des Arts et Métiers. Albert being imprisoned in England, Boyer-Fonfrède turned in 1793 to an unusual technical adviser, Isaac Gouldbroof, who must be one of the very few Jews to have been a skilled mechanic in the English cotton industry. He was to supervise spinning operations, train workers, and supervise their work but, with splendid irony when one thinks of his master's English espionage, 'give neither plan, nor drawing, nor any information whatsoever, and enter no [other] textile, cotton or woollen business during the period of his contract, under penalty of losing two years' wages'. He got £105 a year and a share of profits which could have in the long term given him a salary of 8,500 *livres*, extremely high for the time. Boyer-Fonfrède's general operations, originally conceived on a huge scale, cannot be followed here; they were marked by the use of some English prisoners of war after 1793, and by a massive resort to child labour with a thirteen-hour day. He ran into a series of supply and trading problems and his firm wound up about 1808.[9]

The industrial espionage of Lieven Bauwens is often cited. He does not fit too neatly into our framework. He was Belgian, some of his major activities were concentrated around Ghent, and many of his main achievements were in the years after 1800. But some of his enterprises were within the former boundaries of France. While his industrial espionage was in some ways remarkably blatant and successful, and a seeming example of how readily British technology could be penetrated and stolen, this is by no means the whole story.

Of a noble family which seems to have engaged uninhibitedly in industry and commerce, he was early directed to the family's large tanning enterprise, and at sixteen he was sent to England to the firm of Undershell and Fox, where he stayed three years – it is hardly

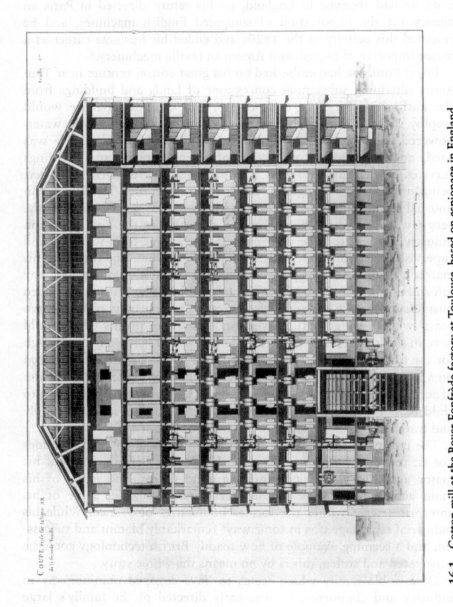

16.1   Cotton mill at the Boyer-Fonfrède factory at Toulouse, based on espionage in England

remarkable if, as Ballot rather strangely puts it, he 'succeeded in unearthing the secrets of the English manufacture'. Back in his native Ghent he built a very large new tannery, and after the annexation of Belgium by France he created another great tannery in Paris. There is no doubt that he travelled extensively as a merchant, and that the war did not immediately hinder that. He had many relations in England, and his brother had a banking house at Hamburg which had a London branch. The Hamburg bank was tied in with a firm which dealt with colonial imports, presumably including British ones.

Bauwens made an espionage trip to England in 1797, accompanied by a relation and business associate, François de Pauw. His plan to obtain English cotton machinery and workers was approved of by the French government, but not financed by them – they no doubt thought he was perfectly capable of paying his own costs. He won over Saul Harding, a London worker, whom he sent to Manchester to buy machines, while he himself also bought machines, and suborned a number of workers including the machine-maker James Hulse of Manchester, Dean, a spinner, James Farrar, a turner, and a factory manager, James Kenyon. He also purchased a small steam-engine from Boulton and Watt and bought large quantities of sugar, indigo and other goods on behalf of his brother's Hamburg house. He therefore had a cover of genuine mercantile activities behind which he could carry on his industrial espionage; long resident in England in his youth, and a frequent visitor afterwards, language would present no difficulty, while he was able to use another foreign banking house to handle some of the machinery dispatched to him. Bauwens's own English espionage was discontinuous, because of his need to attend to his large businesses on the Continent, but he came and went without much difficulty. Harding, for his part, bargained with a Manchester machine-builder and sent machine parts to London.

But the operations were not smooth or uninterrupted. When the first consignment of machines was sent abroad in March 1798, though the machine parts were carefully concealed in bales of colonial goods and put on a Danish ship, they were spotted by Customs and the ship and cargo seized, and the ship's master fined the £100 provided for under the legislation.[10] Lammens, Bauwens's ally with the London banking house, fled the country and Bauwens himself left more sedately. The espionage was not abandoned, but proceeded with greater caution now the English authorities were on the alert in Manchester and in London. A single workman and some machinery were successfully sent off. In

August of 1798 Bauwens came back; while it is often stated that this was his thirty-second (and last) visit to England, this certainly does not mean he had made all those journeys as ones of industrial espionage. Most would be made for trading purposes; if he had spent three years in the English leather trade common observation in that industry might have been as significant as deliberate spying. The cotton trade espionage seems only to have begun in 1797. Bauwens made arrangements with a London publican to house workers, and men were engaged at the high premium of £60 each and the substantial wages of 3 guineas a week. Then there was a delay until all the machinery had been delivered, while the chief conspirators, Bauwens, de Pauw, Lammens (now also returned) and Harding, studied machine plans and, most interestingly, a cut-out cardboard model of one of the cotton machines. After detailed preparations the group prepared to sail from Gravesend in November 1798, but were exposed because of a noisy scene provoked by Harding's wife, who objected to being left behind with her children, and the magistrates were alerted. Harding initially made up some cover story, while Bauwens claimed to be an uninvolved bystander. They got back to London and warned the others involved. Bauwens took eight workers by coach to Yarmouth, and secured a vessel there, and despite bad weather and (it is said) pursuit by English vessels, reached Hamburg on 17 November 1798. He had not told the workers that the spinning factory they were to mount was to be in the enemy country of France. They were naturally upset, and tried to denounce Bauwens to British representatives in Hamburg. But five workers were prepared to stay with him and he managed to get them to Ghent.

However, several boxes of equipment were still to be sent from England. The deserting workmen informed on those who had organized the espionage, and Harding, Lammens and the pub-keeper, Swainson, were arrested, and the boxes seized. They were each sentenced to a £500 fine and a year in prison. Thus Bauwens's ambitious plan had not been smoothly run or a complete success; though he had obtained important machines and skills it was at a heavy cost, even if, as in the case of Boyer-Fonfrède, that cost had been mainly paid in the fines and imprisonment suffered by others. The machines he had smuggled out were large mules with over 200 spindles and all the ancillary equipment for spinning, together with calico-printing machinery and fly-shuttle looms. His first establishment was set up in an old convent at Passy near Paris, and he subsequently built large steam-powered works in and around Ghent, as well as continuing in a large way in the tanning business in both Ghent and Paris. His cotton product was of high quality and carried off the major prizes at the early French industrial exhibitions which were held at the turn of the century. In 1811 he was said to be worth 1.5 million francs, but like some other great industrialists of the Empire period he was unable to stand the British competition which was briefly unleashed when French cotton duties were reduced in 1814. His works were sold, though he avoided actual bankruptcy.[11]

Bauwens, probably because of his familiarity with both commerce and language in England, was able to pick good managers, mechanics and operatives. The fly-shuttle weavers he recruited were able to provide a service under the Consulate by training weavers sent in by the Prefects of Departments at government expense. Twenty fly-shuttle looms were built and sent out to Departments which requested them, and this exercise was even continued after Bauwens gave up the Passy works in 1806. With James Farrar, one of the mechanics he had brought over, Bauwens submitted a collection of machines auxiliary and central to mule spinning to a competitive assessment organized in the Year XI – we can be sure which of the two was the real technologist. In awarding Bauwens 60,000 *livres* and Farrar 10,000, the jury spoke of the Englishman as a 'precious acquisition for France, who deserves government protection'. Thomas Ferguson, another of the Bauwens team, was awarded 2,000 *livres* for his skills in spinning and carding and his qualities in instructing and training operatives. He was an early recruit to the technological training staff of the Conservatoire des Arts et Métiers, where the director, Molard, brought in several leading English mechanics. Ferguson was in charge of the spinning section from the Year XII to the Year XIV, where foremen and even entrepreneurs were introduced to English machinery. It had a short but effective life, apparently declining and closing when good on-the-job training became generally available with the expansion of the cotton factory system in France. J.-B. Say was perhaps the most celebrated pupil.[12]

Another Bauwens employee was John Hulse. In the Year X Molard reported to the Minister of the Interior on an offer Hulse had earlier made to make cotton carding and spinning machines. He had originally been promised a premium of 200 francs on each of the first hundred sets of machines he made within a five-year period, and that he should have a 3,000 franc advance. Molard had closely followed his work on machines destined for display at the Conservatoire des Arts et Métiers. But the Ministry had not yet been able to find the money to pay him even the 3,000 franc advance, and Hulse, who had been dismissed by Bauwens, unjustly in his own opinion, had gone off to Rouen to work for Rawle, the English merchant who, as we have seen, had set up a commercial house there before the Revolution, and then entered cotton manufacture in a big way. Molard, in pursuing the matter, found that Hulse declined proceeding further with the Government's offer, now in the form of an allocation of 6,000 francs for a set of machinery to be placed in the Conservatoire. Hulse said that his machines would have been novel when the Government had first taken an interest in them, 'but since that time a very considerable number of those machines have been made for different people. When I say up-wards of thirty I am within the truth'. Technology in cotton machinery was dynamic not static. In fact 'those made by [other] individuals will be made with all the improvements made by the Application of Practice, while those placed by me in the Depot will remain in their Primitive state'. These considerations

> strike me with far more force as a Practical Mechanic than they possibly can any man who has not had a long experience of the hourly improvements that occur and have occurred from every machine in the Cotton Branch from Practice only and not from any suggestion of the Makers of the Machine.

It would, he said, be improper to take the nation's money in the circumstances!

Molard was not ready to take Hulse's reasons for declining the Government's offer at face value, he believed that his new employer, Rawle, wanted to keep an outstandingly good worker in his firm and not let neighbouring and rival firms obtain and spread the best machines amongst them. But Hulse was making a valid point in saying that textile machinery was continually being improved and that, unless continuously uprated, such equipment could become not the latest technological evidence in an exhibition centre, but a misleading museum piece. Molard, however, thought that the way round Hulse's rejection of the Government's offer was to go to the Bauwens brothers, who would match the original offer of Hulse, but would want 1,000 francs for each of the first fifty sets of spinning-machinery they provided. They would provide an exemplary set for the Conservatoire des Arts et Métiers and mount it themselves, also providing workmen instructors to operate the machines and even one-month crash courses in their use.[13]

It is noteworthy that Molard stated that it was to the Bauwens family that 'France owes the introduction of the most perfect mule-jennies of all those known in our manufactures', which reinforces the point that it was a group of particularly able technologists that they had recruited and brought to France. But on the other hand Ballot is right to point out that there was a considerable hyperbole in their claims to have brought the mule, fly-shuttle and cylinder-printing to France. With their British acolytes they may have set a standard nearer to the 'state of the art' of textile technology across the Channel at the end of the century than did their French rivals, but they did not first introduce these machines and processes to France. He is similarly right to be critical of the supposed facility with which Bauwens had penetrated British industrial workshops and machine technology. It had been very ambitious industrial espionage, but by no means wholly successful, or ineffectively opposed by British manufacturers and magistrates.[14]

Another major industrialist of the turn of the century was François Richard of the firm of Richard-Lenoir who had risen from more humble origins than Bauwens through sheer entrepreneurial drive. He changed from commercial dealings to manufacture in 1799. His technological recruitment was less sophisticated than Bauwens's: 'He had the good luck to get hold of a poor Englishman, Brown [presumably a man who had come to France to take his chance] who designed looms for him which were originally operated by four or five English workers'. In doing this Richard was apparently moving from a smuggling business in English cloths to direct manufacture. He next recruited the mechanic William Bramwells, a Derbyshire man in France since 1792, who had first worked for Thomas Leclerc at Liancourt. He seems to have turned out good mules at considerable speed. By 1810 Richard was in a vast way of business, directing the largest industrial enterprise in France, with well over 6,000 weavers in Normandy and Picardy, 641 mules and water frames at several different factories, and 400 employees at calico-printing. He was an important politician of the industry and government adviser. His concerns suffered many shocks, the Napoleonic duty on raw cotton caused great problems early in 1811, in 1812 he decided to convert much of his operations to worsted, and then, under pressure from creditors, sold part of his empire to a relation. Though still retaining two works as late as 1830, he died impoverished at the end of the decade.[15]

One of the most important men interested in moving to France was William Douglas. He was a major industrialist in his own right in Britain with a famous early Arkwright-type cotton-mill at Hollywell in Flintshire and other works at Manchester. One of the most significant and unusual features of his proposed emigration is that the initiative was his. He was not recruited, he offered his services to France. He was no clever artisan, keen to earn more on the other side of the channel, or dissatisfied with his advancement at home, or bothered by petty debts. He was a major entrepreneur. It is claimed that he followed a first offer to migrate, which was not taken up, with a second and much later one which was, but this is a confusion between two men of the same surname.

William Douglas's proposal to leave England came just before the Revolution. He was apparently motivated by a temporary depression in the cotton industry due to heavy imports of cotton goods by the East India Company. In December 1788 he wrote from Chester to D'Aragon, the secretary to the French ambassador in London. He had just visited his Welsh cotton factories, and sent the embassy two important pamphlets on his cotton manufactures, and two samples of cotton spun by one of his water-powered factories. He boasted that a pound of cotton could produce over 60 miles of thread, as contained in one sample, and 90 miles in another. He and his partner Atherton had a new machine, of which they claimed to be as yet the sole possessors, which could produce yarn of 230 to 250 count, finer than any Indian-spun cotton. He could prove the quality and the great size of his spinning facilities, and the excellence of the machines, and was willing to conduct D'Aragon round the whole plant and show him everything from the opening of the raw cotton to the production of cloth of the highest standard and of many kinds. The tour would include the very latest machines. They would even show D'Aragon things which were not normally revealed to some of their most skilful workmen. After seeing the Welsh works they could travel to their Manchester mills, a mere 2 miles from the town centre, and D'Aragon would also be given a thorough tour of the Manchester neighbourhood so as to provide him with a complete impression of that new industrial world. Douglas said he would also take D'Aragon to see machinery as now employed in the woollen industry, all the easier in that several of his relatives were in that industry. It is interesting that he spoke of the densely populated area round Manchester which 'constitutes so to speak a single village in a 40 mile circuit'.[16] D'Aragon would see things no foreigner had ever seen, and be able to report back to his own government in a way which would be highly creditable to him.

D'Aragon added his own note to Douglas's letter, indicating that this was a man who had already made an offer of services to the French court in the previous November. He emphasized that Douglas owned some of the largest premises and was one of the greatest capitalists in the cotton industry. At this time when England, under the Eden-Rayneval treaty, was unloading huge quantities of cottons on the French market, and when France was sending emissaries on trips of industrial espionage 'where the discoveries made can only depend on a degree of good luck', an opportunity such as Douglas offered should not be lost. The cost of making the remarkable guided tour proffered by Douglas would be trivial compared with the potential advantages. Apparently the proposal was all the more apt in that one of Douglas's correspondents, probably Barthélemy, was being considered for a newly proposed post of French commercial consul in the relevant British industrial provinces.[17]

While in general terms, given the disastrous impact of English imports on the French cotton industry, Douglas's proposition was indeed well timed, in terms of the immediate preoccupations of the French government it was not. A letter was drafted to the French ambassador in England, possibly by Tolozan, which said that the writer had been unable to discuss the matter with Necker, because the latter was totally preoccupied by the preparations for calling the Estates General. The writer's own view was that Douglas could be completely distinguished from

> a multitude of Englishmen who are coming into this country to offer to make cylinder type machines for the carding and spinning of cotton.[18] We have believed them far too easily and the majority have deceived us, for our machines [i.e. the ones they have made for us] do not produce anything near the effects they promised us.

While four cotton factories had now been set up in France, the new English machines were still to be desired in that country, especially those that would produce the finest yarn for muslin.

Douglas's offer should certainly not be ignored, but his price must be ascertained, and also the cost advantages to be gained from his machines. Accurate fact-finding about Douglas's equipment and that already acquired in France was essential. The Government was intending to send to England 'a very intelligent man and above all well trained in the art of drawing and later constructing all the machines he sees'. The writer referred to Le Turc, already well known to Barthélemy, and a particular expert on stocking looms, who had already had a remarkable period of industrial espionage in England. He had in fact just agreed a contract with the Government for a return to England to get information on machinery for carding and spinning cotton, and he could assess Douglas's technology and advise. He could even make a partnership agreement with Douglas to come and work with him in France. Le Turc's activities we will explore later, but it seems that the espionage contract with him was never put into force and the journey not made.[19]

Then there is a gap to the Year X. A man, said to be the same Douglas, arrived at Bordeaux, obtained an introduction to the prefect, and offered to introduce English wool-spinning machinery and finishing equipment – he threw in for good measure a plan for a new cast iron bridge over the Thames! He was invited to Paris, received warmly by some of the main woollen manufacturers and by them strongly recommended to Chaptal, minister of the interior, and of course himself a former industrial chemist and subsequent author of outstanding books on French industry and the application of chemistry to industry. He offered Douglas a factory site, in fact the former great steam-powered corn-mills erected by Périer on the Ile des Cygnes in the Seine at Paris. He first granted Douglas a modest 15,000 *livres* for a set of machines for opening, carding, coarse spinning, fine spinning, shearing and nap raising. As well as developing his own factory on the Ile des Cygnes Douglas supplied large numbers of machines to other manufacturers. In the Year XIII he had already delivered ninety-six machines, and was currently handling orders for thirty-seven.[20] By 1810 he had supplied 949 machines to one hundred factories in forty departments. But it seems virtually certain that the two mentioned Douglases were different men. Two documents in the CNAM archives show that it was a J. Douglas who took out a comprehensive *brevet d'invention* for new woollen machinery and that he was certainly the one based at the Ile des Cygnes. It was his machines which the Ternaux brothers bought from 1803, but subsequently complained of, stating that the Cockerill family had introduced similar but better machines into the Belgian part of French territory.[21] In the second source it is a *James* Douglas who is referred to as having the patent (*brevet*) and who seems to be the object of the attack by the Ternaux, and it was certainly a James Douglas who corresponded with Molard of the Conservatoire offering shearing machines to complete the full set of his 'assortiment' of wool machines.[22]

The later career of William Douglas lies outside the period of this study. He was apparently a member of the Douglas family of whom John Douglas was the most prominent, and had joined with the Smalley family in works at Holywell. John Smalley, an early partner of Arkwright, had broken away to establish a Flintshire works in 1777;

large new Holywell mills were built in 1780 and 1785 and John Douglas had then become a principal in a firm called Douglas and Company or Douglas, Smalley and Company. How far the William Douglas partnership with Atherton was separate is unclear. The family continued prominently in the business; a William Douglas owned the Holywell Twist Company in 1818 with 840 workers, and had another 531 workers at mills at Pendleton near Manchester.[23]

This account of the English transferrers of textile technology to France does not aim to be exhaustive; it has tried to single out the most important instances and individuals and those cases where suborning and the illegal export of machines from Britain were involved, and the laws against what we now call industrial espionage were broken. It also makes it clear there is a small minority of cases where transfers took place without suborning or machine smuggling. Now three final topics will be explored as far as evidence allows: the contemporary French views on the success of their largely illegal acquisition of British technology – illegal that is from a British viewpoint; the extent to which the Revolution and early stages of war held up the process of technology transfer; and, finally, how far the technologists who came to France before 1800 made worthwhile careers for themselves.

The importance of introducing English machinery was not in any way neglected by the French government, particularly the Bureau of Commerce once Tolozan came to head it, but there were frequent misgivings about the success obtained. A memoir of 1787 shows Tolozan had been greatly concerned to see that full advantage was taken of the English machines acquired to card and spin cotton, often at great expense. He had enlisted the services of the Academician Desmarets, and of two other inspectors, to examine the various machines and discover their advantages and disadvantages.[24] They were conscious that the cotton-spinning factories so far set up, Epine, Louviers and Orléans, were basically using the same Arkwright technology, but the Milnes' version of the carding machinery was better. The inspectors realized that the Arkwright roller-spinning machines did not give the best fine thread, gave too much twist for the yarns used in some cloths and were best for warp thread. Fine spinning needed much improvement at this point in time if it was to equal English, but the inspectors were not yet clear about the importance of the mule. They recognized that the twist thread of the Arkwright machines could be combined as a warp with weft from the simpler jenny, but they thought French jennies needed much improvement.[25]

In their search for machines capable of equalling the fineness to which the English were now taking their yarn they confessed that 'the considerable expenditure that has been made on this subject has not been given the necessary consideration, and we have given a little too much trust to foreign workmen, who have neither the proper overview nor the preliminary principles on the manufacture of yarn'. It was recognized that publicity was of the greatest importance, and Tolozan as we have seen formed the plan of setting up a manufacture of his own with the objects of producing cotton for printing (in order to contest imports of Swiss printed calicoes) and to produce cotton suitable for making both plain and ribbed stockings. He was going to seize on the framework knitting machines now being smuggled from England by Le Turc under his supervision. To those and the improved jenny of the Frenchman Lhomond he would add cleaning, opening and carding machines from Milne. Over many of these operations the inspector Lazowski would preside. They were to be mounted in buildings which belonged to Tolozan, on an estate he had acquired at Courrouges in the Barrois, and would serve as a model for other cotton manufactures in Champagne, the three Bishoprics, Alsace and Lorraine. The inspector Lazowski, his associate in the enterprise, was to stay there until all the machinery was in perfect order and product prices were brought lower than those in the rest of France.

It is remarkable that so much effort was being put into a scheme which included neither water frame nor mule, but perhaps capital was the problem. The 12,000 *livres* envisaged seems rather small. But it may have been that the plentiful and cheap labour available in the locality was thought of as a means of setting up an industrial model somewhere between proto-industrialization and a complete factory system. This interesting operation seems to have quickly failed, monumental rows between Lhomond and Lazowski being certainly one reason. But it would have been an enterprise conducted by the head of the Bureau of Commerce, apparently for his own profit, and employing officials or technologists paid or subsidized by the State. It would certainly have comprised all those combinations of public office holding and private entrepreneurship for which the Holkers had been so sharply attacked, and may explain why Le Turc changed from regarding Tolozan as a disinterested patron of his espionage on the English stocking industry to considering him an enemy exploiting machines he had so painfully gained in the hope of employing them directly himself.[26]

On the eve of the Revolution, with a general economic crisis, aggravated, particularly for the large Norman cotton industry, by the flood of English imports under the Eden-Rayneval treaty, there were enquiries into the critical issue of the quantity and quality of machine-spinning of cotton. A meeting of the Bureau of Commerce in 1788 chaired by Loménie de Brienne, which reappraised industrial policy, said that the two chief government preoccupations were those with the manufacture of steel and with spinning.[27] There were serious attempts to compare the progress of the spinning industry in England and France.[28]

It was agreed that English cotton cloths enjoyed a preference over French even when the French made the same articles, because they were cheaper and because the yarn used was superior, and this superiority had become very marked once machine-spinning had started to make its astonishing progress.

> They have marched from invention to invention at a pace so rapid, that French industry, plunged into despair and nearly destroyed, has with difficulty ... followed the path which has been thus shown to it. Twenty years experimentation crowned with the greatest success on the English side, has not enlightened the manufacturers of Normandy

who had clung to the narrow sphere of products in which they had been trained.[29] There was also in the late 1780s and early 1790s some apprehension on the way in which popular resistance, like that which had destroyed the works of Garnett and others in Rouen, would delay the introduction of the new English processes, and workers' fears were increased by the comments of 'ignorant observers who have not realized that these [new] kinds of spinning tend to create a production of new cloths which does not harm older-type manufactures'.[30]

The peak period of anxiety was obviously that of the negotiation and the impact of the Eden-Rayneval treaty of 1786, and the reappraisals made then were often painful. The past attitude of French governments, that the best policy for industry and society was to put the maximum number of hands to work by conventional hand processes, was now in sharp contrast with the English belief that the substitution of workers by machinery would, by enlarging the market, eventually be the best means of procuring increased employment. The manufactures of Louviers, commenting on the difference, were proud of the attempts to settle the English system in their town, but 'while we are quite sure that we have obtained the most perfect machines there are in France, we are a very long way from having achieved the perfection the English have arrived at'. It was not all that simple to get high-quality English workers. 'The good workers make a very good living in England. The language problem is a big obstacle to them, it is nearly always the less skilled and the "mauvais sujets" who decide to come over to France. To invite those of superior talents larger rewards are needed which the individual [businessman] cannot offer.' The imputation was that only large firms and those enjoying privileges and subsidies could manage the transfer to the new English technology successfully.[31]

At a critical period in the Eden treaty negotiations it is remarkable to see that it was the opinions of the elder Holker which were sought, within three months of his death. It is clear that the greatest importance was attached to his views. One problem with the framing of treaty policy was that the two commissioners charged with fact-finding by Calonne, Dupont and Boyetet, were on opposite sides, Dupont enthusiastic for a treaty, Boyetet cautious and suspicious to say the least.[32] In August 1786 a committee of the royal council was called to give a rapid opinion on the duties to be fixed by the treaty. The committee, perhaps intentionally, was not composed of the most relevant and knowledgeable ministers and was pressed for a reply the same day. On the critical subject of cotton Boyetet discovered that though Holker's opinion had been sought, it had not been given to the committee. In fact he claimed that it was only after persistent enquiries, and partly by accident, that he himself had been able to read it, because Dupont was reluctant to have its contents known. Holker was, in Boyetet's view, 'in a better position than anyone else to throw a clear light on the state of this kind of industry in both kingdoms', and it was for this reason that it had been proposed that he should be consulted.[33]

Holker wrote to Rayneval at the end of December 1785.[34] He would do what the minister wanted and obtain a full set of samples of Manchester cloths to examine against French ones.[35] But Holker suggested that the exercise would take too long and be futile anyway, for even if 25 or 30 per cent duty was put on Manchester products they would readily outsell French goods, because English machinery, whether hand, horse or water powered, enabled them to undercut French cottons. To try to compensate this by very high duties would simply lead to smuggling. The only real remedy would be to bring French manufactures to a similar state of efficiency. He gave examples of the enormous savings the English powered carding machines and coarse-spinning machines gave over French hand methods. Where in France there were woman-powered spinning-machines – presumably jennies – they saved two-thirds of the cost of spinning. While careful to point out that he had no personal knowledge of spinning by water-power, Holker thought there must be a further saving, since the British had built mills with 1,000 to 1,500 spindles.

There were now three English-type powered factories in France. None of these should have exclusive privileges; the great thing was to multiply them as they were now rapidly multiplying in Scotland, Wales and Lancashire, where he thought there were already fifteen powered by water. If the French industry was given its head there were many English workers who would be keen to come over to improve their lot; if France delayed potential emigrants would go to other countries.[36] He was himself in negotiation with an emigrant who was able to make water-powered carding and spinning machines – indicating that it was only his illness and death which prevented Holker from embarking on a water-powered factory, even in his sixties. As high duties simply led to smuggling, Holker favoured a complete prohibition on cotton goods made in Britain. This would encourage the setting up of eight or ten more cotton-mills in France in the next five or six years, which, in a state of free internal competition, might then be able to take on the English importer; inefficient privileged mills would be a disaster and lead to mass unemployment if England had to be competed with. As far as woollens were concerned, not only had the English product long been better, but it was founded upon wools which were both superior and cheaper. In fine woollens the superiority was not so much a matter of technical advantage as the complete freedom from regulation in England, and the manufacturer's ability to experiment commercially with his product. The regulation and inspection of French products should end.

Holker briefly remarked on iron foundries and pottery; in both, England had a great superiority and free admission of their goods would ruin the French manufacturer. English manufactures were carried on by men of greater capital, who stayed with the business, French capitalists were less wealthy, and once they had made enough they got out and became rentiers. He ended by defending the move to powered-machine manufacture: it would in the end lead to a greater, not a lesser, employment of workers. But he emphasized forcibly the dangers of allowing the entry of English cottons, because the French could not as yet stand the competition. What happened of course was that Boyetet interpreted Holker's letter as simply a demand for a permanent prohibition on English cottons, while Dupont de Nemours interpreted it as saying that with a few years of wise domestic policy towards the adoption of powered machinery the French would be able to compete with the British.[37]

At the depth of the crisis caused by the crushing superiority of English imports once the Eden treaty was enforced French commentators were astonished that the English could sell cottons so cheaply on the French market, but sure a comparable mechanization was the answer. 'We have set the French workmen to grips with the English workman. It is the combat of a naked man against an armed man and it has the outcome we may expect, and the victory cannot be disputed. Is no resource left to us?' It had to be the introduction of all those machines now in vogue in Britain 'the perfecting of which is the fruit of over 50 years of constant effort and continuous emulation'. It was now up to France to try to catch up on this machinery in a very condensed period, and to concentrate on spinning which constituted 'the triumph of the English manufacture'. The early French spinning factories at Louviers and Arpajon 'are still far below the perfection of the English ones', said another commentator.[38]

Desmarets, in urging that English improvements in the modification and use of hand looms should be followed in order to produce fashionable and quality cloths, insisted that advances in imitation of English textiles should not stop with spinning:

> Because in each trade the English have neglected nothing to economize labour and give a high degree of perfection to their products, we ought in imitating them to embrace the whole succession of their processes, because they are well thought out and intimately depend the one upon the other: but I ought to say that we have only seized on certain parts of the trades, and it is to this bad system that we can attribute the small success we have had up to the present in a number of the English trades which we have tried to introduce in France: let us then devote ourselves to the whole.[39]

Again, after the problems of the Eden Treaty the Chamber of Commerce of Rouen memorialized their Provincial Assembly. They had sent two emissaries, Hurard fils and Rabasse, to England to go through the relevant counties, learn about all the works, bring back samples of the different cloths made, and study the 'genius and the means employed to facilitate and perfect labour', and 'finally reach an understanding of the national character which governs the whole working class'. On their return they made a comparative tour of the Norman works. They concluded that while the late M. Holker was to be given credit for the 'courage, talents and diligence' with which he had begun the making of new cotton cloths at Saint Sever, for the first introduction of English workers, and for their teaching of French trainees which had resulted in the employment of many families, this relatively recent development was threatened, as could be seen by looking at the sample cards of the Saint Sever works and comparing them with those of Manchester. It was pointed out in another document that it was already perceptible that when English experts and workmen had come over in recent times, the French soon became keen to emulate them in the 'instruments' (machine tools) they used and the hand tools of excellent temper they employed. 'It is to these advantages that they owe a large part of their superiority.'[40]

There are some rather melancholy, perhaps too pessimistic, retrospective documents from the administrators who had tried to steer the French cotton textile industry, especially spinning, towards the English path in the years before the Revolution. One of their preoccupations had been to try to provide accommodation in which pioneering technologists, particularly British, could try to develop their new machines and processes until they could become technologically established, and send out the initial batches of machines to French entrepreneurs. The most commonly used accommodation was that in the former Quinze-Vingts hospital in Paris, and with the closing of the Bureau of Commerce this site, which was considered an important attraction and a form of subsidy inducing foreigners to come over, was under threat.[41] We have already shown that Pickford's works was installed there to produce some of the first mules made in France, and he was turning out good machines, so 'it would be very disadvantageous to the progress of our industry to displace this expert (artiste)'.

It was represented that the Ministry of the Interior must make up its mind whether it wanted to continue paying the rents and various expenses and make fresh agreements with a new administration which had taken over the Quinze-Vingts. A house within the old hospital had been specifically allotted for comparative trials of Milne's machines with those of Pickford, and to receive other spinning machines which their builders had sent to the Bureau of Commerce for its verdict. But not only were there the administrative threats to the continued use of the Quinze-Vingts as a centre for new industrial technology, the Faubourg Saint Antoine was a very unsettled district of revolutionary Paris, there were serious disturbances in the hospital itself and threats to burn it down, and it was decided to move these machines to a workshop elsewhere in the city. There Brown, the former inspector of manufactures, paid the rent, looked after the machines for which he had given a proper receipt, and was putting them into production on his own account, while he had agreed to put the machines on view to all manufacturers who wished to set up works using similar equipment.

There had been many complaints about the machines the Milnes had made at La Muette, but the old Commerce administrators believed that it was not the machines themselves which constituted the problem, but the lack of skill in the workers of the firms who had bought them, and the Milnes themselves were not as expert at operating as they were at machine-building. But they had now brought English skilled workers to France who set them up as they should be. Their Arkwright-type machinery was better than that of other English makers now in France, as could be seen at the great factory at Orléans, part of which was to be operated by a steam-engine now under construction. But the Chateau of the Muette, like the Quinze-Vingts, was also under threat. Now made part of the *biens nationaux*, the Paris authorities proposed to sell it off, and all the trouble and expense entered into by the old Bureau of Commerce would be thrown away. If machine-makers were to be moved the Minister of the Interior must sort the matter out. Tolozan not only listed these machines in a letter of 1792, but others which were stored in his own office.[42]

A final retrospective memoir from the administrators of the old regime survives from 1793; they stressed their concentration on spinning inventions, but recorded that the policy 'was in continual danger of being abused, and has often been so by the English technicians who always claimed that the machines which they manufactured were more advanced than those known up to that time'. Only comparative trials could settle these claims. The successive British machines arriving in France were described. The jennies were cheap but mainly useful for yarns of 15 to 24 count. The Arkwright machines were very important but it was claimed that many French craftsmen had tried to imitate them in vain, and instances were given. This type of machine produced yarn at great speed, and was capable of yielding high profits. The Milnes were their main introducers in France, but their success had taken time to establish. This was largely, as other witnesses had indicated, because French operators did not understand how to use them: 'they require an infinite degree of precision, both in the way in which they are set up and in the skill with which they are operated'. The mules had then arrived, but none had been as successful as Pickford's, and 90 count was as fine as the French had achieved with his.[43]

It is not unnatural that the state of technical transfer as related by displaced and dispirited officials of the old regime should convey a sense of incompleteness and imperfect success. In fact things were much more active than they suggested. Indeed the Revolutionary and Directory periods saw not the disappearance of British technological input, but the continuance of much that had arrived during the *ancien régime* and even the arrival of more. Of course we cannot account for all British workers in French textiles, but we know of the principal ones, whose names are attached to the major new enterprises using British technology. We have already shown that there were many active during the last decade of the century. This view has been powerfully reinforced in a recent paper by Serge Chassagne.[44] He points out that the new English machines were fully known about at the beginning of the Revolution. Nor were they the monopoly of secretive manufacturers, for examples existed in the display of key technological equipment exhibited in the Hôtel de Mortagne in Paris. The Milnes were already turning out their Arkwright machinery, Pickford was producing mules – the first probably for the Abbé Calonne at Melun in 1788; Spencer was at work for Morgan and Massey at Amiens. The large works of the Duc d'Orléans were already in train. There was however still some feeling that even large enterprises might be unwilling to embark on the costs of importing new foreign technology without some state assistance. But the potential gains from the new machinery were so large that entrepreneurs went ahead, apparently little deterred by the Revolution.

Chassagne cites Boyer-Fonfrède and Albert, with their suborning of English workers, the arrival of the second of the Collier brothers, the activities of James White, who for some time worked with the immigrant Austrian entrepreneur Pobecheim, John Newton Ford who for nine years worked with the English merchant-entrepreneur Rawle at mills near Rouen. In addition Chassagne lists about twenty men involved in Rouen spinning, of whom we have only dealt with Hulse. There were at least six Irish and several Scots, and many of the men married in France, became settled and remained there to their deaths. From the considerable number of textile workers (often described as 'mecaniciens') listed as 'hostages' after 1803, there was clearly an important additional influx during the peace of Amiens, though that period lies outside this study. Chassagne mentions British weavers who introduced new methods in France in the last decade of the century. In addition to fairly well recorded men like McCloude and Balfe, he mentions the recruitment of prisoners of war into French industry. Twenty-four joined a single firm in the Year III, having sworn not to take arms against France again. There are a number of Irish names among weavers, though they had sometimes worked in Lancashire; a number of these are again known to have married in France. We can presume that both Catholicism and the troubled state of Ireland helped these men to find French civilian life more congenial than the British army.

Chassagne points out[45] that while the Revolutionary decade may have slowed down it certainly did not stop the mechanization of the French textile industry, and the mechanization at this period mainly means cotton. There were six works spinning cotton by machinery in 1789, twelve in 1792, twenty-five in 1796 and thirty-seven in 1799, and there was a much increased pace of expansion in the Consulate and early Empire. More serious than the problems of attracting British artisans and transferring their skills were then, he believes, problems in the supply of raw cotton.

One important qualitative issue, however, needs much more examination. How far were the machines built and installed in France the equals of those being built in England? If somewhere near the British state of the art when they were first erected, did they receive improvement and uprating in parallel with their British counterparts during the war years? Could they be operated as fast? Did they require more maintenance? When they came into competition with British factories in 1814, the French found themselves virtually as uncompetitive as they had been under the Eden-Rayneval treaty, and even in 1825 some of the best British engineering judges were convinced that the technological gap was still great, especially in the quality of machine-building.[46] There was little or no notable French invention in cotton textiles; the obtaining of the British inventions did not prove a source of fertile inspiration to French minds.[47]

What sort of career did the British cotton industry immigrants who entered France before 1800 make for themselves? There were some who came to France primarily as technicians but seem to have had some entrepreneurial ability and ended up as owners of cotton-spinning works or textile machinery works or both. The Collier brothers and James White seem to have been in this category, and for a time at least, John Newton Ford. Farrar seems to have been successful and supported by the Government, and closely associated with Bauwens, at least to the Year XI, but was running his own spinning factory at his death in 1815. There were several others who had lengthy careers as foremen or even factory managers without ever breaking into the big time in business. On the other hand some of the technologists in whom the French government had taken a considerable interest, in some cases promising subsidies or purchasing machines or providing premises, did not end their days in prosperity. Garnett's hard times have already been discussed; it is possible that he may have had an exaggerated view of his own expertise. Pickford was certainly a much more important technologist, and the French government seems to have recognized that he had given important services, particularly with the introduction of the mule. He was recommended for government aid as late as the early 1820s, but he was obviously then of no worth to them.

Wood (still referring to his real name of Theakston) wrote to the Government that the Louviers company with which he had been associated since he introduced Arkwright water-powered spinning there in 1784 had dissolved because of current economic difficulties at the beginning of 1800. They had, he claimed, not given him a salary he could live on, but they had advanced him money from time to time for the upkeep of his family. They had the decency to cancel the debts he thus owed them when they wound up their affairs. But this would not keep his family – a wife and five children who were still too young to work, even though he was an elderly father, sixty years of age. He claimed it would be impossible for him to go back to England because of the harsh treatment he would receive as a skilled worker who had taken his technological skills abroad. (This danger of punishment on the return of expatriate workers was really a myth, but it is hard to tell whether emigrants really believed in it themselves.) He asked the French government for an annual pension for his services in transferring technology. His former employers backed him, pointing out that they had been awarded an exclusive privilege which had been made absurd by its also being awarded to others, and, without naming names, mentioned the rewards given to the Milnes. None of their promises to Wood had in fact been fulfilled, but he had, like them, been a victim of an economy vitiated by the assignats and the maximum, and he had lost 24,000 *livres* which the Louviers company had formerly assured him would accrue to him. The 'small pension' he asked for would be a limited reassurance for foreign workers who served French industry.[48]

While the Milnes remained active in the production of Arkwright-type machines until 1793, their production then fell off, largely due to the availability of the mule. John Milne the father died at eighty in the

Year XII, after which their main machine-building operation stopped. He was receiving a pension of 6,000 *livres*, and this was continued by the Imperial government, but it was later reduced to 4,000 *livres* divided between two sons and two daughters. The family enjoyed a respectable apartment in the Hôtel Vaucanson. This did not prevent a mass of memorials to successive governments in which they pressed continued claims. On the whole they seem to have been treated with considerable generosity. James Milne presented a collection of machines to the government competition of the Year X for cotton-spinning machines, but a poor view was taken of various supposed improvements of detail he had made, and he received only an award of 2,000 *livres*, seemingly a compensation prize. He took over as director of the spinning school at the Arts et Métiers, succeeding Ferguson, but with the spread of knowledge of cotton spinning this was in decline and closed in 1814, and he died in 1816. John Milne junior was briefly involved with wool spinning, and continued to develop spinning-machines for various textiles, of which those for spinning silk waste had some success. He died at seventy-three in 1834, but his widow's residence at the Hôtel de Vaucauson on a small pension tells its own tale.

Another son, Thomas Milne, was memorializing the Government in 1806 proposing to introduce the latest English bleaching methods and the spinning of tow waste and cotton mixtures. He was in a poor way financially, for which he blamed unscrupulous business partners, and was trying to support a large family. He received 600 *livres* from the Government, which would not go far among his eleven children. He recounted his arrival in France at the beginning of 1786 which the Government of the time had arranged with his father, and said that Holker had made an agreement with him to set up a cotton-spinning works. As Holker died in April 1786 this must have been one of his last industrial projects.[49] Ballot sums it all up in a few words: 'all the Milnes died poor'.[50] While undoubtedly mainly responsible for the establishment of the water frame in France, and thus the initiation of the factory system in cotton, the impression is that though they had a high opinion of their own inventive capacity, the Milnes' technical ingenuity was not genuinely creative. They seem to have been consistently bad businessmen, and their main period of success was when they were installed in subsidized premises by government, making machines to order at set prices, and with a regular pension.

Foxlow, the Milnes' relative by marriage, had fairly impressive success, buying up in the Year III the mill at Orléans he had previously directed for the Duke of Orléans. However, by the Year VII he was in some difficulty and cut back on his operations. He needed a sizeable government loan in the Year XI and finally went out of business in 1808, when the concern was sold to his chief creditor.[51] Nevertheless, he had during his period of success owned one of the most valuable units in the French cotton industry.[52] He had, it is important to note, an important mercantile operation in Manchester before coming to France. Some other Englishmen who owned and ran very large cotton firms were similarly merchants by origin. One of the most important was Rawle, a merchant who, as we have seen, established himself at Rouen in 1787, and employed two of the most important English mechanics, Ford and Hulse. As late as 1820 his firm was valued at over 250,000 francs, but by this time he had had to renounce his control of it, having endeavoured to keep afloat by moving to wool spinning. In 1806 he was said to have employed around a million francs in setting up two mills, and an appeal he made for a government loan at that time was turned down partly on the chauvinistic grounds that it was inappropriate to give it to an English spinner at a time when many French spinners were in difficulties, and because of the excessive expansion which English entrepreneurs were considered to indulge in without sufficient regard to capital sources and wartime speculation crises. As late as 1811 Rawle employed 1,500 workers.[53]

Sykes, a merchant of Anglo-Dutch origin, born at The Hague in 1743, resident at Paris since 1777, set up an important works at Saint Rémy sur Avre and later obtained permission to build another at Verneuil. He employed William Aitkin, a very important machine builder whose operations fall outside the period of our study, who first arrived in France during the Peace of Amiens. In the early 1790s Sykes was making use of the labour of young paupers under contracts bearing considerable resemblance to English poor law pauper apprentice indentures.[54] In 1811 his Saint Rémy works was valued at 1.5 million francs. Sykes was succeeded in his business first by his son-in-law the English merchant and banker William Waddington, who was naturalized French in 1816 and died a millionaire, and then by his Waddington grandsons, one of whom had been carefully sent over to England to master the 'mechanic and hydraulic arts'.[55] The Waddingtons had a long and solidly based success. While they had their notable failures – and one must remember that years of wartime difficulty, and brief post-war open English competition, destroyed many of the greatest French textile firms – there seems evidence to suggest that the really ambitious

English enterprises in France were generally directed by men of mercantile background, and that few of the Britons who came to France as technical experts moved into the commercial side of the textile industries.

It is perhaps not as generally realized as it might be that just as there was an important British lead in textile-finishing techniques which preceded by at least three or four decades the importation of the first British spinning-machines into France, so there was a distinct, if shorter, British lead in textile printing techniques. This had been complicated by the French prohibition on cloth-printing within the realm, which was lifted first for silk at the beginning of 1759, and for all textiles by October of the same year, so that the production of 'toiles imprimées' could go ahead openly. The term 'indiennage' was often used, showing that here Europeans were engaged in the import substitution of a particularly attractive Indian product.

The English made several advances in the use of dyes and mordants. Lead acetate, probably discovered in England before 1754, was an excellent mordant for madder which produced reds and lilacs, while in the 1730s and 1740s the use of indigo for blues was made effective by using ferrous sulphate as mordant.[56] After 1759 many Swiss, who had been practising textile printing very successfully, moved into France to provide the skill previously lacking because of the prohibition. The most famous was Christophe Oberkampf. In 1769 he sent his brother Frédéric to Mulhouse, to Basle and to other parts of Switzerland on an intelligence gathering and suborning mission, and a main aim was to see how far manufacturers there had managed to copy successfully the 'English blue'. The dominant elder brother told the younger: 'You must see how they make the English blue: try to visit all the works, even the smallest ones.'[57] On the same tour Frédéric was also endeavouring to acquire the copperplates on which some works in Neuchatel were now relying for printing, again a British invention. Said to have been first introduced by Francis Nixon at Dublin, the inventor sold the technique to a printworks at Merton in Surrey in the mid-1750s and other English works were soon using it. There were attempts to keep the method in Britain, but it spread slowly abroad. A London printer, Louis Beauford (a name that suggests a French, possibly Huguenot, origin) took it to France, to Sèvres, in 1763. This was said to have been done 'under the patronage of the French government', and an English worker called Parsons seems to have been the essential skilled operative. Not only could copper printing lead to a range of new elegant and pictorial designs, but the plates could be made much larger than the existing wood blocks (a yard square as compared with under a foot square), so economizing on labour. Manually operated machines were next introduced, first in a works at Wandsworth in 1760, and these seem to have reached France by 1768. When a firm applied to the French government in 1769 to set up copperplate printing in Alsace they wished to do it 'in the English manner'. The method was taken up at Oberkampf's famous Jouy works in 1770.

Unfortunately, we do not have any details of the suborning of Parsons or any of the industrial espionage which may have accompanied these transfers of technology.[58] However, we can get some insights from the papers of Oberkampf, for many years the outstanding French manufacturer. His interest in English blue has been mentioned, and the reports which his brother made on Swiss and Neuchatel users. His brother also reported on machines for copperplate printing, and may have actually bought engraved copperplates, and he recruited a copperplate engraver. The attempts to keep new techniques to themselves can be seen from the Oberkampf contract for six years with three of his existing printers, who were to develop the copper instead of the woodblock method. They were 'not to disclose any information on their proceedings either by word of mouth or in writing, nor to make drawings of machines or parts of machines, nor to pass on drawings or samples, or let anyone come in'.[59]

Oberkampf came to London in part to buy cloths for printing at the East India Company sales, combining this with a little touring and social life. He spent time examining goods for sale in the shops, and even had some cloths printed for him in England which he could not equal himself. Perhaps his accompanying Pourtalès, the great Neuchatel textile printing 'king', helped him,[60] but he was able to observe the English industry at close quarters, visiting, apparently with little hidden from him, important cotton-printing firms in the London area, those of Robert Jones at Oldford on the river Lea in Essex and of John Arbuthnot at Mitcham in Surrey, noting virtually every part of the process, the use of coal- and coke-fuel and even wage rates. He on one occasion had Arbuthnot as a dinner guest. He extended his London visit to look over five other printing works and a finishers, though some of the printers were on holiday.

From his English trip he learned a great deal: 'if I stay away from home, it is to inform myself about many things that I have wanted to know for such a long time'. And again 'my time will not be lost but used profitably ... the ease I have in visiting the manufactures here and the kindness with which I have been received have made me delay my departure'. Oberkampf did not entirely reciprocate the gentility of his reception in England; he suborned an engraver of Swiss origin who had worked at two of the main London works, and who arrived with his family at Jouy in 1774.[61] Through an intermediary he also tried, but unsuccessfully, to get from a Mr Brown a model of a new machine which may have been a predecessor of Bell's famous cylinder-printing invention. He had shown an interest in the possibilities of such a method as early as the 1760s.

Somehow Oberkampf got information on the Bell machine which he passed to the younger Périer brother, Augustin, who produced drawings, and the brothers made a machine for him over 1787–88, but there were serious teething problems with it when it was built, and it was still being struggled with in 1791. Success was achieved about that time, but the riots against spinning-machines persuaded Oberkampf to postpone using cylinder-printing while there was serious unemployment in the calico-printing industry, and he did not use the machinery until 1796.[62] Even when Oberkampf did not himself introduce English technology he was keen to use it, importing English sheet copper until he could persuade Romilly to provide him with an article of comparable quality, purchasing a calender from Holker at Rouen, and buying one of the first consignments of carboys to leave the Holkers' famous sulphuric acid works.[63]

There is seemingly a good deal more to learn, particularly about the way in which French calico-printers, other than Oberkampf, acquired British technologies: his business has been excellently covered. His experience among the London calico-printers in 1773–74 suggests that they were pretty complacent about their technical lead and consequently not fiercely protective of their operations. That he was prepared to suborn men and import machine models is clear. At least we must recognize that calico-printing, like many finishing processes, was a sector of textile technology where there was already a British lead before the French acquisition of machine spinning later in the century.

PART SIX

French Espionage in Eighteenth-Century Britain: an Appraisal

17 A Case Study in Espionage: Eccentric and Engineer – an Industrial Spy of the 1780s

Espionage is a trade which notoriously attracts practitioners who are not of a common mould, and this was as true of the eighteenth century as it is of the twentieth. The engineer Le Turc was not a man who fitted into norms or had much patience with the regular, the commonplace or the humdrum. He had little money sense; he was no businessman; he read the details of contracts he entered into through a visual filter which permitted him only to absorb the clauses which were favourable to him. He confessed an 'inconstancy' which prevented him following up most favourable career opportunities with a sensible steadiness. If there was a man so constituted as to arouse antipathies in bureaucrats, it was he. Over the last three decades of the eighteenth century, and under both the *ancien régime* and the Revolution, he antagonized important ministers, influential officials, enlightened intellectuals, celebrated scientists, many of whom could have been, and some of whom tried to be, his patrons and protectors. Certainly towards the end of his life his hold on reality had become tenuous and erratic, and he could probably be defined as paranoid.

Why then give any historical attention to a man with these deficiencies? Because there were compensatory qualities. He clearly had engineering ability, which he exercised with some success in the earlier part of his life. In some important observations he showed that he appreciated very clearly and very fully the value of the practical mechanic and the skilled operative, and their indispensability in the mounting of new industrial projects. His critical views of the opinions of the contemporary scientific establishment on industrial matters were sometimes well founded. Like others he found his industrial schemes susceptible to the vagaries of ministries which had a limited understanding of their economic potential or the problems of teaching the skills involved. The fall of administrations affected Le Turc as it did others seeking government favour and finance; his schemes risked losing support which could only be regained by renewed and lengthy lobbying.

In his attempts to achieve the transfer of technologies from Britain his fortunes were mixed. His greatest triumph was in a field which had a military application, and here he seems to have identified the technicians, materials and equipment needed with remarkable accuracy, ensuring a transfer of technology of almost unexampled smoothness. Had he been content to continue his oversight of the extension of that technology, he might have lived in the high regard of both the old and the Revolutionary regimes and died in affluence. As an industrial spy seeking new civilian technologies in Britain he was given an astonishingly wide remit, and this does not seem to be caused simply by his own overambition, but the requests of his government. Before his final departure from England in 1787 Le Turc sent a mass of specimens of English consumer goods and a large number of models and drawings of machines to France. If those which were eventually lodged in the Conservatoire des Arts et Métiers had survived we could make a more critical judgement of what he thought important, but only two or three drawings and a couple of stocking frame parts remain. However, his opinions on British industry, industrialists and workers were often penetrating, and he had a deep sense that what was happening in England was quite exceptional and unprecedented and of long-term consequence for other countries.

Le Turc's early career and background is only sketchily covered; unbearably prolix about many things, he was reticent about his activities before the mid-1770s. Even his forenames (Bonaventure Joseph) do not appear on his many letters and memoranda of explanation, justification and complaint that constitute thick dossiers in the Bureau of Commerce, the Marine and the Conservatoire des Arts et Métiers, though the last institution fortunately recorded them.

Le Turc was born at Lille in 1748, and said he began his engineering studies under the director of fortifications for Flanders. Then he was attached to the Ponts et Chaussées administration in some way, and

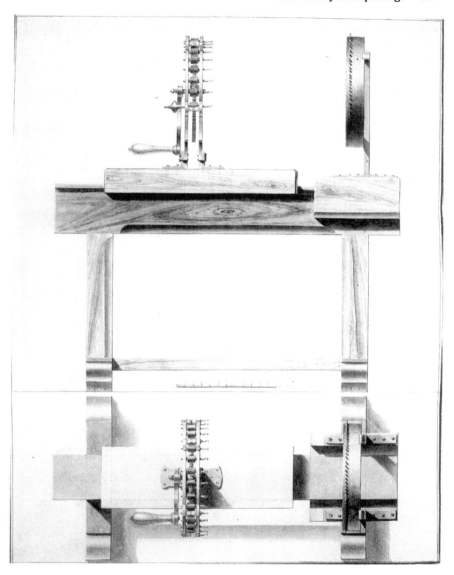

17.1 Design by Le Turc of a machine to manufacture small cords: side elevation and (below scale) viewed from above

claimed to have been involved in important public building projects of the time, including the building of the bridge of Neuilly by Perronet.[1] Certainly he later published pamphlets in England about Perronet's

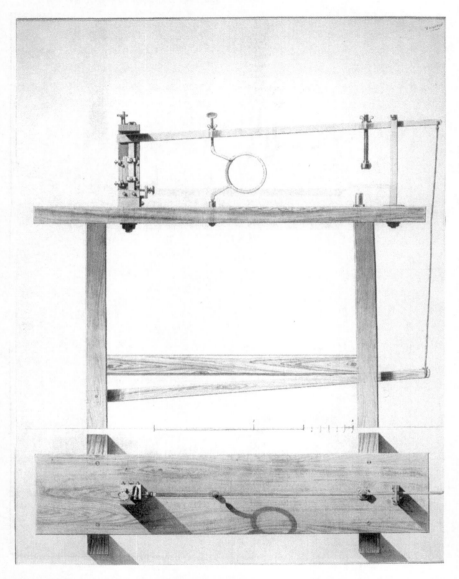

17.2   Design by Le Turc of a machine to make the eyes of needles for use in the
       stocking trade: side elevation and (below scale) viewed from above

methods.[2] Subsequently he was for seven years a professor of fortifications at the royal military school, receiving a small pension when the
establishment was closed. His connections were clearly good, for he

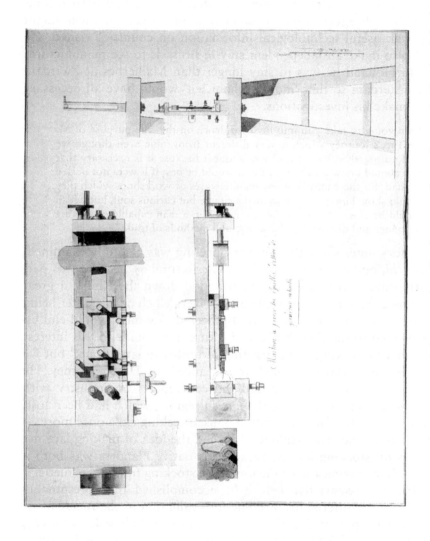

17.3 Design by Le Turc of a machine to make the eyes of needles for use in the stocking trade: details of the design in various elevations and (right) the machine viewed from either end

shortly afterwards (July–November 1776) went to Holland as travelling companion to Malherbes, who found him intelligent, but irresponsible with money.

Malherbes made clear to Vergennes that Le Turc had been recommended by colleagues at the Academy of Sciences as a man who might bring back useful technological information on countries visited. He was also to make an independent stay in Brussels to see manufactures there. In Holland he was to stay longer than Malherbes at Zaardam near Amsterdam so that 'mon mechanicien' would have all necessary time to make his investigations.

> I am going to take you into my confidence on the true purpose of M. Le Turc's journey which is very different from mine even though we will go together. I have told you about it because it is necessary that you should know all about it. But it would be best if it were not noised abroad, for there may be many manufactures or workshops which they would show him if he only seemed a simple but curious soul, but which would be closed to him if they thought him a man capable of making drawings and discovering the secrets and methods of trades.

Malherbes's notes show that civil engineering was carefully examined, as were shipbuilding practices. From later testimony Le Turc was particularly interested in the floating of wood down the Rhine, a great deal coming from the French side of the river. Much of this, after being sawn by a multitude of Dutch wind-powered saw mills would end up by being sold to the French Navy.[3] Le Turc does allude to this interest in the floating, sawing and marketing of timber in later years,[4] but we cannot be sure who sponsored and financed his Dutch journey. He later claimed that he had lodged thirteen reports on industry with government administrators of the *ancien régime*, which had been lost. After his return Le Turc soon found himself seeking exile once more.

He claimed that from childhood he had the idea of making lace net materials on stocking looms, because his native Flanders was both a centre of lace making and of the use of the stocking frame, the 'metier à bas'. He was twenty-five before he accomplished this, presumably about 1773. He offered his machine for evaluation to the Academy of Sciences, who appointed distinguished assessors including de Montigny, Vandermonde and Vaucanson. Here we encounter some of Le Turc's great enmities, perennially pursued; in this case towards Vandermonde. He claimed that Vandermonde had to agree with the approving report of the other commissioners, and to abandon his former support for another inventor of a similar device. Vaucanson being so friendly and supportive to Le Turc increased Vandermonde's discomfiture. According to Le Turc, Vandermonde, a member of the circle of the Duc de Chartres (the later Philippe Egalité) assured the duke that there was much money to be made from the invention, but that Le Turc was 'un homme bizare', impossible to deal with, and that he could have a similar machine made for the duke. While Turgot as controller-general, having himself seen the machine, was awarding Le Turc a subvention and enabling him to set up a works at Vincennes, Vandermonde and the Chartres party were plotting against him. Le Turc became vulnerable because Turgot fell from power at a crucial moment, and though Turgot recommended the venture to his successor, Fourqueux, his tenure of office was very short. The duke sent an engineer in his service together with another member of his circle to view Le Turc's machine. They pretended to want to invest in it, though their true purpose was to give Vandermonde detail of the machine which he had not gained from his original official examination. Though he recruited workers who Le Turc had employed, Vandermonde still did not succeed. According to Le Turc he got one of his workmen, Bidot, to sue him for 40,000 *livres* for unpaid bills, so that the critical parts of the machine could be seized for non-payment. Le Turc believed the influence of the 'prince' (Duc de Chartres) dragged the case to the higher courts. Though the damages were only assessed at 1,200 *livres*, Le Turc claimed that he had lost 30,000 *livres* in previous legal expenses, and had to flee France, threatened with the Bastille. However, the workman Bidot seems to have been skilled and important, and was probably working on commission, not as an employee.[5]

While in Holland with Malherbes, Le Turc claimed his attention was diverted from pursuit of his own inventions to the idea of bringing advanced foreign technology to France: 'I stifled within me the natural inclination I had to invent; thenceforward I had conceived the plan of getting hold of those inventions, which experience had shown to be worthwhile with a view to introducing them in France'. Despite Malherbes's intervention with the prince on their return Le Turc decided that he would either have to give in to him or flee France again. Le Turc's account of the next episodes reads unconvincingly. There was some flirtation with American backers who would accompany him first to London, and then to Philadelphia. Eventually Le Turc arrived penniless in London after first wrecking his machine, which the Orléanist group had tried to impound, and selling up all his property. Once in Britain there were soon complex discussions with De Noailles, the French ambassador, about arranging his safe return to France, providing he immediately abandoned his profession as engineer in England. Le Turc failed to prepare papers they asked for before the embassy left in 1778 at the beginning of the war, and he remained in England until 1783. Meanwhile the Portuguese scientist, Magellan (whom we have met with as an important intermediary in French attempts to secure the Boulton and Watt engine) had tried to join with Le Turc in a venture to launch his lace net machine in England. Warned by a friend that Magellan wanted the machine on behalf of the Vandermonde/Chartres group, Le Turc quickly dismantled one newly erected at Magellan's house, and the onset of war ended this venture. Le Turc then made another machine, but its use was delayed by the industrial espionage activities he became involved in during the mid-1780s.[6]

Around 1780 Le Turc, keeping himself alive by doing hackwork for architects and cartographers, seems to have intended to stay in England. He sought attention by publishing pamphlets in London, one of which advocated building fortifications in England against foreign invasion![7] For five years he pursued various petty commissions in order to support himself. He became more prosperous after devising some improvement in the manufacture of women's hats, and travelled about England a great deal, visiting many towns.

By the middle of 1785 Le Turc proposed to smuggle out an English stocking loom of a type not yet used in France, probably for the ribbed stockings developed by Jedediah Strutt. This was quickly known to Desmarets, the French inspector of manufactures concerned with stocking looms, who called Le Turc 'very intelligent in the knowledge of machines and particularly those of stocking looms'. Desmarets believed that once Le Turc had brought out the frame it would be taken to Spain by the Spaniard Izquierdo 'to enrich Spanish industry with this machine'. Le Turc would be in danger in England once it was known he was shipping machines to France, so Desmarets urged Tolozan, the head of the Bureau of Commerce, and his chief *commis*, Valioud, to negotiate with Le Turc at once. It would be much cheaper to get him to send over machines direct on government account than to pay others to try to copy them in France, and one would have them 'in the state of perfection to which long use has brought them in England'. This was quickly arranged and by early July Le Turc was commissioned to send over English cloth, woollen and patented silk stockings, and a few stocking looms capable of making clothes according to certain samples. There are references to warp looms and velvet looms. There was also a request for the latest patterns of English earthenware.[8]

By 20 July 1785 Le Turc was writing to Tolozan, to set out his career before and during his British exile, and the reasons for it; naturally there might be doubts of the patriotism of one who had spent the war years in England. At the end of his letter Le Turc requested Tolozan's protection, so that he could 'contribute his feeble talents to the prosperity of the manufactures of his own country' – that is embark on industrial espionage on its behalf.[9]

Next month Le Turc was back in England, he travelled to the framework knitting districts round Derby and Nottingham and then to Manchester and Glasgow. He had already set up a stocking loom he had acquired, no doubt to see that it was complete and workable, before sending it to Tolozan, and he was working on another three: if the necessary money arrived he expected to finish the task in October. Meanwhile he sent boxes of goods to Tolozan via a Dunkirk merchant. Le Turc was alert to possibilities of obtaining military technology, as well as civil, and endeavoured to bring the projects of a Captain Whittle for ship design and incendiary shot to the notice of the French navy. They were not interested, but this correspondence may have alerted the navy minister, De Castries, to Le Turc's existence as a spy in England, with important consequences. Already some coded correspondence was being carried on.[10]

The number of looms Le Turc was to send over was increased to five and a sum of 10,000 *livres* was agreed by the Government. By mid-October Le Turc was back in Paris, claiming that he had secured nine stocking looms which could make new products, together with two workers. During his brief stay he was probably negotiating with other prospective companies as he visited various towns in Normandy, including Louviers, where the industrialist Le Camus de Limare, whom we have already met in the contexts of coppering ships and of machine spinning, thought of entering the framework knitting business.[11]

At the beginning of 1786, a year of considerable success for him, Le Turc was very active in London. He sent a short report on English cast steel which he had been asked for. While marginally more accurate than some of the information which had reached France, Le Turc's report was still misleading.[12] There was a heavy shipment of marked boxes to Dunkirk, about the safe arrival of which Le Turc was quite agitated.[13] Framework looms featured prominently and other machines included were probably the attachments which were being developed to produce new patterns of work on existing frames. But a very large number of other goods and models of machines was shipped. The models included one of a whip-making machine in which Le Turc maintained a lasting interest, one of a machine for cleaning wool and raw cotton, others of a spinning-machine, of a machine for making screws for presses, and of a library ladder, possibly of his own invention. But there were many other items, which must have been intended as samples of English products, women's stockings of different qualities, steel watch chains, scissors, buckles. There was a mass of pottery, of every possible kind; some of it Wedgwood. Pottery was used to cover up other items of a more secret nature in the boxes. One box contained English goods which were said to be under patent, an amazing collection, with locks, watch pinions, taps, and shoe black amongst them, and a similar collection of 'other items I do not think they make in France', chiefly particular varieties of fairly common goods. Finally there were a few personal items, like two pairs of shoes for Tolozan! The patented goods were apparently sent to prove some argument which Le Turc was making in a memoir.[14]

He believed that when he had sent another frame and related mechanisms his commitments to the French government would be complete. But workers were needed to operate five types of knitwear machines for different types of cloth. One man already secured could work those for velvet, ribbed and net articles, but it was not likely that one worker could make all the goods 'in a country where labour is so subdivided'. Le Turc realized that he would have to go back to the hosiery districts to find the necessary men. On one commission he could not proceed without more funds. Gun locks could not be bought without buying the guns themselves, and the plainest ones were very expensive.[15]

The most troublesome commission was that from the Spaniard Izquierdo, whose activities in technological transfer we have already mentioned in connection with the coppering of ships and the steam-engine. Here he was ostensibly acting on behalf of the French Rocheguyon company. Le Turc seems to have bought up all the tools and equipment of a framework knitting firm, but could not get final payment from the Spaniard, and was thus left very exposed, having on his hands goods which it was illegal to export but without the funds to get them away. Some care was taken to protect Le Turc in his correspondence with France. It was agreed that his name should not be used in letters sent to him, and that Barthélémy, the chargé d'affaires at the London embassy, should act as postman. Le Turc signed letters 'No. 64', the number of his house in Berwick Street, Soho, a fairly transparent piece of coding. The letter sent to 'M. Le Turc dit Johnson' in early February seems the very nadir of security, but perhaps it had got as far as London in the diplomatic mail. The letters Izquierdo sent were so badly addressed that one was only retrieved by luck from undelivered mail in the post office.[16] Le Turc insisted that it was necessary to send good operatives with machines. He was trying to send two framework knitters over on government account and two on Izquierdo's, but delays in funding meant that he had to house workers himself at his own expense for long periods, while one he had carefully recruited ran away. Money was needed to send off the remaining workers, and especially that 'I should have nothing in my hands which could prove any misdemeanour' as the disappearance of the workers to France might 'make much noise'.[17]

In what he hoped to be his last weeks in England Le Turc made hurried comments or suggestions about a variety of schemes for the recruitment of technologists for France. A skilled cotton-worker had approached the French embassy with the idea of going to France, and Le Turc thought him capable of directing a large cottonworks, but he would need substantial travel expenses and money for the agents who would arrange his passage, and very good wages once he had reached France. Le Turc was also in touch with one of Matthew Boulton's steam-engine erectors. He realized that Boulton was displeased with his former French collaborator Périer who had obtained the plans of the double acting engine by industrial espionage. Le Turc thought that the engine erector would be valuable to have as an expert in cast and wrought iron, as iron was increasingly used in large industrial works. Nothing seems to have come of either of these suggested enticements.[18]

Izquierdo's delays in sending him money put his operations in peril: 'Nothing can express to you the continual danger which the delay of M. Izquierdo puts me in; never in my life have I taken on anything of such a nature, without him ... it would have been impossible that the slightest suspicion should have existed'. Izquierdo had left Paris for Madrid, and Le Turc did not know who would receive the workmen who were being sent over on the Spaniard's account, or the twenty-five chests which were to be dispatched to him. He looked for Tolozan's support if there was chicanery from Izquierdo, and was sending the minister two workers on government account. Le Turc was already beginning to consider what was to be done with the workers, their lodging and working premises. Herein was the germ of the Quinze-Vingts scheme which was eventually to bring him torment and ruin.[19]

Within a few days another knitting frame was being dispatched, and Le Turc was hoping for funds to send over the worker to operate it, and by late March 1786 four other frames were on their way, together with the tools belonging to one of the workmen. Tolozan and Le Turc were greatly concerned to make sure that there was no opening by French customs officers of the boxes Le Turc sent over. This was taken so seriously that the controller-general himself was asked to sign the relevant orders and the boxes were only to be opened in the presence of the Intendants of Commerce after Le Turc's return. Some English luxury goods whose entry was normally prohibited were probably included in these consignments for Tolozan and his friends, though they promised to declare them to the controller-general.[20]

The end of March was frenetic. Le Turc made a trip to Nottingham on the 25th to secure a workman who could make some new fashionable items on one of the looms, a large number of miscellaneous English goods were being bought in London to be taken over to France, and Le Turc was being pestered to add others, like indelible marking ink, flannel, and even chamber-pots. Three workers were successfully sent over the Channel while a fourth ran away at the very last moment. The latter was particularly valuable for fashionable goods, but Le Turc was greatly relieved that he had not persuaded the others to leave 'which could have happened in this land of liberty in 5 minutes', and he sent them off at once to a M. Angelo, 'vice-director of the cabinet of the King of Spain', at Izquierdo's Paris house. Only two of them were for Izquierdo, the other for the Government. One of the workers presents a mystery. He was French, but had been recruited in England, and was very well acquainted with the machines. 'If any accident happens to me' wrote Le Turc, he [Rhambolt] was the one who could set production going without his help. It was presumably the man for whom Le Turc enclosed a letter at the end of the month: 'I present him to you without exaggeration as one of the best workmen of Paris'. But he was at times wrongheaded and hasty and 'has the fault of knowing more about things than those who employ him'. Interestingly, in the traditional accounts of the English framework knitting machinery at this period, it is Rhambolt who is credited with the taking of several machines to France, and Le Turc's part in acquiring, testing, dismantling and shipping the machines was unknown to these writers.[21]

By mid-April Le Turc was back in Paris, and protesting that Izquierdo was exaggerating his own services to the Rocheguyon Company. He was claiming that it was he who had discovered the importance of the loom for ribbed work, when it was Le Turc who had first demonstrated to him the machine, previously unknown in France, on his 1785 visit.

Izquierdo had purchased it and ordered twelve more of the same kind. The other new varieties of loom had nothing to do with the Spaniard, they had been obtained by Desmarets's influence and by Le Turc's use of the funds the French government provided for industrial espionage. Izquierdo had now his original four shares increased to five, and had been made Director of the Rocheguyon Company, while Le Turc had been given a single share, and the Spaniard was getting a free hand to send looms of several different types to Spain. He had also secured for the company the skilled worker named Thomas, who had been sent over at government expense; he was essential for erecting those machines which had been separately brought over on government account.[22]

There followed a rather complex correspondence in which the company tried to get from the Bureau of Commerce a machine of Le Turc's to which they laid claim. They rather brazenly undertook only temporarily to lend Thomas to the Bureau of Commerce for the setting up and trial of one of the Government's machines, and this drew a rather chilly reply from the Bureau. The company was in fact giving up its plans to operate at Rocheguyon and was moving to Popincourt in the Paris outskirts.[23] Le Turc weighed in with the argument that having spent so much money to acquire the English technology, it would be ill advised for the Government to confine it to a single French firm. He proposed that he should be entitled to a version of each of the machines he had brought over so as to set up a machine-building enterprise of his own which would supply such other firms as the Government authorized to enter the hosiery business. He would give up his share in the original company from which he deserved thanks but had only had criticism.

Le Turc vacillated about his desire to return to France. In late May he wrote about wide public knowledge of his operation in England 'which by rights should have been conducted in secret and with caution, I hope you understand Sir, how necessary it is for me to leave at once, so as to take precautions not to be surprised'. Yet Le Turc was still talking of other possible English industrial processes he might obtain, some of which the Bureau rejected; they pointed out that silver plating was already known (these would be the methods introduced by Michael Alcock to produce Sheffield plate in the 1750s) and carpet looms were not needed. Among the other processes and workers Le Turc believed he could get were a loom for horsehair cloth, workmen and equipment for lead shot manufacture, buckle chape makers, a loom to make large gauze shawls with the appropriate workman, and workmen for demonstrating the making of shirt buttons, which could be produced in charity hospitals in France. All this would cost 30,000 *livres*. In the end only the horsehair loom and the buckle chapes interested the Bureau.[24]

Already Le Turc was pressing for accommodation in the former hospital of the Quinze-Vingts charity in Paris, now being used to give subsidized accommodation to the promoters of new industrial processes. He did not want to become an industrial manager 'to put myself in charge of the production of any of these goods and provide close supervision' or to accept any permanent post which might distract him from his real purpose, which was to 'make a gift to my country of such foreign industry as it is in my power to supply it with'. He only wanted to work the imported processes at the Quinze-Vingts until well-capitalized firms could buy his looms, tools and trained workmen, in which firms he would be given a small interest. Once financially secure he would cheerfully resume industrial espionage, and go to England or any other country the administration wished. In this he would no longer be tied to the capricious wishes of any individual (presumably he was thinking of Izquierdo), or to premature disclosure of his operations; only the Government would know of them and 'I would avoid for good this exchange of letters so dangerous when individuals are ready to sacrifice me to their personal interests'.[25]

Le Turc tried to agree the money owed him by the Government before returning to France; there was the cost of the pottery which he had used to cover up the goods in the boxes he had sent over, and the payments for the goods bought in London with a view to their eventual imitation in France. Some items sent over were intended by Le Turc for his own schemes and paid for by him, others were intended by the Bureau of Commerce as industrial exhibits to be displayed in the Hôtel de Mortagne; for these Le Turc was yet to be paid.[26]

Le Turc's efforts to gain suitable accommodation at the Quinze-Vingts for his industrial production and research and for his family were distracted and postponed by the most important commission he received from the Government. This was not from the Bureau of Commerce but from the Marine, and from the Maréchal de Castries as its Minister. In effect Le Turc fulfilled it with astonishing success. Paradoxically, partly by his own fault and partly accidentally, it proved a source of lasting trouble to him, and was an important cause of his later mental unbalance. Initially there was an atmosphere of the self-

interest and intrigue so prevalent in public life at the end of the old
regime. The Rocheguyon Company, no doubt to retain Le Turc's services in the equipping of their enterprise, for which he was supposed to
supply two more frames, tried to ruin his relations with Castries by
claiming that he was about to abscond to Spain, a story all the more
cynical in that a member of their company, Izquierdo, had tried to get
Le Turc to do exactly that.[27]

The industrial espionage that Castries asked Le Turc to undertake
was very important. It constituted the third of the French navy's ambitious efforts to obtain new and outstandingly successful technologies
possessed by the British navy. The first had been the attempts to obtain
the means of manufacturing coke-iron, solid-bored cannon and had
involved the creation of the Indret and then the Le Creusot works. The
second was the attempt to secure the successful technology for copper-
sheathing ships and had involved the creation of the works at Romilly;[28]
the third scheme was to install machinery to make superior standard
blocks and pulleys at Lorient.

The improvements in pulley blocks came from the Taylor family of
Southampton, who experimented with new methods of producing them,
achieved considerable success by the late 1750s, and became long-term
contractors to the navy. They made efficient blocks half the size of
those formerly used. This was an important economy when a 74-gun
warship used around 1,000. The British navy bought 100,000 a year
*c.*1800. A great advantage was the reduced friction of the Taylors'
pulley blocks involving lignum vitae pulleys revolving on carefully
turned iron pins, with flanged bushes (or 'coaks') of antifriction metal,
which were replaceable, but were guaranteed for seven years. The
Taylors greatly improved speed and exactness of production by a range
of machine tools: wooden mandrel lathes for the pulleys, which could
be powered by horse mill or by water; boring machines which themselves used ropes and pulleys to advance the pulleys which were under
manufacture so that straight and accurate pinholes could be bored, and
which also produced starting-holes for morticing; and mechanical reciprocating saws with screws and stops to ensure accurate cutting of
both the pulleys and the assemblies or 'shells' within which they were
mounted. Much was covered by a patent taken by Walter Taylor II's
widow in 1762, but by the early 1780s Walter Taylor III used circular
saws to shape the shells and for morticing, and by 1786 had taken
out a patent for metal bushes which provided internal grooves for
greasing. While the famous Bentham-Brunel-Maudslay development of

block-making machinery at Portsmouth from 1805 marked further advances in organization, design, rigid all-metal construction and more specialized machines, the first great impetus had come from the Taylors. It was their high prices which provoked the navy into sponsoring the later innovations.[29]

The French navy quickly appreciated the importance of the improved technology. Early in 1778 it was stated that the Minister had long been aware of the superiority of English pulleys of recent invention over French ones, and it was proposed to buy from the Taylors a complete set of pulleys for a frigate of twenty-six guns.[30] From 1775 there had been long negotiations with an Englishman called Cole, an English ships' pump maker, who claimed to be able to make the Taylor-type pulleys. The intermediary in the negotiations, a M. de Rosily, a French naval lieutenant who had lived in London, said that the Taylors had spent 30,000 *livres* to establish their invention, and had since made 400,000 *livres*. It was proposed that Cole set up works for pulleys and pumps in the three main French naval arsenals. The pulleys might be more expensive than the French but they would last longer and wear the cordage less. Cole came over to France more than once, and ran up considerable expenses. He seems to have been able to send machinery parts and material through English customs without problem.

Cole's pulleys seem to have been relatively heavy, and not usable for all purposes. His processes were not cheap. He wanted a gratification of 72,000 *livres* and the employment of his nephew at a salary of 5,000 *livres*. There were worries that such a salary would upset French heads of naval workshops with salaries of only 800 or 1,000 *livres*, while security also had to be considered. 'It would not be sensible to station an Englishman in the port of Brest.' Cole's services were considered at the highest level – he was presented to the controller-general and Trudaine de Montigny, the head of the Bureau of Commerce. It is not certain why the scheme was abandoned, but the fall of an administration, that of Turgot, may explain why it faded out in the late spring of 1776.[31] After 1778 the Taylor technology would be hard to get because of the war, but the French navy did not lose sight of it. A memoir of October 1781 rehearsed the merits of the Taylor system, the pulleys being handier, the manoeuvring of ships easier, and one-third fewer men being needed to handle the blocks, which were far more solid and lasting. The phenomenon of interchangeable parts had arrived, each piece of a block 'can be fitted indifferently in place of all the others and replace those which break'.[32] Once Cole had gone back to England those ever-wakeful opportunists, the Périer brothers, stepped in to offer their services. They claimed to have built the necessary machines for Taylor's pulleys, but only furnished the minister with a model. The perfect success they claimed was clearly exaggerated, despite their boast of a high degree of mechanization. In 1781 they were forlornly pleading for the 12,000 *livres* they had spent without the navy giving them any orders.[33]

Le Turc was at Lorient in June 1786, showing that the Marine had already decided where the new pulley-making should be installed. The interest in the Taylor processes was intense. Two different private firms approached Le Turc about the establishment of pulley works in France. Though both companies asked Castries for his consent, he decided to deal only with Le Turc and use him to set up a government works. According to Le Turc the companies then submitted memoirs attacking him, and they also threatened to betray him to the British government. He also received anonymous letters threatening his life once he reached England.[34]

After surmounting problems in London Le Turc obtained some of Taylor's workmen 'without whom the machines themselves would be quite useless'; by 22 August he reached Calais with them and with models of the machinery. The men were amenable enough, but had discovered the joys of wine, and were drinking fifteen bottles a day – from later evidence we know there were only three of them! Le Turc wanted to get the work at Lorient done quickly and to get back to London, and he was able to report rapid progress by the end of the month. By October Castries told the Lorient authorities 'The King's intention is that the new pulley manufacture entrusted to Le Turc should be set up as quickly as can be', old store buildings should be given over to the works, the machines Le Turc required should be bought, and Castries virtually gave the port officials a blank cheque 'to hasten the time when the premises can be put in a state of activity'. Wood required was diverted to Lorient, money Le Turc expended was refunded at once, and advance payment for other expenses approved.[35]

By April 1787 Le Turc had achieved complete success, and sent Castries a careful general account of the production process with drawings. Castries obtained a bonus of 1,000 *livres* for him, payable at once over and above his salary; such a mark of satisfaction he judged good for the service. He hinted at a further rise in salary. Of the English workers, the foreman Rose had received £40 gratuity on arrival in France, and was due a similar amount at the completion of the works; the other two, Dyatt the pulley-maker and Lichfield [Lichfould] the founder received £20 each. To generate a spirit of emulation Le Turc asked favours for French craftsmen and officials who had been valuable to him.

The strongest indication of Le Turc's success was the immediate demand that Taylor-type workshops should be set up at Brest and Toulon. His achievement, rapid, complete and seemingly devoid of the lengthy teething troubles that might have been expected, was in fact a source of Le Turc's future problems. To the navy, the priority was the setting up of more 'pouleries' in other ports, and as Le Turc had been the key figure at Lorient, they wanted him on the spot when the other ports installed the Taylor process. To Le Turc the priority was to set up in Paris a kind of research and development centre, or more precisely a technology transfer centre, where English machines would be erected, viewed and copied for French firms. In this project he believed with an intense and missionary zeal. Anything which diverted him from it was anathema. On the personal front, too, he realized that it was important to close his London house, as there was the danger that the contents might be seized if his espionage activities were realized. But the navy was not greatly concerned with this side of Le Turc's work. To them what we would now call defence industries were all-important.

In May Castries was ordering the ports of Brest, Toulon and Rochefort, Saint Malo and Nantes to each send intelligent young pulley-makers to be trained at Lorient under Le Turc, and apprentices as well; they must be taught 'how to use English tools'. Le Turc's indispensability was emphasized by a collapse of discipline and the production of spoilt pulleys at a time in June when he was away from Lorient dealing with the Bureau of Commerce. Nevertheless the navy would allow Le Turc to go over to England once the *Léopard*, building at Brest, was furnished with pulleys. But they were clear that Le Turc was to remain in their employ, he was simply to have three months' paid leave.[36]

Le Turc spent much of the summer of 1787 in England, selling off the contents of a well-furnished house, though he claimed that much had been sold off by his servants in his absence. He sent more boxes of goods over to France including machines, models and designs for the additional naval pulley manufactures. One box was not dispatched before he left, and Barthélémy at the French embassy dealt with it. This probably contained the cardinal item of circular saws for the Taylor process. Just before he left, Le Turc believed that he was in danger of being betrayed to the British authorities by a fellow Frenchman.[37]

On his return Le Turc proposed that the cheapest way of setting up the Brest and Toulon works would be to use the Lorient works to make the tools and the most demanding machine parts for the other ports. But once the pulley manufacture was set going there it would be necessary to get 'a good edge-tool maker and an excellent turner in iron' to maintain the machines. So he would recruit workers in these trades in Paris to work with the Englishman Rose in the machine building, and then send them on to the other ports. If in future 'one wished to create a workshop for tools of all kinds useful to the Navy, by subdividing the labour, as is the practice of the English, the only way of doing the job well and doing it cheaply', there would be a facility in place, and these arrangements would avoid the need for English workers at Brest and Toulon. In the end Le Turc discovered that he could not find in Paris workers as specialized as those in England, and hired less specialized ones. He remarked on the paradox that in Paris, with highly regulated guilds, master workmen ranged over a wider technical territory than they did in England where there was complete freedom but a more developed division of skill and labour.

In the late autumn of 1787 Le Turc thanked Castries for his protection and promised every effort in the equipping of Brest and Toulon with the Taylor system. The Government was still pleased with him, bonuses he recommended were to be paid to Lorient workers, and a particularly able trainee there was being recommended to head the Toulon works. Le Turc had apparently put in a strong appeal about the dangers he had run in his English espionage and the heavy financial losses which he incurred in his London establishment, and he was to have his salary raised to 7,200 *livres* a year and have a special gratuity of 2,000 *livres* with the king's direct approval. 'I have put your situation before the King and the claims which you have on his favour' wrote Montmorin. 'His majesty wishing to reward your zeal in his service has been willing to grant you the increase in your stipend and the bonus you have requested.'[38]

Direct evidence about the pulley-block operations dies away during the winter of 1787–88; Le Turc claimed in December that after his absences in England to close his house and in Paris to recruit metalworkers, the Lorient works was still running smoothly. With proper support from the administration lignum vitae could replace copper pulleys with savings in weight and cost. By the end of 1787 the Lorient workshop had completed the machinery for Toulon and it was being sent to that port.[39] But as early as February 1788 Le Turc was showing signs of boredom and impatience. He did not like French provincial life and was strongly minded to go to America. He claimed that he was no longer needed by the navy, and his real passion was for the works in Paris where he could install the English equipment he had brought across the Channel. A subordinate official could replace him at naval workshops.[40]

The navy did not think Le Turc was so readily dispensable. Castries, with whom he seems to have had very good relations, had retired and La Luzerne who had replaced him soon deplored the fall off in the quality of pulleys that Lorient was sending to Rochefort. He believed that Le Turc's absence was the problem, and he would require him to go as quickly as possible to Lorient 'to watch over [everything] and direct the whole of the establishment which we owe to him. When this artist arrives at the Port [the treasurer] will pay him the wages due him'. But Le Turc had gone, never to return, and the fury of the naval administrators can be understood. Le Turc believed that they continued to plot against him down the years, and that Monge was later as hostile as La Luzerne had been. He, in turn, took great pains to denounce them as impractical savants who had ruined a navy built up by better men. It must have been particularly galling to the navy when the ambassadors of Tippoo Sultan visited Lorient later in 1788 and wanted skilled workers to go to India to set up pulley-block manufacture, only to be told there were not enough trained men yet for French purposes.[41]

Having quit the marine service without permission Le Turc was now involved with three other issues. One was the knitting frames he had sent over. There were tangles with Izquierdo and the Popincourt Company, and with powerful members of the administration concerning machines and workmen he had sent to France on government account. Another was his negotiations with the Government about a subvention and the lease of premises in the Quinze-Vingts in Paris. The third was an ambitious scheme of 1788 to send Le Turc over to Britain to secure the latest methods of cotton spinning.

Izquierdo having obtained one stocking frame for Spain had been the principal mover with aristocratic or wealthy partners (including the Duc de Rochefaucauld, the Duchesse d'Anville and the financier Lecouteulx), in what we have shown was first the Rocheguyon Company in Normandy, and later the Popincourt Company in Paris. Their original idea had been to get thirty frames for ribbed work from

England, and they later formed the plan of getting Le Turc to make them a hundred more in France.[42]

We have seen that Le Turc obtained the thirty looms for them. It is not possible to follow in detail all the dealings of Le Turc with the Rocheguyon and Popincourt companies; in any case there are many lacunae in the documents. Certainly after a heavy expenditure of over 60,000 *livres*, the implementation of the Eden Treaty was regarded as a fatal blow by the middle of 1787. Early in 1788 the Government was trying to secure the machines of the failing firm, fearing their export to Spain. Le Turc was making desperate efforts to get back his correspondence with Izquierdo which he had sent to officials of the company in order to justify himself and explain his quarrels with the Spaniard. He also wanted the letters back because they dealt with his industrial espionage in Britain and could be used to betray him to the British government.[43]

Le Turc's anxiety is explained because at the end of the year he was on the verge of a major contract with the Government for a spying trip to England to obtain three kinds of spinning-machines. On this a memoir of his survives, but it does not make it entirely clear which machines were to be sought. That for muslin production must be the mule, that for knitwear yarn is presumably the water frame. His demands, successively agreed by Lambert and by Necker, included his secondment to the London embassy: 'this protection is necessary to Sr. Le Turc who will be in continual danger of being arrested'. An advance expense payment of 2,400 *livres* was to be sent to the embassy to allow Le Turc to buy machines or contract with workers. An annual pension of 1,200 *livres* was to be granted to each of his children should he succumb to 'the vengeance of the English who may bear him a great grudge for stealing their machines'. The cordon of Saint Michel and 1,000 *livres* pension would be awarded if his mission succeeded, half transferable to his two sons on his death. The machines once received would be successively sent to his Quinze-Vingts works together with the contracted English workmen. To avoid the accusation of obtaining machines already available in France, he wanted drawings to be made of English spinning-machines already at three French works and placed on file. English workers would be engaged on short-term contract and their pay related to their training of French workers.[44]

The expedition was still on the cards early in 1789. William Douglas, the important cotton manufacturer of Manchester and Holywell, wrote to the French embassy in London in December 1788 offering to show his machines to embassy officials, clearly with a view to his setting up concerns in France. He was worried about current competition from imports of East India cottons. As late as February 1789 it was proposed that Le Turc, still in France, and not yet authorized to make his journey, should be dispatched to Britain on his planned tour, inspect Douglas's machines, and examine his proposal for coming to France. Though Necker was fully informed of the situation it was difficult for officials to see him and get a decision – he was too occupied with the arrangements for the calling of the estates-general. The political and administrative crisis may well explain why Le Turc never made his espionage trip. Nevertheless the contract does indicate the high-water mark in his relations with the Bureau of Commerce, just as the success of the Lorient pulley works had indicated a similar pinnacle of esteem in his relations with the navy.[45]

The graveyard of Le Turc's hopes was the Quinze-Vingts. A mass of petitions, memoirs, complaints and arguments survives about his work there which greatly exceeds the importance of any achievement. As early as 1785 Le Turc had an agreement in principle with the Intendants of Commerce that he would be given a site in those large buildings, and he believed that this would be for life. It would be accompanied by government payment for fifty frames which he would build them for 50,000 *livres*. He was then asked to indicate the buildings he wanted and the modifications needed, so that all would be ready for him after his English mission was complete. But on his return the requisite site had been given to Dauffe, the hardware-maker and mechanical engineer. Le Turc was able to demonstrate his machines to the Intendant of Commerce and various experts in stables attached to the buildings, but returned to England without buildings or grant.

In 1788 Le Turc had some storage facilities at the Quinze-Vingts, for, with the approval of Calonne when controller-general, Vandermonde had organized a break-in of his premises while he was away at Lorient, apparently so that the Government should retrieve some of the English knitting machines Le Turc had brought over, and he put them in the Hôtel de Mortagne. At the same time a whole set of models and samples of English goods which Le Turc had collected over the years was taken. He protested and it was decided that a model of a whip-making machine and two looms should be restored to him, and rather reluctantly Vandermonde had to agree. Vandermonde was clearly involved in some scheme with Rhambolt to employ the English looms.[46]

In December 1788 Le Turc finally got his government subvention. It was not the subsidy he anticipated, rather a loan of 6,000 *livres* over three years. He had expected 12,000 *livres* at once with no need to repay, but it was apparently agreed that once he was operating successfully he would get a further 6,000 *livres*. The Government also gave Le Turc the rent of his premises at the Quinze-Vingts but he decided that they were not altogether suitable. He leased adjoining sections of the building (while airily expecting the Government to meet the bill) and spent a great deal on alterations. In the inauspicious month of July 1789 Le Turc finally invited inspection of his machines, but operators were not available, and it was August before Abeille and Desmarets examined ten machines and ten models for the Bureau of Commerce.[47] While the report was favourable, the delays meant that Le Turc had to sell off materials and dismiss workers. For one as self-centred as he it was not significant that city and nation were in turmoil round him, that government officials were now unsure of their powers, or that the Bureau of Commerce was being wound down. By the middle of 1790 creditors were endeavouring to seize his effects, though the administration of the Quinze-Vingts were trying to get their claim for unpaid rent in first. Eventually his premises were commandeered by the Committee of Public Safety for the use of the Commission des Armes Portatives, some of his machines and tools were thrown into corridors and courtyards to rust, others were seized and put under seal, while another government agency authorized Vandermonde to put some machines in the Hôtel de Mortagne until Le Turc discharged his debt. Hence they were eventually transferred to the Conservatoire des Arts et Métiers. For a time Le Turc had had fifty workers making cockades – a good Revolutionary product – on his looms. He made extravagant claims against the Government for the loss of this business, but he admitted that the workers, presumably unemployed Paris stocking weavers who came to work for him, went off to make the cockades at home once they knew how.[48]

His tirades became increasingly shrill and intemperate. He acknowledged he had risked the guillotine by his angry opposition to the takeover of his premises for arms manufacture; his invective against all naval administrators since Castries and La Touche passed into paranoia as he accused them of having a host of spies and agents attacking his ventures and even plotting with, and causing disloyalty in, his own family. His memorials to successive regimes and ministers met with periods of sympathy and proposals to restore his premises and manufacture, but his listing of more and more enemies, now including Tolozan and Bénezech, his confession that much of his English-type equipment was now rusty and unserviceable, and his admission of failing health made any restoration of his affairs unlikely. Nevertheless as late as the Year VII three commissioners, Abielle, Grégoire and Bardel were appointed to examine his machines, and see what help could be given.[49] However, he died penniless in the Hospice de la Charité in the Year IX.[50]

How can we assess Le Turc's activities as a transferrer of technology, and particularly as an industrial spy? On one achievement there can be little doubt, the transfer of English naval pulley-making methods was extremely successful, the right English craftsmen were identified, and apparently well handled (one was still at Lorient as foreman in 1792). The original Lorient workshop seems to have been entirely satisfactory; Le Turc took a close interest in its installation and made some useful minor modifications in the technology. Le Turc's occasional absences from Lorient in its early operations may have been damaging. But he may have been right to say that craftsmen and foremen could operate the workshops in the various ports without the attention of a senior engineer, once the right equipment for other dockyards had been made at Lorient, taken to its destination and operatives trained, and that attempts to compel him to supervise the other ports were tyrannical.

Of course to him the naval commission was a diversion from his other interest, the diffusion in France of the many new English inventions and new varieties of capital goods and consumers' goods of which he had obtained originals, copies or models. Particularly there was his lifelong and consuming interest in the technology of the framework knitting machine and his commitment to bringing the new English techniques to France. Here it is difficult to measure the results precisely. The collapse of the Quinze-Vingts works and the more and more unbalanced claims of its entrepreneur perhaps produce too negative an impression. There is no doubt that Le Turc made known in France the Derby-rib machine and a whole variety of developments and variants. English authorities tend to ascribe the taking of the various English inventions to France to Rhambolt, but the evidence would indicate that all the many and extensive shipments of machines were made by Le Turc. Rhambolt was certainly one of the workers conveyed to France by Le Turc, who claimed that he had only limited experience of frame-making, though after some delay he was able to assemble frames for Le Turc in London. One contradiction arises from the statement by Felkin that Rhambolt had been in England since 1774 on behalf of the Duc de Rochefoucauld. This seems odd considering the way the Rochefoucauld company during the 1780s was, via Izquierdo, relying on Le Turc to provide machines and workers; Le Turc said that Rhambolt had only been in England three years before he approached him to return. Later the worker was given some of the main frame-making tools and a loom of the Webb-Whittle patent of 1784 which Le Turc had imported, and set himself up in Paris claiming to be the originator of the English machines.[51]

When the Popincourt company collapsed after the Eden Treaty, Tolozan at the Bureau of Commerce endeavoured to pick up the pieces, and particularly to prevent machines being exported to Spain as Izquierdo planned. He secretly financed a Paris master stocking-maker, Germain, to buy up on the cheap the thirty English machines which Le Turc had obtained for the company. Tolozan wanted to set up centres in the provinces, and half the looms seem to have ended up in a concern apparently belonging to Tolozan himself, and in all four centres were supplied. In 1790 it was proposed that a new English loom in the hands of the Bureau of Commerce should be sent to Abbeville to be copied.[52] While, according to Felkin, Rhambolt was rewarded by the Convention for the introduction of the English 'pin' machine of Else and Harvey, it is clear that Le Turc was buying machines from Else while he was in England. From Paris this machine is said to have spread to Lyons, Nîmes and Spain. It is not possible to follow all the complexities, which could only be interpreted by a historian with a knowledge of the intricate technology of the hosiery industry. Yet, despite his own failure at the Quinze-Vingts there seems evidence to suggest that Le Turc's imported machines had a considerable impact on French industry, even if their take-up was spasmodic and ill organized in the chaotic days of the eve and onset of the Revolution, and not significant until the Empire.[53]

How far did Le Turc develop successful techniques of industrial espionage? How far was there a policy for technology transfer behind his activities? How far did he appreciate what was happening to British industry and its potential consequences for France? Despite the legal restrictions Le Turc was able to obtain English workers, machinery, tools, models and samples. His shipment of many cases of equipment and his conveying of a number of workers to France might seem to show that the English laws against the export of men and machines were inoperative or vain. There are, however, many instances where French agents, and particularly their underlings, or the English workers they recruited, were seized or had to flee precipitately. There is equally no doubt that French industrial spies in England were worried about their exposed situation, and this included Le Turc, though he was certainly not timorous by nature. The shipping out via Ireland of the equipment of a complete framework knitting firm was a real, unexampled, coup. His system of directly bribing customs officers, so that his goods crossed the Channel as having been properly examined, worked well. He believed that trying to slip goods past the Customs would, if discovered, endanger agents and put subsequent shipments at risk.[54] Covering machines and tools in boxes with pottery (some of it Wedgwood's expensive pots) would protect the operation, bribed officers could claim they were reluctant to disturb such fragile wares. He believed that his main risks came from insecure correspondence from the French end or unfriendly compatriots in England betraying him to British officials. So far no evidence has been found in British sources about Le Turc's travels and espionage. In his case, a character marked by eccentricity and extravagance was compatible with a trait of secrecy and duplicity. Perhaps his residence in Britain throughout the war of 1778–83, and his acquisition of an elegantly furnished London house – there was even a picture by Reynolds – helped Le Turc's cover.

Over many years Le Turc gave his opinions on the transfer of technology, particularly that between Britain and France, and he indicated how he could himself make a contribution. That contribution he realized was governed by two factors, that of his own predilections and temperament, and that of his contribution as an engineer. Not unnaturally there is some blurring of the two.

He insisted that there was a place for obtaining good models or drawings of machinery in the successful transfer of technology, but the critical element was the skills of the good workman, whether machine-builder or operative. 'It is not with fine words that one is able to get the advantage of machines, but with the rough hands that are used to operating them.' The involvement of a good workman totally changed the commercial advantage of a machine. Having obtained the knitting machines the Government originally sought Le Turc was not satisfied to simply dispatch them to France: 'we have not yet completed the item of the workers, that which is the most essential and which 100 pages would not suffice to explain to you'. Le Turc believed it necessary to come over to France to convince the minister why it was so important. Similarly, once one took a new technology to France

> it is not with words or with drawings that one will make the [French]
> workman, always infatuated with his own method, change it for

another, although superior to his, I know only one means of making this revolution, which is to get hold of clever workmen who may by their example train pupils.

This was essential in obtaining English technology because of their subdivision of labour.

> There is no country where labour is so divided as here. No country, consequently, where the whole of a trade is so difficult to seize hold of. No worker can explain to you the chain of operations, being perpetually occupied with ... a small part: listen to him on anything outside that and you will be burdened with error.[55]

Once specimen machines and men had been acquired Le Turc saw his own role as setting up a kind of research and development organization, or at most a pilot plant, where the techniques of machine building and erection and, quite separately, the training of industrial pupils would be carried on. His plan was to then get large capitalized firms to acquire from government the finished machines and trained workers, the Government would liquidate his debt to them as machines and men were delivered. He was prepared to introduce the technology into such firms, but emphatically not become a works manager or what would later be called a production engineer. This was partly because of his own temperament: 'you know my repugnance to be at the head of a business, however profitable'. He supplied looms asked for and put them in operation. 'That is all they can require of me and I feel I am capable of. It is impossible for me to repeat each day what I did the day before, and above all the detail of a manufacture than which nothing in the world is more boring.' To have carried on with the daily routine of pulley manufacture at Lorient 'would have destroyed my mental faculties and completely paralysed me'. After the heavy disruption of his operation in the Quinze-Vingts in the early 1790s, he suggested a role by which he acted as a technical adviser who would give an impulse to new branches of industry which he thought appropriate, without responsibilities for financial matters 'so that after they are set up I am not obliged to direct the establishments, so that I may devote myself to other enterprises'.[56] In trying to avoid long associations with particular projects and rather involve himself with research and development and consultancies he may, in fitting in with his own character traits, have been envisaging roles for the engineer not consistent with contemporary possibilities.

In the 1790s he was approached by the Government for his views on technological transfer, and whether French or foreign savants could be turned to for the bringing in of foreign industry. He had given much thought to why the transplanting of industry from country to country had been a long and difficult process, but would only comment on mechanical industry, which was within his competence. He was very deprecating about the efforts of scientific men ('gens de cabinet') sent abroad; they believed a few sketches or models could do the trick, they looked down on the practical craftsman, and put too much reliance on their own existing knowledge. However, attracting foreign workers from their workshops and listening to their own accounts of their expertise could be just as unsatisfactory, and French recruiters of foreign labour had frequently been too naïve and trusting. He was even pessimistic about the recruitment of a team consisting of a manufacturer and his workers; they were often liable to make changes in materials and dimensions in their new country which reduced the effectiveness of their processes. He believed a practical engineer with a thorough understanding of the mechanics of the relevant devices, proper machine-builders and trained operatives were needed, and he felt that an engineer who was himself an inventor was the best intermediary – here no doubt he was promoting his own situation.[57]

Le Turc made some highly penetrating observations. We have seen his understanding of the division of labour in England, but he was able to see even wider developments. In his English travels he

> saw with dismay that a revolution in the mechanical arts, the real precursor, the true and principal cause of political revolutions (he meant a changed international balance of power) was developing in a manner frightening to the whole of Europe, and particularly to France, which would receive the severest blow from it.[58]

Le Turc's own efforts to obtain new British industrial processes and transfer them to France had, as we have seen, a very mixed success, and his efforts to exploit some of them were nullified by the difficulties of the times and his own defects. In the activity of industrial espionage, however, he had been immensely active and generally successful. At the peak of his espionage activities he looked forward to another expedition across the Channel: 'It is a hunt which I enjoy and wish to take part in because it is of benefit to my native land.'[59]

18 Laws, Actions and Attitudes in Britain

We will now look at the development of laws against the emigration of artisans and the export of machinery. In the next chapter we will relate this to the attitudes of some major British industrialists. As most of the legislation came in the late eighteenth century and as the industrialists whose views we know lived in the second half of the century, it is best to look at both in successive and related chapters in the latter part of a book which has, as far as possible, respected the chronological flow of events. The 1780s are especially interesting as there was then an unusual amount of evidence. It was a time of discussion and controversy, with the central years of the decade dominated by debate about the proposed revision of commercial intercourse with Ireland, and then by argument about the value and nature of a commercial treaty with France. By these years too, there was a group of industrialists in being whose firms exemplified the greater scale and enhanced technology with which industry was being conducted, and some of the most emphatic in their views, like Boulton and Watt, John Wilkinson, Samuel Garbett, Josiah Wedgwood, Richard Crawshay, commented on the laws protecting British technology from the foreigner, but with some notable variations. Finally we will look at the application of the laws against enticement of workers and the export of equipment, and see whether they were enforced to any significant extent.

While the first general legislation against industrial espionage dates from 1719, and is directed to prevent the suborning of workers abroad, there was already on the statute book an Act to prevent the export of one kind of machinery, the stocking frame. There is little evidence to show its implementation. The stocking frame is perhaps to be regarded as very much an unprecedented, one off, invention, and the product of the genius of one man. It long precedes the later succession of mechanical inventions in textiles which can be traced from the Kay and the Wyatt and Paul inventions of the 1730s, and comes early even in comparison with the long processes of innovation in the coal-using industries which had so markedly altered the British international technological position by the early eighteenth century.[1] The stocking frame invented in 1589 by the Nottinghamshire curate, William Lee, was not long confined to England. Originally it does not seem to have had encouragement in its immediate neighbourhood. It was refused a charter by Elizabeth, and it is generally surmised that a fear that it would cause unemployment was an obstacle both locally and at Court. But Lee was invited over to France and went with his brother and nine workmen to Rouen 'upon allurements of great rewards privilege and honour'. His enterprise there is said to have been disrupted by the assassination of the French king, Henry IV, but he died in France in 1610, though most of the workmen returned soon after.[2]

Returned to London the framework knitting industry expanded, largely specializing in silk products. During 1655–57 the framework knitters approached Oliver Cromwell for incorporation as a chartered company. At that time only a solitary survivor of the original emigrants remained in France, and the petitioners were unconcerned about him. They instanced, however, a workman still under his apprenticeship who had been lured by the Venetian ambassador to settle in that state, but when his frame needed repair it could not be mended there and he returned home. Another man had emigrated to Amsterdam and built frames and employed Dutch labour, but his household was wiped out by plague and no one was left to operate the frames. The framework knitters were grateful that the trade thus seemed to have been providentially preserved for England. Cromwell issued letters patent for the corporation in 1657, a main point apparently being the control of apprenticeship. In 1658 the knitters again petitioned, this time to prevent the export of frames, and they wanted them seized by Customs. There was concern that there had been an Italian order for thirty or forty frames at the high price of £80 each. As their charter had been obtained under the Commonwealth the framework knitters had to have it issued anew under Charles II. It contained the clause:

> The invention being purely English (native born subjects as well as aliens, having by secret means endeavoured to take the art to foreign states, to the discouraging of industrious subjects) no person, whether

freeman or foreigner, denizen or alien shall presume to carry ... any
frame used for making silk stockings, or used in framework knitting,
beyond the seas ...

Officers of the Company could seize frames being exported and have
them forfeited by a Justice of the Peace, half the value of any forfeiture
going to the Company, half to the Exchequer.[3]

The idea that the stocking frame and the skills of frame-making
could be isolated in Britain proved quite unreal. As Chapman says, 'the
real threat was from emigration of artisans and industrial espionage
and the emigration of Catholics in the Commonwealth period'. The
first settlement had been at Avignon, and the settlers were able to
specify and order the metal parts locally and build their own frames,
and there were some groups of workers at Nîmes, Uzès, Alès, Lyons
and Paris. Around the end of the century the French authorities began
to impose arrangements for industrial organization and guild control.
If anything, the export of frames seems to have accelerated after the
Restoration charter; over 400 frames were said to have been exported
between 1670 and 1695, to Paris, Orléans, Rennes, Caen and
Valenciennes, and beyond France to Tournai, Cordova, Seville, Cadiz,
Rome and Messina.[4]

The outcome was the first legislation against machinery export in
1696.[5] The Act referred only to the previous export of 'several' frames,
but this obviously minimized the problem. It prevented export from
1 May 1696 by punishing those who loaded vessels, confiscating the
frames or frame parts at the rate of £40 for each frame or parcel of
parts, half the fine to the Crown, and half to the informer. At the same
time those who bought or sold frames which were to be moved from
place to place within Britain had to give notice of the fact to the
framework knitters' Company within two months or be fined £5.
Felkin's view that the legislation 'immediately caused the practice of
exporting frames to cease' seems highly suspect.[6] It seems more likely
that by the time the legislation was passed there was little point in
inspecting the bolts on the door of an empty stable. In any case there
were many continental sources to which others that had not yet acquired the technology could turn without attempting to get it from
England. The assertion in the petition of the Company for a Bill 'that
the trade of framework knitting might be kept within this kingdom, if
the transporting of frames was effectively prevented; because they can
make them no where else' was quite mistaken.[7] However, when the
series of important new adaptations of the frame, beginning with the

Derby-rib device of Jedediah Strutt, arrived from the late 1750s there was a new wave of foreign interest in English hosiery machinery, sustained by the moves into net and lace making variants. Our account of Le Turc's espionage activities has testified to French and Spanish concern to obtain these new technologies which had caused a great extension of framework knitting.

While it is a matter of some temerity for a non-expert to draw conclusions on an industry which has few specialists, perhaps some may be made. First, the invention of the stocking frame was perhaps the first significant case where there was a major English invention which, once known about, was strongly desired abroad. It was a marked exception to the general pattern of technology transfer up to that time, for England had been overwhelmingly a debtor nation. Certainly in the cases of France and Venice foreign states intervened to get the invention, foreshadowing the eighteenth-century situation where foreign interventions to obtain British technologies were normally state-initiated or state-assisted. The speed and determination with which the stocking frame was carried abroad clearly baffled and strained the credulity of the English users, who believed successively that regulation, proclamation or legislation might prevent it. While it preceded by more than twenty years the first general legislation against industrial espionage, the 1696 Act seems to have had no influence on it; it solely concerned the export of one kind of machine, while the Act of 1719 was solely directed to the emigration of personnel. It was the 1730s before we even hear of government perception that the lack of legislation on machine export might be significant, and 1750 before anything was done about it.

While most of the significant later legislation has been previously mentioned against the context of its first application, it will be useful to summarize it here so as to get a conspectus of the whole. The 1719 Act has been discussed in detail, and needs only the essentials stating. Its main thrust was against anyone enticing any British 'artificer or manufacturer' abroad. The enticer should be fined up to £100 for a first offence and imprisoned for three months and longer if the fine was not paid; a second offence could be fined at discretion and incur a year's imprisonment, continuable until the fine was paid. Emigrant workers who did not return home in six months after being warned to do so by an accredited British official should in effect lose their right to lands and goods in Britain, or to be an administrator or executor; lands and goods could be forfeit to the Crown and the offender would be regarded as an alien, and beyond British protection. Where persons were credibly accused of suborning or of intention to emigrate they had to provide security to attend an appropriate court or if they could not do so be imprisoned until trial. Those workers convicted of making arrangements to emigrate would have to give sufficient security against leaving the country, or be imprisoned until they did.

The coverage of the Act was to be manufacturers or artificers in wool, in steel, iron, brass or any other metal, and watchmakers 'or any other manufacturer or artificer of Great Britain'. While specifically stated trades cover a wide range, one must wonder whether magistrates would be as keen to pursue measures against workmen whose trades were not particularly singled out in the wording of the Act, and whether this is why some other trades were carefully and specifically brought into the terms of later Acts. The Act reflected the fears about the John Law operation of 1718–20 and the way in which suborning or inveigling of workers abroad was at the core of it. As suborning the right workers proved, in the vast majority of cases, to be the *sine qua non* of technological transfer, this explains the continued importance of the Act throughout the century.[8]

Despite the misgivings recorded on the lack of legislation to prevent machines being exported, nothing was done about this until 1750. The failure to mention the existing framework knitting machine prohibition at that time probably means that those two clauses, tacked on to a general act, had been inoperative, perhaps virtually forgotten. The 1750 Act we have shown arose from complaints from the woollen industry, initially the clothiers of Trowbridge, about the threat posed by men who added to the offence of suborning the recent export of 'tools and engines'. Unfortunately neither petition nor legislation indicates what machine export caused concern, but presses and calenders for finishing seem most likely. For the first time, too, we have a proposal to prohibit also the export of 'drafts, models and descriptions' of such equipment, though this was not implemented. The new legislation was seen as an extension of the 1719 Act. It was specifically directed at the seduction of workmen in wool, mohair, cotton and silk, who were added to the metal and other workers of the earlier Act, though keeping the catch-all phrase about workers in other manufactures. The penalty for suborning was smartly increased to £500 per worker seduced, and conviction carried a year's imprisonment and, if need be, further detention until the fine was paid. A second offence would cost £1,000 per worker and two years' imprisonment. Prosecutions had to begin, however, within twelve months of the offence.

The clauses against the export of 'tools and utensils' were in fact confined to wool and silk, cotton being omitted. Foreign export of such equipment was penalized by seizure and by a fine of £200 for each offence. The items involved would be auctioned off, half going to the customs or revenue officer who seized the goods. Shipmasters knowingly conniving were fined £100. Those bringing a prosecution under the Act would get half the forfeitures made, the rest going to the Crown. Anyone suing any individual for wrongful action under the Act was liable to treble costs if the action did not succeed.[9]

The increased importance of cotton manufacture, which at this time still included many cotton-linens, was indicated by an Act of 1774. Beginning with a proposal to revise the 1750 Act,[10] it was decided within a month to concentrate on the export of the 'utensils' of the cotton and linen industries.[11] This reflects the new technology-based growth of the cotton industry as does the almost simultaneous Fustian Act of that year which allowed the printing of home produced cotton-linens, based upon the new situation of the industry following the Arkwright spinning inventions.[12] In order perhaps to achieve some uniformity it was decided to include the silk and wool industries again in the terms of the Act.[13]

The resulting Act nevertheless concentrated on the export of cotton and linen 'tools or utensils', repairing the gap in the 1750 Act, but not touching the offence of suborning, for which cotton and linen had been covered. While the tenor of the 1774 Act was very similar to that of 1750, the penalty on shipmasters knowingly allowing cotton and linen 'tools and utensils' to be put on board their vessels was doubled to £200, as was that for venal Customs officials. A new element was that it was now punishable for anyone to gather together or possess equipment for exportation, not only for the cotton and linen but the silk and wool industries, and if credible information was given to Justices they could seize the equipment and summon and question the persons concerned, confiscating the goods and sending those implicated before Assizes or Quarter Sessions, holding them in the county gaol in the meantime unless they provided proper sureties. On conviction not only should the equipment be forfeited, but the person guilty of assembling it for export fined £200. On such a conviction the person bringing the prosecution would divide the fine with the Crown. The important change here was that steps could be taken against the intending illegal exporter before the actual act of putting the items concerned aboard ship.

The exportation of textile machinery and of the aids to its manufacture were returned to in the spring of 1781, and while other textiles were embraced in new measures which amended and explained the 1774 Act, the marginal heading on one day's entry in the *Commons Journals*, 'Cotton Manufactory', shows where the interest of the House was mainly directed.[14] Basically, it was thought that the penalties provided in the earlier Act and the means of enforcement had proved insufficient. The provisions relating to shipping goods were broadened and clarified. The description of prohibited goods was extended and instead of the 'tools and utensils' of 1774 there was now 'any machine, engine, tool, press, paper, utensil or implement whatsoever' used in the production of woollen, cotton, linen, or silk goods, however named.[15] Now models or plans were clearly specified. This may be thought very belated, for it had been asked for in the petition for the 1750 Act. It may be, however, that English manufacturers and inventors had been rather sceptical about the skills of foreigners and their ability to make good machines from plans without the presence of English artisans – in other words they believed that preventing suborning was the great thing. The fact that some machine-builders had already gone abroad, and the impressive contemporary advances in the quality of draughtsmanship, may have helped to make such a restriction now seem important. The practice of smuggling abroad tools or machine parts packed into innocuous seeming containers of other goods was no doubt aimed at when the Act specified the seizure of all the packets and containers in which suspect goods were found, and all their contents.

Those charged with illegally exporting equipment or plans had to give proper surety to appear in court, and otherwise be imprisoned awaiting trial, and on conviction pay £200, forfeit the illegal goods and papers and other goods packed with them, and be imprisoned for twelve months. The Customs could sell off goods, models and plans they had seized at the point of export, and any other goods with them, half the net proceeds going to the Crown and half to the seizing officer. Penalties against offending shipmasters and customs officials were continued from the previous Act. Where there were attempts to gather and assemble machines, models and plans for export, the offence was more comprehensively described, and anyone who ordered, or had made, machines, tools, models or plans, as well as those who were actually found in possession of them with intent to export, were brought under the Act. Again confiscation, a £200 fine and a year's imprisonment were the penalties. If the fine was not paid imprisonment could be extended.

While in the 1774 Act half the net proceeds of forfeitures under the Act was to go to the person bringing a prosecution under the Act, now it was stated that they were to go 'to the use of the informer', who presumably did not have to bring the prosecution himself.[16] There was the briefest of Acts allowing the export of some hand cards for wool in 1786.[17]

There was one further step to protect the textile industry. An Act of 1782 brought in calico-printing. This was not induced, as might have been expected, by the dangers of European rivalry, but that of the East India Company. The petition pointed to the great growth in the printing of 'Calicoes, Cottons, Muslins and Linens' in Britain, and the strong stimulus to printing from the use of copperplates instead of wood blocks following its invention in 1754. The East India Company had seemingly made a previous attempt to export the metal plates and machines for working them and other blocks and tools, together with skilled workers, in order to be able to print cottons in India by the new methods. Though originally frustrated by opposition from the British calico-printing trade, they now had built a new 'Manufactory of Printing' in India, superintended by British experts. Its products were claimed to be seriously extending the normal and accepted imports (for subsequent re-export) of goods which were 'the original invention and manufacture of natives of the country'. The new type of East India goods of British technique was harming the sale of British manufactured and printed textiles in the export market. There was as yet no legislation to prevent the emigration of workers or equipment in the British textile-printing industry and (as well as some complementary changes in the duties and drawbacks on East India cottons) the British calico-printers demanded action to include textile printing among the industries whose technological transfer was protected.[18] On 8 April the Lancashire calico- and linen-printers added their powerful support, and matters proceeded steadily towards effecting the necessary legislation.[19] This reverted to a concentration on preventing the actual act of exportation of any blocks, plates, engines, tools, and utensils relating to the cotton-, calico-, muslin- or linen-printing trades to any foreign destination. If discovered the equipment was to be confiscated and a fine of £500 levied which could be recovered through the courts.[20]

In the mid-1780s the metal industries were brought under the umbrella of the laws against the export of machinery and tools. The 1719 Act had put some metal trades among those in which suborning was explicitly forbidden, but it was well over sixty years before the equipment of the metal trades was covered. Here the coming of the legislation will be dealt with; the controversial aspects of its utility will be looked at later. The speed with which eighteenth-century Parliaments could act is well instanced here. Leave to bring in a Bill in the Commons was given on 4 July 1785, the Bill passed its third reading on 14 July, was agreed by the Lords on the 19th, and received the royal assent on the 20th of the same month.

Originally directed to prohibit the export of tools, utensils and materials of the 'iron manufactory', which meant the making of goods in iron and did not cover the equipment of primary production, it was quickly modified to take in the equipment for manufacturing steel goods. Very significantly, it was now asked that the seducing abroad of workmen should also be addressed. This strongly suggests that the 1719 Act, which had very clearly singled out workers in 'iron, steel, brass or any other metal' was not being fully applied.

First, the 1785 Tools Act[21] closely specified all exportation or preparation for export of a long list of tools, with a heavy emphasis on stamping machinery, presses (including cutting-out machines), piercing machines, dies for stamping and pressing machines whether cut or not, cast iron rollers for rolling metals, casting equipment, lathes for turning and also for polishing, polishing brushes and metal-cutting shears. There was some coverage of what were materials or semi-manufactures rather than tools, like rolled steel, silver-plated metal, button parts and unfinished buttons. Next the export of some generally heavier machinery or its adjuncts was prohibited, anvils and hammers for iron or copper forging mills, the framework and operative parts of slitting-mills. Then came die-sinking tools, chasing machines, equipment for casting buckles and buttons, polishing brushes, and some items not closely related, like whip-covering machines[22] and glass-pinching tools. There was a final catch-all for any tools or utensils relating to making iron or steel goods, but also the important addition of models and plans of tools and equipment in all these trades. As in previous Acts there were provisions for enforcement. If credible witnesses of export offences testified before magistrates the presumed offender could be summoned, the goods seized, surety for appearance sought if the matter were going to court, or imprisonment until trial if surety was not forthcoming, with the £200 fine and twelve months' imprisonment for the guilty as in earlier legislation. Precedent was again followed in clauses about Customs officers and the £200 fines for conniving shipmasters. Again, similar penalties were applied for those procuring or collecting prohibited goods for export.

Without any reference to the earlier legislation of 1719 there was inserted a clause against anyone contracting with, enticing, persuading or trying to seduce workmen who made iron or steel goods, or who made tools for the manufacture of such goods. Conviction carried a fine of £500 per workman and twelve months in prison; a second offence would attract a fine of £1,000 per workman and a two-year prison sentence.

There are some curiosities in this piece of legislation. It is very clear that it was directed at protecting the light engineering of the Birmingham district, with some relevance also to Sheffield and other centres of metal goods manufacture. Yet there is no mention of the watch tools and specialized machine tools of the South Lancashire trade. Though such a large part of Birmingham manufacture was in copper alloys, particularly brass, they are not referred to, and one has to presume that it was felt sufficient to enumerate the iron and steel tools with which brass and other alloys were worked, while the reference to flasks and casting moulds and that to buckle and button casting equipment would protect brass-founding sufficiently. However, this would not explain why brass-founders were not included in the clause against suborning.

The 1785 Act failed to give sufficient weight to differing views of manufacturers and merchants in the metal trades. These were sufficiently strong to require its modification within the year. An Act of 1786[23] was designed to avoid a situation where there were tools and machines which had apparently become unexportable under the 1785 Act which had previously been part of regular trade and never objected to. It was now enacted that these items could be exported to the British West Indies – indicating that a source of complaint had been exporters to that market – 'or any other foreign part or place whatsoever'.

There follows a list of items still to be excluded from export. This very closely follows the 1785 Act, but there are some differences. Die-sinking tools were not to be sent abroad, but iron or steel dies, listed in the previous Act, are not prohibited. Drilling machines, too, are now left out. Presses with screws less than an inch and a half in diameter are expressly allowed, which was to be a source of future confusion as Customs tended to reject any machine with a screw of more than that size. Some screw-making equipment was now left unhindered, as, very surprisingly, were lathes. On the other hand rolling and slitting machines, with their frames, were specified more closely than in the previous Act, and grooved rollers picked out, no doubt reflecting Cort's recent invention for refining iron using grooved rollers in part of the process. The screws mentioned for both rolling- and slitting-mills will be the large screws with which the distance between rolls could be adjusted. All equipment for casting and boring cannon was brought into the Act. For both rolling- and slitting-mills and cannon-making equipment the export of models was prohibited – plans are not mentioned, perhaps implying that they were less useful.

If there was some relaxation in the tools and machines of the metal trades, the opportunity was taken to widen the Act generally by including wire moulds for paper-making, wheels used in glass cutting, engraving and polishing, and some other glass-makers' tools, potters' lathes of several types and a collection of tools used by saddlers and harness and bridle makers. Some of the actions of pressure groups which led to the modification and extension of the 1785 Tools Act by that of the following year will be looked at later, but the export of rolling machinery to enable the French navy to develop its programme of copper sheathing, the operation of the cannon-boring mills of Indret and the recent completion of Le Creusot must have been well known, as well as the emigration to Russia of key managers and workmen from Carron. Part of the same complex as Le Creusot and under the same company organization was the Verrerie de la Reine, the first attempt to take English flint glass abroad with any degree of success, and this may have influenced the inclusion of glass-cutting equipment.

It may be otiose to take too much notice of all instances of omissions and inclusions in the wording of the two successive Acts – the leaving out of metalworking lathes in the second Act while other key machine tools of the Birmingham toy trade continued to be covered may be an accident of very hastily drafted legislation. One omission from both Acts, however, is remarkable. Files were so important to all early engineering, and the superior quality of the steel and the workmanship of English files so universally recognized, that it is at first surprising that they are mentioned in neither Act. The explanation is simple: their export was so well established, whether by legitimate means or smuggling, that it would have caused far too much trouble to have attempted to prevent it.[24]

These then were the laws to stop the emigration of skilled industrial workers and the export of tools and machines considered valuable in the transfer of British technology abroad. But the existence of law on the statute book does not mean that it is effectively implemented, or that its object is wholly or even partially achieved, that public opinion is generally behind it, or indeed that entrepreneurs in the industries concerned are undivided in their view of the utility, even the desirability, of the legislation.

To examine the Assize and Quarter Session records for evidence on all those towns and districts of England and Wales where there was a considerable presence of technologically innovative industry (let alone their comparable Scottish jurisdictions) over the eighteenth century would require a team effort over several years, and it has not been attempted here. An alternative source is the press, but a local press only came into existence in many major provincial towns around the middle of the century, and it originally consisted of a limited relay of the most significant news in the London press together with local advertisements, though the latter are often of great value to the historian. In their early years the provincial papers were often thin in content even within these limits, and it was only gradually that advertisements increased and controversial correspondence about local issues, and accounts of major local projects and developments, became significant. Because of the bulk of newspaper material, references to the relevant legislation have not been searched for in the press and have generally only been used when they have been cited in secondary sources.[25]

The flow of evidence about British opposition to industrial espionage is very uneven, especially before there was much regional association of manufacturers, even in the most industrially active districts. On the other hand we have seen from the French side that industrial spies were often very worried about their situation. Hyde and De Saudray had, on two quite separate espionage trips to Birmingham, to take refuge in flight. Alcock, trying to get more workers for himself and the French government, had his wife and emigrant workers arrested and, after the later seizure of a large party of workers he had recruited, he seems to have given up his attempts to recruit more English workers. Le Turc, like De Saudray, was a man of courage, but his enjoyment of espionage was continually balanced by fears of arrest for himself, the seizure of technical equipment at the point of export, and of workers whom he was suborning. Jars quickly left a sulphuric acid works once he thought his presence was detected.

In 1764 a spy travelling from Birmingham to London was careless enough to leave two pocket-books containing papers in the coach, and these were handed to John Roebuck, the partner of Samuel Garbett, and like him utterly opposed to industrial espionage. In this case the spy seems to have been a Swede endeavouring to recruit English iron-foundry workers. One of the main suborners, a Mr Downing, was identified, but claimed ignorance of the law and to have made efforts to stop the men recruited once he knew of his offence. The men engaged, who were on the way to take ship for Gothenburg, were sent back to their own district. Lord Stanhope, in replying to Roebuck, requested that the men be required to give security not to leave the kingdom, and that Downing should be prosecuted under the 1719 Act. Downing's suborning had taken place in the Shropshire iron district. In 1766 a workman previously enticed to Holland for iron- and steel-making returned to England to get more workers, and was arrested. In the same year a British worker similarly returned from Sweden to obtain more workers was being held, and his prosecution was being requested.[26] In 1778 a James Homer, described as a labourer of London, but probably the Birmingham man who had been the chief workman of De Saudray, was indicted for seduction of workers.[27] Thus, while the formation of commercial committees in some major manufacturing towns in the 1780s led to an increased interest in enforcing the laws against the emigration of workers and the export of machinery, the relevant laws had not been a dead letter before.

But as the principal manufacturers in the main provincial towns in the late 1770s and early 1780s began to form committees to enable their views to be known more widely and to make representation to Parliament and the Government when those views could be concerted, the pace quickened. The issues important to them included the opposition to the Irish Resolutions of 1785 and the terms of the Anglo-French commercial treaty of 1786. There were some potential consequences in both issues in terms of technology transfer, though they did not bulk large, but in these years other issues which had direct relevance surfaced and engaged the attention of industrialists, like the Tools Acts of 1785 and 1786. As a result, action against exporters of machinery and suborners of workers was undertaken. For a time a General Chamber of Manufacturers was in existence, but eventually foundered on divisions between the interests of those who represented the technologically innovative and commercially aggressive industries and those representing traditional and conservative ones. A useful consequence of the discussion and debates of the period is that they allow us to see the position and standards, indeed sometimes the double standards, of some of the great industrialists of the time, the Wilkinsons, Boulton, Watt, Williams, Garbett, Crawshay, Wedgwood as they encountered the existing laws limiting the transfer of technology, or supported or opposed new ones.

One of the first of the regional organizations of general importance, in part superseding organizations of specialized producers of particular products,[28] was the Manchester Committee for the Protection of Trade of 1774. While it had many other concerns, the Committee 'continued to issue frequent notices in the local newspapers, and was especially active in warning the citizens of Manchester against nefarious schemes of foreigners in their midst, who were suspected of stealing trade secrets'. They issued a 'caution' in January 1775 that 'foreigners, attended by a Person, formerly engaged in the Cotton Business' intended to visit Manchester for espionage purposes. It requested all artisans 'not to admit any Foreigners to a sight of their work, without being introduced by a Gentleman of the Town'.[29] In a report on its activities at the end of 1782 it listed as one of its functions checking the emigration of artisans.[30]

The pottery manufacturers of Staffordshire were closely contemporary in their organization, and Wedgwood was highly influential within it. He had a continual concern with espionage and suborning, including that between British firms as well as that of foreigners. He wrote to his partner Bentley in 1779 about forbidding part of his works to foreigners because he believed they wanted the secret of black basalt ware.[31] He had written a most important pamphlet for pottery workers against their emigration in 1783.[32] He played a leading role in the formation of the Association of Manufacturers of Earthenware. Though this was formally established in 1784, it had been preceded by earlier meetings of potters to concert policy on matters of mutual concern, going back at least to 1773. With Wedgwood usually in the chair it inevitably set its face against industrial espionage, and it also worked to include certain pottery-making equipment within the scope of the Tools Act of 1786. Early in its existence it sought to work with the parallel manufacturers' committees in Birmingham and Manchester.[33] Wedgwood's personal attitude towards the emigration of workers and the export of machinery is discussed later in comparison with that of other leading industrialists.

There had been associations of Birmingham merchants and manufacturers for particular purposes before the 1780s, on the export of button chapes in 1760, on the need to establish an assay office in the town in 1773, on the liberalization of legislation complained of by the American Colonies in 1775, but they had not always spoken with a single voice, particularly on the last issue. There had been well organized and successful approaches to local aristocrats and MPs to act as a regional interest in the support of these Birmingham initiatives. One such successful appeal had been very much the lobby of Boulton and Watt and their close allies, rather than that of the town as a whole – the campaign to extend Watt's original patent by twenty-five years, from 1775 to 1800, by Act of Parliament.

In 1783, however, there was a large Town Meeting with Samuel Garbett in the chair, and it was decided to form a Birmingham Commercial Committee. The immediate stimulus is said to have been a danger that legislation preventing the export of brass might be repealed. Over the rest of the decade a main preoccupation of the committee was the emigration of skilled workers and the export of machinery.[34]

A meeting of 25 January 1785 published its resolutions and they were reported in the press. They thought that there were 'many things of great importance to the Manufactures of this Town and Neighbourhood' on which the Government should be pressured. A restriction on the entry of Birmingham goods into the Habsburg Empire was feared, and the results of enquiries by the British ambassador in Vienna anticipated. It had been learned that the Government was involved in discussions about commercial treaties with France and Spain; there were difficulties in exporting Birmingham goods to several countries and the committee welcomed commerce with those foreign countries which were prepared to fix reciprocal low duties, or even have a free trade in manufacture. But high on the priorities of the committee was industrial espionage. 'There is reason to believe, attempts have been lately made to seduce artists in this Neighbourhood to go to work on foreign countries; and also that artists that have been abroad return here to seduce others.' The Government was to be written to to help prevent this, and an advertisement was to be placed in the Birmingham papers. The advertisement offered a reward of 50 guineas for any information leading to the detection and conviction of anyone suborning workers. The committee went further; they would apply to the Government to enforce that part of the 1719 Act which could make alien and outlaw such workers as exercised their trade abroad 'to the prejudice of the Manufactures of this country'.[35]

The report of this major meeting repeatedly returned to the issue of industrial espionage. They declared 'a spirit of rivalling and supplanting our manufactures is now operating in various parts of Europe, to a degree truly alarming, and our present laws are found ineffectual for preventing our ingenious tools being exported, and our most valuable workmen and artificers from being inveigled away to other countries'. Manufacturers abroad were often favoured by remission of taxes on raw materials, while the British government continued to tax domestic industrial materials without any knowledge of the supportive attitude of foreign governments towards their subjects, or appreciation of 'the inducements which are continually offered (and with some success) to entice artists to leave this kingdom'. These were among the subjects which made it important for manufacturers throughout the kingdom to correspond, concert their views and lobby government, a process in which the pottery manufacturers of Staffordshire were already active. The offer of the reward for information was repeated twice in 1786 and Birmingham manufacturers said they had decided to admit no more foreigners to their workshops.[36]

A powerful motive for the closer association of manufacturers was the general opposition to Pitt's efforts to liberalize trade between Great Britain and Ireland as embodied in the Irish Resolutions. One argument was that lower taxation in Ireland would cause the removal of important English industries there, but the inference sometimes seems to be that the movement might be to foreign countries via Ireland.[37] Additional fuel was added to the fire by the recently strongly opposed excise on fustians, by the contemptuous attitude of the Government to the fustian manufacturers' representations, and the expectation that the newer, rising, industries would be unconsidered in any protection against Irish competition, while old and traditional ones would be.

In early 1785 there were petitions in opposition to the resolutions, from Liverpool, Lancashire and Glasgow. In March Birmingham joined in, emphasizing the need for there to be import duties on foreign iron coming in to Ireland to equal the heavy duties on iron imported into Britain (there was still a need for large imports from Sweden and Russia despite the technical breakthroughs which were about to revolutionize British production) but they announced a forthcoming attack on another front, 'the Petitioners have long hoped for a favourable Opportunity to entreat the House to appoint a Committee to take the State of the Hardware Trade into Consideration, as an Object of National Importance', the outcome of which was the rapid passage of the Tools Act in July. In arguments put before the House of Lords against the Irish Resolutions by James Watt and James Keir, they argued not merely against the movement to Ireland of 'Tools, implement and Machines, invented and made by our Artists, for the better carrying on of their several Manufactures', but that Irish merchants, with a complete disregard for the consequences, would ship them freely to foreign states. They instanced the current danger of shipping cast iron rolls for rolling copper sheathing to France, of sending there and to Germany partly manufactured buttons and plated metal for 'toy' manufacture. Even if the Birmingham manufacturers obtained protective legislation against tool export, as the textile manufacturers had done for their tools and machines, it would be useless. It was doubtful if the Irish parliament would pass effective legislation to prevent Birmingham equipment being passed abroad through Ireland, or an artificer emigrating via Ireland, 'prohibitory law will probably be much less effectively observed in Ireland', while English manufacturers who would be hurt by these actions could do nothing to prevent them. Watt and Keir expected continued technological fertility in England, which should be protected.[38]

During the series of London meetings held by manufacturers in different parts of Britain to organize opposition to the Fustian Tax and the Irish Resolutions the lobbyists decided to form a more permanent organization which would continue when the current protests had achieved their result, and in March 1785 the General Chamber of Manufacturers of Great Britain was formed, in time to make one of the later petitions against the resolutions.[39] Once operative some of its main preoccupations were, as Witt Bowden pointed out, to help manufacturers guard their improvements and inventions from being exported, to maintain vigilance against foreign spies, and to enforce the laws against the emigration of workers.[40]

It was at this point that the Birmingham manufacturers pushed ahead with the lobbying for what became the 1785 Tools Act. At the end of the previous year they had linked pressure on the Government about the terms of a prospective treaty of commerce with France with the problems about the emigration of workmen and the export of tools. They had been particularly concerned when local magistrates had declared themselves unauthorized to summon someone before them who was engaged in suborning a worker to go abroad – possibly because it was not demonstrable that the process of suborning had occurred, possibly because the Birmingham trades had not been specifically mentioned in the 1719 Act and they would not use the catch-all clause as being too vague. When tools were embarked to accompany an emigrating worker a minister had been unable to get Customs to do anything as the tools were not covered by any Act. In July the following year a meeting of the Birmingham Commercial Committee was announced to plan the prohibition of the export of tools and materials which might be injurious to the manufactures of the region, without interfering with the export of materials or products which had been previously exported without opposition. Members were asked to list for the Committee chairman, Samuel Garbett, items which should go in either category. It was made clear that a parliamentary petition and Bill were being promoted. Ten principal manufacturers signed the notice of meeting, with Boulton at the head.

The 1785 Act, as we have seen, passed with great speed and virtually without opposition, but soon there developed a strong resistance to it, and an attempt at repeal the following year. Much of this resistance came from London export merchants. We have shown that the result was not repeal but rather a modifying Act in 1786 which made some concession to the export of certain tools, and clarified the right to export tools to which there had previously been no objection, which the Birmingham committee had conceded from the outset. On the other hand Birmingham industrialists added new items to the prohibited list under the amending Act. The year 1786 was obviously one in which manufacturer action to reduce the dangers of exporting technology was prominent, but another important issue for them was the Eden Treaty. Though the treaty was particularly an object to the industrialists of the 'new' industries – Lancashire cotton, Birmingham region hardware and Staffordshire pottery – there will not be any attempt to examine this most interesting issue here, except where matters relating to the transfer of technology were involved.

The attempts to repeal the 1785 Act are perhaps the first sign of a rift in what had at first seemed a solid front presented by manufacturers in their approach to the Government on policy issues. There seems to have been a willingness on the part of the Birmingham committee to discuss with its critics some agreed modification of the first Tools Act. But a London group replied that they would be satisfied with nothing less than total repeal. Crawshay, the leading spirit in London, was twice told that a public meeting – presumably of the General Chamber of Manufacturers, or a section of it – was being held to discuss the issue, but though well able to attend, he ostentatiously played bowls until the meeting was over. Crawshay, very shortly (1787) to enter iron-making at Cyfarthfa, and to be crucial in supporting the Cort puddling and rolling process until it had achieved commercial success, was still at this time overwhelmingly a merchant. He made much of his excellent relations with Pitt, the prime minister. Garbett felt it only right that those who intended to export tools and equipment should specify them, so that objections could be entered if others could show the export detrimental to British manufactures, but Crawshay and his allies 'declined a Treaty on this plain fair Ground'. Garbett was however consoled that the equipment which was essential to Cort's 'valuable improvement in manufacturing Bar Iron' was covered by the Tools Act.[41] It was somewhat unrealistic for Garbett to hope for any conversion by Crawshay at this stage, for a printed broadsheet had already been circulated in which he and his allies insisted on repeal. They maintained that those export orders which involved an assortment of goods, some of which were prohibited under the Tools Act, would be badly affected. Moreover it would lead to foreigners being all the keener to domesticate the British technologies in their own countries. The Act 'betrays a fearful Jealousy of Foreigners, which we consider as ill-founded'; interfering with particular items within export orders 'is to compel them into an Emulation against ourselves', and cause 'rapid improvement' in their own production of iron and steel goods.[42]

While the Crawshay party put forward this argument, a very powerful counter was put forward from the copper industry, apparently by John Vivian, the leader of the Cornish mining interest. He had been a key figure in the establishment of the Cornish Metal Company in 1785 to monopolize Cornish ore production and create a cartel with Anglesey Mines to control the national market. He said that the prohibition of the export of copper sheet to prevent the French and their allies getting our copper to sheathe their navies during the recent war had had the unfortunate effect of reducing the dependence of other nations on the produce of our rolling-mills with their superior rollers. The Russians, Swedes and Hamburgers had imported British rolls and supplied our enemies with sheathing metal. After the war the British had got back a great deal of the foreign market, 'the Excellence of our Workmanship yet kept us up'. The Tools Act had been 'wisely passed', but the haste in its drafting had led to items traditionally exported without any danger to the economy being included in the general prohibition. But rolls should continue to be included in any revised Act, even though orders from Russia, Sweden, Hamburgh, Holland and France were coming in. Their export would damage not merely the profits from rolling, but the production of the British copper mines which provided the metal for the rolled sheets, and it would also affect the plating industry and other producers of rolled metal products. He described the French attempts to move to a coppered navy, and their need for sheathing and copper fastenings which would have to come from Britain if they could not succeed themselves. He was aware of the great efforts of Le Camus de Limare to establish naval copper manufacture at Romilly and his seduction of English workers, and of his problems in raising the necessary finance. He was now getting the equivalent of £40,000 from Rouen merchants who had been assured by British ironmasters that the Tools Act would be repealed. He gave details of the problems of Romilly where one pair of English rolls they were using had broken and been sent to be recast here, but had been trapped by the passing of the Tools Act.[43]

This evidence was apparently looked at in conjunction with the earlier Watt and Keir evidence on the Irish Resolutions which has been already referred to. This was resurrected and consulted again by the Birmingham group early in 1786. It had referred to the order and shipping of large rolls for copper sheathing in France; the making of such rolls was 'a work of considerable difficulty and has not been performed with success, except by certain workmen in Great Britain, as well on account of the superior properties of the Cast Iron of England for such purposes, as of the skill of the workmen'. We have thus knowledge of some of the evidence gathered by the metal manufacturers who fought a generally successful action against an extensive revision of the 1785 Act by the one of the following year, though we do not know exactly how it was used in the lobbying. Boulton and Garbett were among eight signatories of an advertisement from the Commercial Committee calling a hasty Birmingham meeting in July 1786 about the petitioning of Parliament against the repeal of the first Tool Act.[44]

The Eden Treaty only influenced those concerned with the transfer of technology to a marginal extent. Garbett reported Necker's opinion that a liberal trade treaty between England and France would have one justification as being a 'proper means of learning what foreign manufactures to Establish in France'. Some Frenchmen thought as did Boyetet and Dupont de Nemours, who promised to report to Necker's successor, Calonne, 'on the means to bring over to France foreigners with their industry and even their capital'. Under Calonne's administration there was an 'admiration of British technology and the determination to transplant and foster adoption of "ingenious machines", so that France could rival British production, permeated French preparations for the negotiations'.[45]

The idea that not only technology, but entrepreneurs and their capital, might easily move to France under the more liberal trading atmosphere of the Eden Treaty was not merely a dream of French statesmen, but a fear of some Englishmen.

> There is perhaps no danger arising from the Commercial Treaty more imminent than this – that a number of partnerships will be formed between Englishmen and Frenchmen, for the purpose of carrying on manufactures both in England and France. Thus, France will not only have the benefit of English capitals, but they will send young men apprentices into their houses to acquire the English arts; by which, in a few years, they will be able to transmit them to France.[46]

The French originally pressed the treaty issue on a reluctant British government under the terms of peace at the end of the American War, but once Eden and Vergennes made progress the potential gains to the progressive sectors of the British economy created a more constructive atmosphere. But the French applied some sticks as well as offering carrots. They tried to reduce the large British contraband trade into France. They made *arrêts* to enforce all prohibitions placed on the import of specific British products since as far back as 1687, particularly to include saddlery, knitted goods, cloth, hardware and polished steel. English imports had been injurious because of their attraction for those seeking 'fashion and fancy'. However, the well-to-do were allowed to have 'the liberty of satisfying their taste' by bringing in newly developed goods from abroad which they felt were of higher quality, but only by paying high duties. French shops were no longer to put signs on their premises like 'Magazin de Merchandise D'Angleterre'. However, the French had no wish to cut off their nose to spite their face – polished steel could come in as artisan tools and scientific instruments. Materials like wool and cotton and tin could also come in, and coal, English glue (which the French curiously could never equal), wool shears, and 'other tools and instruments useful in trade'. While some of the damage of this decree was quickly overcome by extra smuggling, it probably had an effect in hastening negotiations.[47]

The French did not only use the stick of import restrictions. Letters patent were issued in February 1786 which invited to France those foreign businessmen willing to set up there the manufacture 'of those kinds of goods whose import we have prohibited'. The Government would agree to their bringing in their tools and raw materials necessary to making such goods, allow them the same advantages they enjoyed in their own countries, and liberty to return home after a period of years. Goods whose producers would be particularly welcome included muslins, prints, cotton and woollen cloths and all kinds of hardware –

the concentration on attracting British immigrant entrepreneurs could hardly have been clearer. They were not expected to come unaccompanied, and not only they but the workers they brought with them were to be exempt from most taxes for three years, from others permanently. The relevant men would be excused entry dues to those guilds of merchants and workers which they were fitted to join, and all payments of duties on foreigners and their property, and they could buy and sell real estate.[48] The inclusion of workers and the specific targeting of English imports must have meant the French were cynically aware that they were inducing both British workmen and those who seduced them to break their country's laws by coming over.[49]

While the terms of the Eden Treaty were generally satisfactory to the cotton, hardware and pottery manufacturers, some industrialists in traditional trades found them less so, and quarrels and divisions occurred in the General Chamber of Manufacturers, which the Government found convenient, because it did not want to confront a powerful and united national industrial lobby. Once the Eden Treaty was signed on a basis very favourable to them there was equally a falling-off in interest in promoting particular industrial policies by the 'new' industrialists, for there was no major policy to urge. Garbett even found it almost impossible to get Birmingham manufacturers to leave their businesses to come to London to assist in listing classified hardware goods under the treaty once their battle on the main terms had been won. The slide of the General Chamber towards insignificance and demise from 1787 is important from our point of view in that opposition to suborning and export of equipment had been one of its main and agreed preoccupations. With its collapse for other reasons a potential national platform and influence was lost to those deeply opposed to the free export of technology.

Other examples will be given when we look at the attitudes of major industrialists towards worker emigration and machinery export – Wedgwood for instance led almost every move taken in the Potteries – but both before and after the General Chamber was available as a focus, the commercial committees or other formal or informal associations in the manufacturing districts continued to try to use vigilance and legal process against technology transfer. In 1781 there was cooperation between Manchester and Leeds, when a foreigner who had come with letters of recommendation to a leading Leeds merchant was found trying to export 'machines lately invented for the improvement of the woollen manufacture': the Leeds men informed the Manchester committee, who alerted the local manufacturers through the newspapers.[50] In 1784 a Mr Lunn of Lichfield was informed on by Reed Algood, who had been told by Rudge, a man Lunn had attempted to seduce, that he had been given his travelling expenses to Ostend, where he would be met by Lawrence Knot, a Birmingham japanner now in Amsterdam. Knot, Lunn and Rudge were to set up a japanning works in Holland. Rudge had left Birmingham to take ship, and had sent on half a ton of unspecified goods which were to be shipped with him. Garbett, as chairman of the Birmingham Commercial Committee, applied to the Home Office to have ships for Holland and Ostend searched as tools to manufacture japanned goods were thought to be involved, and Garbett had a helper who might be able to show where Rudge was staying.[51] A Stockport machine-maker, John Swindell, laid information in 1782 about Wilde, a schoolmaster of Mellor, who had been recruiting a large number of cotton workers, and even a 'common engine maker', which just possibly may mean an erector of Newcomen engines. Their hope was to go to America, even in wartime, and they had sent a negotiator over to see Benjamin Franklin in Paris. They were now about to go to Liverpool, whence they would go to Londonderry, and thence to America by a 'frigate', which may mean they would be picked up off the Irish coast by an American warship. The emigration was frustrated, but not without bad consequences for Swindell, who was ostracized and got into business difficulties.[52]

In 1787 the Birmingham Commercial Committee informed their fellow citizens that

> certain Foreigners, who are at private lodgings in this Town, frequent Public Houses, that they meet and drink freely with Manufacturers [clearly workmen in this context] and ... there is reason to believe that they attempt to persuade workmen that foreign Countries offer better means of Living and enjoy the Blessing of as much personal Freedom as in Old England.

The Commercial Committee would reward any person whose information led to a successful prosecution with the substantial sum of 50 guineas, and they would display 'proper Resentment' to any publicans who allowed foreigners to meet with workmen on their premises. They reprinted a long notice from the *London Gazette*, directed against the emigration of workers, and reciting the 1719 Act and the 1750 Act, and in a suffix mentioning the further legislation under George III, including the textile machinery Act of 1774, and the Tools Acts of 1785 and 1786. In the same year the committee entered a 'caution' in the press about a foreigner of unspecified nationality whom their London contacts had told them was coming to the town to obtain 'employment and instruction for which he will offer a handsome Premium'. They wanted to be told of every local instance of this kind of practice, so that they could protect the town's trade and stop all efforts to procure tools and seduce workmen abroad.[53]

The Manchester industrialists continued to be concerned by machinery export, but sometimes in two minds as to what was the best approach to the problem. In late 1794 the newly formed Manchester Commercial Society worried about the effect of the large current exports of cotton twist, fearing that experience of the quality of this yarn would excite foreigners to obtain the relevant machinery, but soon recognized that prohibition of export would itself inspire an even greater desire to have the relevant mechanism. As this was the machinery of the Arkwright system, and as it had reached France about a decade before, it was doubtful if anything very effective could be done. Perhaps the best was to try to inhibit emigration or machinery export, for the numbers of men able to erect, or teach the operation, of the machinery in France was yet small, and it could be helpful to slow down the export of the latest improvements.[54]

In 1798–99 the Manchester Commercial Society was prompted by intended prosecutions against men exporting machinery and 'inveigling mechanicks' to attempt to ally with the existing Society for the Prosecution of Felons to see whether they could concert action on this kind of prosecution. The partial breaking of the Bauwens conspiracy to obtain workers and machines was certainly the occasion for this alliance. All interested in the defence of the trade of the region were invited to meet on 15 January. In March a Committee for the General Protection of Trade, presumably a joint committee combining the interests of both societies, recorded its pleasure at the good attendance at the January meeting and emphasized the need to enforce the laws, and to raise funds in order to do so. The new body claimed to have been influential in the prosecution of Bauwens's associates Harding, Saul and Lammens. The trial of the last two had already taken place, with a year's imprisonment and a £500 fine each, and with the penalty of further imprisonment if the fine was not paid. Harding had been sent to Manchester by Bauwens as a knowledgeable cotton spinner to buy equipment for cotton spinning and calico-printing which was to be sent on to the export merchant Lammens for shipment abroad. The deception by Bauwens of the ten workers who did get through the net, in telling them that they were going to Hamburg when they were destined for France, was now known. Two men were already back home.

At the trial the judge, Lord Kenyon, had emphasized the importance of avoiding injury to the economic assets of the country at a time when it was engaged in a desperate war: 'The great resources of the country are our manufactures, and the general commerce of the kingdom. If these are to be invaded, and taken from us, – Alas, all is over'. The committee, having reported the outcome of the trial, emphasized the danger from 'wicked, misguided or deluded agents' used by foreign powers to further their industrial espionage in the British industrial regions, 'to pirate her ingenuity and manufactures'. Cotton-workers in every branch of the industry should be 'extremely cautious not to listen to offers, however specious or flattering' which could lead them into heavy punishments. The Acts establishing the criminal nature of workers' emigration and machinery export were finally cited, and a reward for information on such activities promised. There was a very heavy irony in these proceedings. One of the signatures of the members of the Committee which had put the advertisement in the press was that of William Douglas, who had barely ten years before offered to take a senior member of the French embassy round all his North Wales and Manchester works and show him everything without reservation, with a view to moving to France himself. Presumably his fellow signatories knew nothing about it.[55]

19 The Views of Great Industrialists

How did the most important industrialists, the ones we associate with the great advances in technique and scale in the latter part of the eighteenth century, react to the existence of widespread industrial espionage? Did they show a clear and consistent opposition to it? Were they hypocritical or at least grossly inconsistent, as we have seen William Douglas to have been? Were they indifferent to it? Were they self-interested, commercially-minded, and willing to help the foreigner to get British technology if there were something in it for them?

Steadfast in their pursuit of foreign spies, opposed to the export of equipment which might enable the foreigner to catch up on British technical advances, constantly on the *qui vive* about the dangers of the suborning of workers were Wedgwood and Garbett. Wedgwood was particularly important because of his pre-eminence in the pottery industry and the tendency of others in the industry to follow his lead. Like Garbett, Wedgwood was not committed to any purist, high moral ground view about industrial espionage: if there were foreign processes and technicians that would be valuable to us, it was commonsense for us to procure them by means fair or foul. There was a constant and natural, inveterate commercial competition between nations; industrial espionage was really a continuation of existing adversarial trade practices by other means. However, in this kind of warfare between nations patriotism was as much an essential element as in the overtly military kind, and it behoved all who had the national interest at heart, ministers, magistrates, merchants, industrialists, even workers, to join in frustrating the knavish tricks of technologically acquisitive foreigners.

Where of course normal diplomacy might be advantageous to the pottery interest, Wedgwood was happy to support it. There was a discussion between the British government and the French embassy in April 1773 on the grounds that there might be a free importation into France of 'faience de Wedgwood' – which must mean creamware and other popular Staffordshire products – in return for the free importation into Britain of some unspecified French goods.[1] Nothing came of this and the war intervened, but when negotiations for the commercial treaty of 1786 took place Wedgwood was among the stronger supporters, and of course the pottery interest was among the main gainers. But this did not in any way detract from his opposition to the transfer of British technology.

In 1783 he published *An Address to the Workmen in the Pottery, on the Subject of Entering into the Service of Foreign Manufacturers.*[2] He first referred to recent attempts by foreigners to seduce local pottery workers, and he argued that accepting such offers was not only against the national interest, but not as advantageous to the workers as it might seem. He believed that English potters received higher wages than those in other countries, while 'greater care is taken of the poor, when sick or past labour in England, than in any other part of the world', an interesting testimony to the old Poor Law. Nevertheless many workers had been tempted to go abroad from time to time, though usually 'of the looser kind', not easily satisfied at home. He said he would not recount the hard times emigrating workers had often experienced: 'it would look more like romance than real history'. He concentrated on two emigrations organized to the American colonies, to South Carolina and to Pennsylvania, with episodes of shipwreck, epidemic, failure of potteries, failure to pay agreed wages, harsh treatment and poverty. However true these accounts were, they were of course of legitimate migration to British colonies, and the workmen of the Staffordshire potteries would know that there had been long and successful emigration to America, and would not be readily intimidated. Perhaps Wedgwood was afraid that with the return of peace there might be renewed pressure to tempt workmen away to the new United States. In a sense there was perhaps small difference to him whether men went to the old colonies or the new nation; if they set up an efficient production of pottery in either it was likely to reduce the Staffordshire export market.

He then turned to the recent activities of George Shaw, who had left England for France about 1773, and had returned to recruit accompanied by a foreigner 'probably because his employers durst not trust him alone with the money necessary' for suborning. Shaw we have seen was

at the Montereau pottery imitating Wedgwood wares.[3] While Shaw
was offering men double the wages they received in England, Wedgwood argued that these wages, vastly higher than French ones, could
not be paid permanently, that the English workers would be required
to train apprentices, after which they would be dispensed with in
favour of cheap French labour. Wedgwood then did some scare-
mongering about the difficulties they would have in leaving France to
return home if they so wished, especially if they were in debt, the
iniquities of arbitrary government, including *lettres de cachet*, and the
strict border and port emigration controls. More realistically he went
into the problems of cultural acclimatization in a country with a different language and religion, very different from life at home, among
those 'brought up in the same habits of life as yourselves'. They would
also be despised as people who had deserted their own country and
helped to ruin its manufactures. Not merely would they have no support in illness and old age from the Poor Law, they would certainly
suffer from home sickness. If Wedgwood was aware of the pensions
commonly granted to emigrant English workers in France by employers or the state, he suppressed the knowledge. As for Shaw, he had
every reason to live abroad, he was a deserter from the army and must
fear punishment if taken, so his example in working abroad was a
misleading one.

But Wedgwood finally emphasized patriotism. Even if there were
some gain in money from working abroad,

> would it have no weight with you ... that you were ruining a trade
> which it had taken the united efforts of some thousands of people,
> over more than an age, to bring to the perfection it has now attained
> ... Englishmen, in arts and manufactures as well as in arms, can only
> be conquered by Englishmen

and 'the enemy must first gain over some traitors and renegadoes' to
gain a decisive advantage in manufactures. Just in case the words of
warning and patriotic duty had not made their mark, Wedgwood set
out in detail the provisions of the 1719 and 1750 Acts, and the penalties they carried. To offset the stick with a carrot, he offered a 50
guinea award, additional to any awards available under the relevant
Acts, for anyone providing information which would lead to the successful prosecution of a suborner.

In 1784 Wedgwood produced a policy paper on worker emigration.[4]
He advocated the further spread of Committees of Commerce into all
manufacturing counties, districts and large towns throughout Britain,

and regular communication between them on this particular issue, with annual or more frequent delegate meetings. This draft document has some sections scored through. One clause suggested that Parliament be approached to improve the laws so as to make the arresting of offenders easier, as at present it was nearly impossible to organize an arrest 'without giving the party sufficient time to escape'. But deletions make it seem that in fact, without fresh legislation, there were to be extra pressures on, and new instructions to, the revenue officers, particularly to searchers at ports, to look out for and apprehend emigrant workers. They should be returned to their parish of origin, with apprehending customs officers being rewarded. A clause proposed that the native parish pay for the removal home of emigrants who were caught through a special levy, one idea being that those parishioners paying the levy would be much more interested in preventing such unlawful emigration in the first place. This seems to have been abandoned, but other clauses provided for information on revenue officers at each port to be available to all Committees of Commerce, who should pass on relevant details to places as yet without committees, together with abstracts of the key legislation and information on the activities of existing committees.

However, prevention was better than cure, and the commercial committees should set up systems to obtain foreknowledge of attempts to emigrate, for instance offering rewards for strictly confidential information, and following this up by sending for intending emigrants and reproving them and warning them of the dangers if they persisted in their intentions, when they could be dealt with without compunction. Examples of legal action should be published and distributed among workmen, and unfortunate cases of workmen abroad should be made part of the propaganda of Committees of Commerce, whether in the local newspaper or – as we have seen done by Wedgwood – by distributing small pamphlets. Once it was known that workers had left their homes on a journey abroad there should be good intelligence of their intentions, and accurate descriptions sent to revenue officers and principal magistrates at all seaports. A final section of the document was crossed through and marked 'This was not intended to have been copied'. Perhaps its tenor was regarded as being too insensitive, too suggestive of the police state which Englishmen took pride in having avoided and condemned in the absolutist states on the wrong side of the Channel. It provided for descriptions of wanted men by age, complexion, height, tone of voice, any peculiarity of pronunciation, the foot length to be obtained from a shoemaker, other measurements from a tailor. A man's relations and connections should also be given so that a careful magistrate could ask some question about them in interrogation, 'an unguarded answer to which may haply be the means of identifying' the man sought.

Throughout the early 1780s Wedgwood was preoccupied by the problem of industrial espionage. As we shall see with Boulton, he found a problem when he was visited by distinguished foreigners who should be received with courtesy, and whose curiosity to see the most celebrated English industrial firms was probably innocent, though experience showed that there were more sinister instances. In 1784 Wedgwood wrote to Boulton to recommend to him a M. Genet who was to visit Birmingham on a tour of England. A corresponding member of the Academy of Sciences in Paris and highly regarded, Wedgwood knew Boulton would receive him so as 'To impress him with the most favourable sentiments of the hospitality and politeness of your countrymen'. He himself, nevertheless, would arrange that Genet

> shall not be introduced into any parts [of his works] that I deem to be essentially necessary to conceal from intelligent foreigners ... This is a jealousy which I have always thought the interest of my country required of me, though it has sometimes run counter to the inclination I have felt for a free and open communication with ingenious men of another nation.[5]

He obviously expected Boulton to have the same reservations.

In January 1784 Wedgwood wrote to Watt thanking him for his support of a 'little thing I wrote to my brethren in the pottery' on industrial espionage, which he felt was important enough to 'employ an abler pen'. The draft document described above is dated April 1784, so the 'little thing' preceded that. The *Address to the Workmen* is of 1783, and if printed late in the year may conceivably fit the bill, but Wedgwood's appeal to 'my brethren' strongly suggests a paper or printed pamphlet which went to other pottery manufacturers. There may thus have been a third item of limited circulation. At this point Wedgwood was advocating co-operation with government to improve the laws against industrial espionage, an idea which was abandoned in the course of writing the April document, but he was looking forward to the establishment of a national body of manufacturers such as was embodied in the General Chamber of the following year which could combine in preventing 'much of the evil of emigration'. Foreign rivals were now concentrating on suborning rather than competition. 'Our enemies are sapping the fortress they could not take by storm, and this last manoeuvre is, in my opinion, more dangerous than the first ... .' Later Watt wrote to Wedgwood about the visit of the Périer/de Wendel party to Birmingham, where some manufacturers had refused them admission to their works, and about their onward journey to Wilkinson and the ironworks. He did not think they would visit the Potteries, but 'you are warned that they are clever scientific people, and one of them Mr Périer an excellent mechanic'.[6]

In October 1785 Wedgwood wrote to the secretary of the new General Chamber of Manufacturers. He had just met with Watt and other Birmingham manufacturers at Lichfield, who told him of three different sets of spies currently active in the investigation of British machinery. He wanted the chamber to warn manufacturers generally about these 'dangerous guests' by newspaper advertisements and by letters in their correspondence with Lancashire, Yorkshire, and elsewhere. By doing this the chamber would be both protecting the manufacturing interest and strengthening its credit with it. Wedgwood believed the foreign espionage agents were becoming more daring and more persistent. Some of them 'exhibited the greatest show of impudence ever known upon like occasions'. Having met a clerk when trying to visit a works and being turned away by him, they had tried to re-enter when he was not about 'and almost forced their way to the machines they wanted to see'. In another case, having been turned away at one door they tried entering at another telling a different tale. In some cases they pretended to know of improvements to machines they wanted to spy on and so have opportunity to take drawings or obtain models. They were also crafty in going to well-meaning gentlemen to get introductions to local firms, without of course revealing their intentions to spy, or even persuading local gentry to accompany them to the works in the hope that in their company they would not be turned away.

Wedgwood felt that advertisements on this subject by the General Chamber had not been effective enough, that they should appear regularly and obtain a proper national coverage by being inserted in the principal provincial papers.[7] He had just been informed, however, seemingly while composing the letter, that a foreign spy had been taken ill and died at Manchester, and that his companion had been taken for questioning. While it might not be best to add this report to the new advertisement which Wedgwood sought to persuade Nicholson to publish, it might be put into the press as a news paragraph and 'have a good effect upon the other gentry of this kind now in England'.

Perhaps the most remarkable instance of action against foreign industrial spies in which Wedgwood was involved was that of the Dane, Ljungberg. Like a surprising proportion of the Scandinavians gathering industrial intelligence in eighteenth-century England, he was a professor.[8] His efforts were backed by the powerful minister of commerce and finance in Denmark, H. C. Schimmelmann, though he may have been operating on his own initiative for some of the time. Schimmelmann, in a highly complex career, had earlier worked for both the Saxon and Prussian governments during the Seven Years War, and had played a double-dealing part in the administration of the famous porcelain factory of Meissen in wartime and acquired a massive personal stock of porcelain which he sold at Hamburg. After joining the Danish government he had embarked on an ambitious programme of worker seduction from Meissen to Denmark.[9]

Ljungberg's travels in England were said to have taken place over sixteen years, and to have taken the form of three separate journeys, the last of which had itself taken two and a half years. He had earlier brought back drawings of spinning and carding machines and had made them available in both Sweden and Denmark. They aroused more interest in Denmark, where they were mounted in a large building outside Copenhagen, where ironically they were destroyed by the English bombardment of 1807. In 1778 a Danish cabinet instruction had ordered him to England, with a particular commission to investigate spinning-machinery. He was sent abroad again in 1784, on this occasion taking Aachen in his itinerary, where he was to try to recruit a manager for a cloth factory. There is thus no question of the official support, even direction, of Ljungberg's espionage, though he made much effort to seem the honest but curious scientific engineer, and lived openly for much of the time. Boulton wrote:

> I know Mr. Ljungberg very well and I know him to be a very ingenious man and a good chymist. He lived at Birmingham about a year, and was esteemed for his ingenuity, modesty and Gentleman-like behaviour but we all suspected he was employed by the Court of Denmark, to collect such knowledge in this country as might be useful in that.

Boulton had actually given him a letter of introduction to Wedgwood![10]

Ljungberg was arrested in London when the Customs searched his baggage as he was leaving England. Thomas Byerley, Wedgwood's nephew and agent, wrote to Boulton on 21 August 1789 that drawings of machines, tools, and specimens of manufactures had been found, and that the tools export was now contrary to the recent Act. Relevant manufacturers would be approached to see if the drawings and samples should be allowed to be exported.[11] It was some time before Ljungberg was firmly identified as the man who had been bribing workmen to give him drawings of kilns at Wedgwood's works and collecting samples of clays and other raw materials.[12] Wedgwood knew that he had investigated other industries than pottery, and 'has taken drawings of our machinery and manufactures from Cornwall to Yorkshire'.[13] It was a few months later that Byerley was able to tell a meeting of the Committee of Potters, held at Etruria with Wedgwood in the chair, of the correspondence Neale, Spode and he had with the various committees of manufacturers in other parts of the country about the seizure of tools and other articles which Ljungberg had collected in Britain and had tried to export to create industries abroad.

Included with the tools and materials were extensive manuscripts, and it seemed very important that these should be translated to see what they contained. While the Customs had no objection, they were the perfect model of bureaucracy. They insisted that the books be examined at the Customs House 'during office hours, under the inspection of an officer, and at the expense of those who desire it'. To comply, it was proposed that a committee from the various interested groups of British manufacturers should meet in London to make proper arrangements. The business rolled rather slowly on; it was July before it was reported to another meeting of the potters' committee by their chairman, Wedgwood, that a group of industrialists had underwritten the cost of translating Ljungberg's manuscripts, including the firms of Wedgwood, Sons and Byerley, Matthew Boulton, William Parker and Son (flint-glass makers of London); Crawshay, Son and Thompson, Jukes, Coulson (the London founders and engineers) and two more potters, Neale and Spode. They sought the formal support of the potters' committee for the translation and the formation of a committee of subscribers to effect it. Byerley and Neale had been permitted to look at the materials Ljundberg had collected, specimens of the different earthenwares made in England (not very sinister), but also experimental specimens of cobalt and manganese and other minerals, and the fine cloths used for sieving in the Potteries, a collection to 'convey information to other manufactories abroad'.

There was a large bound volume in Danish or German, full of drawings of 'machines and engines', some made in the Potteries, but others from Cornwall, Birmingham, Coalbrookdale, Derby, Manchester,

Leeds, Matlock, Nottingham, and elsewhere, some dated as long ago as 1775. The commissioners would destroy all articles which the British manufacturers did not wish to see exported. The potters were now sure that Ljungberg was the man who had been spying in their area some months before, and bribing workmen to get kiln measurements. However, the committee appointed to arrange the translation of the manuscript book found that industrialists in some towns thought that Ljungberg's collection of material might have been made 'merely for the amusement of a traveller', and were not greatly interested because their own towns had not been visited by him, but the committee urged on them the importance of 'making a common cause of all matters of this nature which relate to manufacturers or manufactories'. In the present case it was obvious that a youngish man without any personal fortune could never have lived in England in some style for years 'merely for his amusement'.[14]

On the Danish side their embassy informed their government in code about Ljungberg's arrest and there was a correspondence between him and the embassy and the British government of a very 'inspired' nature, intended to show his innocence and the unimportance of the material in the packing-cases seized when ready for export, and Ljungberg said he had believed that they did not infringe British law. There is some confusion about the outcome. The Danish embassy paid £300 to get Ljungberg out of gaol on bail, when as all concerned would have expected, he fled the country. This no doubt suited both the Danish and British governments, which seem to have wished to diminish a difficult diplomatic incident. As was provided for under the legislation, part at least of Ljungberg's effects was auctioned off by the Customs, and much was bought on behalf of the Danish embassy.

Certainly cases and documents reached Denmark, and were received by Schimmelmann and another prominent member of the Government, J. L. Reventlow. However Ljungberg, once back at the College of Commerce, not only petitioned the king for £300 for the travelling and other expenses incurred in England, but for the cost of models and technical drawings he had lost in London, and this may have amounted to three-quarters of his property there. Archival gaps mean there is no clear evidence of the effect his espionage may have had on the development of the Royal Copenhagen Pottery, there were already some Danish potteries producing a decent Queen's Ware, if not seriously rivalling British.[15] The outstanding feature of the investigation of the Ljungberg affair and the pressure put on the Customs to act is the influence of the potters led by Wedgwood, and the work of his nephew, agent and partner Thomas Byerley as intermediary.

As consistent as Wedgwood in his opposition to industrial espionage was Samuel Garbett. Said originally to have been a Birmingham brassworker, he became agent to a London merchant house, and his influence grew rapidly thereafter. He was perhaps equally important as Boulton in securing an Assay Office for Birmingham, he was influential in the foundation of the General Hospital, and he led the anti-slavery movement in Birmingham as well as chairing the Commercial Committee as we have seen. On a national plane, he and his son made an enquiry into the Mint, but it was not published for decades. Technologically Garbett's main claim to fame is his development of the lead chamber process for the production of sulphuric acid on a large scale, in which his partner was Dr John Roebuck, who had trained at Edinburgh and Leyden. Originally the partners had operated in Birmingham as chemical consultants and refiners and recoverers of precious metals. They went on to develop the great acid works at Prestonpans in Scotland, and from this they made an even more dramatic investment, being two of the partnership which set up the great Carron Iron Company in 1760. That company played a leading part in the development of coke-iron making north of the border, and this involved the creation of a famous iron-founding business.

Charles Gascoigne joined the firm in its early years, and quickly became a key figure. Of a Yorkshire gentry family, Gascoigne had worked for the East India Company, but met Garbett in the late 1750s, greatly impressed him, and married his daughter in 1759. He undoubtedly was a man of great charm, persuasiveness and speciousness. He became a shareholder in Carron, and a personal assistant to Garbett there. Once in place he determined on complete control, and this involved ousting, cuckoo-in-the-nest fashion, the original partners, including his father-in-law. Roebuck was an inveterate speculator and made heavy investments in the Kinneil colliery, in the course of which he became Watt's patron, partly on the basis that the engine Watt was developing might solve the severe drainage problems. His long-threatened insolvency led to various covert transactions by which he transferred the ownership of their Birmingham business to Garbett, and sold Carron shares to the Garbett family and Gascoigne. In 1773, as we have seen, he sold his right in the Watt steam-engine to Boulton, and he was effectively in the hands of his creditors until his death in 1794.

Under Gascoigne's management the affairs of Carron Company became 'infinitely complicated', and it was in continuous trouble after the Scottish banking crisis of 1772. Garbett was subsequently in financial difficulty until 1782 when he became bankrupt. He had put his Carron shares in trust in 1772 and from 1776 was permanently at loggerheads with Gascoigne. Highly respected in Birmingham, his creditors, headed by Matthew Boulton, let him re-establish himself in acid manufacture and precious metal refining there, and he died at a great age in 1803, leaving the considerable sum of £12,000. But Gascoigne, after tangling Carron's affairs almost inextricably, had gone bankrupt himself, and after long intrigues with Russia involving the export of technology by sending both workers and machinery, went there himself in 1786, became manufacturer of ordnance to Catherine the Great, and died wealthy, having lived 'in splendour'.[16]

This short account of Garbett's long and eventful career has been necessary to explain the nature of his business interests and his strong campaign to prevent technology export, and particularly to Russia. He, like Wedgwood, regarded intelligence and espionage as a normal part of international commercial competition. He simply wished to ensure that his own country came out on top. In 1764 he reported that his son was going to the Low Countries to examine the methods of the main ironworks there, and to France. In the previous year he had been in Norway and Sweden, 'and made some important discoveries which have already been carried into practice and will prove a national advantage'. Next year he would tour iron and steel works in Germany. This he clearly regarded as fair game. For the Swedes in particular were hunting both important entrepreneurs and workmen in Birmingham, and his son had met two English workmen in Stockholm, though they were dissatisfied and probably returning.[17] In 1766 he again appears in Home Office papers, proposing the seizure of an English workman returning from Gothenburg. A little later in the year, and referring to several different problems, Garbett wrote to William Burke bemoaning 'the various encroachments that are making in various ways by foreigners on our manufactures' and 'the little, the very little, attention given by administration to support our manufactures'.[18]

Garbett and Roebuck believed that secrecy was the best method of protecting new technology and invention, and in the case of the lead chamber process they relied on it for twenty years. Joseph Black, the famous chemist, first patron of Watt, and a close friend of Roebuck, told an enquirer that Roebuck 'never dropped the smallest hint to me upon the subject, and I know they are at great pains to keep it a secret as being a very lucrative business. I never presumed to show any curiosity with regard to it'. Needless to say they were not able to stop all leaks, and men who were sacked from the Birmingham or Prestonpans works, or were bribed away, spread the process, and as a reaction in 1771 the partners took out a patent. They were unable to sustain it in the courts, however, an obvious weakness being that they had been employing the process commercially for twenty years.[19]

During the later 1770s there is less evidence for Garbett's campaign against industrial espionage; perhaps the complications and difficulties of his business affairs entirely engrossed him. In the mid-1780s, once he had re-established his business affairs after his bankruptcy of 1782, his campaign was revived, but now, as we have seen, mainly through his role as chairman of the Birmingham Commercial Committee. In 1785 he was, however, concerned in his private capacity about Robert Hickman, the substantial Birmingham manufacturer who had gone to Vienna, and was now working hard to get artisans to join him there. While it was known from an affidavit made by the man himself that the 'ingenious artist' Thomas Bennet had been offered a £500 bribe, £100 a year for the lives of his wife and himself, and a house worth £40 a year, Garbett found himself frustrated because 'the offers were made so artfully that we could not proceed with effect'.[20] In the August of the following year he was writing to Boulton about main articles of the Birmingham 'toy' trade now being made in Russia, and about an eminent Sheffield plate-maker who had left for Paris. Though he was daily informed of suspicions about workers preparing to go abroad, he was despondent about any action from Pitt or the Board of Trade after their failure to respond to representations from Boulton and himself, and he advocated the organization of a lobby of the nobility and principal gentry, presumably those of the West Midlands, to wait upon Pitt.[21]

Despite increasing age Garbett continued to act as chairman of the Commercial Committee until 1790, when a quarrel about sword-making in Birmingham became extremely acrimonious, and effectively split the committee, Boulton taking over the chair for a time. It was less active thereafter, becoming the Commercial Society in 1795, and was virtually moribund by 1798. Garbett apparently refused to hand over the Commercial Committee minute book, which explains how we have to rely on newspaper advertisements and insertions to gather the committee's policies. By the time of his resignation some members were apparently unhappy about his continued obsession with artisan emigration.

That obsession was fuelled by his long-running arguments with Gascoigne, who, once facing inevitable bankruptcy himself, and aware that he could never restore his fortunes in Britain, began to organize a new career for himself in Russia, where, as we have mentioned, he was very successful. To be effective there he needed to send over not only skilled workmen, but some heavy engineering items, like rolls and boring machines. He tried to draw a veil of concealment and trickery between himself and his fellow partners at Carron, blurring the distinction between cannon export, nearly always permitted in peacetime, and regarded as a useful export of a product embodying high-quality British technology, and that of the equipment for cannon-making, which would tend to make Russia independent of British suppliers. Some export items of course would be legal: Carron had already supplied steam-engines to Russia, and iron equipment for blast furnaces (like blowing cylinders and iron pipes) does not seem to be included in any legislation. It may well be Garbett's influence with the Birmingham Commercial Committee which had cannon-making equipment clearly marked out as an illegal export in the revised Tools Act of 1786.

Gascoigne first put the argument to Carron Company that if they did not supply Russia with the equipment others would, and Carron would not receive further Russian orders.[22] He subsequently admitted that he had infringed the law, but convinced the Lord Advocate in Scotland that he had been ignorant of the illegality of his activities. However, Gascoigne managed to persuade Pitt that it would not be illegal for him to go over to Russia, temporarily, to supervise ordnance production, and he tried to persuade his partners at Carron that the Russians would only order from them the machinery and equipment that the law allowed, and not seek to attract artificers. The firm allowed him to go to Russia, as he claimed for some months, but he never returned, and proceeded to try to attract skilled men over to join him, as had been anticipated by Garbett; 'that our workmen are easily seduced abroad is not necessary to prove; it is alas! too well known ... the same inducements which carry Gascoigne from Britain will draw such Workmen after him as he may choose to have'.[23]

During the last stages of the disputes within the Carron Company Gascoigne was held for a short time on the charges brought by Garbett of attempting to send abroad tools and workmen covered by the Tools Act. But the Lord Advocate was sympathetic to him, and put pressure on Garbett and Boulton not to oppose his release, presumably on the basis that he had undertaken not to repeat his offences. Gascoigne was

obviously a master of charm and the manifestation of specious innocence.[24] Garbett felt that there was a perverse consequence of his giving
information on Gascoigne. 'I now see I am to be thought ill of by Mr.
Pitt in this Business.' Despite all he had suffered from Gascoigne, even
Garbett felt the attractiveness of his personality: 'I have always had a
personal attachment to Gascoigne, I am almost ashamed to say that I
still have ... when I can keep my thoughts from his Base Conduct. But
it is that sort of Affection that Fathers have for a very culpable and
peevish Child'.[25]

Interestingly Garbett bracketed John Wilkinson with Gascoigne in
his condemnation – he would have known of the Wilkinsons' involvement with Indret and Le Creusot.[26] He may not have known, however,
that several attempts had been made to entice Watt to Russia in the
1770s, in part because of his acquaintance with iron and cannon
production at Carron, and were finally turned down 'by a hair's
breadth'.[27] Important as was Gascoigne, his emigration was accompanied by others from Carron, particularly Charles and James Baird.
Both, and especially Charles, were to be immensely important in Russian metallurgical industry, Charles being the first major steam-engine
manufacturer in Russia.[28] Gascoigne was of gentry background, while
the Bairds' father had been superintendent of the Forth and Clyde
Canal, so they could not be thought of as workmen, and there was
never any suggestion that the 1719 or later Acts should apply to the
emigration of the gentry or professional classes. Four of the moulders
recruited by Gascoigne, however, were caught and taken off a ship
bound for Russia, and the suborner acting for Gascoigne was prosecuted, but other craftsmen got through and joined him.[29]

The attitude of Boulton to foreign industrial espionage is, to say the
least of it, equivocal. This can be regarded as a matter of indecision or
confusion, or as reaction to different kinds of espionage in different
ways, as befitted their relevance or seriousness.[30] There can, however,
be a sharper verdict, that he was on several occasions guilty of unmiti-
gated hypocrisy, and that his conduct was governed by no higher
motives than the obtaining of a profit and the protection of his own
interests.

A notable inconsistency lies in his backing the move for a prohibition of the export of buckle chapes made in the Birmingham hardware
district, supposedly in the interests of maintaining the hard-won predominance of the region's goods on foreign markets. This was put
forward on the basis that the manufacture and export of buckles was

being held back by the high price of chapes and the difficulty of getting them, that this was the result of a combination among the chape-makers, and that buckle rings were on stock in large numbers, unable to be exported for want of chapes. The final product was thus the result of the work of two quite separate trades, the chapes being made from the output of local iron, which, if inferior to some European irons for some purposes, was superior for this. It was put through slitting-mills, and then forged and filed. A large part of the production was not in Birmingham, but in the adjacent hardware district, later known as the Black Country. Buckles were produced largely in Birmingham itself, mainly of non-ferrous metals and their alloys, often silver plated or gilded, and increasingly of polished steel. Boulton in particular was developing buckles inlaid with glass in imitation of jewellery.

Essentially this was an inter-industry squabble, and as there was little proof of the supposed cartel among chape-makers, there seems to have been a strong desire for dominance by the buckle-makers. Boulton's biographer, usually very generous to his subject, condemns him here: 'It is difficult to imagine a more impudent attempt on the part of one branch of a trade to try and restrict another branch from doing exactly what the first was doing ... [so as] ... to cream off the lion's share of the profit'.[31] While very different views of the ease or difficulty of copying our chapes abroad were advanced to the Commons Commit-tee which considered the matter, subsequent events show that our superiority continued. One cogent argument against the buckle-makers and exporters was that if chape exports were actually prohibited it would 'be an Encouragement to the Workmen to go abroad'.[32]

Dickinson hoped 'that Boulton lived to regret the illiberal part he had played in promoting the Bill'. In fact, with a perfect hypocrisy, we find him doing some years later exactly what he had tried to stop others doing in 1760. In 1781 Joseph Alcock, the elder son of the Birmingham manufacturer who had so notoriously defected to France, was with his younger brother running a Birmingham 'toy' manufacture at Roanne. We have seen that he had visited Birmingham in the late 1770s, had met Boulton and had recommended the Watt engine to the French government. He now ordered a large quantity of buckle chapes from Boulton.[33] In 1767, when Watt first met Boulton, he said that Boulton was making buckle chapes himself, in which he had made 'some ingenious improvements', but, as with so many of Boulton's ventures, it had not persisted.[34] However, he assured Alcock that as merchants 'we ever did and will continue to serve our friends' on the best terms, and he had put the work out to contract, though where Alcock had insisted on maximum prices for types of chape, the quality might have to be adjusted. Boulton would ship the chapes to Ostend. This was an interesting transaction; not only was Boulton completely contravening the policy of non-export of chapes he had advocated in 1760, he was helping an English émigré firm in France to make buckles better than their compatriots could make them, and therefore enabling them to compete better with English buckle exports. Of course in 1781 this was a trade carried out in wartime, involving smuggling through a neutral country, and of an article commonly prohibited by the French in any case, so Alcock was breaking his adopted country's laws; the ease of evasion is conveyed by the insurance of a mere 31*s.* 6*d.* per £100 value.[35] In 1780 there had been a proposal from Michael Alcock junior that he should open a shop in Paris to sell certain kinds of Boulton's more up-market products.[36]

The opposition of Boulton to foreign penetration of the techniques and secrets of British industry is distinctly equivocal. Ostensibly he was sternly against it, and Garbett, as we have seen, tried to use him as an ally in his anti-espionage campaigns, and so did Wedgwood. Occasionally it is Watt who writes to their fellow industrialists, mainly in the Midlands, to warn them of the presence of potentially dangerous foreigners in their neighbourhoods. This may be because as the owner of the outstanding intellectual property of the age, the improved steam-engine, he was very anxious about foreign steam-engine pirates, just as he was about British ones, and therefore likely, in his own interest, to sound the tocsin. Possibly it may sometimes be because his senior partner, Boulton, had requested he write the warning letters when Boulton himself was reluctant to do so for some reason. In 1767 Francis Garbett had requested Boulton's support in the prosecution of a worker bound for Vienna, and conveyed Shelburne's promise that if he did so the Government would foot the bill. But Boulton squirmed out of it; he protested too much about pressure of business, difficulty of coming to London, and the costs of the proceedings, despite Shelburne's assurance on the last point. He had some ulterior motive for failing to prosecute which he would not divulge.

In 1775 it was Boulton and Watt who recommended de la Houlière to John Wilkinson[37] with the most important results for the French iron industry and their naval munitions programme. Before he left Britain de la Houlière understandably wrote a fervent and sincere letter of thanks to Boulton. Not only had John Wilkinson shown him his

Broseley (New Willey) works and toured with him the Coalbrookdale district, but he had sent him on with a recommendation to his brother and partner William at Bersham. While de la Houlière does not spell it out in his letter, it was there that he had recruited William for French service, which led to the founding of Indret and Le Creusot. The French ambassador also seems to have visited Soho about this time, possibly with de la Houlière. The latter writes in the same letter that the Comte de Guines, when Boulton was next in London, would show him how he was carried away with admiration, just as de la Houlière was, with everything that could be seen 'chez vous' (i.e. at Soho) and the ideas that animated his researches and everything that he did.[38] If de Guines did accompany de la Houlière, this could be a good example of Boulton's vulnerability in terms of industrial intelligence where the most important foreign nobility and officials were concerned. He was straining every nerve to spread the fame and admiration of his highest range of products, for instance *ormoulu*, silver and silver plate, and ornamental vases. He based his reputation on them rather than on the more ordinary products of the Soho Manufactory, but in his eventually doomed efforts to make them pay he tried to bring them to the attention of the influential of every nation who were willing to visit Soho.

Inevitably there were among these distinguished visitors some with knowledge which could enable them to report usefully back home on the technological advances embodied in what they had seen, especially about the steam-engine. However, there were limits here; while Watt carried out experiments and trials at Birmingham, and some smaller high-quality parts were made there, the firm's manufacture of complete engines only began from 1796, once the Soho Foundry was in full operation. Both Boulton and Watt were regarded as worthy members of the scientific community, they and James Keir, partner with them in several ventures, were elected Fellows of the Royal Society in 1785. Watt's engine was regarded as a scientific marvel throughout Europe. Consequently they found it difficult to refuse foreigners of a genuine scientific repute the right to visit their premises; indeed they well deserved the right to bask in the glow of their European reputation. But they could not always count on the probity of their scientific visitors either at Soho or at other places where their engines were to be seen, particularly, during their brief life, the extremely prominent and accessible Albion Mills in London.[39] Robinson puts it in a nutshell: 'Internationalism in science could conflict with patriotic duty or self-interest'.[40] At Albion Mills, as we have seen, two members of the Académie des

Sciences, Coulomb and Betancourt, both separately and flagrantly spied, the former under Boulton's nose. Boulton and Watt's greatest error was in finally putting trust in Périer, after several misgivings, as the introducer of their engine into France. It may be speculated that Boulton's constant preoccupation with power made Périer seem the best instrument for promoting the Boulton and Watt engine in France because of his high favour with the house of Orléans and key position in the Paris waterworks company. But from the beginning Périer had no intention of helping to completion, or in the least respecting, their provisional French privilege; he wanted to build Watt engines himself without restriction, and as soon as Betancourt had told him of the double-acting engine he was ready to build that too, without any reference to Boulton and Watt.

One of the most celebrated attempts at espionage on the Watt engine was that of the celebrated Baron Stein. To be famously associated with Hardenberg in the Prussian reforms of the early nineteenth century, Stein had been appointed the director of mines in Prussia's western provinces in 1784 and had embarked on plans for the improvement of the mines of the Ruhr. He had as a technical colleague Eversmann, who had himself been in England during 1784–85 to study the metal-working industries. In 1786–87 Stein himself made a 'mineralogical and technical journey' to England to examine industrial sites. He seems at one point to have proposed ordering a small engine from Boulton and Watt, but the order was cancelled. He got in touch with R. E. Raspe, a German savant and scientist whose early career in Germany had been marked by spectacular numismatic scandals, but who had finally settled in Cornwall as a mineralogist, prospector, and assay master. His lasting fame is as 'translator' of the *Travels of Baron Munchausen*.[41] Raspe knew Boulton, however, and gave him full warning of Stein's intentions of coming to Cornwall, and of his current activities. He thought Stein's order for an engine was just a cover to find out the latest information on the Watt engine. He pointed out that the Prussian government had already been trying to erect a Watt engine, information on which had been obtained by espionage by a man called Buckling, but the engine was proving costly and inefficient. That Stein's likely purpose was espionage was apparent from his bringing with him an 'engineer and modeller', Friederich, who was an expert draughtsman, and Raspe had seen drawings he had made of Watt's latest improvements including rotative motion. Raspe with his usual cunning believed that the best revenge on Stein would be to seduce his young engineer away from him, which Raspe himself was willing to do! 'In other respects Baron Stein is a well-bred, sensible and excellent young Nobleman – If he thinks it a liberal exertion of Patriotism to enrich his Country with useful knowledge in a sly, backstair way, he cannot possibly have an objection to ours if possibly we can turn the tables on him ... '.

Stein's drawings had been made for him at London breweries which used Boulton and Watt engines. There followed a correspondence in which Stein seems to have tried to involve Sir Joseph Banks, the President of the Royal Society, as a mollifying intermediary. Stein drew up a memorial in February 1787 in which he claimed he had tried to get engine drawings to learn if the Watt engine would be worth ordering to implement plans he had in mind. His memorial was specious but quite unconvincing, and showed that, after some disappointments elsewhere in London, he had gained access to the Barclay and Perkins brewery engine. Having got in when most of the men were away at dinner, he was not able to get the information he wanted. He was then referred to a Boulton and Watt employee, Cartwright, who asked for time and money to show an engine and provide information. He pulled the rug very skilfully from under Stein, got hold of the drawings he already had under pretence of rectifying them, took 2 guineas off him and then went straight to Boulton and Watt who happened to be in London. Stein had not only tried to get Cartwright to take him to see Watt engines in Staffordshire and Cornwall, but, according to Cartwright's own statement, had tried to persuade him to go abroad. Even when Stein knew that Boulton and Watt were in London, he made another attempt to see the Barclay and Perkins engine: 'a great deal of it's Effects depends on the perfection of the Work, which could never be so well made by other Workmen' than Boulton and Watt's experienced men.

Boulton in a paper, 'Facts relative to Baron Stein', pointed out that Stein's was the second Prussian attempt at espionage on his engines. He recounted the Buckling episode, Buckling being 'Councelor of Mines of his Prussian Majesty'. He with another Prussian emissary had tried in 1779 to bribe Cartwright, then engaged in erecting the Chelsea waterworks engine, but unsuccessfully. (Clearly there had not been liaison between the two Prussian spying expeditions, or Stein would have kept clear of Cartwright.) The Buckling party then played the other tack and went directly to Soho – one of them assuming a title in order to ensure a reception, perhaps well informed that Boulton loved a lord. But he was away. Watt, however, showed them Soho, and then took them to see one of the canal pumping engines at work, dined them, and showed 'such other particulars as were necessary to Gratify the Curiosity of Gentlemen travelling for amusement'. Next day, however, they returned to Soho in Watt's absence and bribed workmen to dismount an engine so they could see the main parts. Buckling returned to Germany and tried to erect an engine, but despite boasts in European journals that he had gained the secrets of Watt's engines, made a very bad one. He had to come back, inspected Watt engines in Cornwall, had part models made, and after many different attempts did get a workman, but a very poor one, to go back to Prussia.

Banks sent on Stein's 'Memorial' to Boulton, who wrote back, largely destroying the Baron's case on the basis that he was trying to get covert information from workmen when he knew well that Boulton and Watt were in London, and had been surprised while spying on the Barclay engine on a Sunday morning. Boulton said he would not have bothered had he been on his own, 'but finding him with two assistants making their attacks with Bribery and Blacklead pencil' serious espionage was inescapable and had to be opposed. He showed Stein's operation was closely comparable with one by the Duke of Aremburg[42] who in 1782 had sent a man called Fastor to see Boulton who had been very helpful to him, entertaining him at Soho House, and showing him not only a small engine at Soho but large ones in Shropshire. He was repaid by Aremburg having Fastor make a Watt engine at one of his mines and, like Buckling, boast of it in the European press. Again, however, the engine had not worked properly, and Fastor came back to England 'to correct his errors', but the outcome was unknown. 'If I have anything to reproach myself of in my conduct towards Strangers', Boulton wrote to Banks, 'it is in my having been too liberal in showing those things which my duty to my Country and myself required more reservation in.'

To Stein he wrote that having now received a formal enquiry from him about an engine for a saltworks, his first demand was for an exclusive privilege for the Watt engine in Prussia, like the one in France, which in the immediate aftermath of their 1786–87 visit to France Boulton and Watt now believed would be honoured. If Prussia gave such privileges to inventors, Stein could see and negotiate with Watt, now in London. Despite the recent rather disagreeable passage between them, Boulton was willing to advise Stein on a prospective visit to Cornwall. 'If I can promote your views as a Natural Philosopher, as a Mineralogist, or as a Gentleman, I shall be happy. But as a Mechanick and an Engineer you must pardon me if I throw Obstructions in your Way'.[43] That there was something very equivocal in Boulton's attitude to Stein is implied in his remarks to Banks that he had considered calling on Stein to reproach him for his conduct, and tell him that by trying to seduce English workmen he was liable to a £500 fine and imprisonment. But as on other occasions when he did not intend doing what he claimed to be proposing to do, Boulton advanced pressure of business as the reason for not calling on Stein. Remarkably, Stein was subsequently welcomed at Soho.[44] Perhaps Boulton carefully avoided any outright quarrel with Stein as long as there was a possibility of negotiating for a monopoly privilege in Prussia with this rising official and luminary of that state.

Boulton, like Garbett and Wedgwood, while he might sometimes fulminate against, and normally oppose, foreign attempts to get British artisans and equipment, was entirely without reservations himself when it came to obtaining men and tools abroad. This has been very well described by Eric Robinson.[45] He shows that some foreign firms shared with him a rather relaxed attitude about technological theft. One firm from Pforzheim wrote that they bore him no ill will for persecuting them in their espionage in Britain; he was patriotic in attacking them, they were patriotic in trying to take the Birmingham hardware manufacture to their country.

Boulton and Fothergill had two secret foreign partners, John Friedrich Bargum, a Dane, a founder of the Danish Guinea Company, and John Herman Ebbinghaus, a German hardware merchant of Iserlohn, and this gave opportunity for the sharing of trade secrets when appropriate. When Boulton first tried to break into the *ormoulu* trade he turned to Solomen Hymen, a Paris merchant, and tentatively requested him to get some suitable workers, if his principles allowed. He was less hesitantly applied to for a top-quality silversmith and for tools for gold-lace making. Boulton employed a French gilder at Soho, and asked for his father's help in getting tools. A Brussels correspondent bought a lathe for Boulton, an Amsterdam man provided brazier's tools. Boulton used Raspe to search out good engravers in Vienna, Hanau, Berlin and Sweden, and at least one other foreign national helped him in the search. For a time he was able to employ engravers of European distinction, Droz and Kuchler. In 1771 he employed five expert French craftsmen, and other leaders in the Birmingham 'toy' trade, including the most famous, John Taylor, also had highly paid French employees. Boulton picked up one foreign worker indirectly; Kern, a Saxon jeweller, expert at inlaying steel with gold and silver, had been recruited by Orsel, the French merchant and manufacturer in Birmingham, but his bad treatment of the man, paralleled by his later treatment of English workers when he returned to France, saw Kern defect to Boulton and Fothergill. The French and German-run drawing schools in Birmingham may have been primarily established to enable Birmingham manufacturers to produce their fancier and more artistic goods to suit continental tastes, but they must also have been useful cover both for Birmingham men trying to recruit foreign workmen, and for the seduction of English workmen by the agency of foreign drawing masters.[46]

Robinson, as mentioned earlier, believes that Watt had been very seriously tempted to emigrate to Russia. Despite his apparent fierceness against the emigration of British workers (and sometimes, as with Gascoigne, entrepreneurs) Boulton very seriously considered emigrating to Sweden. In 1763 – before he and Boulton had become close friends – Garbett reported to the Home Office that Boulton had been made a very tempting offer by a Swedish Intendant of Commerce. Robinson shows that the intendant was John Westermann, and he visited Soho with the Swedish industrial observer John Alströmer. Both had been recruiting English workers for Sweden, perhaps including those about whom Garbett was agitated.[47] In his master's absence, Farquharson, Garbett's clerk, tried to calm government fears by pointing to Boulton's huge investment in the Soho manufactory, but there seems to have been a persistent attempt by Dr Solander, the Swedish scientist in England (who became secretary and librarian to Sir Joseph Banks, and one of the experts taking part in Cook's voyages in the *Endeavour*), to make contact with Boulton.[48] The authorities had been told of a new Swedish drive, like that of the previous year, to get English workers, and that Solander was involved in negotiations. They wrote to Roebuck in strict secrecy to make enquiries. It was rumoured that Solander had been in Birmingham 'with proposals to one Boulton, whom the Swedes are very desirous of engaging to settle amongst them'. There was even the suggestion that Boulton might be proceeded against under the 1719 Act, but this supposes that the officials concerned knew very little about him at this date, a businessman of his importance would not have been prosecuted for emigration. However, if he had seduced workmen to accompany him it was then possible, and as we shall see this was not out of the question.

Farquharson, in the absence of Garbett and Roebuck in Scotland, wrote that Solander had not been in Birmingham in the last year, and that it was inconceivable that Boulton, now making additions worth £2,000 to the plant at Soho, on which he had already spent £4,000, and having taken Fothergill as partner in the last two years, would be thinking of leaving the town.[49] A little later Farquharson[50] wrote confirming that Boulton was not for Sweden, 'though he has had very advantageous offers made him. On the contrary he would spare no expense to detect any scheme of that kind, which he considers so prejudicial to his country'. Boulton had recently heard from Solander, but had declined having anything to do with him; he claimed that four earlier letters Solander had written him had not been received. This is a little suspicious, for Boulton said on several occasions that embarrassing or potentially difficult letters had failed to reach him.

So apparently we have a pointless scare, a storm in a teacup, a story with no foundation. But Eric Robinson has shown that things were not so simple. Westermann had written to Boulton from Cologne in the autumn of 1763. He wrote in French as a matter of security, no doubt to prevent any clerk in Boulton's office from reading the letter. The letter indicates that the approach about emigration had been from Boulton to Westermann, not the other way round. It said that Boulton had already given the intendant to understand 'That you were virtually committed to set yourself up in some foreign country', providing he could find the convenient resources to carry on a manufacture like that at Soho. The terms Westermann offered Boulton included £500 for travelling expenses for himself *and his workmen*, £1,500 for the cost of a water-wheel and for tools, a generous bounty on exports, and a rich partner. But all depended on Boulton bringing a sufficient and well selected group of workmen. The Swedish government confirmed these terms at the end of 1763. It is impossible that the discussion would have got into this detail unless Boulton had been in earnest about emigrating in that year.

Why the plan went no further is not certain. It may have to do with Boulton's finances. There had been a quarrel with his partner Fothergill in summer 1763. Boulton's financial resources had largely come from the fortunes of his two wives. The first, Mary Robinson, dying in 1759, he had later married her younger sister Anne, also with a good dowry, but the circumstances of the marriage are obscure, because marriage with a deceased wife's sister was contrary to ecclesiastical law. The death of his brother-in-law, Luke Robinson, in 1764 may have had some bearing on the matter if he had had a life interest in some of the family property. Some significant change in Boulton's financial position by May 1765 is confirmed by a letter from Benjamin Franklin which congratulates him: 'Mr. Baskerville informs me that you have lately had considerable addition to your fortune.' There seems reason to suppose that Boulton's patriotism, which he paraded in the following year in the keen pursuit of the workmen who were being suborned for the works at Pforzheim, was very dependent on his self-interest, as dictated by his financial position. His continued spending on the Soho manufactory does not tell greatly in the balance; it reflects his insatiable appetite for prestige, esteem and admiration. Once the Watt steam-engine was fairly launched, it saved Boulton's fortunes, which the fine hardware and luxury goods trade would certainly have ruined.[51]

In 1786 the Calonne administration decided to try to recruit Boulton and Watt. In that year Barthélémy wrote from London to the French foreign minister. He first mentioned the view of British merchants that in the operation of the Eden Treaty the principle the French had pursued of exchanging the products of their soil (e.g. wines) for British manufactures would lead to a damaging decline in the French balance of trade. One means of countering this, 'the effect of which would be inestimable', would be 'the possibility ... of gaining for ourselves the talents of two men, to one of whom especially England owes in large part the success of her manufactures and by consequence her wealth'. The talents of Boulton and Watt were known. Watt was a great mechanical genius. 'I heard, a month ago, the King of England speak of him in the most honourable terms.' It was impossible to see all the great industrial enterprises which his inventions had made possible, without wanting to possess such a clever man in one's own country. There was no hope of getting Boulton and Watt to abandon their British interests – their involvement with the Cornish mining industry would alone prevent it – but they should be brought over on the pretext of reporting on the Machine of Marly, famous but now old and defective, which supplied water from the Seine to Marly and Versailles.[52] This commission and the confidence shown by the Ministry would enlist the genius of Boulton and Watt and the speculative investments of French capitalists and give them 'the prospect and glory of covering with their works a country as fine and rich as ours, I dare think that we might be close to having nothing to fear from British industry'. Such encouragement to Boulton and Watt would induce many English artisans to come to France. The idea of commissioning Boulton and Watt to examine the Marly machine had already been floated, and correspondence was being exchanged.[53]

One other major consultancy was added to that on the machine of Marly. Calonne, the controller-general, had decided to buy La Charité, the great hardware works founded by Michael Alcock, which had reached the point of collapse.[54] This, of course, was a matter for Boulton, perhaps the most celebrated manufacturer in England in this line, but we must remember he had not been commercially successful in it. We have already dealt with his consultancy and report in the account of technological transfer in hardware.[55] In the end nothing came of the Marly project, about which Watt showed little enthusiasm. The conduct of Boulton and Watt was extremely equivocal. They did not make any attack on Périer, and Watt visited his Chaillot works and praised the quality of his engineering. Of more immediate importance than Marly was the question of additional water supply for Paris itself. Here things were complicated by the increasing general dissatisfaction with the water company monopoly and the hostility between Périer and the Baron de Breteuil, the minister responsible for the Maison du Roi and the Department of Paris. The water company was to become the Royal Water Administration in 1788 and the Périer brothers were thrown out.

Having examined the Notre Dame and Pont Neuf hydraulic pumping engines which still helped to supply Paris, Boulton and Watt oddly failed to come up with a clear case for steam-engine replacement, and even talked of an aqueduct supply.[56] They seem not to have wanted an entire break with Périer, perhaps in case he and the water company retained their Paris monopoly. On the other hand they did not tell him about the improved, direct-acting, engine, which he had to learn about from Betancourt's espionage. Perhaps hanging over everything else was the hope they entertained that their good relations with Calonne would mean that their incomplete and inoperative French privilege would be made effective, which was destroyed by Calonne's fall early in 1787. The outcome then was nothing more than 'tractations mysterieuses' as Payen justly calls them, and the ideas that Barthélémy had entertained of a great boost to French industry developing from the Boulton and Watt consultancy proved a pipe dream.

As for La Charité, Boulton claimed that patriotism would prevent his personal investment there, as opposed to giving advice, but it was probably the run-down state of the manufacture, its technical and locational problems, and the need for a high-quality businessman on the spot to direct it that dissuaded him, rather than patriotism.[57] Patriotism, Tann points out, was decidedly missing in Boulton's plans to act as consultant and investor in a proposed Paris copper rolling and coining project of the Monneron brothers in 1791. He told them it was important 'it not being known that I am a partner [or] it may be very injurious to me in this country'. This would be particularly true if British rolls were to be provided, contrary to the Tool Act.[58]

Boulton's position was also equivocal when around the end of the century he negotiated with foreign powers to provide them with his excellent steam-powered mints. Here he used his great lobbying abilities, and in 1799 obtained an Act of Parliament[59] for the export of a complete set of minting machinery for St Petersburg. While the official Russian approach made it difficult for the British to deny a system of great public benefit to a friendly power, it did not find favour in Birmingham, and there was a petition against the Act, but Boulton coolly declared that rolling-mills, steam-engines and other equipment were already known in Russia. Cynically at the same time he was pointing out to the Russians how the advantages of the machines would go beyond coining, and the steam-mill could be used by the Russian navy for rolling copper. Incidentally, he trained A. Deriabin at Soho to run the Russian Mint, and sent him on a long tour through England and Wales, well directed and recommended to the chief manufacturers in many industries. This was extremely valuable experience for the man who was to run not only the Russian mints, but their mines and ordnance factories.[60]

In the case of Denmark, Boulton tried to press the Danes to let him coin for them at Soho at a time when his mint there seemed likely to be out of work because of the difficulty of obtaining British government coining contracts when copper prices were high in 1799 and 1800. But Schimmelmann, the Danish minister, stuck out for the provision of a mint, which as late as the end of 1800 Boulton had declared impossible because the British government would not allow the export of the machinery – even though an Act had just been obtained for erecting a mint at St Petersburg! In 1804 such a project was put in hand, no doubt because it now suited Boulton better commercially. In exporting the basic machinery care was taken to export steel and tools also, including machine tools. No doubt the claim would be made that this was essential to have the means of repairing and maintaining the mint machinery, but it nevertheless amounted to a transfer of British technology in the face of the Tools Acts.[61]

On this evidence there seems no reason to change an earlier verdict that on policy against industrial espionage 'Boulton was a perfect weathercock ... turning wherever his momentary personal interest dictated'. On Boulton as a patriot, Tann is quite right: 'Matthew Boulton was a businessman first, an Englishman second.'[62]

Richard Crawshay was generally more consistent. As we have seen he was usually against any restrictions on exports, and this brought him in opposition to the Tools Acts. He and other London and outport iron merchants felt the Acts sacrificed their interests in favour of the metal goods manufacturers, especially those of the West Midlands. As they hindered the assortment of goods that could be exported, it could affect the placing of whole orders, and mean that such orders would go to Germany or other competitors, who would be encouraged to make themselves the goods hitherto made only in England.[63] In a letter to Hawkesbury putting this view, Crawshay said ninety-nine men out of a hundred involved in trade agreed with him – and that Boulton had authorized him to indicate his agreement – again indicating Boulton's tergiversation. So often he ran with the hare and hunted with the hounds.[64] In 1786 Crawshay had expressed his general opposition to the Acts in a letter to the Lords Commissioners for Trade. 'We cannot forbear to represent to your Lordships that while the absurd Tools Act of the two last sessions remains in force a material part of the benefits of the [Eden] Treaty will be frustrated, a Repeal of it is absolutely necessary on Principles of Sound Policy.'[65] His position was not quite absolute, however, in that his firm supported the investigation of Ljungberg's papers, and the detention of his property and papers had been made under the Tools Acts.

The position of the Wilkinson brothers has become very evident already. They were industrialists and businessmen operating entirely in their own best interests, without shame or hypocrisy. Only rarely, and briefly, could John Wilkinson be involved in any plans for trade organization or lobbying, even though he was regarded as the foremost and most knowledgeable man in the iron industry. He disliked interruptions for any purpose, and wished to get back as quickly as possible to making iron. His works were open to most foreign visitors, and the Périer brothers, de la Houlière, de Wendel, de Givry and Dulubre, among the most important people in French engineering and iron-making, had ready access. The only good description of John Wilkinson's New Willey (Broseley) ironworks, is that of the de la Rochefoucauld party, the young noblemen being in the care of Lazowski, brother to a notable French inspector of industry. Wilkinson sent his clerk to guide them and give them all the information they wanted.[66] John Wilkinson and Thomas Williams, the extremely powerful copper industrialist and monopolist, were close allies in business, and Williams seems to have had an identical open and uncaring attitude about foreign inspection of his works. It was with William Wilkinson that, after visiting John Wilkinson's works, the Périer, de Givry, de Wendel and Dulubre party were taken to see Ravenhead, then in 1784 the world's greatest copper smelter, and thence to the Holywell water-powered plant in Flintshire, where the new cold-rolling process, critical to successful coppering of ships, was operating. It is to their report that modern historians owe much information on these great works.[67] Amusingly, Watt gave Wilkinson warning about the visit of the party, who had not been allowed to see much at Birmingham. He clearly did not know of the intimacy of their connection with the Wilkinsons, especially William, though he was aware that they already knew John. He did not expect that John would be 'very communicative' with the French party, a complete misconception.[68]

We know that Westwood, one of the two joint inventors of the cold-rolling process, was alarmed by the shipment of the critical rolls from the Dee estuary to France, which can only have been by Wilkinson from his Bersham works. The order was possibly a follow-up of the de Wendel visit. Such an export was not illegal, as it just anticipated the Tools Acts, and it cannot have been unknown to Williams, but it seems to have caused no adverse reaction from the copper tycoon, for his business co-operation with Wilkinson was at a peak in the following years, from 1785 to 1787. Finally, John Wilkinson had a good working relationship with another important foreigner, Baron Friedrich Wilhelm von Reden, who had a very successful career as a mining engineer and administrator in Prussia. Reden visited John Wilkinson in 1782, and was with him at Broseley (New Willey), Wrexham (Bersham) and at his North Lancashire mansion at Castlehead. While in the north von Reden was to 'give me a lecture on Smelting Copper in a Blast Furnace'. Similarly William Wilkinson visited von Reden at Tarnowitz, and made trials of smelting lead with coke. It is unlikely that either process succeeded, but at least John Wilkinson supplied a steam-engine at Tarnowitz.[69]

It is only in the case of a handful of major contemporary industrialists that we have worthwhile evidence on the attitude to foreign industrial espionage and machine export, and the maintenance, extension and enforcement of the British laws against them. Consequently dependable generalization is hazardous. But the indications are that there was no firm consensus, for Wedgwood and Garbett were at the opposite end of the see-saw from Wilkinson and Williams. The last two were men of great business power and immense self-confidence, and seemingly believed that no foreign acquisition of technical knowledge and equipment would dent their primacy as industrial leaders.

There was, however, an important difference between a belief that suitable laws might seriously retard the acquisition of British technology by foreign competitors, and the idea that it could be retained for ever, which was rarely held. In 1779 the Lancashire magistrates, after condemning the conduct of those rioting against the new cotton-mills in the belief that they reduced wages, passed several resolutions. These were to be published in the London, Manchester and Liverpool newspapers. One read:

> Resolved that it is the Unanimous Opinion of this Court that it is impossible to Restrain the Force of Ingenuity, when employed in the Improvement of Manufactures. That any Machines, that have been found to effectuate that purpose, become the property of the World. That the Destroying them in one Country, only Serves to establish them in another, and that if the Legislature was to prevent the Exercise of them in this Kingdom, it would tend to Establish them in Foreign Countrys, which would be highly Detrimental to the Trade of this Country.[70]

20   Comparisons I: Industrial Espionage in Britain, France and other Nations

This book shows how the drive for technological transfer between England and France in the eighteenth century is demonstrated by the extent and methods of industrial espionage. But one important point to establish is how far this kind of transfer was largely confined to the two countries under discussion. Were other countries in Europe similarly concerned to acquire British technology by espionage, and did this involve the suborning of workers and the smuggling of machines? It must be said at the outset that comparative study of this subject is in its infancy. The differing extent, coverage and nature of national, local and private archives in European countries is a first great problem. Perhaps even greater is the linguistic one. Few historians command a wide range of European languages, while the problems of reading the archives in some cases, and the precise meaning of contemporary technical terms in others, present additional barriers. It is to be hoped that these barriers will be progressively surmounted by international teamwork, but all that can be said here is indicative rather than conclusive, and in no way does it produce a thoroughly balanced picture, in which the relative extent of the acquisition of British technology by covert means by all the major European powers can be exactly seen.

Some of the best evidence available is for the Scandinavian countries, for Sweden and for Denmark–Norway (a united kingdom at the time with which we are dealing). The Swedish evidence is particularly good, because two well-organized bodies, the Bergskollegium (Board of Mines) from the late seventeenth century and the Jernkontoret (Ironmasters'

Association) after its formation in the middle of the eighteenth century, sent a long procession of observers, well educated and technically informed, to examine the British scene. The Bergskollegium men were, as Lindqvist points out, itinerant civil servants.[1] While they did sometimes observe other kinds of industry and commerce, the Swedes, with their economy heavily dependent, particularly in the export sector, on iron and copper, naturally directed their main attention to the mining of these metals, and to their smelting, refining and manufacturing. This sometimes extended beyond copper to the other non-ferrous metals, tin and lead, and to the mining of calamine and the production of zinc as essential for brass. The Swedes also investigated the making-up of metals, for instance in the growing hardware district of the West Midlands, or the iron manufactures of the North East. There they frequently visited the famous works of the Crowleys, strongly focused on the naval iron market. Increasingly as the British mastered steel production, that too became a preoccupation, much strengthened when the new crucible cast steel was developed in Sheffield.

In the years after the Second World War two British historians of the iron industry first made known to industrial historians in general the interest which the Swedes took in British technology and industrial practice in the last decades of the seventeenth century and throughout the whole of the eighteenth century. The work of Flinn[2] and Birch,[3] largely based on Rydberg, has recently been supplemented by the work of Lindqvist on Triewald and the Newcomen engine, and by articles in a volume of collected essays on technical transfer to Scandinavia, edited by Bruland. There has also been an interesting excerpt by Woolrich from the papers of a Swedish spy of 1759–60. Naturally Birch and Flinn are most concerned with Swedish reports on the British iron industry, Lindqvist and Woolrich bring out their early interest in the steam-engine and their important concern with copper and brass. As we have seen, Lindqvist points out the anxiety of the Swedish authorities, even in the earliest years of the eighteenth century, that there should not be any serious interruption in the succession of official technological visitors to Britain. The news of the Newcomen engine reached them as 'a matter of routine by the Swedish civil service', that is, by 'regular industrial reconnaissance abroad by the Board of Mines'.[4]

One of the first important Swedish visitors was the metallurgist Odhelius who came briefly in 1686 and for about six months in 1691–92, as a part of wider travels. He was acquainted with leading members of the Royal Society. His English section accounts for only fifty-six pages of a very large travel journal, but the copper and brass industry, mining for coal and for calamine, and the manufacture of alum and vitriol are mentioned, as well, of course, as iron. He knew of some of the early attempts at the coal smelting of iron. Christopher Polhem, the greatest name in Swedish technology, came over in 1695, but there is no record of his findings. Cletscher, who came in the following year, was mainly concerned with the English copper industry, showing how quickly the transformation of the English industry, with the discovery of coal smelting and the accompanying expansion of Cornish mining, was picked up in Sweden. Silfvercrantz, conducting a six-year European tour, was in England in 1702, and made a visit to the famous Crowley works. Wallerius in 1710 had a special interest in the manufacture of iron goods, particularly in Birmingham, but as yet no evidence is available from his reports. More or less contemporaneously Svab was here, concentrating on the copper industry, whose output he believed was already half that of Sweden, formerly so dominant in European trade. On a later visit he commented on the casting of Newcomen engine cylinders at Coalbrookdale, shortly after Ticquet had reported on it for France.[5]

Swedenborg, whose comments on the Newcomen engine we have already mentioned, was here during 1710–12, and on several later occasions. He endeavoured in vain to witness some of the experiments of the Wood ironmaster family at Whitehaven, and was able to record the use of coke in iron smelting in his famous *De Ferro* of 1734. Alströmer had a very long time in England, first settling in 1707 as a businessman. He succeeded, and took out English citizenship, being Swedish consul here for two short periods. He kept surviving travel diaries which are said to be ambitious and valuable, but have not been translated. Kahlmeter, a Bergskollegium official, spent a total of four years in Britain during the period 1718–30, and was at one time in regular correspondence with Alströmer. Schröderstierna, a professor, was a member of the Bergskollegium for thirty-three years. His daybook covers an extensive tour of British centres of industry and trade. His account of Birmingham and the West Midlands is particularly rich and there are now moves to make this available in English; part of his report on the English iron industry has already been translated by the late Professor Flinn.[6]

Fairly close on Schröderstierna's heels came Angerstein, between 1753 and 1755, a particularly famous reporter. He had previously visited Russia, Hungary, Italy, Spain and Portugal. His travel journal is

900 pages long, and has valuable illustrations. Very early he visited one of the coal-fired cementation steelworks in Birmingham, and button and brass works there, and he toured the region three times. While he concentrated to a considerable degree on iron, with an extended account of the Coalbrookdale district, and another on the Crowleys' various works in the North East, he explored widely, including for instance Worcester pottery and Kidderminster carpets. His credentials were very strong, in 1753 he was appointed Director of Steelworks at the Jernkontoret, the powerful Swedish ironmasters' association which had been founded in 1747. 'There can have been few industrial sites of importance, or processes employed, particularly in the metallurgical industries, not described by Angerstein', writes Flinn.[7]

Having the very important asset of Dannemora iron, almost always used in Britain for conversion to steel, the Swedes naturally took a keen interest in English steel-making, and quickly understood the importance of Huntsman's new crucible cast steel. Johan Robsahm, one of two brothers running a steelworks in Sweden, came over in 1761 to investigate the process. Though he was received hospitably by Huntsman, the inventor would not tell him how to make the critical crucibles, even refusing £50 for the secret. However, Robsahm did not confine himself to Sheffield, but looked at the ironworks at Coalbrookdale, the industries of the hardware district, and glass at Bristol and Newcastle. He managed to spend his £50 to advantage by bribing a Wednesbury erector to build a steam-engine in Sweden, so satisfying a supplementary request by the Jernkontoret conveyed to him *en route*. The next enquirer, Andersson, was especially interested in the relationship between coal and the British iron industry. His observations were recorded in two parts, one giving details of some ironworks of particular interest in England, Wales and Scotland; the second, written much later, was a long account of British processes, now clearly more advanced than Swedish.[8]

The British iron industry was on a new and dynamic technical path which a coal-less Sweden could not emulate, and Britain was now also the world leader in copper, with a superior resource in ores, as well as coal-based technologies. These extended, like those for iron, from smelting through the gamut of production to the manufacture of producers' and consumers' goods. Once completely established the revolutionary transformation of the two industries reduced the need for further exploratory travels by Swedish experts.

Bengt Ferrner does not seem to have a direct connection with either of the two official bodies which sponsored most of the Swedish tours we have mentioned. He was an astronomer at Uppsala University from 1751 and professor of mathematics at the Karlskrona naval academy from 1756, in which year he was elected to the Swedish Royal Academy of Sciences. In 1765 he became a permanent secretary and counsellor to the king, Gustav III, being ennobled in 1766. He was clearly a man of great talents and, not untypically for senior European academics of the period, became tutor to Jean Lefebure, son of Jean-Henri Lefebure, a wealthy merchant of Huguenot origin. The father dominated the Swedish copper trade with France, and acquired the largest Swedish brassworks in 1759. Ferrner accompanied the son on a lengthy European tour from 1758 to 1763, which included a British tour during 1759–60. His extensive journal is available in a modern Swedish edition. There is, however, an English translation of that part of the journal which deals with observations on Bristol, Bath and their environs.

This shows, in the clearest manner, that Ferrner was charged with obtaining intelligence of the non-ferrous industry of the region, and that he was supposed to spy quite intensively to obtain the workers needed. He was particularly interested in processes for making zinc for brass. He bribed men who were able to guide him to works without themselves being knowledgeable enough to understand what he was after. He went to drink with workmen in pubs over the Christmas holidays, when they would hopefully be at their most talkative and relaxed, but failed to get worthwhile information. Though he found a man who would take him into the copper and spelter works at Crewshole near Bristol, he was warned that 'there is a strict supervision here', and on his attempt to enter the works he found himself betrayed, was followed, and was finally met and upbraided by the foreman, who told him 'that all workmen were strictly instructed that it was entirely forbidden to show any foreigner the least part of the new works'. However, Ferrner persisted, consulting with Lefebure before he acted, influencing workmen with drink and bribing a foreman. The foreman's information was incomprehensible without entry into the relevant works, which with much secrecy, subterfuge and some disguise was eventually accomplished. The foreman was willing to emigrate to Sweden, but only for double pay, and the outcome is unclear.[9]

Ferrner made two attempts to penetrate the works of Champion at Warmley, where some of the spelter processes had originally been obtained by espionage from Holland, and a few Dutch workmen were still employed. As we have several times seen in cases of French firms which were highly secretive about methods they had themselves obtained by espionage and suborning in Britain, Champion was fiercely protective of his purloined techniques; even workmen's wives were shut out, and their husbands forbidden to talk to them about their work, while no other workman from other parts of the works 'may put a foot inside that door'. Ferrner managed to get to see a rolling and slitting mill, believing that the owner, being a Quaker, 'therefore kept no secrets' – a misleading generalization which would not have covered Huntsman or the Darbys. His attempt to get into a tin plate works seemed to be going well and an intermediary was about to admit him into the plant at night, only to inform him at the last minute that the manager had learned of the plan and, concerned 'to prevent any foreigner from approaching the works', would be on the lookout all night with a loaded gun. However, Ferrner hoped to secure the son of his accomplice for a Swedish firm.[10]

Despite the growing technical divergence of the British and Swedish metal industries the technological tours did not die out entirely. Broling was financed to study metals in Britain between 1797 and 1799, producing a three-volume report of over 1,000 pages, though not published until the second decade of the next century. He took a particular interest in John Wilkinson's very new cupola furnace. So did Svedenstierna, in Britain in 1802–03.[11] Unusually, for part of the tour he travelled with a French mining engineer he had met in London. Topics outside the metals are treated, though iron predominates, for he was a servant of Jernkontoret. Unusually too, an English translation of the tour exists, taken from an 1811 German version of a Swedish publication of 1804. This in turn is a less specialized version of a scholarly book which eventually saw the light in 1813. According to Fritz, though Svedenstierna's tour was cut short by the ending of the Peace of Amiens, it did result in the use of the cupola furnace in Sweden in 1805, though founded on minimal observation by him and using charcoal fuel.[12]

The Swedish efforts at industrial espionage in Britain over the eighteenth century came nearest to challenging those of the French. They should probably be assigned second place, though the comparison is not a straightforward one. The Swedish authorities had a more steady and administratively better organized system of surveillance of British technological developments than had the French, certainly before the elder Trudaine came to dominate French industrial policy at midcentury. They were very conscious that there was a continuing pattern of technical change in Britain, and they endeavoured to monitor it regularly by sending observers who were highly qualified, and instructing them to report in minute detail, which inevitably meant massive travel journals. While some of the Swedish visitors spread a wider net, all concentrated, and some very strongly, on the metal industries. Within them there was further concentration, particularly on iron and copper, for the technical changes, increasingly focused on the use of coal in British smelting and manufacturing, were impinging on Swedish European dominance. The Swedish superiority was first overcome in copper. In iron the severity of the technological problems of conversion to coal-fuel, combined with the costs of labour and wood-fuel in the existing British charcoal iron industry, and expanding home and export markets for iron goods, meant that a large part of these British markets was captured by Swedish bar iron. Around 1750 at least half British iron needs were supplied by imports, and here Sweden predominated. Bar (i.e. wrought) iron accounted for 60 per cent of Swedish exports at this time, and 55 per cent of that was sent to England. The reason for Swedish interest in the British iron industry is obvious and highly justifiable. The need for information was all the greater because the situation was undergoing fundamental change.

The invention of coke-pig in 1709 was initially most significant in its effect on the gradually growing market for engineering castings. It hardly affected the immediate, and increasing, demand for Swedish bar iron. But the British ability to convert coke-pig to wrought iron after 1750 was a major change. The arrival of methods enabling the iron industry to carry out that conversion with coal, first by the stamping and potting methods of the 1760s, and then by puddling and rolling from the late 1780s, was decisive. In the second half of the 1790s imports began to fall, and were now not much more than a third of the British market, as home production grew rapidly. Even so, the Swedish element no longer predominated in British imports. There Russia had gained the lead in 1765, and subsequently sent more iron than Sweden had done.[13]

There were, as we have seen, several French visits of intelligence and espionage which lasted some months, in the odd case over a year. The visits of Jars and Faujas de Saint-Fond are obvious instances. But long and thorough visits, sometimes over years, resulting in very long travel journals and reports, with a careful and detailed survey of large parts of one or two industries are typical of the Swedish case rather than the French one.[14] Le Turc of course stayed about eight years in Britain, but for most of that time he was merely an exile; only after the American

514   *Industrial Espionage and Technology Transfer*

war did he become an industrial spy. As compared with the Swedes the French were much broader in their interests. They had a very wide textile sector, covering all the range the British possessed, if with a different balance. They were interested in chemicals, glass, ceramics. They had a coal industry, if much smaller than the British. While their interest in metals was not so consuming as the Swedes', naval rivalry led them into a great plan to acquire a coal-fuelled iron industry. Without being a significant primary producer of copper, they were desperate to get the technology of naval copper. This spread of interests led to a greater number of points of attack on British industries.

Some of these were *ad hoc*, and came from individuals, partnerships and companies which wanted to know more about British methods in their industry and to obtain them by espionage if they seemed appropriate for transfer to France. The State might simply be involved in the provision of passports, and a recommendation to the embassy in London, in the hope of providing some diplomatic help if espionage ran into accidents and discovery. Alternatively, the State itself might dispatch spies with the plan of helping firms or industries, singly or collectively. In either case the implication commonly was that new, worthwhile processes obtained from Britain might be subsidized, and the costs of suborning and transporting men, and of buying and importing equipment be borne by the Government. Present evidence would indicate that while individual Swedish expeditions of intelligence and espionage were often longer, at more regular intervals and more thorough in their coverage than the French, the latter were more numerous in total and wider in their industrial distribution.[15]

How far were the Swedish travellers concerned with collecting the best industrial intelligence that they could get without breaking English laws; how far were they involved in industrial espionage? A verdict here is not easy. But it seems reasonable to presume that if they wanted to maintain a steady, long-term, invigilation of British industrial development, the Swedes would not carry on a reckless, precipitate, or injudicious campaign of entering industrial premises where strong precautions were being taken to prevent it, because this would put industrialists and magistrates on the alert. It would mean not only that the traveller who was detected would have to leave the country, but subsequent Swedish travellers seeking to gather industrial intelligence would be continually under suspicion and debarred from works and mines.

Schröderstierna seems to have endeavoured, with great success, to strike up friendships with industrialists, dining them and dining with them, and being taken to see works by them. In his case, and that of most of the other Swedish visitors, they were men of not merely technical, but some scientific background and, given the great popularity of scientific lecturers in the industrial towns, their scientific interests may have been something of a passport.[16] Of course when opportunity and the importance of the British technology seemed to make covert investigations worth while, the bounds would be overstepped. Of Angerstein a modern authority writes 'he was not unacquainted with the method of spying to find out things not given to him voluntarily'.[17] One of the last of the succession of Swedish industrial travellers, Svedenstierna, made a specific statement that his investigations would 'go no further in the matter than the rules of hospitality allowed'. He planned his itinerary and enquiries by 'the assiduous study of guide books' and the systematic use of letters of introduction from the Swedish consul-general in London and several distinguished scientists he met there.[18] On the contrary we have seen Ferrner, a Swedish professor closely connected with a private firm in the copper and brass industry, involved in the most brazen attempts at industrial espionage in the Bristol area. Perhaps he was less inhibited because he was not on the staff of the Bergskollegium, and would have been cheerfully disavowed by the Swedish government. A Swedish industrialist seems to have acted independently in suborning Shropshire ironworkers.

The negotiations for Boulton's proposed migration to Sweden, as we have seen, were conducted with a senior Swedish official who visited Soho with Alströmer, and some later correspondence passed through a Swedish merchant house in London. Also involved in these negotiations was Dr Solander, an eminent Swedish scientist, then resident in England. He became secretary and librarian to Sir Joseph Banks, the President of the Royal Society, and was a scientist on Cook's *Endeavour* voyage. He more than once took part in schemes to seduce English experts to his native country. The best generalization that can be made is that while the long continuance of official Swedish visitations of British industrial sites could not have been maintained without considerable discretion, and some of these industrial voyagers specifically claimed that they did not spy, some did when it was important enough and they thought it safe enough. Other Swedish citizens outside the Bergskollegium and Jerkontoret spied and suborned without conscience, and it was only the limited range of Sweden's resources and of her industrial base that restricted her to the second place in espionage, behind France.

The other Scandinavian power, Denmark–Norway (two countries under the same crown at the period we are concerned with) had a history of espionage and seduction in Britain which is less well known than the Swedish, but not unimportant. There had been from the late seventeenth century a presence of mercantilist ideas, which included plans for import substitution. A Commercial College was set up by Frederick IV, but this collapsed, only to be revived in the 1730s. Then Count Otto Thott produced a mercantilist plan for industry which involved the development of textiles, glass and iron. Between 1730 and the late 1740s about sixty manufacturers from Britain, Holland and Germany were brought in, but problems with charlatans amongst them, as well as a lack of raw materials, capital and skilled indigenous workers, were discouraging. It was rare that well-qualified people with enough capital could be persuaded to leave their homes and settle in an unknown foreign country. Equally it was difficult to predict in advance how useful foreign artisans would be: they might be desirous of picking up premiums and subsidies without having anything significant to impart.[19]

In 1750 John Smith, an Englishman already living in Denmark, smuggled a model of an English calender into the country, claiming, like many French industrial spies of the period, that he had risked his life to do so. Workers who made particular parts of the machine he mounted in Denmark were kept ignorant of the work of those who made others. Smith's workers took an oath not to divulge the secrets and he obtained for himself the sole right to use the machine. In 1765 a 'public utility' fund was set up to subsidize travel abroad by experts and craftsmen, but the travellers had to make reports on their findings, and if new machinery resulted in Denmark, it had to be open to viewing by others. A specific travel fund was set up in 1795 and an 'industrial fund' in 1797, the latter under the Commercial College, which also supported the work of Nordberg which we will now examine.[20]

In a number of cases Denmark was willing to welcome Swedes who had experience of the British situation. Nordberg who had originally gone to England about 1760, interested in general advances in production and technology, returned to Sweden in 1775 with the plan of setting up a 'Manchester' factory for spinning and weaving, but did not get the encouragement he had hoped for, and eventually in 1779 he was invited by the Danish College of Commerce to set up a similar works in that country. There he met Ljungberg, whom we have already met. He too was Swedish and had left for England as Nordberg returned. He also received a poor reception on regaining Sweden, and similarly moved to Copenhagen, where he joined up with Nordberg. They set up a new cotton factory where Ljungberg was for a time in charge of spinning and Nordberg of weaving and finishing. The establishment seems to have had a very fluctuating existence. In 1784 it had carding engines, thirty spinning-machines, a calendering department and a printing works, an Englishman, John Dalton, being in charge of dyeing and printing. It built up to 800 employees and was supposed to have a major national training function. But there was difficulty in keeping up with English practice. A new spinning-machine was smuggled in in 1785, but could not be made to operate properly, and in 1787 Nordberg returned to England for more spying, smuggling out drawings of carding and spinning machines from the West of England woollen industry.

The problem seems largely to have been the lack of expertise for building machines in Denmark; Nordberg spent time studying metalworking machines in Birmingham and Sheffield. His machine-making was financed by the Government on his return: 'the workers were quite inexperienced for such tasks, and there was much trial and error with the more intricate metal parts'. Continuing problems forced Nordberg into another espionage visit to England in 1791. In the mid-1790s he endeavoured to found a fully integrated water-powered cotton factory outside Copenhagen, which was however sold off in 1798. Difficulties persisted in obtaining card lengths for the carding machines and in finding qualified people to maintain machines in general. In the same year Nordberg set up a textile machinery works in Copenhagen with government support, but the machines made were still defective, and a fourth espionage trip to England took place in 1799. Bankrupt in 1806, Nordberg was able to resume business until his death in 1812. His son Charles proved more successful in supplying cotton machinery in both Denmark and Norway. This tortuous progress seems to reflect a repeated underestimation of the difficulties of transfer, a failure to appreciate the extent to which mechanical engineering skills had come to underpin British textile machine-making, and a mistaken reliance on the obtaining of drawings and of some key parts which could more easily avoid the British anti-espionage legislation and its enforcers than could the smuggling of complete machines. At any rate, there was a reluctance or inability to obtain the full range of key machines and the appropriate skilled men to teach their operation and build others.

However, Nordberg introduced the jenny, water frame and mule to Denmark, and within one or two decades of their adoption in England. The fly-shuttle which arrived in the 1790s was slow in adoption because of general worker opposition and wage disputes.[21]

Amdam has recently opened up a formerly obscure topic, the transfer of British glass technology to Norway by industrial espionage.[22] The first Norwegian glassworks were set up 60 km west of Oslo in 1741, run by the Norwegian Company formed in 1739 by Norwegian and German entrepreneurs, with the King of Denmark an investor and patron. From 1751 the majority shareholding was Norwegian and from 1776 the firm was state owned. To a great extent Denmark and Norway formed a common market for its product, but Norway's greater wood-fuel supplies determined the works' siting. Foreign glass was banned from 1760, and the Company produced all kinds of glass except plate, having a monopoly privilege for both countries. Altogether at various times the firm ran seven glassworks, building three between 1756 and 1766. By the middle of the century it was the leading producer of high quality crystal in Scandinavia.

Window glass was naturally a major product, and it is here that information on industrial espionage is most plentiful. There had been some rather haphazard attraction of French workers before mid-century, a Frenchman, Fillion, arriving via Sweden, while de Mohr had come to Norway as far back as the 1690s as a result of a crisis at Saint Gobain, but failed to establish plate glass. The Norwegian privileged company's works remained small until the arrival of Caspar Hermann von Storm in 1753. In seeking to expand it might have seemed natural to turn to the German cylinder-blown glass method, but it was decided to go for the crown method which gave a superior but dearer product, a process originally developed in France, but taken to England in the 1560s, and subsequently adapted to coal-fuel. It is interesting that the Norwegians decided that the English crown glass industry was the one to be imitated. However, crown glass was determined on only after the recruitment of cylinder-glass makers from Pomerania and Mecklenberg had been considered. Von Storm was enthusiastic about the 'highly perfected factories' producing crown glass in Britain. Amdam points out that 'Britain's leading role in the industrial field had at this time begun to be recognized by the rest of Europe'.

Morten Waern was selected as the industrial spy to recruit workers from Britain, and to learn about working processes, furnace construction and fuel costs.[23] During 1754–56 he travelled in England and

Scotland. He concentrated on Newcastle, Leith, Hull, Liverpool, Bristol and London, but claimed to have visited all the glasshouses in England and Scotland. He did his best to conceal his purpose, and like so many spies he was worried about his letters being opened in the post, tried to communicate his findings via Scottish business houses and used a code to cover the names of individuals in his correspondence. He also endeavoured to reduce risks by only recruiting workers who were not bound to their masters.

Nevertheless he was arrested in London in the summer of 1755, accused of trying to obtain the composition of crystal and of window glass, and of suborning workers to emigrate. Imprisoned for a month in Newgate, he was bailed, an operation in which the Danish ambassador was involved, and then fled to France. Once in France Waern took the opportunity of visiting their glasshouses, including Saint Gobain. He had taken great care to investigate the Scottish kelp industry as a source of alkali, but it was from France that in fact he recruited kelp-burners. Five English glassworkers suborned by Waern reached Norway as he was arrested in England, and they were sent to Hurdal 80 km north of Oslo to construct the first window glass factory. Though Amdam believed they came from Newcastle, at least one, Joseph Pyne, was from Bristol, and his contract survives. Pyne agreed with Storm 'to go from [Bristol] over sea to Norway and when there work as a gatherer in the crown glass way or as a finisher in bottles … after the Bristol method'. He undertook to train Norwegian workers or apprentices and generally help out in the glassworks. He agreed to be faithful to his employers and 'sober in my business' and to accept the giving of three months' notice on either side. He would have free passage to Norway, 21 shillings a week, a free house and fuel. If there was no work for him he would still get half wages.[24] Waern also secured two Liverpool makers of crystal glass: one wonders if they were able to make flint glass without a coal supply. It was information about their recruitment which had led to Waern's arrest. It is interesting that a Danish official policy to attract foreign workers, launched in 1753, sensibly included the provision of funds to enable workers to repay loans from their employers in their home countries.

The Danish–Norwegian plan to establish a domestic glass industry was initially a matter of national technological prestige rather than commerce, and there was no profit until the end of the 1780s; to 1759 sales did not cover more than 5 per cent of cost in any one year. Large warehouse stocks accumulated, including crown glass, and only the ban on glass imports in 1760 helped matters. Little window glass was used outside the towns.[25]

Another Danish initiative, partly above board, partly clandestine, has been described by Christensen. Jesper Bidstrup had studied maths, astronomy and physics at Copenhagen University, and also trained under Ahl, a Swedish instrument-maker suborned to Denmark. Bugge, the director of the Observatory, wanted to advance the career of his protégé Bidstrup as a successor to Ahl. He sent him to England quite openly in 1787, hoping that he might use the influence of Sir Joseph Banks at the Royal Society to apprentice Bidstrup to one of the leading London scientific instrument-makers like Jesse Ramsden. Magellan, whom we have met in the steam-engine context, was also approached to help. But Bidstrup was only able to get into the workshop of a subcontractor to the leading makers, paying a premium for training, but able to make machines for himself. He began, however, to ship to Denmark not only tools and instruments he had made, but British machine tools he had purchased. At a later stage he had his own small London workshop, but sold few instruments. He had some major successes, one being the shipment of a machine for glass grinding weighing half a ton, and like French illegal exporters he shipped some steel goods mixed with other commodities and in different ships to Hamburg and Copenhagen. Bidstrup determined to return to Denmark, concerned by the arrest of Ljungberg and believing that he was also under suspicion. After a short delay due to illness, he took ship from Yarmouth, taking lathes and a cupola furnace with him. Though he set up a machine workshop in Copenhagen on his return, his early death probably meant that it was never seriously put to work.[26]

The Danes made considerable efforts to keep an eye on British naval advances, and between 1708 and the end of the century about twenty naval officers spent time in England for that purpose, often staying a year or two. One actually joined the Royal Navy. Most reported on naval dockyards, some also on private yards building for the navy; there were occasional accounts of industrial centres. They may have been fairly open observers, one was elected to the Royal Society, another to an agricultural society. The general verdict of Christensen is that the intelligence-gathering of Norway–Denmark was less centralized and organized than that of France. While there were interesting initiatives backed by government, there was no consistent overview or consistent policy like that of Trudaine. The espionage of the Danish Admiralty was, however, something of an exception. The lack of good information and good planning on the civilian side is perhaps best illustrated by the situation where an important ironworks near Oslo received a large subsidy from the Danish crown to erect plant for steel-making and send a 'Mr. Kaas' over to England to recruit workers, though two British workers at a different firm were already making crucible cast steel as a result of industrial espionage they had organized in England.[27]

While it would not be possible to survey here industrial espionage in Britain in the eighteenth century by every European country, it must be made clear that Scandinavian countries were not the only ones to parallel France. One or two further examples may be enough to put the French example in perspective. Freudenberger has supplied very useful material for Austria. He emphasizes the role of the skilled worker teaching by example, what is sometimes referred to as the 'non-verbal' means of transferring technology. There was a large element of government sponsorship and recruitment of foreign workers, and even when private individuals supplied the initiative, there was an important measure of government assistance. Some English workers, as well as Dutch, had been recruited in 1715 for the important Waldstein woollen-mill, which was intended as a means of upgrading the work of local peasants to achieve the higher grades of cloth. The idea of import substitution was very much to the fore, there was further recruitment of cloth experts from Belgium and western Germany, and a major effort to establish a silk industry. Out of a total of about thirty-six silkmasters in Vienna about 1800, thirty-one had come from Paris or Lyon.

The 1760s saw an important influx of British metalworkers. A main recruiting agent was the cook to the Austrian embassy in London, the target being principally button and buckle makers and steel-makers. Given the high reputation of Styrian and Carinthian steel in Europe, the search for English steel-makers is an interesting reflection on a change in technological leadership. The steel-maker Welch, and three others, Grove, Johnson and Craighill, were directed to a state mining and metal concern at Graz. There were problems on either side, complaints of poor treatment and of the poor discipline of local labour by the English, complaints about the laziness, drinking and gambling of the English by the Austrian authorities. Tempted to send one Englishman back home, the Austrians decided against it, so as not to deter other English workers who might wish to come. The steel and the iron goods produced were of low quality, and there was discussion of restricting the import of similar products into Austria.

A Thomas Lightowler, probably a machine-maker from Birmingham, arrived in Vienna in 1768 to make a pressing machine for the production of the English glazed cardboard in which we have seen the French deeply interested because of its importance in cloth finishing. Despite a government subvention he did not make a good machine. Though his daughter was married to the secretary of the Court Commercial Council he seems to have fallen into disfavour. However, a Thomas Lightowler later had great success as a button-maker, and given the flexibility of Birmingham machine-makers it may very well be the same man. The problem is that he was said to have emigrated only in 1780 and to have recruited more English skilled workers via Hamburg in the same year. Whether the original immigrant or a later one, possibly from the same family, the second-mentioned Lightowler must have done well, for he was ennobled in 1794.

The Austrian embassy cook continued his valuable suborning activities in 1766, recruiting Thomas Rosthorn, the foreman of a London button-making firm, and a chief workman, George Collins. Their plans were discovered and they had to leave hastily. The men were well received in Austria, pensions were offered, as were free accommodation and fuel, and a premium for each apprentice Rosthorn trained. The Government paid for the necessary machinery and tools and the travel costs of Rosthorn and his family. Rosthorn could not find a sufficiently skilled Austrian die-maker. An English worker sent to find one in England absconded with the suborning money, and there was thus a delay in getting a qualified English expert. With Rosthorn, as with other men producing in Austrian conditions, there were for some time problems in selling a product which was dearer than the British imports, and there were proposals to inhibit the sale of foreign buttons. However, Rosthorn eventually succeeded. His sons continued to expand and diversify in the metal trades after his death in 1805.

One of the Englishmen Rosthorn recruited was the Birmingham manufacturer Robert Hickman, originally engaged for the essential die-making. His recruitment of additional workers in Birmingham was done with skill, so that even Garbett was unable to prevent it. He was joined in Vienna by his brother William, a Birmingham button-maker who had been selling his goods in Germany. Robert Hickman returned to England in 1785 to obtain more workers, putting in the usual claims that his mission had been very expensive and that his life had even been in danger. There was a fierce debate between the families of the two Hickmans about the credit for establishing button-making in Austria;

William's family said that the main achievement had been his, and Robert had been a poor manager.

There was an Austrian assault on the new British textile technology of the late eighteenth century paralleling that on the metal trades. At the very end of the century the Vienna Loan Bank in 1799–1800 commissioned Karl George, Baron von Glave-Kolbielski, of Prussian origin, and formerly active there and in Poland, but latterly engaged as a propagandist for Austria, to go to England to engage English textile factory workers. He was chased out of England, but had directly or indirectly recruited a number of English workers in Hamburg, of whom John Thornton was the most important, and he also used a London agent to engage skilled workers. The operation was a very tangled business. But Thornton was highly successful, in 1811 he was operating one of the largest cotton factories on the Continent, certainly the largest in Austria. Apart from supervisory staff it employed 1,133 men and 1,156 women workers and 800 machines, which from 1808 had included mules and water frames. He was ennobled in 1812.

There were, as we have seen, British attempts to prevent the outflow of workers to Austria, though this seems to have increased the difficulty of recruitment without preventing it when there was a sufficient resolve on the part of both enticers and enticed. On at least one occasion there was an attempt to get workers to return. In 1769 the British ambassador to Austria called together all the British workers in Vienna, and read to them the terms of the 1719 Act, under which they could lose legal rights in Britain, including those over any property they owned or inherited, if they did not return home after being notified. The proceeding caused considerable annoyance to the Austrian government, but no other consequence is recorded.[28]

Russia took a strong interest in British technology in the eighteenth century. Peter the Great made a famous visit to England in 1698 and particularly concerned himself with navigation and shipbuilding with the object of creating a powerful navy. He was attended by senior British naval officers, notably Rear-Admiral Lord Carmarthen, who advised on the recruitment of master shipwrights, and of a limited number of British officers. There began the practice of training Russian naval officers on British ships which gained momentum from 1706. Some officers so trained became admirals, Kozlianinov becoming commander of the Russian fleet in 1788 during the war against the Swedes. Inevitably these officers were well informed on technical advances made in the British navy.[29]

The generally friendly relations between Britain and Russia during the eighteenth century, commercial treaties and growing trade, made for a friendlier reception to Russian industrial travellers and trainees than was given to the French, whose country was so frequently an enemy. A commercial treaty of 1734 included a provision whereby the British government promised a welcome to Russians coming to study trade processes.[30] This was very valuable, but did not of course mean that all British industrialists would allow Russians to see their works without restraint. There was some falling-off in the Russian government's industrial interest in Britain between Peter the Great and Catherine the Great, but it then revived strongly. For instance, John Perry was recruited under Peter for various hydraulic works including canals; after a considerable hiatus Catherine sent several young engineers, notably Korsakov, to investigate British canal-building. On the best examples of British canal-building to examine he had the advice of Smeaton. But he also visited ironworks like Carron, where cannon-boring was then shut off from him, but he had better success with Wilkinson, whose new blowing machinery and cannon-boring machinery he saw. He had lengthy and helpful meetings with Smeaton. Boulton arranged for him to tour Birmingham manufactures, Wedgwood gave him introductions to industrialists. English instrument-makers went to Russia, first under Peter, later under Elizabeth and Catherine.[31]

In the 1770s and 1780s there was an emphasis on large-scale production and heavy industry. When the great metalworks at Tula were due for renovation two celebrated experts, Surnin and Leont'ev were sent over in 1785. They had two years' education here in English and drawing and other subjects related to their understanding of the technology they would investigate. In 1787 they set off on tour, Birmingham and Sheffield being particularly important to them, but they were advised by the ambassador not to pay too much attention to the 'toy' trade, rather to concentrate on industry essential to armaments. Surnin and Leont'ev gained enthusiastic support from the famous gunmaker Henry Knock, who developed a standard musket for the British army and improved firearms for the navy. He was extremely friendly to Russia, and according to Surnin 'told me without the slightest evasion all the secrets of his trade', and he said that he was indebted to Knock 'for all my success, for my visits to the most important factories, for information about and export of various useful machines which were of the utmost secrecy'. Surnin returned to Russia in 1791, he took plans of machines with him and had made arrangements for the smuggling of the machines themselves, despite the Tools Acts. Knock had apparently made advances towards rifles with interchangeable parts, and ones which could have their locks readily disassembled and reassembled. Surnin was important in reforming the Russian arms factories on his return, especially in a great reorganization of Tula. Leont'ev was also an overseer there in 1806.[32]

Another Russian mechanic of great practical gifts, Sabakin, came to England in middle life, but underwent a similar preliminary training here to the men we have just mentioned, including in English and mathematics, before setting off on his industrial tour. This included Newcastle and Edinburgh, and he then went on to Boulton and Watt in Birmingham. An introduction from the Russian ambassador meant that he was cordially received, but 'they were more prepared to entertain me and take me through the gardens [at Soho] than through their works and factories and [there], I expect, they gave warning in advance what was secret and where I should be taken'. However, he saw much of interest, but was afraid to give attention to particular machines in case 'such attention might make them suspicious of me'. On his return he wrote short articles on steel-making in Birmingham, on steam-engines, road-making techniques, and stoneware manufacture, and made improvements and mechanical inventions in his native region and at the industrial administrative centre of Ekaterinburg. He was emphatic about the craft element in technological transfer, teaching his compatriots 'how to make English instruments and apparatus which they did not know about'. He later worked under Deriabin.[33]

Samuel Bentham, brother of the philosopher Jeremy Bentham, was important in the expansion of the Russian navy, and particularly in the necessary shipbuilding. He records the efforts of Potemkin to attract skilled men in a variety of trades and professions to Russia, while he himself was particularly concerned to bring in shipwrights, boat-builders and sailcloth weavers for the Crimea, but also technicians for the immigrant colony at Krichev in Belorussia and for Siberia.

This brief account of Russian attempts to master British technology is all that can be undertaken here. However, we have already recounted the British concern about Russian apprenticeships in 1719, the great efforts of the Russians to obtain the services of Watt, the training of Deriabin at Soho (which went beyond the strict necessities of his future supervision of the mint Boulton built for St Petersburg) and the very important seduction of Gascoigne, the Bairds, and a considerable number of workmen from Carron in the 1790s. The attitude of the British authorities was relatively relaxed, even indulgent, towards Russian attempts to acquire our technologies, particularly as compared with French ones. But individual industrialists put their own strict limits on what Russian industrial visitors could see, draw or purchase, and hindered their suborning of workers when they thought it prudent.[34]

While our sample of other European countries seeking new technology from Britain in the eighteenth century has been defective and based merely on accessibility of evidence, it does throw light on the French situation. In the first place it shows that France was not alone in recognizing new areas of British technological superiority, and concerned to secure the relevant technologies for herself. Though there are cases of attempts by individuals and firms to obtain the technologies, in all the countries examined the main drive for acquisition came from the State. The State sent individuals or small teams to investigate British industries and to bring back all the information and – where possible – equipment they could. Despite the British laws none of the countries ruled out industrial espionage, though there were some differences in attitude between them. Official Swedish observers exercised discretion and moderation so as not to damage long-term intelligence-gathering, though Swedes independent of state or trade institutions were not so careful. The British government attitude to Russia was distinctly indulgent, though that of individual British industrialists varied from the secretive to the welcoming. Garbett's efforts to prevent the exodus of men and machines from Carron ironworks had less than enthusiastic support from either local or national authorities. Where France was to some degree exceptional was in the very wide range of British industries and technologies which she subjected to industrial espionage, the assiduity with which it was carried out, and some emphasis on what we now euphemistically call 'defence' industries. These would reflect the preoccupations of a century when, despite some Anglomania among intellectuals, the two nations were mostly in opposition, politically, economically and militarily, national rivals, natural enemies.

21 Comparisons II: the Balance of Transfer between Britain and France

With some exceptions, for instance the case study of the spy Le Turc, our accounts of French industrial espionage in Britain and the technology it acquired have mainly been given in relation to particular industrial sectors. However, before we try to arrive at a balance of espionage-driven technology transfer between the two countries three further notable French tours or expeditions should be looked at. They are those of Lescallier and Forfait, of Faujas de Saint-Fond and of the de la Rochefoucauld brothers. They have the useful quality of illustrating the varying degree of espionage in different tours devoted to intelligence-gathering. At one end of the spectrum there is a tour apparently merely seeking education and enlightenment ('innocent espionage'), at the other an expedition of straightforward spying on British naval technology, with the intermediate case of a savant with a genuine programme of scientific investigation but with the intention of finding answers to some industrial questions. In the first and third there are, however, interesting nuances which make the final verdict on them less simple than might at first appear.

Pierre-Alexandre-Laurent Forfait and Daniel (baron) Lescallier were two highly regarded naval administrators sent to England in 1789–90 to get the latest information on the state of British naval technology. Forfait was in his thirties, Lescallier in his forties. Forfait was an 'ingenieur constructeur de marine', he had worked at Brest, had seen active service at sea, and by 1786 was a highly paid 'ingenieur en chef' and in charge of administration at Le Havre. After his English visit he was briefly a member of the Legislative Assembly, subsequently ran into trouble with the Revolutionary administration in 1793–94, but was then restored to favour. He was briefly in charge of forests for naval supply, and then much involved with Bonaparte's costly and abortive plans of 1798 for an invasion of England with flat-bottomed boats. He was responsible for the shipping of the Egyptian expedition, and was for a short time navy and colonial minister under Napoleon, and a continued advocate of an invasion of England. Though he remained a *conseiller d'état* his career failures during an appointment at Genoa led to disgrace in 1805.

Lescallier had spent five years in England between the ages of thirteen and eighteen, had a perfect command of the language, and, despite the periods of war with England, was fundamentally an Anglophile. He began as a naval administrator in Saint Domingo in 1765, returned to France as a sub-commissioner of ports and arsenals, and in 1770 was sent by the navy minister to England, Russia and Sweden. He published a well-regarded dictionary of Anglo-French naval terms in 1777. Following colonial administrative posts of rising seniority he was in 1790 a member of the naval committee of the Constituent Assembly. After his English expedition of 1789–90 he became an important official on the colonial side of the navy ministry, but was an English prisoner from 1793 to 1797, having been captured at Pondicherry. A *conseiller d'état* in 1799, he was later colonial prefect at Guadeloupe. After another brief capture by the British he was consul-general in the United States of America until 1815, but was out of favour after the Restoration.

The two men sent over to England in 1789 by the French navy were therefore already highly experienced, and their quality was demonstrated by their future careers. However, their espionage had a mixture of advantages and disadvantages. Lescallier had English friends with whom he had had very open and helpful relations on his previous visits, a good command of the language, an almost unique mastery of naval terminology, and he had published a standard work on ships' rigging. Forfait was an expert on ship construction. But they had been sent over as winter came on, and reduced daylight hindered their observations, also restricted by days of unremitting rain. Forfait was ill during much of their short visit. They found that the navy yards were completely closed to them.

The last problem was not as severe as it seemed. There were important yards, for instance for the Greenland trade, and for the East India trade at Blackwell, where ships of the highest strength and standard were under construction. In war the demands of the Admiralty meant that such London yards (and others in the provinces) had to build ships of considerable size for the Admiralty, so that there was nothing significant in naval shipbuilding practice which was unknown to them. Indeed the French observers believed the East India constructors were less hidebound (or rule bound) than the royal yards, and good new techniques were developed there which were later taken up in the royal ones. There was virtually no inhibition at all about visiting the yards for Greenland and East India vessels. Some of the owners of these great private yards were already intimate personal friends of Lescallier, which made access especially easy. The naval gun parks were often separate from the yards, and there was little difficulty in getting to see them. Where individual contractors made equipment for the navy, even when under patent, their premises were often accessible when naval ones were not – as Le Turc's penetration of Taylor's works at Southampton has demonstrated. There could have been advantages in seeing yards beyond those close to the capital, but the spies had not been given time, and had to regard their visit as a 'first journey which can be regarded as a trial which can show the possibilities of getting the greatest advantages from one or more later journeys', ones with better advance planning, and with enough time and at a better season of the year.

Perhaps as a result their discoveries were not earth-shattering. They made the interesting general observation that while French naval constructors were regarded as being better theoreticians than the British, the latter had been 'plus savants que les nôtres' in their progress in the actual building of ships. The two Frenchmen paid a good deal of attention to the details of coppering, finding that the British used sheets of a different dimension, and that they used paper and coal tar between the sheathing and the vessel, though there was also some placing of sheathing directly on the hull, in the belief that it would stay more firmly in place. They discovered that the British had made further developments in block and pulley design, and they took back with them some with cast iron pulleys running on copper bearings for testing in France. While the report has some valuable general observations it does not seem to contain outstanding espionage material. However, it may have been readily accepted as preliminary, and a follow-up seems to have been frustrated. Forfait was 'just about to carry out for the French admiralty a mission in England of the highest importance' when he was diverted by his Revolutionary duties in 1791 on being appointed to the Legislative Assembly.[1]

A very knowledgeable French visitor was Faujas de Saint-Fond. His account of *A Journey Through England and Scotland to the Hebrides in 1784*[2] would seem chiefly to be the report of a notable mineralogist, particularly concerned with his studies of basalt and volcanic evidence, but nevertheless with a general interest in coal, and a natural wish to talk to congenial scientific spirits. This made Birmingham, then home to William Withering, James Watt, Joseph Priestley and Matthew Boulton (all members of its Lunar Society) a most interesting place to visit.[3] But he was attached to the inspectorate *Des Bouches à Feu* with its concern to convert French industry to coal fuel. It was natural therefore that he should applaud Wedgwood's Queen's Ware (so prevalent that in travelling over vast distances of Europe one was served upon it at every inn), while regretting that the Montereau potteries in France were not able to imitate it perfectly – though run by Englishmen – and would only do so when they also could employ coal in making it.[4] In visiting Newcastle Saint-Fond remarked on glassworks which were in 'buildings with hardly any appearance', but whose cheapness made it more attractive to invest in them. 'Architecture is a plague in establishments of this kind', a quiet criticism of the Verrerie de la Reine, which he had mentioned earlier in referring to the taking of the British flint glass industry to France.[5] But the question of espionage came up once he visited the great Prestonpans works for sulphuric acid. Speciously he claimed that it was only his acquaintance with a German scientist who was planning a chemical factory nearby which took him there. However, he went into detail about the security precautions, the high wall around the premises 'which does not even let the chimney tops of the works be seen'. Even the harbour where ships brought in sulphur (and no doubt shipped acid out) was surrounded by walls of great height. Next his German friend Swediaur took Saint-Fond and his party to Carron 'where it is impossible to obtain admission without very strong recommendations'. A note to an acquaintance of Swediaur's in Carron Company drew the reply that names, titles and home addresses of the visitors would first be required. They were admitted, but escorted round by an official who warned that they would not be able to see cannon bored, because methods unique to Carron Company were being used, though Saint-Fond doubted if they were any more sophisticated than the steam-powered ones William Wilkinson had installed at Le Creusot. He was impressed by the coking and by the progressive improvements in ore selection over the years. The regularity of operation and the system of the charging of the

45-feet high, cylinder-blown blast furnaces clearly fascinated him, the charging and tapping being governed by the chiming of an on-site clock.[6]

There seems little of espionage in this. But Saint-Fond writes:

> while directing my whole attention to so interesting and complicated a manufactory, I was obliged to trust to my memory for retaining the facts; for *it may be presumed that I was not at liberty to take notes of them in writing* [my italics]. I was therefore obliged to take up part of the night in drawing up an account of my observations.

We clearly do not have all these observations in the *Journey*.[7] That Saint-Fond's tour was not purely personal or scientific is confirmed by the espionage report of Forfait and Lescallier a few years later. They refer to the new British process for extracting coal tar: 'M. Faujas de Saint-Fond ... made with this design a voyage to England and visited the works of Lord Dundonald' [the inventor of a tar extraction process]. On his return Saint-Fond made a small-scale trial of coal tar manufacture in the Jardin du Roi 'in the presence of M. le Ml. de Castries', the navy minister.[8]

The memoir of a tour by the young brothers François and Alexandre de la Rochefoucauld, almost coincidental with that of Saint-Fond, can generally be regarded, as Norman Scarfe's title has it, as of 'innocent espionage'.[9] Their father, the Duc de Liancourt, was an enlightened aristocrat, keen on agricultural improvement, but also on the creation of industrial employment on his estates, where he established an industrial school (*école des arts et métiers*). He had recruited the young Pole, Maximilien Lazowski, as travelling companion to his sons. It is worth noting that one of Lazowski's brothers was a prominent inspector of industry, who was involved in some of the textile manufactures, including framework knitting, which were the personal concerns of Tolozan, the director of the Bureau of Commerce. After the elder of the Rochefoucauld brothers had made a tour of France, the two brothers and Lazowski spent a year in Sussex,[10] where they met Arthur Young, who had taken them on a short local agricultural tour, leading to firm friendships between Young, the young aristocrats, and their tutor, which in turn led to their family's useful support of Young's later French tours. In the following year, 1785, the three made a second British tour, with a specialization on the industrial centres.[11]

The information contained in the narrative is remarkably good coming from non-specialists. On the Leicester stocking manufacture François has to give up in his description of the operation of the frames: 'I'm in no position to describe what I saw, and could only begin to explain it if I had a simple stocking frame in front of me: yet I examined it for half an hour with the greatest attention.' Their relative, the Duc de la Rochefoucauld, was about to be involved in a company, originally on his estates, and using English knitting machines smuggled out by the spy Le Turc, which may shade the innocence of this piece of espionage. The best non-technical minds were and are readily confused by the stocking frame.[12] The party went on to see the famous silk-mill at Derby, with the technology of the machine-throwing of silk stolen from Italy by the Lombe family, and installed in 1719, one of the last major transfers of technology from Europe as the balance tilted in Britain's favour. The current owner, Swift, was operating an attached cotton-mill, to which the Frenchmen were at first denied access. But when Swift arrived on the premises he said that 'seeing we were foreigners ... [he would admit them] ... though he would certainly not admit an Englishman'. François knew of the reluctance of English industrialists to admit outsiders. 'I find that it is very courteous of them to show their processes to strangers (foreigners) who can do no harm to their business; or at least very little harm, and a long time in the future, by establishing these processes at home.' Inspection by compatriots 'might do them real, immediate, and serious damage'. He thought the carding engines employed were more developed than those he had seen at the Holker works at Oissel. Swift seems to have been using variant versions of Arkwright machinery to avoid patent dues. François was particularly struck by the precision of the iron and brass parts of the spinning-machinery.[13]

The party were only able to get a superficial view of steel-making at Sheffield, but an accommodating manufacturer took them to see silver plating and button-making, which was much better than that at Amboise, at the works run by Sanche and Hyde. One factory owner, Yonge, showed them all his workshops and had the workmen themselves explain each process.[14] At Manchester their main contact was the celebrated doctor, Thomas Percival, an important figure in the history of public health, and a key figure in the foundation of the famous Manchester Literary and Philosophical Society. Percival warned the tourists that they would have difficulty in approaching Manchester factory owners, because a Marquis de Crillon had been active in espionage there and the constables had seized a packet of machine components from him, naturally putting the industrialists on their guard.[15] They had a good opportunity to see ribbon looms, but this was not new technology. They went on to Worsley and the Duke of Bridgewater's mines, his canals overground and underground, and the Barton Aqueduct, but these were well-known industrial monuments open to the view of all Europe.[16] In Warrington they were only able to get limited information on flint glass and copper works; they were not kept out, but had no expositor available. François intelligently remarked of the making of flint glasses: 'you feel that it is the precision of the workman's hand that produces the quality of the work'.[17]

In many ways their best account of an industrial district is that of what is now known as the Ironbridge Gorge, and particularly Coalbrookdale and Broseley.[18] At Coalbrookdale they first admired the engineering wonder of the age, the iron bridge itself, only opened at the beginning of 1781. They then met and conversed with two senior workmen. One had worked on the bridge as Abraham Darby III's senior pattern-maker, and had a mahogany model of it. In turn he introduced them to a senior furnaceman, who explained the working of the old furnace, the first iron furnace in the world to have been fired with coke (1709), from which the members of the iron bridge had been cast about sixty years later. They saw the forge stage of iron production and the stamping and potting process which allowed a conversion of pig iron to wrought iron by an entirely coal-using method. They marvelled at the casting of great steam-engine cylinders, pipes and accurately made iron gears, things which they knew had not been accomplished in France, and which they knew Périer had had to import from England in the first place for the Paris waterworks. While John Wilkinson was ill, he gave the Rochefoucauld party every facility at Broseley[19] and they were taken round by his manager. The resulting description is the only good one of Wilkinson's New Willey works. They knew of the Wilkinson involvement with the Indret cannon plant. They were given an estimate of forty as the annual number of steam-engines produced in the Gorge. Later they saw Wilkinson's works at Bradley in the Black Country,[20] and quickly appreciated that the operation of both blowing engines and hammers by steam-power freed the iron industry geographically from water-power sources.

At Birmingham they had letters of introduction to Joseph Priestley. He in turn provided others to two manufactures, but thought them hardly necessary, understandable when it was the premises of Henry Clay, the great maker of japanned paperboard, and those of Boulton which were involved. Clay took them round his works himself. Neither Boulton nor Watt was in residence at Soho, but whoever showed them the premises was clearly an employee of Boulton, for the Watt steam-engine, the duplicating machine and what seems to be the Argand lamp were all ascribed to his inventiveness. Their descriptions would have been fuller if both partners had been in residence, and there can be no doubt that Boulton, with his love of a lord, would have done the honours himself had he been available.[21]

Here, therefore, we have three well-recorded parties of visitors to Britain which each had a keen, if very different, interest in industry. Lescallier and Forfait were here as military-industrial spies, highly knowledgeable, and in Lescallier's case, with good English connections. Their important conclusion was that through contacts with private shipbuilders building for the navy, or with private firms supplying equipment which was of high quality or even under patent, they could circumvent the very tight security at the royal yards. Yet they do not seem to have produced much intelligence of electrifying importance; allotted little time at the wrong season this was not their fault, and a follow-up was frustrated. The journey of Faujas de Saint-Fond is deceptive, in that his genuine mineralogical interests were in fact a partial cover for his official interest in the further exploitation of mineral fuel in French industry. His visits to Prestonpans and to Carron were not as fortuitous as he unconvincingly suggests, and Lescallier and Forfait show that he was under instructions to investigate the new English coal tar, which he demonstrated on his return.

There was indubitably a large purely educational element in the tour of the de la Rochefoucauld brothers and their tutor. But their investigations were not entirely disinterested. In giving a good deal of attention to the stocking industry they may have been aware of the efforts of their relative, the Duc de la Rochefoucauld, to acclimatize the latest improvements in the English stocking industry through Le Turc (his estates were inherited by their branch of the family after his murder in 1794). Their father was already trying to set up workshops in Liancourt and the surrounding villages for 'a manufacture of linen and stuffs mixed with thread and cotton'.[22] Their position in the first rank of French aristocracy was able to open British factory doors to them, and it is interesting that the information they gained influenced one brother to emulate British technological advances. About 1795 Alexandre set up on a property of his in the canton of Mello (L'Oise department), a cotton enterprise which occupied several hundred workers. The spinning was mechanized, probably using jennies, and the weavers produced muslins and quilting 'in the English manner'. He had secured at great expense the services of Macloude to supervise the concern. In 1798–99, however, output was still not great, though it was hoped that peace with Austria (1797) would improve trade. But the firm could not make progress in its original ambitious form, and in 1811 there were only thirty people working in the outbuildings of the château at Mello, with no machine production. Some of the intelligence gathered by Alexandre de la Rochefoucauld had therefore been applied, if not very successfully.[23]

Having completed our survey of French efforts to learn about, understand, and (if need be) obtain by espionage British technological advances, what conclusions can be drawn? First, what was the balance of transfer between Britain and France? The weight of evidence of technological transfer to France in the present work would leave little possibility of doubt. Here we are talking about an 'eighteenth century' which may be defined as running from the end of its first decade to the end of the chronological century. The end of the first decade, which saw the discovery of the coke-smelting of iron and the development of the Newcomen engine, decisively marks the point beyond which the British began a technological leadership which they did not lose until the second half of the nineteenth century, and then gradually and partially.

The situation about 1710 was a new one. There is no question that Britain had been a technological debtor until late in the seventeenth century. In the sixteenth century France, or the Walloon part of The Netherlands, had been of the greatest importance as a source for the blast furnace and the indirect process in the charcoal iron industry and for the crown and broad processes in flat glass. The very vocabulary of these industries once they had been transferred retained strong traces of their French origin.

Perhaps the most important of all the inputs from abroad in terms of the rapid stimulation of British industry was the introduction of the 'new draperies', the manufacture of lighter textiles, generally cheaper, with a wider range of weaves and patterns. They were often mixtures of wools of different types or of wool with other fibres, so there were not only wool-worsted mixtures, but ones involving mohair, silk, linen and cotton. A key element in these changes was the immigration of Flemish and Walloon weavers driven out of The Netherlands by religious persecution or by the fear of warfare and tumult, and attracted not only by the congenial Protestantism now taking hold in England, but by a country with the advantages of high-quality wools and a cheaper cost of living but a good standard of living. The immigrants flowed in from the 1560s onwards, and found themselves well received. Of course they were not able, even where strongly established, as in Norwich or Canterbury, to keep their secrets and specialities to themselves, at least for more than a generation. Once the English became producers of the new draperies they rapidly became innovators, developing a bewildering range of cloths and of finishes, the finishes too in their original form frequently being continental imports. By the mid-seventeenth century they constituted half exports, and much more than compensated for the decline of demand for broadcloth. By 1700 newer cloths of all types constituted half our cloth exports by value. The notable thing here is the evidence of a great new commercial and technological resilience. Englishmen had not simply absorbed new practices from The Netherlands and then carried on with them much as they had been introduced: they had gone on to develop these ideas and methods in a way that changed the whole nature of customer choice and demand, and so altered the industry and its ability to export. Even in traditional cloths like kerseys there were continual modifications, and there were efforts to establish English-type kersey manufacture in Leiden, Bruges and Hondschoote from the middle of the seventeenth century.

There was emigration of English workers both in the older declining branches of the cloth industry and the newer English expanding ones, and we see here the first signs of government opposition to worker emigration. In 1591 the Privy Council took sureties to prevent a West of England man from providing 'instructions or advice' to foreigners to make any English cloths, and from persuading or procuring the emigration of workers. They put pressure on him to bring back weavers and other English workers who had gone to Pomerania. Even before religious persecution of Puritans could have been a strong incentive, and certainly from the Laudian period, there were largish emigrations of cloth workers from Kent, Suffolk, Norfolk and other places to Holland and the Palatinate. Here their possessions of skills valued abroad obviously assisted the emigration. The distractions of the Civil War meant that at its end many of the disaffected or those whose trade had been damaged sought relief abroad. The City of London Committee on Trade reported to the Council of Trade in 1651 'our workmen are enticed or enforced beyond seas to become teachers or servants to strangers in the art of clothing'. Leiden was a particular gainer, as were Poland, Silesia and Prussia.

Particularly from the late seventeenth century a wide range of English cloths were being imitated in The Netherlands, and increasingly in France from the turn of the seventeenth century. There does not seem to be a tide of worker emigration, in many cases it was a matter of imitating English cloth styles or weaves or mixtures rather than any fundamental technical change being needed. But these transfusions of fashionable production did mean that markets were cut back or lost for some sections of the English cloth industry, so that it was well for the industry that the late eighteenth century saw the creation of a new native machine technology. As Kerridge says, 'the time had come for England to start a fresh round of innovation'.

The new draperies certainly marked an important transfer of technology to England from the nearer parts of Europe. It constituted a major instance of our technological indebtedness. But the new methods had been embraced remarkably quickly, and indeed turned into a fertile basis for our own adaptations and innovations, so that there is nothing surprising in the fact that a considerable element in the Law scheme of 1718–20 was devoted to taking English woollen manufactures to France.[24]

The Law scheme, and the accompanying British recognition that there were now important areas of technology in which Britain had a leadership which it was essential not to lose, marked an even more remarkable transition for another reason. The second great period of persecution at the end of the seventeenth century, decisively marked by the revocation of the Edict of Nantes, drove out a large number of Huguenots into Protestant or tolerant states. This exodus, perhaps 200,000 in all, of which 40,000 came to Britain, contained many industrial entrepreneurs and skilled workers.[25] Despite Charles II's Catholic leanings and James II's open Catholicism, English public opinion was so strongly sympathetic to the immigrants that they were freely permitted to enter this country, and allowed to bring in their possessions duty-free. Under William and Mary not only was protection continued 'but we will also do our endeavour in all reasonable ways and means so to support, aid and assist them in their several trades and ways of livelihood as that their living in this realm may be comfortable and easy to them'.[26] Just as the English attempted to bring back their workers from France after the Law scheme, Louis XIV appreciated the loss of skill caused by his bigotry and in 1686 sent experts to England to persuade the Huguenots to return, but only about 500 did.[27] The industries most assisted by the immigration were paper, silk and linen.

Brown, blue and white paper was being made in England before the Huguenot immigration, but the white paper particularly was not of the best quality for printing or writing. The story of the achievements and experiences of the Huguenots is complex, their significance hard to assess.[28] By 1686 a large group of Huguenots and English investors set up a company of white-paper makers which was given a fourteen-year monopoly, extended by another fourteen-year period from 1690, this time only for more expensive white paper. The French concern at the loss of skilled workers in the trade led to strenuous efforts by the French ambassador, Barillon, to get experts and skilled workers to return home.[29] Coleman's verdict is that the company did make improvements in the quality of English white paper, but it had given up business by 1698.[30] A similar company operating in Scotland with certain privileges, went out of existence having let two of its mills in 1703. War, tariffs and excise complicate the position; there was a scattering of Huguenots working at mills outside the two companies. But there seems to be little doubt that the Huguenots contributed to a real qualitative improvement in products of the paper industry already established before their arrival.

Another famous Huguenot immigration was that into the Spitalfields district of London. There was already silk production in England and a Spitalfields textile industry before they arrived, but they greatly stimulated the silk industry and turned Spitalfields into a Huguenot colony. Their contribution seems to have been greater skill, and perhaps even more a capacity for design,[31] which was kept up, though perhaps in a declining way, by their remaining contacts with the French industry. But dyeing and finishing, ribbon-weaving, and throwing were all improved.[32] However, we must not forget that water-powered, mechanized silk throwing was introduced at Derby by Sir Thomas Lombe during 1719–21, and that this was a transfer of technology from Italy. Further large mills were gradually added, generally in the provinces, and provided material for the production of stock products of the industry in new centres like Coventry and Macclesfield. The innovation and vigour of the Huguenots of Spitalfields probably fell off in the first half of the eighteenth century;[33] there is no suggestion of Huguenot influence in the success of the English watering process, which as we have seen constituted a reverse transfer in the silk industry, when John Badger took it to France in the 1750s.

The Huguenots made their greatest single impact on the Irish linen industry. This was very much in decline in the mid-seventeenth century despite efforts of Strafford to revive it in the 1630s and Ormonde in the 1660s, Ormonde's efforts including attempts to bring in Huguenots. In 1697 William III enticed the Picardy Huguenot, Louis Crommelin, at that time a refugee in Holland, over to Ireland, settling at Lisburn near Belfast. He originally brought in twenty-five families from Holland and France, which eventually extended to 500 families, and brought in large numbers of spinning wheels and looms. Land was drained, superior flax seed imported, improved growing and harvesting methods introduced, and new techniques introduced into bleaching. Encouraged by both the British and Irish parliaments the industry gathered pace remarkably; linen cloth exports valued at £14,000 in 1701 were averaging over £750,000 in the early 1750s.[34]

While there were imports of Huguenot skills in gold and silversmithing, and there were celebrated Huguenot gunmakers and watchmakers, particularly in London, these were important additions to the national pool of skill rather than bearers of important novel technologies; in the last two and particularly watch-making, England was entering its own golden age of industrial leadership. Of course France was not the only source of British technological indebtedness in the seventeenth century, the Dutch made great contributions in hydraulic engineering, in the copying of their Delft ware and salt-glaze pottery, in some preparatory and finishing methods for fine woollen cloth and, of course, in agricultural techniques. South Germany and the Tyrol supplied most of the knowledge behind the first great effort to give Britain a copper and brass industry in the late sixteenth century and early seventeenth century.

However, the fact that the Huguenot immigration of the late seventeenth century is so well known a theme of political and religious as well as of economic history has given it a great historical significance. This tends to imply a continuing British condition of technological indebtedness at this period and dangerously overshadows the time when, as dramatically illustrated by the Law scheme of 1718 and the consequent legislation, the balance was decisively changing. That scheme marks the first moment when there was an unusually early and perceptive appreciation by a foreign power of the new skills Britain had to offer, and an equally new and strong apprehension in Britain of the dangers of the exports of those skills. The major technological divergence between Britain and other nations which largely explains the change of balance is that of a coal-fuel technology, so often referred to in earlier chapters, and this will be again examined in our next and final chapter.

The subsequent eighteenth-century transfers of British technology to France have been looked at in great detail in this book. To what extent were they balanced by eighteenth-century transfers of French technologies to Britain? There were such transfers, but there is no way in which they can be regarded as equal and balancing. We have fairly strictly taken 1710 to 1800 as the period studied for the transfer of English technology to France, so it is reasonable to stick to that period for the reverse process. There are three important cases of transfer. One, the cast plate glass industry, we have already looked at in detail.[35] The casting process was entirely a French invention, and was developed to the point of commercial viability by them, in contrast to the blown plate process which they had acquired by suborning Venetian workers. We have seen that, many decades later, the British gained the cast process by suborning French managers and a small number of workers. After the greatest difficulty it was naturalized, it being essential in Britain to secure the conversion of the process to coal, while the French at home narrowly and simultaneously failed to do the same thing. The British, however, through Watt, added a new element, machinery which could polish glasses by steam-power. However, there is no question that they took the central casting techniques from the French.

Similarly, chlorine bleaching came from France. There is the important qualification that the discovery of chlorine and its bleaching properties were the work of the famous Swedish chemist, Scheele. But it was Berthollet who, as part of his work for the French government, developed the bleaching liquid which came to be known as 'eau de Javelle', which was quickly available to French industry, and particularly textiles. Berthollet very remarkably took a very liberal and ethical scientific position on his discovery, seeking neither to gain for himself industrial profit, nor to take a narrow nationalist position, and he made the discovery available to James Watt, who had relatives in the bleaching and dyeing business, during Watt's industrial consultancy visit to France in 1786–87.[36]

The story of the introduction of chlorine bleaching into Britain is extremely complicated, and there were even claims by Charles Taylor, an eminent Manchester cotton manufacturer, bleacher and dyer that he embarked on chlorine bleaching on the basis of information supplied by Scheele to the important Irish chemist Richard Kirwan. However, Berthollet was unquestionably the great influence. In the 1780s the Frenchmen Bourboulon de Bonneil and his colleagues Mathew Vallet and Hugh Foy, who came from the Javelle works in France, based themselves in Liverpool. They erected bleaching plant for manufacturers not only in Lancashire but in Scotland. They then seem to have made the important introduction of potash into bleaching liquor and later the partners were early users of lime water as a substitute for potash. Bonneil and Vallet had petitioned Parliament in 1788 to have an extended patent for their bleaching process (and for a soda one), but an extensive campaign organized in Manchester, Glasgow, Birmingham and London had their scheme thrown out. While the basic chlorine bleaching process was clearly a technological transfer from France to Britain, there was a rapid auxiliary invention here, when Charles Tennant patented and developed a bleaching powder in Scotland, probably the discovery of his partner Charles Macintosh. The powder had the advantage of portability and hence enjoyed improved distributive qualities.[37]

Finally, while the Turkey (or Adrianople) Red process had been keenly sought by many European dyers, and it was not of course a European development, it seems that the French were earlier to domesticate it successfully, particularly at Rouen. The Frenchmen Louis Borelle and Pierre Papillon seem to have been responsible for introducing improved methods in Manchester and Glasgow. However, British dyers had sent investigators to Turkey, and a Greek expert had been brought over. There had been continual experiment here as in France, and frequent (if not very successful) attempts to put dyeing on a scientific basis.[38] While in mid-century the French had commonly made reference to the superiority of British empirically based dyeing, by the end of the century they may have had the edge after the successive labours of Dufay, Hellot, Macquer and Berthollet, an array of scientific talent patronized, encouraged and supported by their government.

On careful examination one major French contribution falls outside our period. In the last two decades of the eighteenth century there was considerable experiment in both Britain and France to produce soda from common salt. Various techniques with some success but a limited output were developed in Britain, particularly by James Keir in the Midlands and Lords Dundonald and Dundas and William Losh on the Tyne. It is interesting that Dundonald is said to have sent Losh to Paris in 1791 to improve his knowledge of chemistry. The difficulty and cost of obtaining barilla, the soda-yielding maritime plant found in Spain, made industrialists in both countries keen to achieve an 'artificial' soda. Nicholas Leblanc, surgeon to the Duke of Orléans, experimented during 1784–88 to produce the celebrated process to which he gave his name, which received a fifteen-year *brevet* (patent) in 1791. He was then making it at Saint Denis near Paris. When Spain joined her enemies there was a strong campaign by the Committee of Public Safety for France to become self-sufficient in soda. A scientific commission in 1794 again reported favourably on the works of Leblanc and partners, called La Franciade, at Saint Denis. But the execution of the Duke of Orléans and the seizure of his effects by the State led to a tangled situation which plunged Leblanc into poverty, and though he made efforts to produce soda by an unspecified method after 1801, and in 1805 was awarded (but did not receive) some compensation for his losses, he killed himself at the beginning of the following year.[39] Others in France began to use his process at the very end of the century, but there is no indication that there was any attempt to transfer his process to Britain during the war years. The 'French plan' was utilized by Losh after a visit to France in 1815, and by Tennant at Glasgow. However, the efforts of Muspratt and Gamble on Merseyside in the 1820s, coinciding with the removal of the salt excise, are often regarded as marking the take-off of the British Leblanc soda industry.[40]

Therefore while this famous process, so dominant in the heavy chemical industry for much of the nineteenth century, had thus been invented in France before the Revolution, it cannot be considered among French transfers of technology to Britain before 1800. The major French techniques which came to England in the eighteenth century were consequently few. Chlorine bleaching was crucial to the great expansion in the European textile industry in the nineteenth century, but once chlorine was known, and its whitening properties, it would have developed somewhere with no great time-lag: its rapid development in France in the late 1780s is nevertheless a testimony to the French predominance in chemistry at this period. French dyeing improvements were an important acquisition by Britain, but perhaps best viewed as a lengthening of the strides already being made by a rapidly advancing textile industry. Plate glass was an up-market product of French industry, but its technology did not have important side-effects on other branches of glass-making, or outside that sector. Put these against the great range of techniques in metal-working, textiles, glass, steam-power and other industries which came over from Britain to France, and one end of the technological see-saw bangs heavily on the ground, while the other rests high in the air. That some of the small host of transfers to France did not take well, or if taken were not acclimatized to the point where there were some indigenous improvements, does not detract from the fact that they were seen by the French as eminently desirable, potentially critical, and therefore to be sought by means open or covert, implying industrial espionage.

22 French Industrial Espionage in Eighteenth-Century Britain and Technology Transfer: an Evaluation

How effective were the French efforts at industrial intelligence-gathering and espionage in eighteenth-century Britain? How far did they result in transfers of technology? Was the technology transferred fully equal to industrial practice in Britain?

On a superficial view it could be claimed that the French obtained whatever British technology they wanted, and that they often acquired it speedily. The collapse of Law's financial schemes implied the dissolution of the industrial enterprises he had brought from Britain and there is little evidence of permanent technological gain from them, though there is evidence of continued French interest in British technology. This is indicated by the welcome given to some of the principals of the Law scheme who returned to France, and by the travels in England of French inspectors of manufactures like Ticquet and Morel. The late 1740s and early 1750s saw a quickening of French acquisition of British technology. In the cases of Kay, Alcock and Holker there were pressures driving them from Britain as well as attractions to France. Kay took the fly-shuttle there before it was well established in England. Alcock may have come over of his own accord, but he was encouraged and subsidized to bring over additional workers from Britain, and the Birmingham ornamental hardware techniques were permanently established in France, if at a lower qualitative level, and there were later French rival importers of the relevant processes. Holker introduced English methods in the spinning, weaving, bleaching, dyeing and calendering of cotton and some woollens, involving the suborning of English workers and the introduction of some British equipment. Badger introduced the watering of silk, with the importation of key calender parts organized by Holker. Naval technologies relating to the coppering of ships, the rolling of copper and the production of cold-rolled bolts were the object of quite notable espionage, as was the new technology in the production of ships' blocks and pulleys. In these cases it is remarkable how quickly the Marine established the existence and importance of the British technology which was eventually acquired, and how well the needful espionage was mounted. The technology of coal-fired bottle glass was not very sophisticated, and it was gained by the French at the beginning of the eighteenth century: we have no knowledge if espionage was involved. It was certainly heavily, if not efficiently, involved in the obtaining of the technology of flint glass in the last years of the old regime after many contretemps.

With remarkable speed the great English textile spinning inventions were brought to France, the jenny by Holker fils at the end of 1770, the water frame and the mule in the early to mid-1780s. The globe and lead chamber processes of sulphuric acid production were the subject of espionage by Jars and Holker fils in the 1760s and soon in large-scale production, the first by 1768 and the second by 1772. There was no need for espionage to obtain the Newcomen engine, introduced in France by its proprietors in 1726, little more than a decade from its first successful working in England. Nor was there for the original Watt engine, introduced by Boulton and Watt themselves within a decade of its patent, though espionage was involved in acquiring the double-acting engine. The solid boring of iron cannon was brought to France by the brother of the inventor, with the inventor's encouragement, and their co-operation was essential to the first introduction of the coke-smelting of iron with steam-powered blast, iron-railed ways and all the appurtenances of the most up-to-date English ironworks. Thus baldly stated it would seem that the technology of the British industrial revolution was neatly boxed and dispatched to France within a short period after its invention, and almost as if it was a normal cargo of the packet boats.

This seems a perfect confirmation of the celebrated case put forward by David Jeremy, when looking at the evidence after 1780, that the

British attempt by legislation to 'dam the flood' of the export of technology had failed. However, the difference in period between Jeremy's classic paper and the present study must be emphasized, for in part he covers the period 1825–43 when the export of some machinery from Britain was prohibited, but not the suborning of workers, while we are only concerned with the years to 1800.[1]

But the issue is a complicated one, even if we concentrate only on the French evidence. There were some cases where British technology failed to be transferred at all, or so poorly as to make no impact, as with the production of cementation and crucible steel with coal-fuel. Iron puddling was not successfully established in France before the Restoration. Even where the French state brought great influence to bear because of the armaments implications, as in the coke-smelting of iron, the failure to transfer effectively was immensely costly and constituted a humiliating deterrent to further innovation of the kind in the medium term. Flint glass production was taken to France, but only after great cost, and a comedy of errors, and with mediocre results. But even when some types of technology were successfully transferred, to the extent that the equipment copied in France worked to a worthwhile extent, and represented an advance on previous French methods of production, this did not mean that French practice equalled British practice. For instance, the owners of the Louviers cotton-mill were forced to confess in 1787: 'We are far from the perfection the English have reached.'[2]

The sub-British standard of technology transferred from that country and operated in France was a frequent problem and two reasons for it were advanced. One was the quality of suborned workers. In the 1780s it was recognized, as it had been much earlier, that it was difficult to suborn the best English workers. They could do very well at home, especially in a cotton industry that was expanding at great speed, and in which the possibilities of supervisory posts and good pay were strong, and where a few could even break through into management. There were sufficient arrests of suborned workers to dissuade the more cautious, while the belief that, once emigrated, workers would not be allowed to return, or could do so only under severe penalties, however mistaken, was often held. It was advanced by English workers in France and by French masters and administrators. The legal position that, before any sanction could be imposed, emigrated workers had to have received a six months' warning from the English diplomatic service abroad, and then to have ignored it, was clearly not understood.[3]

French industrialists and administrators were very doubtful that the best British workers were normally recruited. There were good examples, like Adam Tinsley at La Charité, or Le Turc's block-makers at Lorient, or Hulse or Ferguson in the cotton industry, where expertise was unquestioned, as was the men's respectability. But there were many who were undisciplined, 'mauvais sujets', and there were times when their French masters regretted they had ever sought them out and suborned them. This feeling was, of course, all the stronger when it was felt that the workers had exaggerated their knowledge and expertise, and the plant they had set up worked badly, not comparably to the English models, and was in continual need of modification and repair. Tolozan, the Director of the Bureau of Commerce, the best person to have an overview of the situation, had complained of the many Englishmen 'coming into the country to offer to make ... machines for carding and spinning cotton. We have believed them far too easily, and the majority have deceived us, [the machines made] do not produce anything like the effects they have promised us'.[4] It was true that English workers were independent and self-willed beyond the experience of their potential continental employers. This did not mean that they were ungovernable if well treated, and the independence made them the more easily detached from their original English employers, and the more ready to betray the secrets of their machines. Dupont de Nemours put it most strongly:

> One can keep the secrets of a German works because German workers are docile, wise, and content with little. But English workers are haughty, quarrelsome, risk-takers and greedy. There is nothing easier than to suborn them and when a machine produces some gain for English industry the French government can always be master of it in six months [because they would know of it from the patent].[5]

One certainly can only marvel at the adventurousness of British workers, which must have been a great advantage to those endeavouring to suborn them. There may have been cases where debt or harsh masters provided a propulsive element which matched and indeed increased the attractions of high pay, pensions and other amenities they were promised in France. But for men to travel great distances, to settle in another country with a different language and, for most, a different religion, with a very different diet and countless other strangenesses of custom affecting daily life, and then to bring over, in many cases, wives and children to join them, required a readiness to face change which is quite remarkable.

There does seem to be some justification for Dupont de Nemour's resort to national characteristics to explain the readiness of British workers to face challenges, to take a gamble. In the case of the original group of artisans brought in by the elder Holker, there is no doubt that he was bringing in men who were Catholics, and often of a Jacobite persuasion. In his paper to Trudaine setting forth his recommendations for the suborning of workers as the means to the transfer of technology, he again recommended the recruitment of Catholics. There does not seem to have been any long-term consistency of French government policy, however. There were a considerable number of Irish among the later immigrants, particularly in textiles, and this sometimes reflects recruitment of former textile workers among Irishmen in the French army, or prisoners of war from the British forces, though a few of the Irish cotton workers seem to have had some earlier experience as immigrants into South Lancashire. The Irish would overwhelmingly be Catholic. A pro-Catholic bias no doubt lingered in the Holker-influenced centres like Rouen and Sens, though there is little indication that it was general. But there is one instance, that of La Charité, where there are statements that Michael Alcock and some of his workers had feeling stirred up against them as Protestants.

This, however, was part of a situation where there was a conspiracy to discredit and remove Alcock by French associates. His sons embraced Catholicism, no doubt reflecting their wish to avoid such problems. Thereafter there is silence on the subject, and an absence of references to Catholicism as a desideratum in the recruitment of technologists. It is possible that where British Catholics were recruited by French industry they may have felt more at home and integrated better into the new communities they entered, but no direct research has been done on this. However, the large number of British workers that could be detached from their original homes incontrovertibly argues for their having a strong sense of their own worth, a willingness to take risks and face change, a reluctance to stay in one place, however familiar, if there was the hope of better things elsewhere. From the viewpoint of their new French masters there was a downside to this. Willingness to be recruited was matched by unwillingness to accept what they thought harsh or unfair conditions in France, and a disposition to be awkward and obstreperous if they disliked their situation, to move on and change employers or go back home.

One of the main problems in managing English workers was to deal with their drunkenness, several examples of which have already been encountered. Naturally this may be especially noticeable in the workers who went abroad, who may have been particularly inclined to drink, for there was a frequent connection between drink and debt. A regular toper was more likely to be unthrifty, fall into debt and, if the debt was to the employer, become effectively bound to him. It was a common situation in Britain that a worker could only change his job if a new employer who wanted his particular skills was willing to take over his debts from his existing employer. An invitation from a foreign employer could break this fetter of indebtedness either by a bribe which could enable the worker to pay off his debt, or simply by providing the means of flight.[6] Suborning was invariably accompanied by the promise of higher wages in a cheaper country, giving promise of more drink. Of course the drink–debt link was not universal. Sober workers in Britain could find themselves in difficulty because of a slump in trade, sickness in the family, the costs of a wife's pregnancy and childbirth, or just too many children to maintain, to give familiar examples.[7]

It was not only French employers who found problems with English workers, and drink prominent among them. The Swiss Johann Conrad Fischer, founder of the famous Schaffhausen engineering firm, visited England first in 1794 (when he briefly worked in London) and several more times before a final visit in 1851. He advised other Swiss against employing English workers.

> Not only do they cost a damned lot of money but they are often intoxicated. English workers who are efficient and well behaved can earn a very good living at home. It is not uncommon to come across English workers in foreign countries who are far from competent in all the branches of their trade.[8]

However, from prime minister to ploughman Britain was a hard-drinking society; Wesleyanism and evangelicalism only began to make their sobering impact late in the century; as with the block-makers who surprised Le Turc, heavy boozing and excellent workmanship were sometimes compatible.

A most important difficulty in using suborned English workers to transfer technology to France was the craft nature of virtually all the technology that was attempted to be transferred. This meant that written descriptions and plans and drawings were only marginally useful. They might convey the nature of a new process, though with different exactness in different industries: it was easier to explain a machine, at least in principle, than it was a metallurgical process. To enhance the difficulty, even in machine-based methods it was rarely possible to obtain the drawings owned by entrepreneurs and managers, and we have seen several instances where foreign spies tried to make drawings hurriedly, covertly, and in anything but ideal conditions.

The wisest heads throughout the century believed it was the migration of the craftsman, not the obtaining of descriptions and designs, that transferred technology. 'The arts never pass in written form from one nation to another; only the eyes and practice can train men in this work', wrote Mignot de Montigny in 1752.[9] Le Turc, thirty years later, made the same point: '[It] is not with words or with drawings that one will make the [French] workman, always infatuated with his own method, change it for another, although superior to his.' Clever foreign workmen had to be found who could train French pupils, but the problem in getting them from England was made very difficult by the subdivision of labour and the consequent specialization of workmen who were each expert in only one part of the productive process.[10]

Chaptal, whose experience as a scientist, industrial chemist, and minister responsible for industry, gave him a unique view of French industry, and who wrote two classic industrial studies, one on the application of chemistry to industry [*La Chimie Appliqué aux Arts et Manufactures* (1807)], certainly believed that French deficiencies in copying British industry were largely due to the failure to master the intricacies and knacks of crafts:

> We have seen several kinds of industry establish themselves and prosper in England, and render other nations subservient to their products over many years, we have made every effort we could to obtain for ourselves such manufactures, but in importing the machines, in putting dependence on various transmitted techniques, did we really believe that we had naturalized these crafts in every particular? Can we believe we possess all the immensity of detail, all those knacks [*tours de main*] those habits which are the soul of industry?[11]

David Jeremy, describing the transmission of British technology to the Philadelphia region, stresses the non-verbal (i.e. non-verbal and non-graphic) nature of the transfer to that district, and shows that machines and models not accompanied by a skilled mechanic were rarely successfully employed.[12] Akos Paulinyi, recently writing of the Prussian experience, has pointed out that personal contact is still important in technology transfer today and that it was even more critical earlier.

> The dependence was much stronger during the first half of the nineteenth century, as the overwhelming bulk of British technology was

not intelligible through written (or printed) information or through drawings published in Britain. Hence it was very difficult to communicate technical knowledge or acquire technical skills outside the production process itself (i.e. outside the technical action).[13]

The need to import craftsmen to make any real use of machines, plans or drawings was therefore virtually absolute.

To the extent that British law dissuaded the law-abiding, responsible, sober and securely employed craftsmen from leaving home, and it was the footloose, undisciplined, restless men, fond of their drink, who went abroad, there was likely to be a reduction in the quality of their craftsmanship, and a lower quality in their product.

There is the difficult question of how many English technologists went over to France in our period. ('Technologist' is here used as an anachronistic term to encompass entrepreneurs, managers and artisans – there was no significant recruitment of the unskilled or low skilled.) Bellefonds who looked into the situation in detail would only offer a guesstimate of 400 technicians (*techniciens*) and 1,000 workers (*ouvriers*) between 1715 and 1815.[14] There are problems here: it seems that the distinction between technicians and workers is doubtful. Few unskilled workers were recruited, so the distinction between 'technicians' and 'workers' is hard to maintain. The suborned virtually all claimed to be skilled, though whether the quality of their work and the suitability of their dispositions justified their recruitment is a different matter. Where the recruited man had something of a leadership role among a group of skilled workers recruited for a particular industrial unit, or where he created difficulties or problems, he is often named and can consequently be identified. The question of how many other immigrants there were in the background is often difficult to answer. Generally we are talking of small numbers whenever we have serious evidence.

Indeed the remarkable thing is how few men, if well chosen, could impart a major technology. For instance there were three for the important Taylor block and pulley processes; there were probably never more than a dozen English workers of either sex at La Charité; Kay seems to have had few English outside his own family for fly-shuttle or hand card production, and had difficulty in keeping his own sons. The one really large immigration was that of the Law scheme, preceding the Act of 1719, and there were probably 200–300, which would include some wives and children and some apprentices. As this event has only recently been rediscovered it cannot come under Bellefonds's total. If there were about 200 workers at Romilly, and they were originally all English, this would be the one other large immigration.

Again our examination of the transfer of technology ends in 1800 while Bellefonds's continues to 1815, and includes the considerable influx under the Peace of Amiens. Many, probably most, of the British in France at the end of the peace in 1803 were overtaken by the rapid British declaration of war, and were seized as hostages ('otages') and held by the French until 1814. While some were held in camps, those who had come to France for industrial purposes were generally allowed to return to work; some of course had come to France long before 1802. An incomplete survey by Audin showed that the hostages included seventy-five commercial men, and at least 316 manufacturers and artisans. This included a minimum of 177 textile workers, a few being released prisoners of war, and about sixty of them are given as 'mechanicien'. It is known that a minimum of twenty-four of the textile workers had arrived during the peace of Amiens, but this will not account for all the arrivals in that period.[15]

Precision is impossible, but even including the Law scheme immigrants, and excluding those after 1800, modifying Bellefonds's total for 1715 to 1815 to 1,000 for 1710–1800 would seem generous. However, any idea that all the immigrations of British workers into France constituted part of a steadily increasing total is misleading. The legal restrictions on their return seem to have been virtually inoperative, there are no known instances of their property in Britain having been seized or their being officially deemed alien. There seems to have been a belief among some emigrants that they would be unable to return home, but their assertions to this effect may have been partly intended to impress on the French authorities the moral responsibility they had for the immigrants' continued employment, protection and generous treatment. Certainly large numbers went home. The workers of the Law scheme of course returned home with British government assistance, and only a handful of the major technicians returned to France later. The highly skilled Green family left La Charité and returned home; Kay's sons reappeared in England; de Saudray recruited men successfully, but he was not then able to employ them properly and one group certainly went home as a whole. The flint-glass makers recruited for Saint Cloud were mostly persuaded to return home by British diplomatic officials under the terms of the 1719 Act, very few were employed after the firm moved to Le Creusot. Romilly copper works, however large the original recruitment, had only three or four British technicians remaining in the early nineteenth century. However, despite the mixed fortunes in France of some of the original purveyors of the machine technology of textiles, mainly cotton, that sector seems to have constituted a continued market for skilled British workers. But there can be no doubt that several hundreds, perhaps over 400, of British technological emigrants to France in our period returned home.

Good craftsmen demand good tools; the English workers in France found themselves facing problems here. There is not a significant literature on the economic history of hand tools, and for present purposes we have to rely on occasional references. The first group of workers brought in by Holker in the early 1750s began by buying the materials to make their own tools before they could make anything else, not finding French ones serviceable. This was still the same for Wood when he came to work for the Louviers textile entrepreneurs in the 1780s. He wrote of the 'difficulties he has experienced in establishing in a country where everything had to be created a machine [water frame] so complicated are inexpressible ... [He] has been obliged to make with his own hands the tools and instruments proper to work on the different pieces of mechanism'.[16] The tools of their suborned expert, Spencer, who ran their machine shop, and was capable of making 160 spindle mules, were bought up by his employer Morgan and Massey (themselves long settled in France) in 1791, possibly because of his death or return home. Though they had brought other workers and mechanics over, there was some doubt if more machines like Spencer's could be made.[17] When the Chamber of Commerce of Normandy reported critically on the effects of the Eden Treaty, they recorded as one favourable sign the good effects on tool production of the immigration of English workers into Normandy:

> We have already noticed that the residence in our works of several English experts and workmen inspires us with a taste for the perfection of the tools they use and the excellent tempering of their tools. It is to this advantage that they owe a great deal of their superiority.[18]

The skills which the French sought to steal, and the British to protect, were of course ones in which Britain had a lead, or possessed exclusively. Why had Britain developed this important differential in skills, and in tools? A main cause was the new and unprecedented direction which Britain had taken in technology. This new direction was well enough understood among industrialists, their managers and the most intelligent workers, but it was not articulated by political and economic writers of the eighteenth century, almost certainly because it was not fully comprehended by them.

This is not the place to discuss the general theory of technological change, which itself is currently entering a period of fundamental reappraisal.[19] Here it is simply argued that the achievement of a technology based on the extensive use of a low-cost energy source, and the ready availability of materials on which that energy could be employed, were basic to British industrialization.

Though its use as a domestic fuel long predominated, coal began to be used in the Middle Ages as an industrial fuel for purposes like lime-burning and brewing (as early as 1264), especially where there was inexpensive water transport from collieries to the industrial sites. It became widely used by smiths in preference to charcoal. In the late sixteenth and seventeenth centuries the rising price of wood accelerated the industrial use of coal, and dyers and bakers took to it. The availability of a cheap fuel with a certain supply was an aid and often an incentive in the establishment of new industries like the boiling of soap and sugar, and there was a turning from wood to coal in the making of glass, bricks, tiles and pottery. Of great importance was the new use of coal in smelting the non-ferrous metals, copper, lead and tin, towards the end of the seventeenth century, and in brass-making at the opening of the eighteenth century. The success and importance of Britain in non-ferrous metal production, in European and even world terms, in the eighteenth century is strangely neglected. Some north-eastern and Scottish salt-pans were burning coal as early as the thirteenth century, though some inland centres continued to use wood or turf, and Cheshire salt-pans were only converted to coal in the mid-seventeenth century. Not only did coal replace wood as a fuel for brewers over much of the country in the sixteenth and seventeenth centuries, one of the first uses of coked coal was in malting, from the middle of the seventeenth century.

Coal made great strides in the auxiliary industries of textiles; dyers and hatters had long adopted coal according to a statement of the 1570s. It was also used in kilns for the drying of flax and yarn, in cauldrons in which wool and other textiles were cleaned, and to heat hot presses for cloth. The rising industries for elementary chemicals like alum and copperas for use in the textile industry, and saltpetre used in gunpowder, were based on coal in the seventeenth century. The making of glass with coal-fuel alone was established by a long-running patent from 1614. Brick-making with coal went back to the fourteenth century, but results were not always good until improvements in kilns were made in the seventeenth century. As we have seen the technology of the smelting and refining of iron with coal-fuel presented the most obdurate technical problem, and its use in smelting was only partly solved in 1709, even if a superior cast iron was thenceforward available. The production of wrought iron with coal was only achieved by progressive improvements in the second half of the century.

The great credit for placing coal at the centre of the history of British industrial growth belongs to John Nef, though there were mistakes in timing and emphasis in his analysis, and these have now been carefully and fairly corrected by Hatcher.[20] There seems no reason to follow Nef in his overemphasis of the 1540–1640 period, while his idea that there was an inventive hiatus in the conversion of industry to coal between 1640 and the conventional industrial revolution of the eighteenth century is the reverse of the truth. By 1700 British industry had predominantly moved to a coal-fuel technology. This was not merely a matter of using coal as fuel where wood and charcoal had been used in a similar way. Nearly always there had to be adaptation, in the metal and the making of boilers, in the construction of grates, in the design of furnaces, in the selection of refractory materials and their embodiment in hearths, furnaces and crucibles, in the design of ventilation and draught systems, notably exemplified in the modification of the 'air' or reverberatory furnace as used with coal-fuel, or the cones within which the furnaces of some coal-using industries operated.

This had two general effects. The continued need for innovation in order to use coal at all meant that technical change became regarded as customary, and its basis became not only modification of the old, but distinct invention. A substantial part of industry became accustomed to living with novelty. The new coal-fuel technologies sometimes modified existing crafts, which were learned and passed on as the ancestor crafts had been, and sometimes created new ones which were soon similarly transmitted. The new skills were not embodied in drawings and manuals, and to gain their advantages you had to acquire the craftsmen, which the past chapters have continually instanced and insisted on as the prime means of transferring technology. The range of new specialized crafts meant that other countries seeking to acquire the new coal-based technologies faced problems in identifying the subdivisions of processes and the specialized craftsmen needed to be recruited for each stage of production and for the building of plant and equipment.

Wrigley has well demonstrated that there was a major change in Britain from an 'organic' economy in which wood-fuel and agriculture-based raw materials were the foundation of industry, to a new-model economy, a 'mineral-based' one, in which coal was the overwhelming fuel source,[21] and eventually, through the steam-engine, a source of mechanical energy. Of course all this would have been fragile if the reserves of coal in the ground had not been immense, if their variety had not been great, if they had not been remarkably widely distributed in Britain, so that once turned to they seemed inexhaustible. A variety of specific coal types was available for the special needs of different industries, a point which can hardly be sufficiently emphasized. With incremental transport improvements in waggon-ways, roads and canals to add to the existing facilities of the coastal trade the mines were able to answer potential demands at acceptable cost. Given the shift towards a mineral-based economy Wrigley points out 'that the old constraints on the scale of output fell away, unit production costs declined continuously across a wide swathe of industries, and both production and productivity could rise without knocking against the ceiling present in the earlier system'.[22]

The early experience of cost-saving with coal-fuel meant that technological ingenuity was given a programme, a target to aim for, a line of direction which past gains indicated could be followed with considerable optimism. This meant that innovation was no longer regarded as random, occasional, fortuitous, but a rational process in which many could participate. This concentration on a growing coal-fuel technology gave British industry a 'focusing device' of the kind identified by Rosenberg, which meant the technological effort was far more effective than if it had been scattered weakly round all those sectors of industry where some limited technological innovation seemed feasible.[23]

Since Ticquet in 1738[24] there had been those who urged the French government and its officials that it was important to follow Britain in the use of coal. Of course the Holkers had done so, and Jars, and there had been an important initiative by Grignon in 1779 who proposed, and eventually got, a small inspectorate to examine the fuel use and needs of France, record those places where fires and furnaces were used in industry, and avoid the danger of wood-fuel scarcity by moving to coal.[25] This fear of wood famine had long haunted France. It was present in the thinking of Faujas de Saint-Fond, attached to the inspectorate, as he toured England and Scotland in 1784. The great push in its operations was the major fuel enquiry administered by Baron de Dietrich in 1788,[26] which was in progress as the country's central and provincial administration began to lose its grip, and had no consequences once Calonne had fallen and all his schemes became anathema to his successors.

It is not always easy to see how far French administrators were enthusiastic about coal merely as a replacement fuel if wood became scarce,[27] and how far they recognized that coal was, as it were, the carrier for a new technology. Calonne, however, with his concept of Le Creusot as the exemplar, the display centre in France of new British technology, with its coke-smelting of iron, flint-glass manufacture, and steam-power (all new technologies based on coal and inseparable from it) was very much on target.

While it cannot be fully developed here, one factor central to the development of a coal-fuel technology in Britain is passed over by most economic historians – with the major exception of Wrigley,[28] and constitutes an inexplicable silence in their narrative. In terms of any possible demand in the eighteenth century Britain was remarkably provided with industrial raw materials. She possessed large quantities of all the non-ferrous metals, lead, copper, tin and the calamine to make zinc for brass, while France was much less endowed, especially in tin and copper. Britain was well supplied with the mordants for dyeing, particularly alum and copperas, and with fuller's earth. Fireclay, often overlooked, but of the greatest importance, was frequently found in coal measures, while some of outstanding quality was found in the Stourbridge district. Without good firebrick efficient and durable furnaces could not be built, without fireclay of the first quality crucibles good enough for flint glass, or particularly cast steel, were not possible. France had, as we have seen, a qualitative and a quantitative deficiency in steel. Britain was well provided with china clay, as there were vast deposits in Cornwall.[29] As a well-informed technologist wrote in 1787:

> Great Britain receives more benefits from the bowels of the earth than perhaps any other nation under heaven, as may be at once discovered by taking a cursory view of her abundant magazines of most excellent coals, and her most numerous, rich, and various mines of the precious and useful metals ... Coal in particular is now become of such immense consequence to our cities and populous countries, to our forges and other manufactories ... that it was impossible for us to arrive at such eminence, and impossible for us to support our present flourishing state of society without it; and we are as much indebted to the other parts of the mineral kingdom, for the materials of our staple commodities which are so widely diffused in the numerous channels of our commerce.[30]

The quantity, and above all the quality of British wool was envied in France, a superiority from the old 'organic' economy which continued into the period when industrial activity was increasingly mineral based. France thus had other resource handicaps, beyond the obvious one of the poorer endowment and geographical distribution of coal, which reduced any advantages which could be obtained by the best industrial intelligence and the most daring espionage. The acquisition of skills from Britain was made the more difficult because the French had to try to comprehend all the complications of a coal-fuel technology within a mineral-based economy. This was a world new to them, even if it had been developing in Britain over a couple of centuries. Just as difficult was the acquisition of machines.

It has been seen that the basic knowledge of new British technology was often taken rapidly to France. It has been shown that as the technology was increasingly embodied in machines, particularly in cotton textiles from the 1760s, so examples of the British machines were taken to France. If it had been possible freely to import in quantity as many machines of every type as were desired, there would have been a greater likelihood of French workshops and factories being founded which were perfectly qualitatively equivalent to their British exemplars. The only obstacle, which would have been gradually overcome, would have been the training of men and women to work the machines, for which English managers and skilled operatives would have had to be suborned (though entailing problems we have already discussed) and this was of course done. But it was only possible to obtain a small number of machines, by stealth, disassembled, and concealed by splitting them between other cargoes. It was not possible to ship a factory-full, whatever the inefficiencies of British magistrates, constables, or customs officers.

As late as 1824 the *Parliamentary Report on Artisans and Machinery* produced strong evidence reflecting continuing machinery problems for the French. By this time large works managed by Englishmen were making textile machines and even steam-engines in France. But the London engineer John Martineau pointed out that important costs for these firms were the high wages of the English craftsmen they used for their superior work. He believed that the critical thing was that 'the difference does not only consist in the quality of the workmanship but in the quantity a man can manufacture in a given time'. A related problem was that iron, the main raw material, was 100 per cent dearer than in England. Questioned, he said that a factory to make machines could be established quickly in Britain 'because we have such facilities of obtaining tools of every description, in France it would take a considerable time'. While at the English-run factories at Charenton and Chaillot the workmanship was as good as English, the materials were not.[31] The celebrated engineer Galloway thought that there was no question that French machine manufacture was improving, especially over the last few years. Some French makers, particularly Callas, made quite excellent machines, though they were more costly than English. Nevertheless, Britain generally made better and cheaper machines, 'most of the raw commodities from which machines are constituted, are cheaper in England; secondly our coals are less expensive, and we possess many facilities in machines and tools for machine-making which are not anywhere else than in this country possessed'.[32] Another notable engineer, Donkin, said he was aware that the 'mechanical arts' had greatly improved in France, but 'there is still the same relative difference between us that there was fifty years ago'.[33]

A Mr Alexander, who had a close acquaintance with the French cotton industry, said 'a machine made in England is certainly superior in certain metals, as cast iron, steel and brass, and generally better finished'. Sixty machines could be made in England while ten of the same kind were made in France.[34] As late as the *Report* of 1824 there were several statements that it was still not possible to make good machines abroad from drawings and models alone. While one outcome of the 1824 enquiry was that it was found useless to try to stop the emigration of artisans (and quite inequitable when British capitalists could set up works abroad as they wished) the other was the usefulness of the continuation of the prohibition on the export of textile and other machinery, because its mass export would have made a present to France and other countries of a technological leadership which we still possessed, and which their copying of British machines did not yet eliminate.

The mass of evidence given in preceding chapters and the clear balance in the transfer of technology between Britain and France, means that some contemporary quotations about inventive achievement in the two countries can be dismissed as aberrations not requiring serious refutation. One is the view of a Swiss calico-printer that the English 'cannot boast of many inventions, but only of having perfected the inventions of others, whence comes the proverb that for a thing to be perfect it must have been invented in France and worked out in England'. The continuous flow of seekers of new and better technology who entered France from England (with only the merest trickle in the opposite direction) cannot be squared with the suggestions that France was more inventive than England.[35]

There is no suggestion that Frenchmen were inherently less inventive than Britons. If one can regard the establishment of new scientific knowledge as a type of invention such a nonsense is immediately exposed by the contemporary record of French achievement. Nor can the French be thought of as being lacking in technological imagination: D'Auxiron's concept of the steamboat, Cugnot's of the locomotive, Mongolfier's of the balloon, are testimonies to the very opposite. Mongolfier's idea was marvellous, but had little utility. Cugnot's and D'Auxiron's were ideas of genius, but unfortunately some decades ahead of the technological knowhow that was necessary for fulfilment. They both vainly attempted to push further, indeed too fast, the contemporary British achievements with the steam-engine. Périer, too, had prophetic ideas on the development of the steam-engine. But in technology an idea often had to await the ability to control and work materials, and the opportunity to use critical components, perhaps unexciting in themselves, but essential to its realization.

That within the limits of the new coal-fuel technology the French were on new and unfamiliar territory can be seen from their failure to make any independent advance with the steam-engine between 1789 and 1815, and their failure to make significant developments of the new British textile technology over the same period, where metal quality and working were critical for the key parts. Similarly they failed to make blister or crucible steel with consistent success, while enormous expenditure on coke-iron and flint glass produced very limited results. Outside those limits they could often be technologically as creative as other nations: witness their great progress in silk, fine ceramics and plate glass. In the last, as we have seen, they had success as long as they were employing wood as the fuel, but were not able to consolidate the advantages of conversion to coal, and did not obtain the advantages of steam-powered grinding and polishing for many decades. It is noteworthy that in sulphuric acid production, where their chemical expertise was able to come into play, they did significantly improve on the British technology they had adopted.

The work of the French government in trying to promote technological advance was critical, as has been seen throughout this book. One of the institutions on which it much relied was its Academy of Sciences, whose connection with the Crown was very different from that of the

Royal Society in England, where the relationship was much more one of a detached patronage. Here we are only concerned with the Academy as it related to transferred technology. From 1699[36] at least the duty of the Academicians was formalized; they were to advise the Government on new industrial schemes or equipment or processes about which it wished to be assured before issuing letters patent to inventors or, more significantly, granting privileges, especially where these involved remission of taxes or direct subsidy by the Crown.

Sometimes these enquiries were handled by small temporary groups of commissioners chosen from the Academicians on the basis of the supposed relevance of their scientific knowledge to the technical subject to be decided. Sometimes alone, or as part of such groups, the Government turned to those Academicians who had been given long-term commissions to advise, examine and frequently to experiment and research in particular industrial areas. We have seen Dufay, Hellot, Macquer, Berthollet in this role, all with reference to the dyeing and bleaching of textiles, and the last three also to ceramics, though this did not exhaust the matters on which they were called to pronounce. In these particular areas the scientists certainly did use their chemical ability to make some important advances. But in other industrial sectors Academicians were not always able to make a significant contribution. Metallurgy was one, and we have seen that steel in particular was a marked failure, and this despite the discovery by Berthollet, Vandermonde and Monge of the carbon content distinction between cast iron, wrought iron and steel. The production of good small, trial quantities of metals or alloys for academics to assess had little relevance to the ability of the manufacturer who submitted them to make good quality materials on a large scale. While a learned horologist and a brilliant mathematician might have some sensible things to say about a new English textile machine, in the end it was imported skills in manufacture, assembly and operation which were necessary for its success. The good record of some Academicians as advisers was in part due to their efforts to introduce rationality into industrial production, but in the case of two of the most successful, Mignot de Montigny and Desmarets, it was mainly their long experience as commissioner or inspector, combined with commonsense, assiduity and outstanding powers of observation which enabled them to help textiles and paper. They both were expert in identifying the important processes, skills and technologists, English and Dutch, needing transfer to France if something like an equal efficiency of production was to be achieved.

Some other negative factors were involved in the reliance on the opinions of Academicians. It often took some time to assemble the supposedly expert team and arrange the examination of the new process and equipment to be appraised, and sometimes more than one panel was necessary, all of which put back the time when the new industrial activity could be mounted full scale. If the report of the Academy commission was unfavourable, the inventor or introducer of the new industrial method or machine would rarely accept the decision as final and there would follow a long and increasingly complex correspondence as the intending innovator tried to get it reversed. If the decision was favourable, this would open the door to new discussions about what subsidy, concessions or privileges would be awarded the innovator, which could itself be a lengthy process. Changes of administration could cause major disruptions here, as with de Saudray and Le Turc. All this tended to delay the business of introducing new technology. It tended too to cast a shadow over innovations which were not officially approved by the scientific establishment. Again, it tended to inhibit the innovator from seeking a full commercial capital from the outset. It postponed the moment when he had simply to rely on the consumer to try out and to approve his product, a test which was inevitable anyway.

The place of the Academy in the central establishment of the State meant that innovators had almost invariably to prove their innovations to Academicians in Paris, whether that was the sensible place or not. All these problems had their effect. There was by the Revolution a large cohort of the frustrated and aggrieved among inventors and innovators, the last including some transferrers of technology, who believed that their efforts had been seriously affected by theoretically biased, impractical Academicians. Among the most eminent leaders of this movement, as we have seen, was de Saudray, and it was an important reason for the dissolution of the Academy in 1793.[37]

From the late 1740s there was a change of emphasis at the Bureau of Commerce from the mainly regulatory approach to industry to an approach which looked more to improvement and 'amelioration', and the function of the provincial inspectors themselves tended to reflect this shift, though it was sometimes limited by the age and conservatism of industrial inspectors, and even by that of some of their superiors in Paris. Some industrial towns with very traditional products and markets were firmly attached to the regulatory system and did not welcome innovation.

Where the Bureau of Commerce officials endeavoured to evaluate the possibilities of new industrial development proposed on the initiative of French subjects, they employed a sophisticated system of bureaucratic investigation and enquiry which has been splendidly and sympathetically described by Harold Parker. When it came to their assessment of French industry in comparison with that of England, the level of understanding seems to have fluctuated. Daniel Trudaine, advised by men of his choice, like John Holker, Gabriel Jars and Mignot de Montigny, was more accurate in his views than the intendants of commerce in 1781 who felt, in Parker's words, that:

> French industry seemed to be doing all right. If England appeared to be ahead in some industries (hardware, cottons and woollens) France was front runner in silk and was catching up in paper and chemicals. No doubt French industrialists would soon overtake the British in woollens, cottons and hardware, and the French economy would continue to advance in a sound, balanced development.[38]

The evidence of the later 1780s showed this to have been a delusory optimism, but when the Bureau of Commerce was abruptly closed in the next decade its remaining officials were apparently infected by a pessimism which was nearly as far off target.

The evidence reviewed over the previous chapters is so extensive and conclusive that there need be no further discussion on the overwhelming importance of industrial espionage in the transfer of technology from Britain to France in the eighteenth century. Similarly it needs no emphasis that the French state was deeply involved with that espionage, as well as with general intelligence-gathering. Espionage was generally instigated by the State, though of course often prompted by individuals with industrial interests. There were also what might be called in-house promptings from members of its own industrial inspectorate, or from Ministries other than Commerce, particularly from the armament demands of the Marine. Even where, as with Camus de Limare and naval copper, or Martin and textile machinery, there are instances of espionage being initiated and carried out by individuals, their actions were based on a correct belief that the State would help by subsidizing the new technology while it was being naturalized in France (including compensating for the costs of suborning workers or obtaining machinery) and that they would be given the advantages of privileged manufacture.

However, the more liberal regime that took over at the Bureau of Commerce in mid-century with the arrival of Trudaine and Du Gournay was increasingly disinclined to go beyond subsidy to newly transferred industry, and was against conferring national monopolies or even regional ones, and this policy was made official by an *arrêt* of 1762. There were increasing and important exceptions to this policy under Necker, and some were seemingly made because the securing of the new English cotton technology, and the inauguration of factory production in textiles were thought so important that those attempting these things deserved special protection and encouragement. As we have seen, Necker could be quite Thatcherite in his views on industrial independence, and the cotton firms that briefly benefited from exclusive privileges were soon complaining that their monopolies in fact conflicted with rights conferred on other firms or were being disregarded. In the run up to the Eden Treaty the need for at least ten French spinning factories was being advocated by Holker, quite incompatible with exclusive privileges to any. The Milnes were being given facilities to make Arkwright machines for whoever wanted them.

There had been relatively short periods of intense persecution, usually religious, which drove skilled Walloons in the sixteenth century, and Huguenots in the late seventeenth, into refuge in other lands, taking important industrial technologies with them. But the main method of taking technology from one European country to another in the eighteenth century seems unquestionably to have been industrial espionage. It is beyond the scope of this book to examine industrial espionage in the medieval or early modern world or, even, for the eighteenth century, to take more than a cursory view of espionage by countries other than France. It is hoped that others will follow up these themes; for our purpose it is sufficient to have demonstrated the centrality of espionage in technology transfer between Britain and France in the eighteenth century.

The examination of the essential role of the industrial spy in technology transfer, the study of the statesmen and officials of the acquiring country, and their understanding of the need for transfer, the appreciation of the attitudes of industrialists and technologists in the country suffering the theft of its industrial knowhow and equipment, all require an understanding of the situation, abilities and feelings of individuals. In our day the mind of the spy, his reaction to the hostile world in which he operates, his fears and personal triumphs, have become the stuff of media entertainment and some of the most widely read fiction. His eighteenth-century predecessors often had similar feelings. To write the history of industrial espionage in the eighteenth century is one means of restoring the thoughts and activities of human beings to the centre stage of industrial history, from which a generation of writing dominated by economic analysis has largely banished them.

Notes

Notes for Introduction

1. C. Ballot, *L'Introduction du Machinisme dans L'Industrie Française* (Lille-Paris, 1923), p. 437. 'Following their usual practice, the royal government sent abroad experts [*hommes de l'art*] to study the secrets and filch them as needed.'

2. It has been argued by Karel Davids for Holland that at the peak of her technological prowess between 1680 and the early eighteenth century the country was virtually an open society for technological transfer. It was only during the last decades of the Dutch Republic, apparently from about 1770, that there was serious opposition to industrial transfer and industrial espionage. This indifference may have been partly due to the non-unitary constitution of the Dutch state as the United Provinces, partly to a deep complacency induced by an age of the 'embarrassment of riches', and perhaps by a far more liberal trade policy than that practised by most European countries. No central or provincial agency of the Republic, except the Amsterdam Admiralty, organized journeys of inspection to learn about technological advances abroad. See K. Davids, 'Openness or secrecy? Industrial espionage in the Dutch Republic', *Journal of European Economic History*, vol. 24, no. 2 (Fall 1995), 333–48.

3. *Introduction du Machinisme* (1923).

4. W. O. Henderson, *Britain and Industrial Europe, 1750–1870* (1st edn Liverpool, 1954; 2nd edn Leicester, 1965).

5. P. Mathias, 'Skills and the diffusion of innovations from Britain in the eighteenth century', *Transactions of the Royal Historical Society*, 5th series, vol. 25 (1975), 93–113; D. J. Jeremy, 'Damming the flood: British government efforts to check the outflow of technicians and machinery, 1780–1843', *Business History Review*, vol. 51 (1977), 1–34; J. R. Harris, 'Saint-Gobain and Ravenhead', originally published in 1975, and 'Attempts to transfer English steel techniques to France in the eighteenth century', originally published in 1978, both now republished as Chapters II and III of *Essays in Industry and Technology in the Eighteenth Century: England and France* (Aldershot, 1992). For conferences, the International Economic History

566

Conference, Berne, 1986; Society for the History of Technology Conference, Sacramento, 1989; European Social Science History Conference, Amsterdam, 1996. The Société Française d'Histoire des Sciences et des Techniques devoted its 1996 Lyon conference to 'De la diffusion des sciences à l'éspionage scientifique et industriel'. There will be a theme on 'Inventions, Innovations and Espionage' at the International Economic History Conference in 1998. The two books referred to are: K. Bruland, ed., *Technology Transfer and Scandinavian Industrialisation* (Oxford, 1991) and D. C. Christensen, *Det Moderne Project, Teknik & Kultur i Danmark-Norge 1750–(1814)–1850* (Gyldendal, 1996).

6. B. Freemantle, *The Steal: Counterfeiting and Industrial Espionage* (London, 1986), pp. 63–74.
7. For the examples of coke-iron solid-bored cannon, naval copper and naval pulley blocks, see below, Chapters 11, 12 and 17.
8. R. Fagliot, 'Paris puts spies back in business', *The European*, 29 August–4 September 1996.

Notes for Chapter 1

1. For the earlier, apparently inoperative, Act of 1696 against the export of knitting frames, see below, p. 455; for the change in technological balance, below, p. 535 seq.
2. *Commons Journals*, 17 January 1719.
3. *Commons Journals*, 27 January 1719.
4. M. W. Flinn, *Men of Iron, the Crowleys in the Early Iron Industry* (Edinburgh, 1962), p. 72.
5. *Commons Journals*, 2 February 1719.
6. *Commons Journals*, 6 February 1719.
7. *Lords Journals*, 5 March, 9 March, 14 March, 19 March 1719, 4 April, 9 April, 10 April, 11 April, 13 April, 14 April, 15 April, 17 April, 18 April 1719.
8. 5 Geo. 1 c. 27.
9. *Journals of the Commissioners for Trade and the Plantations*, March 1717 to November 1719.
10. PRO, State Papers (hereafter SP) 35, 14 fol. 43; Petition of the Manufacturers of Iron, fol. 44.
11. So far no detailed documentation has come to light showing Law's motivation or how his ideas developed. The evidence used here largely derives from obvious sources in British state papers which seemingly have never been reviewed, though Law's biographer, H. Montgomery Hyde, clearly referred to the episode (*John Law: the History of an Honest Adventurer* [1948], p. 123, and for the 1703 proposals, p. 45).
12. SP 35, 25 fol. 105.
13. SP 35, 25 fol. 72.
14. G. B. Hill (ed.), *The Memoirs of The Life of Edward Gibbon*, (1900), p. 16.

15. SP 35, 25 fol. 105.
16. There is additional detail in another Douglas letter, SP 35, 26 fol. 11.
17. SP Foreign, France, 164 fol. 2.
18. SP Foreign, France, 165 fol. 231.
19. Ibid.
20. SP Foreign, France 166 fol. 99, 9 Jan. 1720.
21 Ibid.
22. SP Foreign, France, 167 fols 287, 386.
23. SP Foreign France, 169 fols 87, 145. The only French documentation as yet found for the Law works is an undated paper of 1720 concerning payment of about 300 French and English persons at the Harfleur works and 150 at Charleval (*sic*). The first works was said to need 4,000 *livres* a week and the second 2,000, but only 1,000 and 500 were apparently granted, to be paid over by a Sieur Arbuthnot. (Archives Départementales (subsequently AD) Seine Maritime C1047).
24. SP Foreign, France, 169 fol. 87 Sutton to Craggs, 30 October 1720.
25. SP Foreign, France, 169 fol. 145 seq.
26. SP 35, 25 fol. 125.
27. SP 35, 25 fol. 63.
28. SP 35, 25, Douglas to Townshend, 15 February 1720; letter from artisans, 25 March 1720; SP 35 26, Douglas to Carteret, 10 April 1721; list of payments, 20 April 1721; SP 35, 27, Barnes to Carteret, 12 June 1721.
29. SP Foreign, France, 169 fol. 268; SP 35, 78, fol. 85
30. SP 35, 30 fol. 55, petition of James Reith, watchmaker.
31. See L. Stewart, *The Rise of Public Science* (Cambridge, 1992), pp. 371, 377–8.
32. *Calendar of Treasury Papers 1721* vol. 239, p. 45; SP 35, 25 fol. 48.
33. SP 35, 26 fol. 32.
34. See below, p. 33.
35. SP 35 fol. 30, 31, 103.
36. Affaires Etrangères, Correspondence Politique Angleterre, p. 341; SP Foreign, France, 78 166 fol. 170, Pulteney to Craggs, 5 March 1720. There has been no attempt in this study to examine the technology of ship design and shipbuilding in England and France and make comparisons, as this would be beyond the author's competence. In the period covered by this and the next chapter there were two prominent French naval constructors sent to England to examine our building of warships, Blaise Geslain in 1729 and Blaise Ollivier in 1737. Geslain's instructions survive and certainly involve espionage, and while Ollivier's do not exist, it seems that he was concealing his true identity as a royal shipwright and sending information back by clandestine channels. He was able to spend time with master shipwrights in the British navy yards, though there were limits to the information they would impart. Neither Geslain's nor Ollivier's report was made serious use of by the Marine. It is interesting that both were interested in the use of steam trunks for bending timbers though this was not consistently adopted by the French until the end of the century. Yet Ollivier had a model of a stoving oven in his office! Geslain was ordered to investigate British sheathing

methods, later so important (below p. 262) and the French navy was already very interested in English cutters, as it continued to be until at least the 1780s. In the mid- to late eighteenth century French ship design was often thought to be superior to, and more scientific than, British; in this aspect French technology may not get its full due in this work. For the French investigators of British practice in the early eighteenth century see D. H. Roberts, *Eighteenth Century Shipbuilding* (Jean Boudriot Publications, Rotherfield, East Sussex, 1992), a quite magnificent introduction to and translation of, Ollivier's report. I would like to thank him for a valuable correspondence. The only espionage by French naval officers dealt with in this work is that of Lescallier and Forfait in 1790 (below), p. 527.

37. AN F12 1325 A/B.
38. See below, pp. 293–6.
39. For the transfer of technology in steel, see below, Chapter 9.
40. J. R. Harris, *Industry and Technology in the Eighteenth Century: England and France* (inaugural lecture, University of Birmingham, 1972), p. 9. There is a discussion of the balance of technology transfer in Chapter 21, below, p. 535.

I am grateful to Professor Jan Blanchard and the publishers to be able to use extensively in this chapter a paper which originally appeared in *Industry and Finance in Early Modern History: Essays presented to George Hammersley* (Franz Steiner Verlag, Stuttgart, 1992).

Notes for Chapter 2

1. Archives Nationales (hereafter AN) F12 1325A. The son's subsequent career is outlined in J. J. Bootsgegel, 'William Blakey, a rival to Newcomen', *Transactions of the Newcomen Society*, 16 (1935–36), 97 seq.
2. PRO SP 35, 26 fol. 11.
3. *Journal of the Commissioners for Trade and the Plantations* 7 March, 15 June 1721; PRO SP 35, 27, Barnes to Carteret 12 June 1721, 25 September, 5 October, 17 October, 7 December 1722, 29 January, 4 October, 24 October 1723.
4. *Journal of Commissioners for Trade*, 20 February 1724; A. P. Wadsworth and J. de L. Mann, *The Cotton Trade and Industrial Lancashire, 1600–1780* (Manchester, 1931) 121–3.
5. *Journal of Commissioners for Trade*, 20 November 1724.
6. Ibid., 2 March, 31 May, 4 August 1725.
7. AN F12 682.
8. Wadsworth and Mann, *Cotton Trade*, p. 124.
9. W. O. Henderson, *Britain and Industrial Europe 1750–1870* (2nd edn, Leicester, 1965), 11.
10. AN F12 682.
11. See below, p. 293.

12.   Julien Le Roy, introduction to 1737 edition of H. Sully, *Règle Artificielle du Temps*; AN F12 1325, which gives correspondence between Calonne and leading watchmakers in 1786 when a large enterprise in Paris was proposed. Berthoud wrote that horology began to flourish in Paris under the Regency:

> This Art owes part of its perfection to the celebrated Sully the English Artist who established it in France. He is the author of the *Règle Artificielle du Temps* printed in 1717, and of a very good work entitled *De la mesure du temps en mer* (On the Measurement of Time at Sea) printed in 1726. Among artists who were his contemporaries one may above all mention Julien Le Roy, for whom the love he had for this Art has much contributed to its Perfection ... we owe to Julien Le Roy several fine Memoirs on Horology, printed as a sequel he provided to an Edition of Sully's *Règle Artificielle du Temps*.

13.   PRO, SP 35, 61.
14.   PRO, SP 36, 20.
15.   SP Foreign France, 78, 194.
16.   Engines for extinguishing fire, not steam-engines.
17.   SP 36, 20.
18.   Jean Hellot (1685–1766) was a chemist attached to the Academy of Sciences from 1735 who succeeded Dufay as head of the department of dyeing and as an inspector of manufactures in 1739. He had been badly affected financially by the Law bubble of 1720, but had travelled extensively in England. He encouraged experiments and developments in dyeing in Normandy and Languedoc, including trials to discover the secret of the elusive Adrianople red. He was also consulted by the Government on matters of metals and mining, including steel innovations and the assessment of coal from different mines. He advised the elder Trudaine on the important mining law of 1744. He published a treatise on the dyeing of wool and translated and extensively edited the major German work on metallurgy by Schlutter. He had a responsibility for the technology of porcelain at Sevres developing a 'Hellot blue' for a service ordered by Louis XV. He advised on the enquiries to be made by Gabriel Jars in his metallurgical travels in England (below, pp. 224–5). He is said to have been much keener on laboratory work than the field enquiries that some of his wide responsibilities indicated, like examining mine workings. As early as 1740 he was elected a Fellow of the Royal Society of London. See A. Birembaut and G. Thuillier, 'Une Source Inédite, Les cahiers du chimiste Hellot', *Annales* (Mars–Avril 1966), pp. 357 seq.; P. Minard, 'L'inspection des manufactures en France, de Colbert à la Revolution', doctorat nouveau régime, Université Paris-1 Panthéon-Sorbonne (December 1994) 3 vols, pp. 477–8.
19.   AN O1 1293.
20.   Ibid.
21.   AN F12 739. D.-C. Trudaine had not authorized Morel's English journey as Bellefonds suggests, but he knew of it; Trudaine only became effective in the Bureau of Commerce in 1744. X. Linant de Bellefonds, 'Les Techniciens Anglais dans L'Industrie Française au XVIIIe Siècle', doctoral thesis, University of Paris, 1971, p. 30.

22. AN F12 739.
23. See below. For the Jubié family see C. Ballot, *L'Introduction du Machinisme dans L'Industrie Française* (Lille-Paris, 1923), pp. 304, 306–9, 312, 327, 329; for Jubié's visit to England in 1747, see Bellefonds, 'Les Techniciens Anglais', pp. 30–31.

Notes for Chapter 3

1. A. Rémond, *John Holker, Manufacturier et Grand Fonctionnaire en France au XVIIIᵉ Siècle 1719–1786* (Paris, 1946). For a brief assessment of Holker, J. R. Harris, First Chaloner Memorial Lecture, 'A Lancashire Jacobite in French industry', *Transactions of the Newcomen Society*, 64 (1992–93), 131–42.
2. She did not die in about 1740 as stated in the article on Holker in the original *Dictionary of National Biography* but was still alive in 1760. See below, p. 68. For the father's occupation, H. T. Crofton, *A History of the Ancient Chapel of Stretford, Chetham Society*, 51, New Series (1908), p. 158.
3. For the social and occupational background of Manchester officer recruits see P. K. Monod, *Jacobitism and the English People 1688–1788* (Cambridge University Press, Cambridge, 1989), pp. 332–6. He inclines to the view that many of the officers from the textile trades, if not themselves gentry, had gentry connections. F. J. McLynn, *The Jacobite Army in England, 1745. The Final Campaign* (Edinburgh, 1983) pp. 98–100, regards Holker as the best officer; he is however mistaken in following Rémond's statement that Holker was at Culloden.
4. Service Historique de l'Armée de la Terre (hereafter SHAT) Archives, Vincennes Xᴮ⁷. I owe this and subsequent references to this source to the late Margaret Audin.
5. See below, and p. 141.
6. B. G. Seton and J. G. Arnott, *The Prisoners of the '45. Scottish History Society, 3rd Series* (1928), vol. 1, pp. 94–9, vol. 2, p. 288. There seems to be some confusion about Moss; he cannot have turned King's Evidence as said in vol. 1, p. 99. According to A. P. Wadsworth and J. de L. Mann, *The Cotton Trade and Industrial Lancashire, 1600–1780* (Manchester, 1931) p. 196, Holker and Moss were partners in a calendering business in Manchester, this would not really contradict Moss's description as a woollen draper (Monod, *Jacobitism*, p. 532; Seton and Arnott, *Prisoners*, pp. 98–101).
7. PRO, SP 36, 84.
8. L. Dutens, *Mémoires d'un voyageur qui se repose* (London, 1806), vol. 2, 99–103. Holker said on this occasion that he was captured at Carlisle.
9. SHAT Archives, Vincennes Xᴮ⁷.
10. F. J. McLynn, *Charles Edward Stuart* (Oxford, 1991), pp. 397–9, 406–7, and his 'Unpopular front; Jews, radicals and Americans in the Jacobite world view', in *Royal Stuart Papers XXI* (Huntingdon, 1988), pp. 8–9. I am grateful for Dr McLynn's help.

11. Rémond, *Holker*, p. 43; AN F12 739, Morel to Terray, 1771.
12. AN F12 739.
13. In his first approach to Trudaine concerning Holker in 1751, Morel claimed that he had already obtained information from England and Ireland about flax-growing, beer and cider making, the construction of dams and the manufacture of linen. S. Chassagne, *Le Coton et Ses Patrons, France, 1760–1840* (Paris, 1991), pp. 45–6. Morel perhaps lost favour with the Trudaines because of his severity in imposing the manufacturing regulations too harshly on the local producers, for which Holker, now his superior, gave him a friendly but strong warning in 1767. See P. Minard, 'L'inspection des manufactures en France, de Colbert à la Révolution', doctorat nouveau régime, Paris 1 (1994),
14. Rémond, *Holker*, p. 25.
15. Chassagne, *Le Coton*, pp. 45–6.
16. Ibid., pp. 25–9.
17. For Hellot, see above Chapter 2, n.18.
18. Chassagne, *Le Coton*, pp. 38–4.
19. Sometimes referred to as the Havards.
20. X. Linant de Bellefonds, 'Les Techniciens Anglais dans L'Industrie Française au XVIIIᵉ Siècle', thesis, Faculté de Droit, Paris (1971), pp. 30, 51, 126, 132, 190.
21. Chassagne, *Le Coton*, p. 46. This was almost certainly an overstatement, but whether a deliberate one, or genuinely reflecting Holker's beliefs, is impossible to tell.
22. De Gaumont, Intendant of Finances, had picked on Trudaine as a suitable husband for his orphan niece, Marie-Margaret Chauvin, and as successor to his office, but Fleury did not assent to the promotion until Trudaine had proved his worth.
23. H. T. Parker, *The Bureau of Commerce in 1781 and its Policies with Respect to French Industry* (Durham, NC, 1979), pp. 101–2.
24. 'Eloge de M. Trudaine' (this was largely prepared by his son). *Histoire de l'Académie Royale des Sciences* (1759, Première Partie 1778), pp. 261–91. See also E. Chouiller, *Les Trudaines* (extracted from the *Révue de Champagne et de Brie*) (Arcis sur Aube 1884), pp. 11–19.
25. AN F12 1411A, D'Haristoy to Trudaine, 31 December 1752.
26. According to Chassagne, *Le Coton*, p. 47. But a letter attached to a document of August 1753 suggests that Peter Morris 'coupeur des Cannelés' got a bonus of 200 *livres* in that year. See also list of workers at the manufacture and the calender royal at Rouen 30 October 1754. See also AN F12 1411A.
27. Holker's original plan was to land in Holland and await his recruits there, but bad weather caused his ship to come into Ostend. AN F12 1411A, De Montigny to Trudaine(?) 4 January 1752. By that time he said that he had exhausted the 7,000 *livres* and was in debt to Morel who had paid for his living costs in Paris.
28. This is the usual spelling, perhaps a version of the common Lancashire name of Tyrer.
29. Possibly a French spelling of another common Lancashire name, Houghton.

30. AN F12 1411A. Document attached to letter of Morel, 23 March 1752.
31. Chassagne, *Le Coton*, p. 47; AN F12 1411A.
32. AN F12 1411A. Letter of 15 August 1752 to Intendant. Calendering and hot-pressing were often done on the same premises. 'The calender was a kind of mangle in which a large and heavily weighted box, up to ten tons, was, by means of a horse or a man-powered [tread] mill, drawn across the two or more cylindrical rollers that pressed the cloth down on to a flat table ... hot-presses ... were heavily-built screw presses with two iron or steel plates, the lower of which formed the top of a rectangular furnace, while the upper one was often double and filled with hot charcoal [later coke]'. Hot-presses, or more usually calenders, were used for 'watering' fabrics, and by 1716 special cut-brass rollers had been developed in England to give particular patterns to cloth subjected to this process (E. Kerridge, *Textile Manufactures in Early Modern England*, Manchester University Press, Manchester, 1985), p. 173.
33. Chassagne, *Le Coton*, pp. 46–9; AN F12 1411A, letter of De La Bourdonnayer, 9 September 1752.
34. Given his refugee condition he would have nothing to invest. For details of these transactions see AN F12 1411A, draft *arrêts* and associated documents.
35. Possibly the *arrêt* surviving in AN F12 1411A is not a public one.
36. AN F12 1411A. *Arrêt*, Versailles 19 September 1752, agreement of partners 31 October 1752; Chassagne, *Le Coton*, pp. 49–51.
37. Chassagne, *Le Coton*, pp. 51–2.
38. AN F12 1411A.
39. Florence M. Montgomery, 'John Holker's mid-eighteenth century Livre d'Echantillons', in (ed.) V. Gervers, *Studies in Textile History in Memory of Harold B. Burnham*, (Toronto, 1977).
40. A similar arrangement was made with Wilson the leather currier, who was first employed at Saint German en Laye. Chassagne, *Le Coton*, pp. 52–3. For Morel's reports, Chassagne, *Le Coton*, pp. 50–53; for his claims, AN F12 739.
41. While written in the third person it is evidently his own composition.
42. See below, p. 457.
43. See below, pp. 96, 140.
44. P. Boissonade, 'Trois Mémoires relatifs a l'amélioration des manufactures de France sous l'administration des Trudaines (1754)', *Révue d'histoire économique et sociale* (1914–18), p. 68 seq.
45. There were four other inspectors-general. The Inspectorate of Manufactures had been founded by Colbert in 1669 with the primary duty of enforcing the regulations for the quality control of manufactures, which in effect meant textiles, and inspectors were usually assigned to generalities. There were partial reorganizations on several occasions before the Revolution. At the beginning of the century there were forty inspectors, sixty to seventy at the end of the 1750s, around forty during the 1770s and sixty-five at the end of the Ancien Régime. In 1730 Orry placed two inspectors-general at the head of the corps, who were to make tours of inspection through the country, one taking the north and the other the south. The duties proving too onerous, in

1736 three inspectors ambulant were given the task of training and reporting (another being added in 1742) while the inspectors-general became supervisors of the system, residing in the capital. In 1746 Rouillé became head of the Bureau of Commerce and abolished the ambulants, creating two more inspectors-general. The senior inspectors-general sat in on meetings of the Bureau, the younger toured, but the system was not well maintained, and in 1756, at the time of Holker's appointment, only one remained in office. With the administration of the elder Trudaine, the inspectors-general were normally appointed because of outstanding expertise which they could bring to the industrial scene, Holker himself and later his son, Vaucanson and Desmarets, were examples here, while others like Cliquot de Blervache and Dupont de Nemours were brought in for their commercial advice. Believing the existing team were too pressured to fulfil all their functions, Calonne in 1784 again recreated four posts of inspectors ambulant. In the late 1780s the inspector-general posts were allowed to fall in, at least partly because some of them had been occupied by economic liberals, and there were six ambulant posts when the Bureau and the inspectorate were closed in 1791.

At the beginning of the century there had been four 'inspectors of foreign manufactures' whose duties were really of customs enforcement and the control of foreign imports at certain ports. Their functions were finally transferred to the Farm General in 1736, and the inspectors ambulants replaced them. In giving Holker a title similar to the one previously used was there an attempt to camouflage his industrial espionage function? The organization of the industrial inspectorate is well covered by P. Minard, 'L'inspection des manufactures', thesis citation, pp. 42–105.

46. AN F12 147. Trudaine to D'Argenson, 29 April 1754.
47. AN F12 148.
48. Rémond, *Holker*, pp. 81–2.
49. AN F12 740, Holker asks for arrangements for a pension to his widow; below, p. 144.
50. See for instance AN F12 740 and AD Hérault, C2525–6, Trudaine to Saint-Priest 28 May 1756.
51. AN F12 1341 from which all references to this report are taken.
52. He was in Troyes on 18 May 1755; AN F12 1442 for Badger, F12 674 for visits to Cambrai, Saint Quentin and Valenciennes.
53. AN F12 674. Later his son was more critical of the commercial practicality of Vaucanson's machines.
54. Alcock was turned to for advice on the Saint Etienne industry in the following year, but he proved difficult to persuade to find time, men and machines for Saint Etienne. He seems not to have visited the town and reported on it until December 1757 and he could not be convinced that Saint Etienne would have been a better centre for his own operations than his factory at La Charité-sur-Loire. For Alcock, see below, pp. 180–81.
55. AN F12 1315B.
56. AN F12 1315B.
57. AN F12 1349.
58. AN F12 1365, Trudaine to Holker 8 February 1762.

59. AN F12 1365.

60. AN F12 740.

61. AN F12 1365, Holker to Trudaine, 3 August 1762. He ended by dismissing very summarily some unspecified ideas of the chemist and academician Hellot (the important government technologist) on bleaching. For the espionage of John Holker II in Britain, see below, Chapter 6. For Hellot, above, Chapter 2, n. 18.

62. AN F12 1330, letter of Holker 21 November 1762.

63. AN F12 1366.

64. AN F12 562.

65. Ibid., letter of Ruste 28 February 1763.

66. Ibid., letter of Ruste 6 June 1763.

67. AN F12 1455, Holker to Trudaine, Paris 12 January 1759, and from Sens, January 1760. AN F12 562, letters of Ruste 6 June, 11 July, 14 July, 24 September 1763. Two personal and critical views of an inspector's function, those of Huet de Vandour (1762) and De Latapie (1773), are worth examining, but may not be very typical (AN F12 560). A reappraisal of the work of the eighteenth-century inspectors, especially in relation to industrial and technological development, was overdue, but has very recently been made by Minard (above, n. 45).

68. P. Vayssière, 'Un pionnier de la révolution industrielle en Languedoc au XVIIIe siècle: John Holker', *Annales du Midi*, 79 (1967), 269–86.

69. A version exists in AN F12 557.

70. AD Hérault, C2525–6, which shows Holker had been carefully introduced. He had also supplied a calender to a *manufacture royale* at Le Puy in 1758; AD Hérault C2623, Trudaine to Saint-Priest, July 1758, 4 October 1759; Report of Inspector Rodier November 1759.

71. *Mémoire instructif sur la fabrique, les apprêts, dégraissage et blanchissage des bayettes et autres lainages anglais* (Paris, 1764).

72. Vayssière, 'Un pionnier', pp. 272–3. However the average pay rose considerably before the Revolution.

73. AN F12 557.

74. AN F12 557. In a document of the early 1760s Holker gave his firm opinion that 'Workers here [in France] are not as well nourished as those in England and it can be therefore presumed that they are not able to stand up to hard work with the same strength and liveliness (AN F12 1365). Subsequent quotations are from AN F12 557.

75. AN F12 557; Vayssière, 'Un pionnier', pp. 279–80.

76. These areas of English superiority before the classic textile inventions of the sixties and seventies of the eighteenth century need more emphasis in accounts of the English textile industry.

77. Vayssière, 'Un pionnier', esp. p. 282 seq.; AN F12 557.

576 Notes for Chapter 4, pp. 81–7

Notes for Chapter 4

1. AN F12 824, Kay to Tolozan 5 August 1779.
2. A. P. Wadsworth and J. de L. Mann, *The Cotton Trade and Industrial Lancashire, 1600–1780* (Manchester, 1931), Ch. 12. H. T. Wood, 'Inventions of John Kay', *Journal of the Royal Society of Arts*, 60, (82) (1911). For the legal difficulties and delays experienced by Kay, C. McLeod, *Inventing the Industrial Revolution* (Cambridge, 1988), p. 60.

    There has been a recent careful reinterpretation of the effectiveness of the main invention of Kay, the fly-shuttle, by A. Paulinyi ('John Kay's flying shuttle', *Textile History*, 17, (2), 149–66, 1986). Paulinyi shows that the doubling of output with the shuttle was an excessive claim by historians; that a 50 per cent increase in production was more realistic; that it was not suitable for all textile products; that a considerable knack was needed to operate the shuttle successfully; that failure to acquire this skill properly led to frequent breakdowns which weavers tended to blame on the technology.

3. A. Rémond, *John Holker, Manufacturier et Grand Fonctionnaire en France au XVIIIᵉ Siècle 1719–1786* (Paris, 1946), p. 36; AN F12 20.
4. Wadsworth and Mann, *Cotton Trade*, p. 459.
5. AN F12 20.
6. Wadsworth and Mann, *Cotton Trade*, p. 460.
7. AN F12 20.
8. AN F12 993.
9. AN F12 992.
10. AN F12 1442. The better English in this letter suggests Kay had help in writing it!
11. X. Linant de Bellefonds, 'Les Techniciens Anglais dans L'Industrie Française au XVIIIᶜ Siècle', doctoral thesis, University of Paris, 1971, p. 149; AN F12 993.
12. Wadsworth and Mann, *Cotton Trade*, p. 461.
13. AN F12 992.
14. The problem of reduced durability of the new as compared with the old cards seems to have been removed by some improvements (AN F12 992).
15. 'On cessa de la lui payer sur ce qu'il refusa de guider des ouvriers dans la construction d'une nouvelle machine pour faire des cardes' AN F12 992, Mémoire du S. Jean Kay ouvrier Anglais.
16. Bellefonds, 'Les Techniciens Anglais', pp. 149–50; Wadsworth and Mann, *Cotton Trade*, pp. 461–2.
17. AN F12 1315A, De Montigny to Trudaine 3 October 1757.
18. AN F12 992. Falkener's work as an accountant was not counted by Kay.
19. AN F12 992.
20. AN F12 992, Kay to Trudaine, 6 May 1761.
21. Wadsworth and Mann, *Cotton Trade*, p. 461; Bellefonds, 'Les Techniciens Anglais', p. 143.
22. Here Kay exaggerated somewhat, the inspector-general retired in 1756; F. Bacquié, *Les inspecteurs des manufactures sous L'Ancien Régime* (1927), p. 369.

23. AN F12 992.
24. See W. H. Chaloner, 'The textile inventor, John Kay' *Bulletin of the John Rylands Library*, 48, (1), (1965) 9 seq., including a statement from John Kay's son, 'Frenchman Kay' as he was called from his long residence in France. [See also AN F12 992: 'His means of support having been taken away from him he approached the Duke of Bedford ... and made known to him the wish he had to return to his native land. The Ambassador enabled him to go there'.]
25. Wadsworth and Mann, *Cotton Trade*, p. 462.
26. Letter of 27 November 1765, Wood, 'Inventions', p. 79.
27. AN F12 992.
28. Ibid.
29. The carding invention surfaced again at the Society of Arts in 1774 in a curious way, when a correspondent in New England drew their attention to card-making machinery used by a Joseph Pope of Boston. They told him they had already seen a better machine, that of John Kay senior. Interestingly they consulted John's son William about the matter, and he later approached the Society for a premium. While acknowledging the development of the machines to be his father's, he claimed to have materially improved them, and to have made them of iron and steel, while his father's were largely wooden. He said his father had never made any for sale (this may have been true for England, but certainly not for France), but that he himself now did, and had reduced the price of cards. In the end the Society gave him 50 guineas. His father would have been enraged, if he ever learned about it. Wood, 'Inventions', pp. 80–81.
30. AN F12 824; AN F12 992, including Holker to Trudaine de Montigny, 2 February 1766.
31. Wadsworth and Mann, *Cotton Trade*, pp. 463–4.
32. AN F12 824, Kay to Necker (?) 17 August 1779.
33. AD Seine Maritime C912, letters of 24 August, 16 December, 19 December 1771.
34. AN F12 824; Wadsworth and Mann, *Cotton Trade*, p. 464.
35. AN F12 824.
36. AN F12 993; Bellefonds, 'Les Techniciens Anglais', p. 252.
37. See below, p. 98.
38. *Williamson's Liverpool Advertiser*, 7 February 1766.
39. AN F12 1442, from which most of the material used here derives.
40. G. Bussière, 'Une Famille anglaise d'ouvriers de Soie à Lyon', *Revolution Française*, July (1907), 25 seq: Bellefonds, 'Les Techniciens Anglais', p. 158 seq. Watering was not new in principle. Kerridge shows it was used in pressing in producing a glazed finish on worsted tammies in the seventeenth century while mohairs, watered cloths made from grosgrain yarns were well established in Norwich in the 1630s. The name 'mohair' was simply a variant of the word 'moire' the French name for watering, suggesting they may have had precedence in the process. It was certainly practised in France as well as England at this period. Evelyn saw the watering of grosgrains and camblets at Tours in 1644 and in London in 1652, where it may have been introduced by

a Huguenot. 'But the system of watering by calender developed in England proved superior to that used in Lyons and possibly in Tours' (E. Kerridge, *Textile Manufactures in Early Modern England* (Manchester University Press, Manchester, 1985), pp. 53–4, 129, 173. The superior British watering envied in France in the middle of the eighteenth century applied to silk.

41. AN F12 1442.
42. Bellefonds, 'Les Techniciens Anglais', pp. 157–8. The calenderer was probably John Smith.
43. Bussière, 'Une Famille anglaise', 32.
44. AN F12 2400, *Addresse à L'Assemblée Nationale, Pour Le Sieur Badger, Moireur à Lyon* (Lyon, 1791).
45. AN F12 1442, including letter of Kay, probably to Trudaine de Montigny, Paris 23 October 1753.
46. Ibid., Badger to Trudaine 23 December 1753.
47. Bussière, 'Une Famille anglaise', 35.
48. AN F12, 1442 Badger to Trudaine de Montigny (?) 23 January 1754.
49. AN F12 1442, Parsons to Holker 4 April 1754; Holker to Trudaine de Montigny (?), Rouen, 11 April 1754.
50. Ibid., Holker to Trudaine de Montigny (?) 16 January 1754; letter of Badger 26 March 1754.
51. Ibid., Badger 5 June 1754 (? to Trudaine de Montigny).
52. Ibid., same to same, 23 July 1754.
53. AN F12 1399, letters of Vial and Rey to Trudaine, 1758. They were claiming additional remuneration, but Trudaine rejected their demands.
54. AN F12 740, 1442.
55. Bellefonds, 'Les Techniciens Anglais', p. 166.
56. Bussière, 'Une Famille anglaise', 38.
57. He was of a family of recent nobility which had ties with trade and the iron industry, and he was to go on to even greater office.
58. AN F12 1442, Flachat to Trudaine 9 December 1754.
59. For the defective iron plates as a problem see Bellefonds, p. 162.
60. Scot had been in Lyons since 1736, had converted to Catholicism in 1740, married a French girl, and brought up his son Claude as a Frenchman.
61. AN F12 1442. Scot was not the first interpreter, one Charoni had been the original one, but had been untrustworthy and a troublemaker and dismissed, see Bussière, 'Une Famille anglaise', pp. 38–9. The document drawn up by Holker is undated, but Bellefonds gives it as being of 13 September 1756, though Bussière shows the Lyons silk manufacturers still discussing the matter on 16 September. Bellefonds, 'Les Techniciens Anglais', p. 169, Bussière, 'Une Famille anglaise', pp. 40–41, 303–6.
62. Bussière, 'Une Famille anglaise', p. 313.
63. Additional work was done on the calenders in 1760 costing nearly 5,000 *livres*, AN F12 149.
64. Seguin complained that his English associates were violent, and he feared for his safety as long as he lived with them; Bellefonds, 'Les Techniciens Anglais', p. 170.
65. AN F12 2400.

66. AN F12 1442, Holker to De Montigny 16 May 1761.
67. Bussière, 'Une Famille anglaise', pp. 316–25; AN F12 2400; Bellefonds, 'Les Techniciens Anglais', pp. 169–71.
68. This extra pension is mentioned by the Badgers in the 1791 pamphlet, but Bellefonds does not refer to it, but to a 6,000 *livres* gratification in 1778. There may be some confusion here, or two separate grants.
69. Bellefonds, 'Les Techniciens Anglais', p. 171.
70. Edward A. Allen, 'Business mentality and technology transfer in eighteenth century France: the Calandre Anglaise at Nîmes, 1752–72', *Technology and History* (1990), 8, (1), 9–23, esp. 16.
71. Bellefonds, 'Les Techniciens Anglais', pp. 173–5. Mrs Badger had been to England to deal with family affairs in 1762 (AN F12 149).
72. Bellefonds, 'Les Techniciens Anglais', p. 169; AN F12 1442, Choiseul to Trudaine 1 January 1760.

Notes for Chapter 5

1. X. Linant de Bellefonds, 'Les Techniciens Anglais dans L'Industrie Française au XVIIIe Siècle', doctoral thesis, University of Paris, 1971, p. 191.
2. S. Chassagne, *Le Coton et Ses Patrons, France, 1760–1840* (Paris, 1991), pp. 54–5; Bellefonds, 'Les Techniciens Anglais', p. 191.
3. AN F12 740; For Holker's attempts to display his achievement to Trudaine, F12 24; for site development and the mounting of looms, F12 1455, Holker to Trudaine 12 January 1759. For Falkener, above p. 86.
4. Chassagne, *Le Coton*, p. 69 seq. The coming of the jenny will be discussed with the general acquisition of the new English textile machinery in the 1770s and 1780s, below, p. 134.
5. A. Wadsworth and J. de L. Mann, *The Cotton Trade and Industrial Lancashire* (Manchester, 1931), pp. 486–8.
6. Chassagne, *Le Coton*, pp. 68–72.
7. For Alcock and La Charité, below, p. 175. Here, though, Trudaine soon had the conviction that Saint Etienne might have been a better site. The question of whether the French state was well advised to try to establish fertile oases in industrial deserts, or on the contrary to encourage greater investment and newer technology in areas where industries were already well established is a most interesting one which needs more debate. Just before the revolution the Bureau of Commerce was against the introduction of more new industry in Normandy on the theory that the province was over-developed!
8. AN F12 675.
9. See below, p. 176.
10. AN F12 675.
11. Subsequently increased, AN F12 25.
12. AN F12 674, 675; a worker called Torrens, probably also Irish, was briefly at Bourges (Bellefonds, 'Les Techniciens Anglais', p. 198).
13. According to Lesage's later statement of 1790 the English experts demanded

a salary bonus of 40 *sols* on each piece made, which was ruinous; AN F12 1373.

14. Chassagne, *Le Coton*, pp. 126–8; AN F12 675.
15. Chassagne, *Le Coton*, pp. 128–34; AN F12 676A.
16. Chassagne, *Le Coton*, pp. 134–6.
17. A. Clow and N. Clow, *The Chemical Revolution* (1952), pp. 130–36.
18. Clow and Clow, *Chemical Revolution*, pp. 136–7.
19. See below, p. 232.
20. Clow and Clow, *Chemical Revolution*, pp. 133–43; J. G. Smith, *The Origins and Early Development of the Heavy Chemical Industry in France* (Oxford, 1979), pp. 5–7; B. Faujas de Saint-Fond, *A Journey through England and Scotland to the Hebrides in 1784*, ed. A. Geickie (Glasgow, 1907), vol. 1, pp. 174–5. The Roebuck and Garbett patent was overthrown in the law courts.
21. Smith, *Origins*, p. 15.
22. Smith, *Origins*, p. 8.
23. For the monopoly see C. C. Gillispie, *Science and Polity in France at the End of the Old Regime* (Princeton, 1980), pp. 50–7.
24. Written Terney in some of the relevant documents.
25. AN F12 1506, Brown's proposals, n.d., and Holker to Trudaine 13 (?) October 1764.
26. Ibid.
27. Ibid., Holker to Trudaine 19 January, Holker to Trudaine de Montigny 5 February; draft *arrêt* 3 February 1765.
28. For Holker's support for them with the local Intendant in the Fécamp venture, AD Seine Maritime C129.
29. Saltpetre could come from Lorient, Britain or Holland. AN F12 1506, Holker letter of 4 June 1766; revised draft *arrêt* of 18 June.
30. Smith, *Origins*, p. 90; AN F12 740.
31. See below, p. 232.
32. AN F12 740.
33. Smith, *Origins*, p. 9.
34. This suggests that when the younger Holker went to Brussels Murry rather than Brown may have been his target.
35. For this and the following paragraphs, AN F12 1506. For the later career of Murry (or Murray), Smith, *Origins*, p. 15.
36. AN F12 1506, esp. letters of 13 April, 7 May 1768.
37. The duty was raised greatly in 1770, Smith *Origins*, pp. 10–11. AN F12 1506, letter of Trudaine de Montigny 12 May 1768; of Holker senior 5 July; Memoirs of 8 July; Trudaine de Montigny to Holkers 27 August.
38. AN F12 1506, Holker to Trudaine, 8 May 1769; Trudaine to Holker, 14 May 1769.
39. Smith, *Origins*, pp. 10–53, and information kindly supplied by Professor Chassagne.
40. Smith, *Origins*, p. 195.
41. Smith, *Origins*, p. 54 seq.
42. Smith, *Origins*, p. 98–100. For the visit of William Losh 'the father of the

alkali trade in Great Britain' to France see Clow and Clow, *Chemical Revolution*, pp. 100, 104. Only in exports did the British lead.

43. T. C. Barker and J. R. Harris, *A Merseyside Town in the Industrial Revolution: St. Helens 1750–1900* (Liverpool, 1954; Cass, London, 1959 and 1993), pp. 225–39.

44. AN F12 879. The Holkers were involved with the chemist and chemical manufacturer J.-F. Demarchy in another controversy over their vitriol production. This was arbitrated by a panel of the Academy of Sciences, headed by the famous chemist Pierre-Joseph Macquer; R. Hahn, *The Anatomy of a Scientific Institution: the Paris Academy of Sciences, 1666–1803* (Berkeley, CA, 1971), p. 70. Demarchy is described by Gillispie as 'apothecary and would-be chemist, pornographer and would-be poet, who boasted of having committed incest with his mother before entering on the life-long quarrel of his marriage' (*Science and Polity*, p. 330).

Notes for Chapter 6

1.   For this and subsequent paragraphs, AN F12 2427.
2.   See below, p. 208.
3.   See below, p. 224.
4.   See below, p. 175.
5.   See below, p. 430. Also P. W. Bamford, *Privilege and Profit*, (Philadelphia, 1988), ch. 2, p. 28 *seq.* for an excellent account of this trade.
6.   Patent rights were readily presumed by Frenchmen to be exactly equivalent to their own grants of monopoly privileges to manufactures.
7.   AN F12 2427. The instructions for the 1767 tour were discussed by both Trudaines.
8.   Ibid.
9.   There are two oddities about Holker's letter; he thought that the machines derived from Northamptonshire rather than Lancashire, probably because that was the county from which his son had written about them. He also seems to have believed there was a 10 per cent bounty on English cotton exports.
10. AN F12 2427, 1338.
11. Apparently a French rediscovery of the timber-bending process which May had demonstrated to them half a century before? Above p. 25.
12. For security at Prestonpans, above, p. 115.
13. AN F12 2427, travel instructions to Holker II; Holker to Trudaine de Montigny, 20 January 1768, 6 October 1770, Holker II to Trudaine de Montigny 2 January 1771, 2 June 1772, to Bruyard, 19 June 1772, to Trudaine de Montigny, 4 August 1772.
14. Internal evidence shows it cannot be before 1767.
15. AN F12 661.
16. AN F12 1352.
17. AN F12 2427.

18. G. Lewis, *The Advent of Modern Capitalism in France 1770–1840: the Contribution of Pierre-François Tubeuf* (Oxford, 1993), chs 1 and 2.

19. AN F12 2427. J. R. Harris, 'Skills, coal and British industry in the eighteenth century', ch. 2 of *Essays in Industry and Technology in the Eighteenth Century: England and France* (Aldershot, 1992).

20. We have no evidence of John Holker II's involvement with a Rouen pottery. However he was the director in 1774 of a pottery at Montereau run by Clark, Shaw and Company. His father in his proposal for an appointment as inspector-general in 1756 had already mentioned the existence of an English type pottery there (above, p. 61). A petition from Clark and Shaw to Trudaine de Montigny of 10 October 1774 says that they had set up their pottery under his protection, which indicates that it was a revival of the one existing in 1756. This was one founded in 1745 by the faience merchant Mazois and Chapelle, a modeller from the Vincennes porcelain works, for creamware manufacture. It had an English partner, John Hill. It was after Mazois' death in 1774 that John Holker II took over. Clark and Shaw made it clear that they were imitating the Queen's Ware of Josiah Wedgwood. They had got two more workers from England, so that with the Clarks, father and son, Shaw and the new man, all with wives and children, there were seventeen English now at Montereau. In the petition they asked that their manufacture 'a l'instar de celle d'Angleterre' be given a number of privileges, including ones about workers' contracts and the seducing away of their apprentices by other firms. They asked for an 800 *livres* subsidy for ten years. Trudaine referred to the younger Holker, who said he had suggested to Clark and Shaw that they petition the Government and stated that he and Antoine and Robert Garvey, the Rouen merchants, had jointly supplied the firm's capital of 40,000 *livres*. The firm received its *arrêt* on 15 March 1775. In 1780 Benjamin Franklin, as ambassador of the United States at Paris, ordered a large quantity of Montereau tableware for his embassy, the first ever ordered for an American mission, almost certainly for a Fourth of July celebration. After the deaths of some of the English partners the work was in the hands of John Hall (alias Hulme) in 1792, presumably related to the textile expert originally brought over by John Holker senior. It was leased to Christopher Potter after Hall's death and continued to operate through the nineteenth century and into the early twentieth. It is interesting that Clark and Shaw were faced with a technological problem in 1774, that of retraining suborned workers used to coal fuel in England, to use charcoal instead. I am grateful for information supplied by Ellen Cohn and Claude-Anne Lopez as editors of the *Papers of Benjamin Franklin* at Yale, some of which has been helpful in other parts of this work, to Gaye Blake Roberts, curator of the Wedgwood Museum, and to M. Jacques Bontillot of the Musée de la Faience de Montereau. For the Clark, Shaw and Holker II correspondence with Trudaine de Montigny, AN F12 1489A. Josiah Wedgwood's views on Shaw and his suborning appear below, p. 479. There is no evidence of the Holkers' involvement in Rouen potteries, though there were sixteen faience workers in the Saint Sever suburb in the late eighteenth century, and they appear not to be involved in the large but short-lived coal-burning works of

William Sturgeon, an Irishman. This was financed by his wealthy English wife, Henrietta Wentworth. This Saint Sever works became a *manufacture royale* in 1781. Sturgeon was insolvent by 1785 and, like other local potters, was put out of business by English imports under the Eden-Rayneval treaty. See M. G. Vanier, 'La Manufacture Royale de Faience Du Faubourg Saint-Sever à Rouen', *Extrait des Actes du 81ᵉ Congrès des Sociétés Savantes, Rouen–Caen 1956* (Paris, 1956), p. 389 seq.

21. AN F12 659A.
22. AN F12 657, 676A. In this year he was raised to the rank of inspector-general. AN F12 740.

Notes for Chapter 7

1. As late as 1768 he tried to plot a Jacobite rising. See below, p. 169.
2. Holker and his first wife had become naturalized French citizens in January 1766.
3. Holker's work was said to have supported 80,000 jobs.
4. AD Seine Maritime, C1205, Memoir of 18 August 1775. Baron de Sénévas, *Une Famille Française du XIVᵉ au XXᵉ Siècle* (Paris, 1929) esp. pp. 327–30.
5. This seems mainly to be an attack on the younger Holker; AN F12 676B.
6. There is a very useful short biography of Roland by Charles A. Le Guin, 'Roland de la Platière, a public servant in the eighteenth century', *Transactions of the American Philosophical Society*, New Series, 56, pt 6 (1966).
7. However, he should be remembered for taking the first steps to establish a national museum in the Louvre, to set up national archives and a national library. See Le Guin, 'Roland de la Platière', p. 123.
8. Ibid., pp. 5–9.
9. Ibid., pp. 10–13.
10. Ibid., pp. 13–18.
11. Ibid., p. 31: 'Without ever having seen it, I was the first to bring in the machine for spinning cotton, which we considerably improved.'
12. Ibid., pp. 48–9.
13. Considering Holker's part in the '45, the daring nature of the escape, and Holker's later political and industrial espionage expeditions to England this was a most gratuitous insult.
14. *L'Art du Fabricant de Velours de Coton* (1780), Introduction, pp. 1–30. For Milne at Rouen see below, p. 363.
15. Le Guin, 'Roland de la Platière', p. 49. Brown was inspector at Caen from 1780 to 1784, inspector for the generality of Paris 1784–87 and inspector ambulant from 1787.
16. *Lettre d'un Citoyen de Villefranche à M. Roland de la Platière*, (n.d.) pp. 1–54. I am indebted for access to this, and the two other pamphlets cited below, to the Municipal Library of Lyon.
17. Ibid., pp. 4–9.

18. Ibid., p. 11.
19. This claim is unsubstantiated, but Holker may have made some improvement on existing practice.
20. *Lettre d'un Citoyen*, p. 15.
21. Ibid., pp. 20–22.
22. This statement in a publication obviously sanctioned by him is another proof that Holker never made any claims to have been at Culloden.
23. *Lettre d'un Citoyen*, pp. 22–6.
24. Ibid., pp. 26–7.
25. Ibid., pp. 29–30.
26. Bibliothèque National; naf 6242, ff. 55–6.
27. *Lettre d'un Citoyen*, p. 30.
28. Ibid., pp. 31–5.
29. Ibid., pp. 35–7.
30. Ibid., pp. 39–40.
31. *Réponse à la Lettre d'un soi-disant citoyen de Villefranche* (n.d.) seems certainly 1781.
32. Ibid., pp. 1–5.
33. Ibid., p. 21.
34. Ibid, pp. 24–7.
35. Ibid., pp. 34–6.
36. Ibid., pp. 45–6.
37. *Lettres imprimés a Rouen, en Octobre 1781*.
38. Ibid., pp. 1–3.
39. His French second wife certainly was not, sometimes acting as a secretary to her husband.
40. *Lettres imprimés*, p. 3.
41. Ibid., p. 4.
42. Ibid., p. 5.
43. J. R. Harris, 'Saint Gobain and Ravenhead', *Essays in Industry and Technology in the Eighteenth Century: England and France* (Aldershot, 1992), pp. 60–61, 71.
44. *Lettres imprimés*, p. 7.
45. Ibid., p. 11.
46. There is a further letter which Roland wrote to Montigny on the same day: Ibid., 'Quatrième lettre', pp. 15–18. This shows his anxiety at having upset Montigny and major Academicians, and there is another one which he wrote to Fougeraux de Bondaray which tries to excuse the embarrassment he had caused to those who had let his 'Introduction' be published, though he still tried to justify himself. Ibid., 'Cinquième lettre', pp. 19–20.
47. Le Guin, 'Roland de la Platière', p. 56.
48. AN F12 650.
49. Le Guin, 'Roland de la Platière', p. 56. Roland's professional rebuffs were connected with his bitter attacks in his *Dictionnaire* on the inspectorate which he had been so eager to join. See also AN F12 661.
50. A very useful source is the series of *The Papers of Robert Morris*, seven volumes of which have been edited for the University of Pittsburgh Press by

E. J. Ferguson and subsequently by J. Catanzariti. Morris was important as Superintendent of Finance from 1781 to 1784 and virtually first minister in the Continental Congress. He obtained major French loans in 1781 and subsequently Dutch ones. He founded the Bank of North America. However his influence had greatly declined by 1783. There were doubts about the probity of some of his early financial dealings with Congress. After the war he tried to set up a deal with the farmers-general for France's tobacco supply and then entered into enormous American land speculations, which collapsed in 1797, leaving him with debts of $3 million. He was in a debtor's prison from 1798 to 1801 and then lived on charity until his death in 1806. See vol. 1 Intro., pp. XVII–XXX. Volume 7, pp. 272–5, has a long and informative editorial note on John Holker and his relations with Morris. The second major source on the Holkers and America is the John Holker Papers (1777–1812) in the Manuscript Division of the Library of Congress. This is a massive source of over 4,000 items, many individually large and carrying, *inter alia*, a great series of correspondence and accounts. Through the kindness of Mr Chuck Kelly of the Manuscripts Division I have been able to make a quick and superficial survey of twenty-five volumes of archive on microfilm. However, there is not any large correspondence between the younger and elder Holker down to the latter's death in 1786, though there are a few useful early letters which are evidently from the father.

51. John Holker Papers, vol. 8, Letters of Tolozan 17 November 1779 and Montaran 20 February 1780.
52. E.g. Le Couteulx brothers to Holker, John Holker Papers, vol. 1, n.d. 1778.
53. John Holker Papers, vol. 2, esp. Holker senior to Holker junior, November 1779.
54. For a list of American and French merchant houses with which Holker was connected see *Papers of Robert Morris*, vol. 7, p. 266, n. 5.
55. *Papers of Robert Morris*, vol. 2, p. 77. Extract from R. Morris's Diary.
56. *Papers of Robert Morris*, vol. 5, p. 366 and vol. 7, p. 277.
57. Some of these transactions were large. In December 1781 Morris in his official capacity asked Franklin in Paris to pay John Holker senior 100,000 *livres* for clothing, apparently imported from France, on his son's account. *Papers of Robert Morris*, vol. 3, p. 333.
58. Ibid. vol. 4, pp. 134–5; for army and navy stores contracts, p. 497; vol. 7, p. 46. Holker had to give a bond of $200,000 as security for one major army contract as partner in Parker, Duer and Holker.
59. John Holker Papers, S. Breck to Parker 5 July 1784.
60. John Holker Papers, letter from Rouen 1 June 1784. His father had been deeply concerned for his return for some time; *Papers of Robert Morris*, vol. 7, Matthew Ridley to Morris 20 November 1782, and see p. 276 n. 9.
61. In 1789, he received $43,646 specie value for the $405,100 paper value burned at his house. These certificates, in his name, were jointly owned with the French firms of Le Couteulx and Ferdinand Grand. *Papers of Thomas Jefferson*, J. P. Boyd (ed.), (Princeton), vol. 17, p. 288.
62. John Holker Papers, vols 34–5. 'Observations of MM. de Fontenay'.

Includes a copy of a letter to the younger Holker of October 1790. He is said to be then in France.

63. Affaires Etrangères, Correspondence Politique Angleterre, p. 458, letter of Holker, Dieppe, 18 August 1780, and his letter of 15 September 1780.

64. This would be the highly eccentric Earl-Bishop (who fancied his talents in secret diplomacy and espionage) possibly on his visit to Paris early in the American War of Independence.

65. Affaires Etrangères, correspondence cited.

66. PRO *Calendar of Home Office Papers (1770–1772)*, p. 254, 22 July 1772.

67. *Thomas Jefferson Papers*, vol. 8, pp. 304–5 and note. Holker wrote to Jefferson on 18 July 1785 'J'ai eu la satisfaction pendant deux jours de posseder ici notre venerable ami le Docteur Franklin. Il a supporté le voyage d'une manière surprenante'. See also Carl van Doren, *Benjamin Franklin* (New York, 1938), pp. 722–5. There are several indications in Franklin's papers of the very friendly basis of his acquaintance with Holker and his second wife. I am deeply indebted to Ellen Cohn for information and references, which include items relating to Holker senior and James Milne and to Holker junior and the Montereau pottery, and come from the ongoing edition of *The Papers of Benjamin Franklin* at Yale. References include vol. 25, p. 141; vol. 26, p. 674; vol. 27, pp. 183–4, 324; vol. 30, pp. 436, 560, 601–2, 609–15; and items from vols 31 and 32, currently in the press.

68. E.g. *Jefferson Papers*, vol. 7, p. 579, Holker, Rouen, to Jefferson 22 December 1784; vol. 8, p. 67, Holker, Rouen to Jefferson 29 March 1785.

69. *Papers of Robert Morris*, vol. 3, p. 373. Letter of 11 December 1781; vol. 4, p. 245, letter of 16 February 1782.

70. AN F12 1455.

71. Affaires Etrangères, Correspondence Politique Angleterre, p. 65, Dupont's Fourth Memoir on the Treaty of Commerce.

72. F. McLynn, 'Unpopular front; Jews, radicals and Americans in the Jacobite world view', *Royal Stuart Papers XXI* (Huntingdon, 1988) pp. 8–9; F. McLynn, *Charles Edward Stuart* (Oxford, 1991), pp. 397–9.

73. C. C. Gillispie, *Science and Polity at the End of the Old Régime* (Princeton, 1980), p. 424.

74. S. Chassagne, *Le Coton et Ses Patrons, France 1760–1840* (Paris, 1991), p. 56.

Notes for Chapter 8

1. For detailed references see 'Michael Alcock and the transfer of Birmingham technology to France before the Revolution', chapter IV of J. R. Harris, *Essays in Industry and Technology in the Eighteenth Century: England and France* (Aldershot, 1992).

2. H. W. Dickinson however did refer to the mint–toymaking connection (*Matthew Boulton* (1937), p. 13) but unfortunately this has not been pursued. It is hoped to investigate this further.

3. AN F12 1315 A, Holker to controller-general 18 May 1756; Harris, 'Michael Alcock', p. 117–23.
4. AN F12 1315A, 1315B; AD Nièvre, IC 12.
5. *Birmingham Gazette*, 7 February 1763.
6. 'Par son génie et son activité (il) peut être regardé comme un excellent sujet', AN F12 1315A.
7. Ibid.; AD Nièvre IC 11.
8. AN F12 1315A.
9. Ibid.
10. J. R. Harris, 'Michael Alcock', pp. 162–3.
11. This he continued to do after he left.
12. AN F12 1315A.
13. The problems of getting La Charité sufficiently advanced to be able to go to the assistance of Carrier at Saint Etienne are discussed in AN F 12 1315A, Holker to Trudaine, early May 1758.
14. L.-J. Gras, *Le Conseil de Commerce de Saint-Etienne* (Saint Etienne, 1899), p. 21.
15. Above, p. 68.
16. AD Nièvre, IC Alcock to Dodart 22 April, 8 May 1763.
17. AD Nièvre IC 11.
18. AN Minutier Central XXIX, p. 441 29 February 1757.
19. AN F12 1316; see also AN F12 1315A and F12 1315B.
20. The remaining partners now admitted that Sanche and Hyde had deliberately worked as the tools of one investor (presumably Billard) to throw out Alcock. After Hyde had converted from Protestantism to Catholicism, they had conspired to incite religious feeling against Alcock as a Protestant.
21. See below, p. 215.
22. AN F12 1315A, 1315B.
23. J. R. Harris, 'Michael Alcock', pp. 152–5.
24. See below, p. 187, for de Saudray's operation.
25. Birmingham Public Libraries, Boulton Papers, Ingram to Boulton 11 March 1774.
26. See below, p. 502.
27. Birmingham Public Libraries, Boulton Papers, Argand to Boulton 13 September 1786; Incoming letters P1/19.
28. Holker hoped they would get the privilege for manufacture, being 'sufficiently unfortunate in having lost by the caprice of their Father the works at La Charité', AN F12 1315B, Holker to Trudaine 11 June 1765.
29. Birmingham Public Libraries, Boulton Papers, Box 1 26, Ingram to Boulton, 11 March 1774.
30. 'pour y terminer quelques affaires de famille', Affaires Etrangères, Mémoires et Documents, Angleterre 523, Trudaine de Montigny to Rayneval, 20 June 1777.
31. AN F12 1315A, Holker to Trudaine, 6 March 1760; Affaires Etrangères, Mémoires et Documents Angleterre 49, memoir of Trudaine 4 January 1752.

32. AN F12 722, Opinion of the Deputies of Commerce, 10 February 1784. One important result of Joseph Alcock's meeting with Boulton on his 1777–78 visit was his immediate communication of the importance of the Boulton and Watt engine to the French government. See below, p. 300.
33. E.g. C. Ballot, *L'Introduction du Machinisme dans L'Industrie Française* (Lille-Paris, 1923) p. 484.
34. Harris, 'Michael Alcock', pp. 153, 155–7.
35. Harris, 'Michael Alcock', p. 131.
36. He also served as a member of a military commission to Turkey.
37. The best general source for de Saudray's life is the *Procès Verbal de la 100ᵉ Séance Publique de L'Athenée Des Arts* (Paris, 1834) which contains a long obituary by Mirault.
38. Ballot, *L'Introduction*, p. 485.
39. AN F12 1316.
40. Vergennes wrote to the Ambassador in London telling him – for his eyes only – of the secret nature of de Saudray's business, that there might be steps to thwart him and harm his plans, and that he would want the ambassador to protect him if necessary. AN F 12 994.
41. AN F12 1316.
42. Ibid.
43. In September 1777 de Saudray wrote to Tolozan 'You are aware Sir, how many changes this business has gone through by passing so frequently from hand to hand', AN F12 1316.
44. AN F12 2232.
45. AN F12 1316.
46. AN F12 1316, 994.
47. AN F994, Vergennes to De Fourqueux 20 August 1777.
48. Rightly or wrongly the commissioners believed that Le Cour had worked in Birmingham during his time in England, though he does not seem to have ever made that claim explicitly himself, and it would have been a very useful point to make in his various propaganda statements.
49. AN F12 994, Montigny to de Saudray 18 October 1777, and to Duc De Nivernois (? October) 1771.
50. AN F12 994, Memoir of 16 December 1777.
51. Matthew Boulton traded with Orsel, père et fils, of Aix en Provence, possibly a branch house of the firm. A. E. Musson and E. Robinson, *Science and Technology in the Industrial Revolution* (Manchester, 1969), p. 220.
52. According to de Saudray they had a turnover of 1.5 million *livres* on their business and 800,000 *livres* worth of property.
53. AN F12 2232 memoir of 15 July 1782; F12 1316, memoir of 1779.
54. AN F12 1315B, Memoir of Orsels to Calonne.
55. AN F12 994, Memoir of De Saudray, 14 December 1784.
56. AN F 12 994, de Saudray to Calonne 14 December 1784. As at the time of Boulton's visit to France in 1786, the Abbé Calonne seems to have acted as his brother's intermediary.
57. AN F12 994, Receipt of Vandermonde 24 September 1784. For the Hôtel de

Mortagne, see A. Doyon and L. Liaigre 'L'hôtel de Mortagne après la mort de Vaucanson', *Histoire des Entreprises*, (11), May 1963.

58. AN F12 994, De Saudray to Tolozan 14 December 1784.
59. Ibid., Report on new memoir of de Saudray.
60. *Procès Verbal de la 100ᵉ Séance Publique de l' Athenée Des Arts* (Paris, 1834); *Moniteur Universel*, 17–20 July 1789, 2 October 1791; printed pamphlets of de Saudray of 21 July 1789, of 18 December 1789 (Etat de mes Services) and of 1790; AN F 12 994, Bailly to Necker 4 September 1790; Michaud, *Biographie Universelle*, New Edition (n.d.), see Saudray or De Saudrais. Under the Empire de Saudray became a Chevalier of the Legion of Honour.
61. For the Lycée des Arts, and its distinction from the Lycée, see W. A. Smeaton, 'The early years of the Lycée and the Lycée des Arts', pt II, 'The Lycée des Arts', *Annals of Science*, 11 (1955), 309 seq. See also R. Hahn, *The Anatomy of a Scientific Institution, the Paris Academy of Sciences, 1666–1803*, (Berkeley, CA, 1971), pp. 185–6, 193, 217–18, 232–6.
62. Below, p. 431.
63. AN F12 994.
64. Probably at the time of the dissolution of his company in late 1777 or early 1778, an inventory of the imported English tools and materials was made, amounting to over £770 sterling, of which £197 was in copper goods to be enamelled, £60 for a pair of rolls and their iron mounting, £100 for unfinished plated work, and £250 in dies and related equipment. Some of the equipment seems to be for watch case manufacture. Lathes, a press and files were among the tools. The men who valued the tools were James Arbuckle and Charles Grey, which gives us the names of at least two of the workmen brought over. AN F12 1316.
65. AN F12 1309.
66. AN F12 1316.
67. AN F12 680, F12 107/8.
68. Musson and Robinson, *Science and Technology*, pp. 220–21.
69. AN F12 1315B, Orsel to Calonne, n.d. 1785.
70. AN F12 1315B.
71. L. Bergeron, *Banquiers, négociants et manufacturiers parisiens du Directoire à l'Empire*, (Paris, 1978), p. 21.
72. *Commons Journals*, 20 March 1759.
73. *Commons Journals*, 22 April, 1 May 1760.
74. See below, p. 210.
75. C. Ballot, *L'Introduction*, p. 487.
76. Ibid.
77. Gournay, *Tableau de Commerce* (1789, 90); AN F12 1317, 2250.
78. Harris, 'Michael Alcock', pp. 158–9.
79. A French prohibition on British hardware imports was imposed in 1785 to concentrate British government attention on the affair of the commercial treaty. It seems to have had little practical effect.
80. Ballot, *L'Introduction*, p. 487.
81. Harris, 'Michael Alcock', p. 160.

Notes for Chapter 9

1. For additional detail and references see 'Attempts to transfer English steel techniques to France in the eighteenth century', Chapter III of J. R. Harris, *Essays in Industry and Technology in the Eighteenth Century: England and France* (Variorum, Aldershot, 1992).
2. *Les techniques métallurgiques Dauphinoises au Dix-huitième siècle* (Paris, 1961).
3. R. A. F. Réaumur, *L'art de convertir le fer forgé en acier* (Paris, 1722), p. 16.
4. AN F12 1315B.
5. AN F12 1302; 1315B.
6. *Birmingham Gazette*, 4 July 1785.
7. Harris, 'Attempts to Transfer', pp. 146–7.
8. AN F12 1316.
9. Harris, 'Attempts to Transfer', pp. 149–50.
10. AN F14 1311, Harris, 'Attempts to Transfer', pp. 87–8. For Jars, below, p. 222.
11. For this and the following paragraphs, Harris, 'Attempts to Transfer', p. 88 seq; Leon, *Les techniques*, pp. 29–30.
12. Harris, 'Attempts to Transfer', pp. 90–91.
13. For the Sanche steel venture, Harris, 'Attempts to Transfer', pp. 91–6.
14. AN F12 107/8.
15. Harris, 'Attempts to Transfer', p. 97 seq.
16. B. Gille, *Les origines de la grande industrie métallurgique en France* (Paris, 1947), p. 97.
17. Harris, 'Attempts to Transfer', pp. 111–12, nn. 61, 63, 75.
18. F. Le Play, 'Mémoire sur la fabrication de l'acier en Yorkshire', *Annales des Mines*, 4th Series, 3 (1843), 583–626.
19. For the views of Arnaud, Saint-Bris and the Jacksons, and the perceptive later comments of Le Play, Harris, 'Attempts to Transfer', pp. 102–8.

Notes for Chapter 10

1. He is described as an entrepreneur and landowner of Lyon by C. C. Gillispie, *Science and Polity in France at the End of the Old Regime* (Princeton, 1980), pp. 427–8.
2. See Gillispie, *Science and Polity*, but the evidence of the Eloge mentioned later in the paragraph suggests that it was only after studies in drawing, mathematics and chemistry that the serious fieldwork began.
3. He also taught the students German.
4. AN F14 1311, Konig to Trudaine 29 April 1753, passed by Trudaine to Hellot.
5. Francois Guillot-Duhamel.
6. Above, p. 570, n. 18.
7. Jean Hellot, *De la fonte des mines et des fonderies*, 2 vols (Paris, 1750–53).

8. AN F14 1311, 10 May 1756.
9. Jars, *Voyages métalurgiques*, vol. 1 (Lyon, 1774) p. xviii, vol. 2 (Paris, 1780), p. viii.
10. AN F14 1311. Important in drawing the attention of British scholars to the existence of Jars's tour of 1764–65 was Jean Chevalier's paper 'La Mission de Gabriel Jars dans les Mines et les Usines Britanniques en 1764', *Transactions of the Newcomen Society*, 26 (1947), 57 seq.
11. See above, pp. 36–7. The initials on the instructions may well have given the impression that another J. H., John Holker, drew them up. He was involved, as we will see, but in a different way.
12. 'This title, I believe, is the most advantageous one I could have when in a foreign country, they would suspect less an inquisitive member of an Academy, than a technical man (homme de l'art)'. AN F14 1311, Jars to Trudaine ? May 1764.
13. Jars, *Voyages*, vol. 1, p. xxiii.
14. Perhaps a throw-back to the claims of Dud Dudley.
15. One of Hellot's official jobs was to examine coal samples from the French coalfields to determine their utility.
16. AN F14 1311.
17. AN F14 1311. Some of the instructions as finally issued came from some observations on Jean Hellot's draft by another official, probably De Montigny of the Academy. There is a D. M. initial, and Mignot De Montigny was one of the experts most consulted by Trudaine. Bacquié seems to be mistaken in saying Jars's instructions were 'pleins de conseils pratiques dus à Holker', no doubt thinking Hellot's (J. H.) initials were Holker's. Some of the enquiries about English file manufacture which Jars was asked to deal with came from a M. de Labelouze.
18. AN F14 1311, letter of 30 July 1764.
19. AN F14 1311, Jars to Trudaine 12 May 1765.
20. See below, p. 344.
21. AN F14 1311.
22. It can be argued that the very strong French interest in file-cutting machines, much stronger than that in England, was due to their inability to match the English hand skill. J. R. Harris 'First thoughts on files', *Journal of the Tools and Trades Society*, 3 (1985), 27–35.
23. See Jars, *Voyages*, vol. 1, pp. 229–30; T. S. Ashton, *An Eighteenth Century Industrialist: Peter Stubs of Warrington, 1756–1806* (Manchester, 1939), pp. 3–4; E. S. Dane, *Peter Stubs and the Lancashire Hand Tool Industry* (Altringham, 1973), pp. 2–5.
24. *Voyages*, vol. 3 (Paris, 1781), pp. 72–5.
25. See below, pp. 271–4.
26. Jars, *Voyages*, vol. 3, pp. 72–8, 217–19.
27. Ibid., p. 106. Jars's observations on Birmingham are more limited than might have been expected, but he recorded the intensive use of machinery and the high degree of specialization reducing labour costs.
28. See Jars, *Voyages*, vol. 2, plate 14 for Newcomen engine, p. 530 seq. for lead industry, p. 542 for the water-column engine.

29. Jars, *Voyages*, vol. 3, p. 309 seq.
30. Below, p. 238.
31. Jars, *Voyages*, vol. 1, pp. 235–7.
32. Jars, *Voyages*, vol. 1, p. 250.
33. Jars, *Voyages*, vol. 1, pp. 265–9.
34. Jars, *Voyages*, vol. 1, p. 280. H. W. Dickinson and R. Jenkins, *James Watt and the Steam Engine* (Ashbourne, 1927, reprint 1981), pp. 24–6.
35. Jars, *Voyages*, vol. 1, pp. 270–4.
36. J. E. Rehder, 'The change from charcoal to coke in iron smelting', *Journal of the Historical Metallurgy Society*, 21, (1), (1987).
37. Jars, *Voyages*, vol. 1, pp. 274–8.
38. Apart from the *Voyages Métallurgiques*, there are some Affaires Etrangères references, e.g. Mémoires et Documents, Angleterre, 49, reports of May and June 1765, and several reports in AN F14 1311.
39. According to Gillispie (*Science and Polity*, p. 60) Lavoisier won the vote of the Academy by a very small margin; according to Jars's brother in the introduction to the first volume of the *Voyages Métallurgiques* (1774), the votes were even ('Intro.' p. XXV). This is taken from the Eloge of Jars given by the permanent secretary, Fouchy, to the Academy, 25 April 1770.
40. A letter of 9 January 1769 survives instructing Jars to go to Dauphiné to look at the steelworks of Rives and the blast furnaces supplying them, and all other furnace industries there, but it is not clear if this journey was made.
41. Jars, *Voyages*, vol. 1, p. 227.
42. Le Play was both the country's Chief Mining Engineer and Professor of Metallurgy at the Ecole Royale des Mines so his access to the archives cannot be disputed. *Mémoire ... des fers à acier* (Paris, 1846), an offprint of the *Annales des Mines*, pp. 102–3; 105.

Notes for Chapter 11

1. AN F14 1311, Jars's report dated Besançon 10 October 1768.
2. C. C. Gillispie, *Science and Polity in France at the End of the Old Regime* (Princeton, 1980), p. 435; see also F. Bacquié, *Les Inspecteurs des manufactures sous L'Ancien Régime* (1927), pp. 45, 46.
3. This somewhat exaggerates the conversion to coke smelting in Britain by this date. G. Jars, *Manière de préparer le Charbon minéral pour le substituer au charbon de bois dans les travaux métallurgiques* (Lyon, 1770).
4. See above, p. 228.
5. AD Hérault, C2703, Bertin to Saint-Priest 25 September 1770. For a more recent version of Bertin's view, C. Ballot, *L'Introduction du Machinisme dans L'Industrie Française* (Lille-Paris, 1923), p. 441, 'La mort de Jars enleva à la nouvelle industrie (coke-iron) son apôtre le plus fidèle et le plus éclairé'.
6. AN F12 1313/14.
7. *Des bouches à feu.*

8. Ballot, *L'Introduction*, pp. 441–7. Stuart and his partner knew of the existence of English processes to convert coke pig to wrought iron using reverberatory furnaces, but claimed the product was poor.

9. Ballot, *L'Introduction*, pp. 448–9.

10. See AN F12 1300, F14 4261. The report was translated into English by the late Professor W. H. Chaloner: *Marchant de la Houlière's Report to the French Government on British Methods of Smelting Iron Ore with Coal and Casting Naval Cannon in the Year 1775* (Sheffield, 1949), five pages, unpaginated. Reprinted from *Edgar Allen News*, December 1948, January 1949.

11. H. W. Dickinson and R. Jenkins, *James Watt and the Steam Engine* (1927), 1981 edn, p. 43.

12. See below, p. 491 seq.

13. Chaloner, *Houlière's Report*, n.p.

14. As Jars had noted, above, p. 234.

15. No. 1054 of 1773.

16. Bronze cannon had been made by boring from the solid for some time, first on the Continent by Maritz and others, and later at Woolwich by the Verbruggens.

17. Chaloner, *Houlière's Report*, n.p.

18. See W. H. Chaloner's excellent short paper 'The brothers John and William Wilkinson and their relations with French metallurgy 1775–1786'. This translation of a French paper of 1956 appears in his selected essays *Industry and Innovation*, D. A. Farnie and W. O. Henderson (eds), (1990). For the letter from the French ambassador, de Guines, see T. S. Ashton, *Iron and Steel in the Industrial Revolution*, 2nd edn (Manchester, 1951), p. 46.

19. AN 127 AP7. Possibly because of his difficult handwriting this officer's name is sometimes given as Serval, but the reading of Secval, as given by Denise Ozanam, 'La Naissance du Creusot', *Revue d'Histoire de la Sidérurgie*, 4 (1963) seems to be right. See also AN F14 4504.

20. Sometimes industrial trials were arranged on wholly unsuitable sites so that they could be readily inspected by commissioners of the Academy, whose approval was often essential to privilege and subsidy.

21. Ballot, *L'Introduction*, p. 450.

22. While in English money these sums were roughly £600 and £2,000, they may be compared to what was considered the high remuneration of an Inspector-General of Manufactures at 8,000 *livres*.

23. AN 127 AP 7, letter of 3 July 1778.

24. The supervisory role of Secval was not entirely concluded and he was still dealing with Wilkinson at least as late as April 1779, though it is stated that his quarrel with Wilkinson meant that no one was any longer following Wilkinson's operations well enough to be able to carry them out without him. AN F12 4500.

25. AN Marine B3 653. Further research seems to be needed, particularly a proper analysis of AN 127 AP 7.

26. 'Il decrivit le Procédé Anglais et rassura pleinement le Ministre sur le pretendu mistère de cette fabrication', AN F14 4504.

27. AN Marine D.3/34. Mémoire sur Indret.

28. AN F14 4504.

29. Port de Lorient, Service Historique, 101/47.

30. AN Marine D3/34.

31. AN Marine B3 771; B. Gille, *Les origines de le grande industrie métallurgique en France* (Paris, 1947), pp. 193–6; AN F14 4504.

32. AN F14 7866.

33. AN Marine D3/34.

34. AN D3/38, Memoir of Wendel; D3/34 'Observations sur le projet de conditions proposées par M. Wilkinson'.

35. AN Marine D3/34.

36. The only effective monopoly of the Wilkinsons was of course for the high quality cylinders of Boulton and Watt engines (AN F14 4505).

37. AN Marine D3/34.

38. Ibid.

39. AN F14 4504.

40. AN Marine D3/31.

41. AN Marine D3/33. Letter of W. Wilkinson 3 July, 1781.

42. W. A. Chaloner, 'The Brothers John and William Wilkinson', pp. 24–5; AN Marine D3/34.

43. AN F12 4504.

44. Baron P. F. de Dietrich *Description des Gites de Minérai et des Bouches à Feu de la France, Tome Premier* (Strasbourg, 1786), reprinted Paris–Geneva, 1986, Avant-Propos, pp. XIII–XVI. I am most grateful to M. Edouard Schloesing and M. Gilbert de Dietrich for access to material on Baron P. F. de Dietrich and for making available this elegant reprint; see also AN F12 680.

45. For the extremely complex finances of Le Creusot, see D. Ozanam, 'La Naissance du Creusot', *Revue d'Histoire de la Sidérurgie*, 4, (1963) pp. 103–18.

46. B. Gille, *Origines*, p. 30. See also N. Rambourg's *De la surabondance et excellence des mines et usines de fer en France* (Paris, 1823), p. 10.

47. For the failures of Le Creusot see D. Woronoff, *L'industrie sidérurgique en France pendant la Révolution et l'Empire* (Paris, 1984) especially pp. 336–9. While a James Watson of Sergeant's Inn was offering what may have been some of Cort's new refining technology to the French in 1784, in practice no progress towards converting pig iron to wrought with coal was made before 1800 (AN F12 1300). For the short-lived attempt to develop Le Creusot by the English firm Manby and Wilson from 1826 to 1833 see W. O. Henderson, *Britain and Industrial Europe*, 2nd edn (1965), pp. 56–7. For the permanent revival of Le Creusot and its successful later history see J. B. Silly, 'La reprise du Creusot', *Revue d'Histoire des Mines et de la Métallurgie*, 1, (2), (1969). A detailed account of the works at Le Creusot just after they began operations is given by C.-B.-E. Guyton, *Mémoire concernant L'Etablissement de la Fonderie Royale du Creusot en 1786*, F. Courtois (ed.), (Le Creusot, 1876).

48. See below, pp. 504–5.

49. Chaloner, 'The Brothers John and William Wilkinson', pp. 28, 31.

Notes for Chapter 12

1. For the predating see A. H. John, 'War and the English economy, 1700–1763', *Economic History Review*, 2nd series, 7, (3), 1955, 331; for a general discussion of copper sheathing and its relation to the technology and markets of the copper industry, see J. R. Harris, 'Copper and shipping in the eighteenth century', *Economic History Review*, 2nd series, 19, 550–68 (1966) reprinted in *Essays in Industry and Technology in the Eighteenth Century* (Aldershot, 1992); and the subsequent papers of R. J. B. Knight, 'The introduction of copper sheathing into the Royal Navy 1779–1786', *The Mariner's Mirror*, August 1973, and G. Rees, 'Copper sheathing; an example of diffusion in the English merchant fleet', *Journal of Transport History* (1971).
2. J. R. Harris, *The Copper King* (Liverpool and Toronto, 1964). The discussion of the introduction of sheathing here, pp. 45–50, is partly superseded by the article of 1966, cited in note 1 above.
3. Harris, *Copper King*, p. 49; Birmingham City Library, Boulton and Watt Collection, Boulton to Watt 10 June 1785.
4. Affaires Etrangères, Correspondence Politique, Angleterre, p. 458.
5. Harris, *Copper King*, p. 554.
6. AN Marine D3 30.
7. In Britain William Collins, one of the two inventors of the cold rolling process, brought out and patented a sheathing metal in 1800, which may have been an anticipation of the later Muntz metal. In France a M. Beaubourg of Bordeaux brought out a new sheathing metal in 1785.
8. For this experimental period see AN Marine, D3 30.
9. AN Marine D1 8, Mémoires et Projets No. 45.
10. AN F12 1222, 29 Thermidor An 13.
11. Writing twenty-five years later, the proprietors did not separate the development of sheathing production from that of bolt production, though the latter was the object of later technical transfer, as the English bolt process was not fully established until 1784. I am most grateful to M. J. F. Belhoste of the Direction du Patrimoine in the French Ministry of Culture for most helpful correspondence and the provision of key transcripts from French archives.
12. Below, p. 308.
13. AN Marine B3 803.
14. He approached the Government in 1780. Guy Richard, 'Les fonderies de Romilly-sur-Andelle', *Actes de XVIIIè Congrès National Des Sociétés Savantes, 1963* (Paris, 1964), p. 452, suggests that Le Camus had certainly learned about the British rolling process by the end of that year, and may have gained the knowledge by the outbreak of the war. But J. F. Belhoste and P. Peyre in 'L'une des premières grandes usines hydrauliques: les fonderies de cuivre de Romilly-sur-Andelle', *Actes du IVè Colloque National sur le Patrimoine Industrielle* (Beauvais, 1982), pp. 15–16, are the first to reveal the wartime espionage. Le Camus obtained government authorization for his works by a decree of 23 April 1782; AN F14 4348.

15. Birmingham City Library, Boulton and Watt Collection, Boulton and Watt Letter Books, vol. 8, p. 418.
16. See below, p. 274.
17. Boulton and Watt Letter Books, vol. 8, p. 417, Watt to Reynolds 3 February 1784.
18. Ibid., p. 419.
19. See below, p. 344.
20. Harris, *Copper King*, pp. 60–84, 52, 141, 173–4, 178. Also information from the late Janet Butler whose study of John Wilkinson deals thoroughly with his copper interests. She shows that Wilkinson made important experiments with copper smelting, endeavouring to use a blast furnace. Though unsuccessful, they anticipated much later practice. Janet Butler's papers have recently been deposited at the Library of Ironbridge Gorge Museum.
21. From whom the writer is descended.
22. AN T591 4 and 5, De Givry papers for this and the following paragraphs. Harris, *Copper King*, pp. 168–9.
23. See M. H. Jackson and C. de Beer, *Eighteenth Century Gunfounding* (Newton Abbott, 1973) for the Verbruggens at Woolwich. The elder Verbruggen, Jan, had died in 1781.
24. AN T591 4 and 5, De Givry papers.
25. AN F12 1308.
26. Possibly for Indret?
27. National Maritime Museum, ADM BP5. For John Dawes, see Harris, *Copper King*, pp. 35, 68–9, 150–52.
28. Port de Lorient, Archives Maritimes, E4 108, 1785.
29. Mona Mine Mss. (University College of North Wales, hereafter UCNW, Bangor) 3544, section headed 'Rochefort'.
30. See below, for Vivian's views on the Tools Acts.
31. *Supplement Au Journal de Normandie*, No. 97 bis, 399.
32. AN F12 1365.
33. Belhoste and Peyre, 'L'une des premières grandes usines hydrauliques', p. 16.
34. AN F12 677C.
35. Arthur Young, *Travels in France*, M. Betham Edwards (ed.), (1889), pp. 126, 310.
36. AN F12 1313.
37. This information on the Harrises comes from SHAT archives at Vincennes, and was given me by the late Margaret Audin, who was kindly making enquiries on my behalf before her death. The John Victor Hariss and the Victor Harris, listed as 'serrurier' and 'tourneur en métaux' at different dates are probably the same person. For English workers in the Year 13 see also AN F12 1313. The man variously given as Grimpret and Grimperet in documents of 1817–18 was then said to be in charge of the whole works and to have been so since its foundation. Of what English name this is a corruption is not clear. AN F14 4348.
38. For his use of the industrial spy Le Turc in Britain, see below, Ch. 17.
39. Le Camus died in 1793; Richard, 'Les fonderies', p. 453.

40. Belhoste and Peyre, 'L'une des premières grandes usines hydrauliques', pp. 16–22.
41. Gilpin, Joshua, *Journal and Notebooks, 1790–1801*, Division of Public Records, Pennsylvania Historical and Museums Commission, notebook 44, (?) April 1798.
42. AD Seine Maritime C2111, Report of the sessions of the Provincial General Assembly of the generality of Rouen, Nov.–Dec. 1787. A plea that the Romilly venture 'should not be under the English yoke and at the mercy of their envious efforts' is in ibid., 8M3.
43. Mona Mine Mss. 3544, UCNW Bangor.
44. AN F12 1313.
45. For Dobson's earlier imprisonment and fine in England when returning to learn more about puddling, C. Ballot, *L'Introduction du Machinisme dans L'Industrie Française* (Lille-Paris, 1923), p. 507.
46. *Annales de l'Industrie, Description des Expositions des produits de l'Industrie Française* (Paris, 1824), vol. 2, pp. 209–10. This covers reports on national industrial exhibitions down to that of 1819.

Notes for Chapter 13

1. S. Chassagne, *Le Coton et Ses Patrons, France 1760–1840* (Paris, 1991), p. 410.
2. For general accounts of the revised views of the Newcomen engine, see L. T. C. Rolt and J. S. Allen, *The Steam Engine of Thomas Newcomen* (Hartington, 1977) *passim*. The revisions by Allen of Rolt's views in the earlier memorial volume version (*Thomas Newcomen, the Prehistory of the Steam Engine* [Hartington, 1963]) are most significant. See also A. E. Musson and E. H. Robinson, 'The early growth of steam power', *Economic History Review*, 2nd Series, 11 (1959); J. R. Harris, 'The employment of steam power in the eighteenth century', *History*, 52 (1967); J. S. Allen, 'The introduction of the Newcomen engine from 1710 to 1733', *Transactions of the Newcomen Society*, 42 (1969–70); and the important survey of J. Kanefsky and J. Robey, 'Steam engines in 18th century Britain, a quantitative assessment', *Technology and Culture*, 21, (2), April 1980. For a personal appraisal of the changes of view on the Newcomen engine, J. R. Harris, 'Recent research on the Newcomen engine and historical studies', *Transactions of the Newcomen Society*, 50 (1978–79) 175–80.
3. E. S. Ferguson, 'The steam engine before 1830', in M. Kranzberg and C. Pursell (eds), *Technology in Western Civilization*, 2 vols (Oxford, 1967), p. 248.
4. A. Smith, '"Engines moved by fire and water", the contribution of Fellows of the Royal Society to the development of steam power 1675–1733', *Transactions of the Newcomen Society*, 63 (1991–92), 229–30. This is a preliminary summary of a paper delivered to the society. The full version has just

appeared in ibid., 66 (1994–95), 1–26. See also Rolt and Allen, *The Steam Engine*, p. 55.

5. Rolt and Allen, *The Steam Engine*, p. 46.

6. J. R. Harris, 'The early steam engine on Merseyside', *Transactions of the Historic Society of Lancashire and Cheshire*, 106 (1954), 110.

7. Triewald may possibly have known Ridley before he came to England. For Triewald see S. Lindquist's brilliant study, *Technology on Trial, the Introduction of Steam Power Technology into Sweden, 1715–1736* (Uppsala, 1984) *passim*, and especially pp. 197 seq, 208–10.

8. G. J. Hollister-Short, 'A new technology and its diffusion: steam engine construction in Europe 1720–c.1780, Part 1', *Industrial Archaeology*, 13, (1) (1978), 9 seq.; and his 'The introduction of the Newcomen engine into Europe', *Transactions of the Newcomen Society*, 48 (1976–77), 11 seq.

9. G. J. Hollister-Short, 'A new technology, Part 1', 14.

10. Lindquist, *Technology on Trial*, p. 213, my italics.

11. Ibid., p. 13 seq.

12. Ibid., pp. 26–9.

13. Hollister-Short, 'A new technology, Part 2', *Industrial Archaeology*, 13, (2) (1978), 116.

14. Lindquist, *Technology on Trial*, pp. 118–21.

15. Probably the published prints of Beighton of 1717 and of Barney of 1719.

16. Lindquist, *Technology on Trial*, p. 124.

17. His italics, ibid., p. 137.

18. Alan Smith points out that the arrival of English workmen is probably marked by the Marquis's import of 300 bottles of English beer a few weeks later. 'The Newcomen engine at Passy, France, in 1725: a transfer of technology which did not take place', *Transactions of the Newcomen Society*, 50 (1978–79), 205. I am grateful to Mr Smith for voluminous information and helpful discussions over many years.

19. The above account of the engine is based on his study in *Transactions of the Newcomen Society*, 50 (1978–79), 205–17. For the Fresnes engine, C. Ballot, op. cit., 385.

20. The engine as first built was based upon an engine at Liège of which the Fresnes mineowners had obtained plans by espionage. However it did not work well, and the English engineer Saunders, who had already built engines in Belgium, had to be called in to alter it. It had an English cylinder (Hollister-Short, 'The introduction of the Newcomen engine', 12–14).

21. Hollister-Short, 'A new technology', *Industrial Archaeology*, Part 1, 19–20; Part 2, 122.

22. B. Gille et al., 'La Machine à Vapeur en France au XVIIIe Siècle', *Techniques et Civilisation*, 2 (1951), 154.

23. AN Marine, G 110. Mémoires et Projets; Machines, Vol. 6, 104 seq.

24. Ibid., Letters of Stephen Glover, Le Roy fils, D'Hérouville, Thomas Stephens (11 April, 28 July, 4 August, 11 August, 21 August 1758).

25. Gille et al., 'La Machine', 156–7.

26. For Périer, the great authority is Jacques Payen, whose masterly *Capital et machine à vapeur au XVIIIe siècle* (Paris, 1969) covers the introduction of

the Boulton and Watt engine in detail. See ch. 3, *passim*, especially p. 100 seq.

27. W. H. Chaloner, *Industry and Innovation: Selected Essays*, D. A. Farnie and W. O. Henderson (eds) (1990), p. 60. He shows that William Wilkinson had made the first connection with the Paris Water Company by soliciting orders for cast iron pipes for the Wilkinsons works before May 1777.
28. AN F12 2205.
29. AN F12 2205, Mémoire sur une nouvelle machine à feu, Paris 15 January 1778. Boulton is described as operating by steam 'un tel nombre de fabriques de quincaillerie Angloises, qu'elles forment presque une petite ville'.
30. H. W. Dickinson and R. Jenkins, *James Watt and the Steam Engine* (Ashbourne, 1927), pp. 146–8. It is made clear that he hoped to make this project the basis of achieving rotative motion.
31. AN F12 2205.
32. He is credited with the first use of the term 'specific heat'. A. E. Musson and E. Robinson, *Science and Technology in the Industrial Revolution* (Manchester, 1969), p. 126. Of him Watt wrote to Black (J.W.P., W/5, Birmingham City Libraries, n.d. *c.*1780) 'Magellan at London ... was our agent in the French business, is I believe a Carthusian or Benedictine monk, by profession a dealer in and retailer of philosophy, and perhaps a spy, however thus far he has acted honestly and honourably by us'. I owe this reference to Margaret Jacob.
33. One wonders what the reaction of Boulton's fellow manufacturers in Birmingham would have been had they known of these proposals!
34. AN Marine G110, Magellan, London, to D'Hérouville, 17 April; same to same, London 24 April; Boulton and Watt to Magellan, 2 May 1778.
35. AN Marine G110, D'Hérouville's observations on the proposals of Boulton and Watt, n.d.
36. AN Marine G110, Boulton to D'Hérouville, 2 June 1778.
37. Ibid., D'Hérouville to D'Angivilliers, 14 June 1778.
38. Ibid., letter of Magellan, London, 17 July 1778.
39. Ibid.
40. Ibid., 'List of Steam Engines of which part has been seen by Mr. Jary'.
41. Ibid., Boulton (Soho), to Magellan, 22 August 1778.
42. Ibid., 16 October 1778.
43. Ibid., Jary to D'Hérouville, n.d.
44. Ibid., Tolozan to Magellan 13 December 1778; Boulton, Redruth, to D'Hérouville, 16 October 1778.
45. A contemporary writing about Périer described his character as 'à la fois insinuant et entreprenant', see J. Payen, *Capital et machine*, p. 105.
46. Boulton and Watt Collection, Birmingham City Library, Box 3, Périer and Motteux bundle 1777–1786. Périer to Boulton 29 October 1778; two documents of January 1779; draught letter B. & W. to D'Hérouville 9 January 1779; MBP 248/204, Watt to Périer 25 January 1779.
47. AN Marine G110, Magellan (London), to D'Hérouville 13 January 1779.
48. AN F12 2205, letter of D'Hérouville 12 February 1778, when unable to walk for gout.

49. He is no longer heard of when Watt revived his bid for another *arrêt* in a letter to Genet, probably of 1783 or 1784. Henry Francis Du Pont Colln. of Winterthur Mss. Group 2, Series E. Eleutherian Mills Library, Wilmington, Delaware. 'Exposé de l'affaire de Mrs. Boulton and Watt rélativement aux Pompes à feu'. Though undated this is written after peace returned between England and France, and at an early stage of the Albion Mills steam corn-mill project.

50. He had himself plans to install a Watt engine at a coal-mine he ran in Burgundy, and he believed the coal there would coke well and so could be used, as Wilkinson and the Carron Company did, to smelt iron. He would employ his engine to work a cylindrical bellows for a blast furnace as well as pump the shallow mine.

51. Boulton and Watt Collection, B & W, Box 2/15/11, Le Camus to Boulton, 28 December 1778.

52. See J.-C. Périer, *Sur les machines à vapeur* (Paris, 1810), pp. 10–12.

53. For the sending of engines to France see the late W. H. Chaloner's 'Hazards of Trade with France in Time of War, 1776–1783', a highly entertaining essay reprinted in his *Selected Essays; Industry and Innovation*, D. A. Farnie and W. O. Henderson (eds) (1990), ch. 4, p. 59 seq.; for the elder Périer and Jary in England, pp. 60–62. Payen (*Capital et machine*, p. 212) records the elder Périer's statement that he visited England five times; visits in 1777 and 1784 were, however, certainly in peacetime. A letter of introduction for the younger Périer says he was coming over with a Mr Wilkinson, presumably William Wilkinson, engaged as we have seen in developing French naval armaments. He would be pleased to see 'ce que Birmingham contient de curieux en manufactures'. B & W, Box 3/9/266, letter from Paris 5 February 1782.

54. See above.

55. MBP, 248/203–7; Chaloner, op. cit., 63.

56. The American passports came from Benjamin Franklin's 'Court at Passy'.

57. Chaloner, *Industry and Innovation*, pp. 62–70; see above.

58. J. R. Harris, *The Copper King* (Liverpool, Toronto, 1964), p. 46.

59. B & W, Box 3/9/14, French Business 1777 to 1786, Périer to Boulton, Paris 3 May 1779.

60. Chaloner, *Industry and Innovation*, pp. 69, 74 n. 71, for Watt's statement that the 'scruples' of the Chepstow officer had seemed likely to prevent the voyage. 'However ... by a proper dose of the golden powder his eyesight has been cleared, and they have seen matters in a very different light.' A memorial to the French government, when they were seeking confirmation of their exclusive privilege for their engine in France, shows that Boulton and Watt knew perfectly well that some of the materials exported with engine orders were for the great munitions works at Le Creusot, and this when the two countries were at war. This attempt to curry favour with the French government amounted to a gross lack of patriotism, even treachery. BCA Matthew Boulton Papers, 234, Letter Book G1, 159a.

61. Payen, *Capital et machine*, pp. 124–5.

62. Ibid., pp. 125–7.

63. Ibid., p. 151.
64. See below.
65. J. P. Muirhead, *Life of James Watt* (1859), p. 267; J.-C. Périer, *Sur les machine à vapeur.*
66. Henry Francis Dupont Collection, Eleutherian Mills Library, Group 2, Series E, n.d. This presumably derives from the papers of Pierre Samuel Dupont de Nemours, which may suggest a date after the beginning of Calonne's administration in 1783 in which he was very influential; it certainly is after the return of peace in that year, but before the first large payment towards Boulton and Watt's bill in February 1784. A 'Memorial on the Part of Boulton and Watt of Birmingham' written during their French visit of 1786–87, and handed in to Genet for the controller-general petitioning that the exclusive privilege granted by their earlier *arrêt* should be made effective by letters patent from the king, shows that they were persuaded by John Wilkinson that if they furnished drawings and directions for an engine for 'Blowing the Great Iron Furnace at Mont Cenis' (Le Creusot) and permitted him to provide other engines for France, it would be regarded favourably by the French government in relation to their privilege (BCA Matthew Boulton Papers, 234, Letter Book G1, 159a).
67. B & W, Box 20/13/14, Watt to Wilkinson, 6 February 1784.
68. The last hope of an engine privilege was raised as a result of Boulton and Watt's industrial consultancy journey to France in 1786–87, 'we have ... good reason to expect that our privilege will be confirmed, notwithstanding the efforts of our old friends' [Périers?]. B & W, M II 4/2/1. Watt to Annie Watt, 7 January 1787. The fall of Calonne probably extinguished these hopes.
69. In the same letter Boulton calls them 'two French Hospital Academicians'. For the background of hospital reform, and Coulomb's mission in Britain, C. C. Gillispie, *Science and Polity in France at the End of the Old Regime* (Princeton, 1980), p. 244 seq., esp. 255.
70. B & W, Box 20/13/14, Boulton to Watt, London, 25 June 1787; Payen, *Capital et machine*, pp. 127–31; for the Coulomb report in full see Payen's *Documents IV*, p. 267 seq. This is a very detailed and sophisticated report, and as Payen says, the first description available in France of the new system of steam engine with separate condenser. Coulomb was thus very well placed to assess the Albion Mills engine.
71. Payen, *Capital et machine*, pp. 157–64. Périer actually took out a 'brevet d'importation et de perfectionnements' in 1792 to protect his monopoly. Betancourt made early attempts to establish the relationship between steam pressure and steam temperature (ibid., p. 157).
72. Ibid., p. 105.
73. 'Watt pense alors (1777) que même si les Français retrouvent par eux-memes le secret des nouvelles machines, ils seront de tout façon incapables d'executer des cylindres sans l'aide de Wilkinson' (ibid., p. 104).
74. Périer had been a most active member, and involved in many commissions of enquiry into new industries, inventions etc. (ibid., pp. 163, 35–9).
75. Ibid., p. 176.

76. Dr Reed Geiger (University of Delaware) is completing research on this question.
77. J. Tann and M. J. Breckin, 'The international diffusion of the Watt engine, 1775–1825', *Economic History Review*, 2nd Series, 31, (4), November 1978, 543, 561–4.

Notes for Chapter 14

1. For those inflows see Eleanor S. Godfrey, *The Development of English Glassmaking 1560–1640* (Oxford, 1975), especially ch. 2, 'The revival of glassmaking in England 1569–1590', p. 16 seq.
2. Godfrey, *English Glassmaking*, ch. 3, 'The transition to coal', p. 38 seq.; J. R. Harris, 'The origins of the St. Helens glass industry' in *Essays in Industry and Technology in the Eighteenth Century* (Aldershot, 1992), p. 195 seq.
3. Godfrey, *English Glassmaking*, pp. 119, 126–8, 133.
4. Ibid., pp. 150, 228–32.
5. See her careful review of the evidence in C. McCleod, 'Accident or design, George Ravenscroft's patent and the invention of lead crystal glass', *Technology and Culture*, 28, (4), October 1987. For the use of louvred roofs instead of cones in the late seventeenth-century glasshouses I am indebted to Wendy Evans of the Museum of London.
6. Warren C. Scoville, *Capitalism and French Glassmaking* (University of California Press, Berkeley, CA, 1950), p. 11 seq. Scoville's is still the best general account of the eighteenth-century French glass industry.
7. J. R. Harris, 'Saint Gobain and Ravenhead', in *Essays in Industry*, pp. 55–8.
8. Scoville, *Capitalism*, pp. 12–13.
9. Ibid., p. 13.
10. AD Hérault C2761; AN F12 1486.
11. AN F12 25/26.
12. AN F12 680.
13. AN F12 20.
14. Scoville, *Capitalism*, p. 14.
15. *Encyclopédie ou dictionnaire raisonné des sciences des arts et des métiers*, vol. 17 (Neufchatel, 1765), p. 102 seq.
16. There had been a quite abortive scheme to make flint glass as early as 1725 connected with an immigrant called Dromgold, but he misled his partners and when they eventually set up the Sèvres glassworks no flint glass was made there. James Barrelet, *La Verrerie en France* (Paris, 1950), p. 107.
17. AN F12 1300.
18. His own spelling. The name gets mangled by French contemporaries.
19. AN F12 1486. A well-composed letter, perfect in grammar and spelling, suggests a man of good background and education.
20. Ibid. There was also a quarrel between Koenig and his banker in 1777.
21. For a general view on the superiority of English optical glass, AN F12 721.
22. AN F12 2276: Ecomusée du Creusot, photostats of Archives Nationales

documents. Macquer mentioned the examination of St Louis white crystal by the Académie des Sciences, only described as 'nearly approaching' the best English pieces.

23. AN F12 1486. This source is used for the subsequent account of the financial, technical and managerial problems of the Saint Cloud glassworks.
24. The visitor was Adam Walker, writer, lecturer and inventor, quoted in J. Lough, *France on the Eve of the Revolution, British Travellers' Observations 1763–1788* (1988), p. 81. Parker was an eminent London glass manufacturer. See below, p. 485.
25. AN F12 1486.
26. AN F12 1489B. Quoted in Collection Mercier, Ecomusée du Creusot.
27. AN O¹ 3795, letter of Le Breton 25 February 1785.
28. Article in the *Journal de Paris*, 13 March 1808, quoted by Marie-Anne Demonfaucon, 'Récherches sur la ville du Creusot et sa population de 1787 à 1836', typescript at Ecomusée, Le Creusot.
29. Dietrich, *Description des gites de minérai et des bouches à feu de la France*, T.1, Avant-Propos, XIII–XVI; AN F14 4505.
30. AN F14 4504.
31. AN O¹ 3795 and F14 4505.
32. Quoted in J. Lough, *France* (1988), pp. 106–7.
33. E. R. Prosser, *Birmingham Inventors and Inventions* (Birmingham, 1881, reprinted Wakefield, 1970). Meyer claimed that the second patent was a renewal of the first, AD Seine Maritime, C2120 139).
34. For problems at the glassworks at Petit Querilly near Rouen, AD Seine Maritime C2120; there is a rather vague letter of support for Oppenheim from Berthollet in 1785, he seems to refer to more than one member of the family (AN F12 2425). The Birmingham firm of Boulton and Fothergill were creditors of Oppenheim, but were oddly reluctant to join other creditors in forcing him into bankruptcy at the end of his operations in England.
35. The Director of the crystal works at Gros Caillou in Paris was appealing to government because of inability to produce at economic prices in the Year XII (AN F12 2425).
36. Barrelet, *La Verrerie*, p. 110. For Belesaigne, AN F12 1489A. Why he should have been recruited by the minister responsible for royal buildings after the foundation of the Verrerie de la Reine, is curious. Perhaps it indicates dissatisfaction with the product of the Le Creusot glassworks.
37. For a fuller comparative study of the plate glass industries of France and England see J. R. Harris, *Essays in Industry and Technology in the Eighteenth Century: England and France* (Aldershot, 1992), ch. 2, pp. 34–77, 'Saint-Gobain and Ravenhead'. Where not otherwise referenced the sources for material in the present section may be found there.
38. There is an outstanding work of scholarship on the Saint Gobain company by the late Claude Pris, to whom the writer is deeply indebted for valuable discussions and help, cut short by his early death. The thesis of 1973 at the University of Paris IV was made available by the Service De Reproduction Des Thèses, University of Lille III, in three volumes in 1975. For access to

the rich archives of the Saint-Gobain Company I am greatly indebted to the kindness of M. Dominique Perrin.

39. T. C. Barker, *Pilkington Brothers and the Glass Industry* (1960), pp. 44–5.
40. Below, pp. 355–6.
41. For the early British attempts to obtain the technology of casting plate glass, Harris, *Essays in Industry*, pp. 41–2.
42. Ibid., p. 42 seq.
43. Ibid., pp. 48–54. The complexities of excise difficulties have been omitted in the present account.
44. Ibid., p. 66.
45. Ibid., pp. 55–8.
46. Ibid., pp. 58–64; for the importance of the 'Historique', J. R. Harris and C. Pris, 'The memoirs of Delaunay Deslandes', *Technology and Culture*, 17, (2), 1976.
47. The same term was used in England as in France, because of the French origin of the English glass industry.
48. Archives, Saint Gobain, C2.
49. *Gore's Liverpool Advertiser*, 29 April 1790.
50. Archives, Saint Gobain, marked 'notes of my nephew Henry Saladin on the manufacture of plate glass in Lancashire'.
51. Pilkington Archives, Minutes of British Plate Glass Co., 11 November 1818.

Notes for Chapter 15

1. MacLeod has established that during 1660–1800 English 'patentees showed a consistently greater interest in improving the quality of products and in saving capital'. C. MacLeod, *Inventing the Industrial Revolution: The English Patent System, 1660–1800* (Cambridge, 1988), ch. 9, p. 158 seq.
2. For this legislation see below, p. 460.
3. S. Chassagne, *Le Coton et Ses Patrons, France 1760–1840* (Paris, 1991).
4. I am most grateful to Phyllis Giles for checking my findings and providing me with important additional data from her extensive knowledge of the Stockport district in the industrial revolution.
5. R. Glen, 'The Milnes of Stockport and the export of English technology during the early Industrial Revolution', *Cheshire History*, 3, (1979), 15–21.
6. There is no discrepancy here if the 'friend' who directed James Milne to Holker was one of his English correspondents and agents in the Manchester district; the price promised by Holker for the machine confirms this.
7. An English print of this patented device is attached to the file 'As sold by Milne, Robinson and Place of Manchester'.
8. AN F12 1340.
9. Ibid., letter dealt with by Blondel, n.d.; C. Ballot, *L'Introduction du Machinisme dans L'Industrie Française* (Lille-Paris, 1923), pp. 64–5, who cites a retrospective document by John Milne II, but written in the 1830s, long after the events; Chassagne, *Le Coton*, pp. 191–2.

10. AN F12 1340, James Milne to Necker 2 February 1780.
11. We ignore here the question of whether, or how far, Arkwright's inventions were his own – his patents were of course overturned in the English courts. R. S. Fitton, *The Arkwrights, Spinners of Fortune* (Manchester, 1989), ch. 5, p. 117 seq. There may be more originality to the Milnes than they have been credited with. Some drawings of their machines show important modifications of the original Arkwright machinery, particularly at the roving and final spinning stages. These drawings made at the Conservatoire Nationale des Arts et Métiers at the beginning of the nineteenth century are in the Portfeuille Vaucanson there, Dossier 13571.172, 172.1 to 172.16. See Figure 15.1, pp. 378–9
12. Chassagne, *Le Coton*, p. 199 seq.
13. Ibid., pp. 206–10; Ballot, *L'Introduction*, pp. 66–8. Apparently the roving machine was operated by four-year-old children, the fine-spinning machine by children of six to eight years old.
14. For Hall see below, p. 384.
15. 'Auberkamp'.
16. AN F12, 2195 and 1338. While the letter written by Holker on 27 May 1783 was being sent on to Tolozan on the 29th, it is addressed to 'Monseigneur' which would not be the usual style for Tolozan, so Parker must be right in giving the original recipient as D'Ormesson, the controller-general: H. T. Parker, *An Administrative Bureau during the Old Régime: the Bureau of Commerce and its Relations to French Industry from May 1781 to November 1783* (University of Delaware Press, Newark, 1993), p. 80.
17. Men who later used the aliases of Wood and Hill.
18. AN F12 2195.
19. Chassagne, *Le Coton*, pp. 192, 216; A. Rémond, *John Holker, Manufacturier et Grand Fonctionnaire en France au XVIIIᵉ siècle 1719–1786* (Paris, 1946), pp. 156–9. X. Linant de Bellefonds, 'Les Techniciens Anglais dans L'Industrie Française au XVIIIᵉ Siècle', doctoral thesis, University of Paris, 1971, p. 212 suggests that the visitors were Wood and Hill and that they came from Ulverston, but that cannot be right because Ulverston is far more than 6 miles from Holker's native Stretford (just possibly from Urmston?). AN F12 1338.
20. While his carding engine had not fulfilled all expectations in 1781, some of his other machines were said to have been useful at Sens, and he was allowed to keep some in order to work on their improvement. The inspector Roland de la Platière had examined the carding engine. AN F12 1340.
21. AN F12 1340. Ballot, *L'Introduction*, pp. 49–50, 54; Chassagne, *Le Coton*, p. 71.
22. AN F12 1338.
23. Archives, Conservatoire des Arts et Métiers (subsequently CNAM) U697.
24. It could not have been anticipated that he would within a few years be the Revolutionary Minister of the Interior, responsible for French industry, and the boss of his former tormentor Tolozan until the closing of the Bureau of Commerce.
25. AN F12 1328.

26. AN F12 1342.
27. This in itself seems to make it very unlikely that they were Holker's visitors of that year.
28. R. S. Fitton, *The Arkwrights*, pp. 141–3; A. E. Musson, *The Growth of British Industry* (New York, 1978), pp. 88–9; J. de L. Mann, *The Cloth Industry in the West of England* (Oxford, 1971), pp. 134–5.
29. Ballot, *L'Introduction*, pp. 82–5; AN F12 2195. Professor Chassagne, however, tells me that he doubts the evidence about Hill's age. Hill's age, if correct, reduces the value of his management experience.
30. Chassagne, *Le Coton*, pp. 216–18.
31. Ballot, *L'Introduction*, p. 84. For his relationship with the industrial spy Le Turc, below, pp. 434–5.
32. Chassagne, *Le Coton*, p. 216.
33. AN F12 2195, Wood to Minister of the Interior, Year X.
34. Chassagne, *Le Coton*, p. 218.
35. Ibid.; Ballot, *L'Introduction*, p. 85; CNAM U1580.
36. AN F12 1338, letter of Vandermonde 1 July 1784.
37. Ibid., report of 14 June 1785. In calling the Arkwright system a 'filature perpetuelle', Brown was close to the future French name of 'continu'.
38. French commentators nearly always regarded English patents as being similar to their own system of state monopolies.
39. A point later made by Dupont de Nemours (see below, p. 547). In fact Arkwright's patents were being overthrown in the British courts (R. S. Fitton, *The Arkwrights*, ch. 5).
40. AN F12 2195, report made at the Louvre 4 May 1785.
41. Ballot, *L'Introduction*, pp. 69–71.
42. Ibid., pp. 71–3.
43. AN F12 1339.
44. For the number of 'assortiments' built by Milnes at La Muette see Chassagne, *Le Coton*, p. 194; for works using new English machines founded in the early revolutionary period, Ballot, *L'Introduction*, pp. 91–2.
45. F. Bacquié, *Les inspecteurs des manufactures sous L'Ancien Régime* (1927), p. 57; AN F12 2384.
46. Above, pp. 183–4.
47. These were always called 'mul(e)-jennies' in France, though this name was only occasionally used in England.
48. Ballot, *L'Introduction*, p. 87, has Lecler as first involved in bringing Pickford over after the original contact by Brown; Bellefonds, 'Les Techniciens', p. 223, says the recruitment was by Charles Clark, son of Lecler, on a trip to England in 1787–88. Chassagne thinks that the Abbé Calonne instigated his move to France, *Le Coton*, p. 185. Pickford certainly seems to have made some machines at Melun for the Abbé, CNAM U343.
49. Lecler was given a grant of 6,000 *livres* in September 1788 for the costs of a journey he had just made to England to get machines to card, prepare and spin cotton, and 6,000 *livres* more if the machines lived up to his claims for them. AN F12 107.
50. Ibid.

51. AN F12 1341; Ballot, *L'Introduction*, pp. 87–8.
52. AN F12 1341, document approved 29 April 1791 and signed by Pickford. This may have removed Pickford's anxieties, for in the previous month he had been concerned because the funds of the old commerce administration on which he had been able to draw had been annulled by the National Assembly. Ibid., letter of 26 March 1791.
53. The inspectorate having been abolished by October 1791; Bacquié, *Les inspecteurs*, p. 352 seq.
54. AN F12 2384.
55. Below. As early as May 1791 the Paris mob was enraged at the spinning-machines in the Quinze-Vingts because of their threat to employment, and threatened to burn them, Ballot, *L'Introduction*, p. 21.
56. AN F12 2384, 4783.
57. AN F12 2218; Harris, *Essays in Industry and Technology in the Eighteenth Century* (Aldershot, 1992), p. 105; CNAM D423.
58. Chassagne, *Le Coton*, pp. 70, 243, 257; Ballot, *L'Introduction*, pp. 86–7.
59. Desmarets and Molard in 1791; AN F12 1339.
60. AN F12 1342, 1411A.
61. A handwritten brochure on a new spinning-machine, said to be the work of 'Spens' at the works of Morgan and Massey at Amiens, is in the CNAM archives (U533). The letter quoted above is U655 in the same series. Massey seems to have been fully integrated into French revolutionary politics. In June 1792 he wrote to the President of the Bureau of Consultation at Paris in his capacity as Deputy of the Departement of the Somme in the National Assembly. He was paying testimony to the work of McCloude (CNAM U543).
62. This may be specious; the Arkwright patents were overthrown in November 1785, so if Garnett had not left England he could have made and sold machines with impunity.
63. AN F12 1340, esp. Hall to Tolozan 13 August 1787 and Garnett to Tolozan 24 October 1787.
64. This agreement as far as the wool-spinning machine was concerned is said to have been backed by the controller-general in October 1787, but this seems to conflict with the evidence of the commission of enquiry as set out here and a letter of Garnett's of 24 October. The agreement is referred to in a later enquiry about Garnett's machines in 1792, also in AN F12 1340.
65. AN F12 1340, esp. letters of Garnett 24 October and Hall 11 November 1787.
66. Ballot, *L'Introduction*, pp. 55–6; W. Reddy, *The Rise of Market Culture. The Textile Trade and French Society, 1750–1900* (Cambridge, 1984), pp. 58–60; Chassagne, *Le Coton*, pp. 188–9, who gives some additional detail; AN F12 1340, esp. undated memoir by Garnett; CNAM U535; U644.
67. AD Seine Maritime, L438.
68. AN F12 1007; CNAM U162.

Notes for Chapter 16

1. Rémond, *John Holker, Manufacturier et Grand Fonctionnaire en France au XVIIIᵉ siècle 1719–1786* (Paris, 1946), p. 99, says that he was sent by Holker, who was of course involved with this firm, to other centres, but I have not seen any archive reference which would connect them. C. Ballot notes McCloude's presence in France in 1788 (*L'Introduction du Machinisme dans L'Industrie Française* (Lille-Paris, 1923), p. 249) but Chassagne has him in France from 1783, three years before Holker's death, so one cannot rule out the possibility of Holker giving directions to him.

2. AN F12 1411A, F12 107/8. He had continued to get his 30 *livres* a week at Sens, but the authorities had failed to pay his rent. In March 1789 he had demanded a gratuity he claimed was due to him for introducing the fly-shuttle into France. The Malloy ('Mallois') brothers similarly claimed to have initiated the use of the fly-shuttle in France at Louviers in 1787, but Kay's introduction of his own invention twenty-five years before was of course on record. Ballot, *L'Introduction*, p. 249.

3. AN F12 107/8.

4. CNAM U1 and 543; S. Chassagne, *Le Coton et Ses Patrons, France 1760–1840* (Paris, 1991), pp. 254, 256–7. The Mello factory was set up about 1795, originally employed several hundreds, but in 1797–98 was still not at full output. It was not very successful, and only employed 20 workers, and those unmechanized, in 1811. It had closed by 1828. See N. Scarfe, *Innocent Espionage, the La Rochefoucauld Brothers' Tour of England in 1785* (Woodbridge, 1995), pp. 255–6.

5. CNAM U213.

6. CNAM U213; Chassagne, *Le Coton*, esp. pp. 244–5, 309, 355.

7. W. O. Henderson, *Britain and Industrial Europe*, 2nd edn (Leicester, 1965), p. 25.

8. For Albert see *Précis Historique pour Charles Albert, Intimé, contre Bernard Boyer-Fonfrède, Appelant* from which the quotations have been taken. Probably first published in 1797, this was reprinted in 1834. Gillian G. Gregg has provided an account of the background of this document and of its contents: *The Précis Historique of Charles Albert (a Story of Industrial Espionage in the Eighteenth Century)*, Lancaster Museum, Monograph, n.d. See also Chassagne, *Le Coton*, esp. pp. 220–21, 265–70, and CNAM U113, U120.

9. Chassagne, *Le Coton*, pp. 220–29. For Gouldbroof, p. 223.

10. See below, pp. 459–60.

11. Ballot, *L'Introduction*, pp. 99–103; Henderson, *Britain and Industrial Europe*, pp. 25–6.

12. Ballot, *L'Introduction*, pp. 118–19; CNAM U95.

13. AN F12 2195, correspondence of Molard and Hulse, An IX.

14. Ballot, *L'Introduction*, pp. 102–3.

15. Ballot, *L'Introduction*, pp. 103–12; Chassagne, *Le Coton*, pp. 230, 233, 265, 271, 326, 361–2.

16. Note the title of J. Aikin's famous contemporary work, *A Description of the Country from Thirty to Forty Miles round Manchester* (1795).

17. AN F12 2195.
18. A curious parallel between the large cylinders of carding engines and the very small ones of the Arkwright water frame.
19. AN F12 2195 and AN F12 2204; below, p. 445.
20. In the Year XII he had been granted French citizenship.
21. William Cockerill was delivering machines at Verviers in 1800 (Henderson, *Britain and Industrial Europe*, pp. 107–8; CNAM U182, U140).
22. Though one always hesitates to question the authority of Ballot, the Douglas of 1788 was not the same man who entered France in the Year X. See also CNAM U158.
23. Ballot, *L'Introduction*, pp. 182 seq., 199–200; Henderson, *Britain and Industrial Europe*, p. 63; R. S. Fitton and A. P. Wadsworth, *The Strutts and the Arkwrights, 1750–1830, a Study of the Early Factory System* (Manchester, 1958), p. 194. I have had very helpful advice from Douglas Farnie on this problem.
24. This seems to be a different survey from that carried out in the same year, when Tolozan got Lazowski, Buol and Brown to produce an account of the cotton-spinning machines then extant in France; Chassagne, *Le Coton*, p. 185.
25. They recommended Lhomond, the French inventor of an improved jenny, but the great interest shown in his machine seems to have come to nothing.
26. AN F12 1342; see below, p. 445.
27. AN F12 107/8.
28. See reports on the state of wool and cotton spinning in France in AN F12 1338 and the memoir on the present state of cotton spinning in F12 1341, which indicate that the matter was discussed at the highest level in the Bureau of Commerce, and that the findings were approved by the controller-general. These include papers preserved showing the latest unofficial estimates of the progress of machinery in Britain, mainly based on No. 72 of the *Annals of Agriculture*.
29. AN F12 1341. 'Mémoire sur l'état actuel de la filature des Cotons' presented to Bureau of Commerce in 1790.
30. Ibid.
31. AN F12 1342.
32. When Dupont submitted 284-page reports there was clearly the possibility of confusion among officials.
33. E. Boyetet, *Second partie du recueil de divers mémoires relatifs au traité de commerce* (Paris, 1789), p. 84 seq.
34. Internal evidence shows that this was in fact his second letter.
35. Boyetet said in a footnote that this would not have really helped Rayneval, who was clueless in such matters.
36. He cited Prussia, Spain, Portugal and Holland as interested in getting British cotton workers.
37. A paper of 'remarks on the observations made to the Committee of 9 Aug. 1786' puts Dupont's case. 'The letter of M. Holker which has been read to the Committee, establishes in the clearest fashion that it is possible for us to maintain a competition with England, as long as we spread through every

cotton manufacture the ingenious machines which the English use', and avoid exclusive privileges. It ends, 'doubtless it is more comfortable to inhabit an old house, whatever it is like, than to make repairs to it; but when circumstances have forced you to take the hammer to it, with a little expense and work everything will sort itself out, and one will find oneself better lodged'. Affaires Etrangères, Com. Politique. Angleterre, 337 and Mémoires et Documents, Angleterre, 65. The Calonne Papers have a memorandum on the contemplated treaty of commerce with England, annotated by Calonne. On cotton the writer says 'it would be ... interesting to check on the advantage which the English manufactures have over the French ones; one knows that the late M. Holker had collected details on this issue, no one knew better than he the state of this industry in England, and in France; his advice should be of the greatest weight'. PRO, Calonne Papers PC 1/123 no. 15. For the negotiations of this period, the best source is the articles of M. Donaghay, particularly: 'Calonne and the Anglo-French Commercial Treaty of 1786', *Journal of Modern History*, 50, (3), September 1978, supplement, D1157–84 esp. D1171–2; *idem*, 'Textiles and the Anglo-French Commercial Treaty 1786', *Textile History*, 13, (2), (1982), 205–2.

38. AN F12 658A.
39. AN F12 1411A, May 1790.
40. AD Seine Maritime C1092, C2120.
41. As well as textile processes some space was used for a brief but unsuccessful diamond-cutting enterprise based on Amsterdam methods, and other space was given to Dauffe, who attempted to rival British products in polished steel, and installed some machine tools. Le Turc, as we will see, also set up workshops to produce and operate English stocking frames (below, pp. 446–7). The much encouraged but unsuccessful spinning-machinery of the Frenchman Barneville, later operated by his son, was also housed there.
42. AN F12 1340; 1342.
43. There were some final items left with the Bureau at its demise; a leather-piercing machine for use in the manufacture of hand cards, which the Milnes claimed to have invented, was transferred to the Hôtel de Mortagne and the care of Vandermonde. Some cards to be mounted on carding machines which had been made by Pickford had been specially ordered from England by Leclerc (Clark) of Brive. These carding machines were supposed to be designed for the needs of jenny spinners. The carding equipment, left to rust and woodworm in the old offices of the Bureau, was sold off. AN F12 1340.
44. S. Chassagne, 'L'innovation technique dans l'industrie textile pendant la Révolution'. *Histoire, Economie et Société* 1ᵉ trimestre 1993, issue devoted to 'Entreprises et Révolutions', directed by François Caron, 51–61.
45. Ibid., 59–60.
46. Below, p. 558.
47. For French acknowledgement of the superiority of English spinning around the turn of the century based on the superiority of their machines, see Chassagne, *Le Coton*, p. 263.
48. AN F12 1295, letters of Wood and of Defontenay and Decretot to Minister, Ventose, Year X.

49. AN F12 2196. This may be the proposed venture into powered cotton manufacture which Holker referred to in his letter to Rayneval about the Eden treaty negotiations, above, pp. 410–11.
50. Ballot, *L'Introduction*, pp. 74–7.
51. Ibid., pp. 72–3.
52. Chassagne, *Le Coton*, p. 334.
53. Chassagne, *Le Coton*, pp. 307–10; idem, 'L'innovation technique', p. 54.
54. Chassagne, *Le Coton*, pp. 294, 237–8; Ballot, *L'Introduction*, p. 95.
55. Chassagne, *Le Coton*, pp. 294, 546–7.
56. S. D. Chapman and S. Chassagne, *European Textile Printers of the Eighteenth Century* (1981), pp. 12–13.
57. S. Chassagne, *Oberkampf, un entrepreneur capitaliste au siècle des lumières* (Paris, 1980), pp. 67–8.
58. Chapman and Chassagne, *European Textile Printers*, pp. 13, 18, 131–3.
59. Ibid., p. 131; Chassagne, *Oberkampf*, pp. 69–70.
60. 'Cet homme à la grande main ici comme chez lui'. Chassagne, *Oberkampf*, p. 118.
61. Whether the enticement of a Swiss national would have contravened British law is doubtful.
62. Chassagne, *Oberkampf*, pp. 159–60; Chapman and Chassagne, *European Textile Printers*, p. 140.
63. Chassagne, *Oberkampf*, pp. 71, 73, 141; Ballot, *L'Introduction*, pp. 290–91.

Notes for Chapter 17

1. AN F12 677C, Le Turc to Tolozan 20 July 1785.
2. *Description des fermes sur lequelles on ceintre actuellement en France les grand arches des ponts*, par Mr Le Turc (London, 1781): *Description du camion prysmatique de Mr. de Perronet*, par Mr Le Turc (London, 1781).
3. See P. Grosclaude, *Malherbes, témoin et interprète de son temps* (Paris, 1961), pp. 520–21; see also pp. 519, 522–4, 526–7.
4. CNAM U216, Le Turc to Citoyen, 14 Nivose An 3.
5. AN F12 677C, Le Turc to Tolozan 20 July 1785. Bidot is recorded as 'mechanicien' to Alexander I of Russia in An 10 (CNAM U216).
6. There is information on this period of Le Turc's life in his printed memoir *Au Directoire Executif*, Paris, 30 June 1797. See p. xxii for the quotation at the beginning of the paragraph.
7. *Instructions Patriotiques et Militaires Adressés aux Anglois*, Par un Citoyen du Monde (London, 1780). The motto 'Ubi bene, ibi patria' on the title page perhaps reflects Le Turc's ambivalent loyalties at this time.
8. AN F12 2204, Desmarets to Tolozan 21 June 1785. For the possible Spanish destination of the first loom, CNAM U216. Also AN F12 677C, Tolozan to Le Turc, 2 July 1785. Izquierdo was probably associated with Le Camus de Limare, see C. Ballot, *L'Introduction du Machinisme dans L'Industrie Française* (Lille-Paris, 1923), pp. 274–5. A mention of a loom obtained for

Le Camus de Limare is made in an undated memoir of Le Turc's: 'Observations on English knitwear' (F12 677C). The connection between Le Camus de Limare and Izquierdo is mentioned in F12 2204; Le Turc, Lorient, to Comte de la Touche 25 January 1788.

9. AN F12 677C.
10. AN F12 677C, letters of Le Turc, 14 and 16 August and 1 September 1785. Bureau of Commerce to Le Turc, 11 September 1785, to De Castries 15 September 1785, De Castries to Tolozan 22 September 1785.
11. AN F12 2204, *Bon* of 4 October 1785; F12 677C n.d. Observations on English knitwear; ibid., Le Turc to Bureau 16 October 1785.
12. AN F12 677C, Mémoire sur l'acier fondu, 27 January 1786.
13. AN F12 677C, letter of Le Turc, 27 January 1786.
14. Ibid., letter of 17 February 1786.
15. Ibid., letters, 20 February 1786, 17 March 1786; F12 2204, letter of 26 January 1786.
16. Ibid., Barthélémy to Tolozan, 28 January 1786, Anon. to Le Turc, 'dit Johnson', 3 February 1786; letters of Le Turc, 26 and 31 January 1786.
17. Ibid., letter of Le Turc, 20 February 1786.
18. Ibid., Le Turc to Tolozan, 28 February 1786.
19. Ibid., Le Turc to Valioud, 3 and 6 March 1786.
20. Ibid., Bureau to Le Turc, 10 March; to Izquierdo, 15 March; letter of De La Roche, 15 March; Bureau to Gravier, 17 March; Le Turc to Valioud, 17 March; Bureau to Le Turc, 17 March 1786.
21. Ibid., Le Turc to Valioud, 21 March and 24 March; tradesmen's bills, 25 March, 27 March; Le Turc, to Valioud, 28 March 1786.
22. Ibid., letter of Le Turc, 13 April 1786. There are variant spellings of the worker's name, e.g. Rhambault. For Rhambolt see S. D. Chapman (ed.), *Felkin's History of the Machine-Wrought Hosiery and Lace Manufactures*, Centenary Edition with introduction by S. D. Chapman (Newton Abbot, 1967), pp. 105, 108, 113, 403.
23. Ibid., letter of Le Turc, 13 April; Deliberations of Rocheguyon Company, 2 May, Bureau to Darthenay, 5 May 1786.
24. AN F12 2204, letter of Le Turc, 18 May; F12 677C, letter of Le Turc, 11 June; Tolozan(?) to Le Turc, 4 June; letter of Le Turc, 13 June; Le Turc, Lorient, 18 June; letter of Le Turc, 25 July 1786.
25. AN F12 677C, two letters of Le Turc, 13 June 1786.
26. AN F12 2204, memoir of Bureau, 13 June 1786.
27. AN F12 677C; letter of Le Turc, 25 July 1786; F12 2204, undated letter 1786, Le Turc to Tolozan.
28. See above, Chapters 11 and 12.
29. See J. M. Pannell, 'The Taylors of Southampton: pioneers in mechanical engineering', *Proceedings of the Institute of Mechanical Engineers*, 165, (1955), 924 seq; K. R. Gilbert, *The Portsmouth Blockmaking Machinery* (HMSO, 1965); H. W. Dickinson, 'The Taylors of Southampton: their ships' blocks, circular saw and ships' pumps', *Transactions of the Newcomen Society*, 29, (1955), 169 seq. Particularly valuable is C. Cooper, 'The Portsmouth system of manufacture', *Technology and Culture*, 25, (2), April 1984, pp. 182–92.

30. AN Marine B1 87, document of 23 February 1778.
31. AN Marine G108, file beginning 'Le Sieur Cole, Mechanicien Anglais: Proposition fait à Monseigneur'.
32. Ibid., memoir of 15 October 1781.
33. Ibid., ff. 50–53.
34. For earlier pulley-making at Lorient, Geneviève Beauchesne, 'Le port de Lorient après sa cession au Roi, 1770–1789', *Révue Historique des Armées*, (2), (1980), 45 seq; AN F12 677C, letters of Le Turc, Lorient, 16 June, 18 June 1786; Marine B3 788, letter of Le Turc, 13 November 1787.
35. AN F12 677C, letter of Le Turc, Rennes.
36. AN Marine D2 31, Le Turc to De Castries, 27 April 1787, with drawings; Establishment at Lorient for Taylors' English pulleys; Archives Maritimes, Lorient, E4 114, letters of De Castries, 13 October, 15 October, 31 October 1786, 22 April, 5 May, 19 May, 16 June 1787. AN F12 677C, letters of Le Turc, Lorient, 30 September, 20 October 1786, 24 March 1787.
37. Archives Maritimes, Lorient, IE4 116; AN Marine B4 788, letters of Le Turc, 3 and 12 September 1787, Barthélémy to Le Turc, 3 September 1787.
38. Archives Maritimes, Lorient, IE4 118; AN Marine B3 788, letters of 30 September 1787; F12 1340, document of 15 October 1787.
39. AN Marine B3, letter of Le Turc, 7 December 1787; F12 677C, letter of Le Turc, 30 December 1787.
40. AN F12 677C, letters of Le Turc, 30 December 1787, 4 February 1788.
41. Archives Maritimes, Lorient, letter of La Luzerne, 30 August 1788; AN Marine B3 803, Henevart to La Luzerne, 27 October 1788.
42. AN F12 677C, letter of Le Turc, 4 September 1786; F12 1401/2, memoir of 22 February 1788; F12 2204, Le Turc to Comte de la Touche, 25 January 1788.
43. AN F12 2204, letter of Le Turc, 16 August 1788, with associated dossier; F12 677C, De Moley to Tolozan, 7 May 1787; F12 1401/2, memoir of 22 February 1788.
44. AN F12 2204, Tolozan to Barthélémy.
45. AN F12 2195, W. Douglas to D'Aragon, 8 December 1788; letter to Marquis de Luzerne, 2 February 1789. For Douglas, see above pp. 403–4.
46. There are several accounts of these events, see particularly AN F12 2204, Report of 15 Prairial An 2; Report of 4 Nivôse An 3; Report of 13 Brumaire An 5; Report of 24 Fructidor An 7; printed memoir to Directory 30 June 1797; Memoirs and Observations 19 Ventose An 2. Also annotated memoir of 23 October 1788; letter of Le Turc, 17 July 1788; letter of Vandermonde, 27 October; Vandermonde to Boutin, 5 November 1788; memoir of Bureau, 23 October; letter of Le Turc, 27 October 1788. Over 1788–90 Le Turc was on several occasions used by the Government as a commissioner to report on new or recently imported machines.
47. AN F12 2204. See 'Bon' of Necker, 11 January 1789; letter of Le Turc, 1 July 1789; unsigned letters of 22 July, 23 July, 28 July; memoir concerning Sr Le Turc (n.d.), dealing with developments of 1789–90.
48. AN F12 2204, Le Turc to Citoyen Ministre, 3 Pluviôse An 2; Minister to Administrators of Quinze-Vingts, 30 Germinal An 2; CNAM U216, Le Turc

to Molard, 6 Floréal An 2; Turfin to Le Turc, 13 Floréal An 2. For the Hôtel de Mortagne see A. Doyon and L. Liagre, 'L'Hôtel de Mortagne après la mort de Vaucanson', *Histoire des Enterprises*, (11), May 1963, 5 seq. A good brief account of the transition from the Vaucanson collection to the Conservatoire des Arts et Métiers, is that of A. Mercier, *Un conservatoire pour les arts et métiers* (Paris, 1994), pp. 13–25.

49. AN F12 2204, report presented to Minister of Interior, 27 Fructidor; Minister to Le Turc, 30 Fructidor An 7.
50. CNAM U216, correspondence of Prairial An 10.
51. CNAM U216, Le Turc memoir, 1 September 1793; S. D. Chapman (ed.), *Felkin's History of the Machine-Wrought Hosiery and Lace Manufactures* (Newton Abbot, 1967), p. 113.
52. AN F12 1396, Tolozan to Blondel, 4 August 1792 and related correspondence; declaration of Lazowski, 7 June 1791; F12 1397, decision of Bureau of Commerce, 13 May 1790; Tolozan to Intendant of Picardy, 10 July 1790. For Tolozan's own interest in textile production, above, p. 372.
53. Chapman, *Felkin's History*, p. 105; S. D. Chapman (ed.), *Henson's History of the Framework Knitters* (Newton Abbot, 1970 edn), p. 317n.
54. AN Marine B3 788, Le Turc to M. le Comte, 12 September 1787.
55. AN F12 677C, letter of Le Turc (? to Tolozan), 4 September 1786; Le Turc to Ministry, 4 October 1785; memoir of 27 January 1786.
56. AN F12 677C, Le Turc letters of 13 June, letter from Lorient, 18 June 1786; F12 2204, Le Turc to Citoyen (? 1791).
57. CNAM U216, Le Turc to Citoyen, 14 Nivôse An 3.
58. AN F12 677C, Le Turc to Citoyen Ministre, 5 Fructidor An 7.
59. AN F12 677C, Le Turc to (? Tolozan), 4 September 1786.

A version of this chapter appeared as a paper in *Icon, Journal of the International Committee for the History of Technology*, 1 (1995).

Notes for Chapter 18

1. J. R. Harris, *Essays in Industry and Technology in the Eighteenth Century* (Aldershot, 1992), introduction, *passim; idem, Industry and Technology in the Eighteenth Century*, inaugural lecture, University of Birmingham, (1972), pp. 6–7.
2. S. D. Chapman (ed.), *Felkin's History of the Machine-Wrought Hosiery and Lace Manufactures*, centenary edn (Newton Abbot, 1967), pp. 53–4.
3. Chapman, *Felkin's History*, pp. 63–70.
4. S. D. Chapman, 'The genesis of the British hosiery industry 1600–1750', *Textile History*, 3, (1972), pp. 13–14; Chapman, *Felkin's History*, p. 71.
5. 7 & 8 William III c. 20.
6. He states that the penalty for moving frames was £10 (in fact it was £5) and that frames were to be numbered to control their movement. This is not prescribed in the Act, though it may have been ordered by the Company.

7. They admitted that proclamations under Charles II and James II had not worked.
8. 14 Geo. I c. 27.
9. 23 Geo. II c. 13.
10. *Commons Journals*, 26 April 1774.
11. Ibid., 5 May 1774.
12. Ibid., 6 May 1774, petition of Jedediah Strutt and Stephen Williams.
13. Ibid., 12 May, 13 May, 16 May, 20 May 1774; 14 Geo. III c. 71.
14. Ibid., 5 April, 1 May, 7 May, 10 May, 16 May 1781.
15. The term 'press' would cover calendering equipment; the paper is clearly not meant to cover plans, which are separately designated, but may cover the paper in the glazed cardboard which we have seen was important in pressing, and had been much desired by French manufacturers.
16. 21 Geo. III c. 37.
17. 26 Geo. III c. 76.
18. *Commons Journals*, 14 March 1782.
19. Ibid., 8 April, 5 April, 6 April, 7 April, 13 April, 14 April, 17 April, 18 June 1782.
20. 22 Geo. III c. 60.
21. 25 Geo. III c. 67.
22. See above for Le Turc's interest in these.
23. 26 Geo. III c. 89.
24. The 1786 Act was made perpetual as part of an Act of 1795; 35 Geo. III c. 38.
25. The writer has surveyed Liverpool newspapers from 1756 to 1820, and has supervised the construction of an index to the material on the metal trades in the Birmingham press 1740–99, but in both instances before he had a specific interest in technology transfer. However, a few references have resulted.
26. PRO Home Office SP 37, 5, 107, 18a–b, 203; *Calendar of Home Office Papers, 1764*, 1339.
27. PRO King's Bench 29/437.
28. Or ones formed on a temporary basis, to deal, for instance, with threatening excise regulations.
29. *Manchester Mercury*, 24 January 1775.
30. A. Redford and others, *Manchester Merchants and Foreign Trade 1794– 1858* (Manchester, 1934), pp. 2–5.
31. R. Reilly, *Wedgwood* (1989), pp. 138–9; Wedgwood Mss, Keele University, E26, 18912, 1 August 1779.
32. J. Wedgwood, *An Address to the Workmen in the Pottery on the Subject of Entering into the Service of Foreign Manufacturers* (Newcastle, Staffs, 1783). See below, p. 479.
33. R. Reilly, *Josiah Wedgwood, 1730–1795* (1992), p. 259; V. W. Bladen, 'The Association of Manufacturers of Earthenware (1784–6)', *Economic History*, supplement to the *Economic Journal*, 1, (1929), 356–67. The association seems to continue after 1786 as the Committee of Potters with Josiah Wedgwood still in the chair, and was active against industrial espionage in 1790

(below, p. 485); a general meeting of Manufacturers of Earthenware chaired by Josiah Wedgwood II met to fix prices in 1814.

34. Birmingham City Library, Local Studies Archives, 240078, Anon., *An Account of the Manner in which a Standing General Commercial Committee was Established at Birmingham* (Birmingham, 1784).

35. Of course the workers would have to be given six months' notice for their return.

36. Birmingham City Archives (subsequently BCA), 358810, Reports of the Meetings of the Commercial Committee, 25 January, 1 February 1785; G. H. Wright, *Chronicles of the Birmingham Chamber of Commerce 1813–1913 and the Birmingham Commercial Society 1783–1812* (Birmingham, 1913), *passim*; *Aris's Birmingham Gazette*, 23 January, 18 September 1786.

37. See the plans of Le Turc, above.

38. This document seems to have been again considered in Birmingham in June 1786, but it is clearly evidence given before the Irish Resolutions were passed in August 1785. They were not implemented because they had been reduced to a form unacceptable in Ireland. 'Exportation of raw materials: James Watt and James Keir', BCA, B & W, n.d.

39. *Commons Journals*, 26 May 1785.

40. W. Bowden, *Industrial Society in England towards the End of the Eighteenth Century*, 2nd edn (1965), p. 169 seq.

41. BCA, MBP, Samuel Garbett Box 1, Garbett to Boulton, 19 June 1786. It is doubtful if Crawshay would have been happy to see Cort's grooved rollers exported once he was deeply involved with the development of the new process.

42. Ibid., Report of meeting at Batson's coffee house, London, 25 April 1786.

43. BCA, MBP, Samuel Garbett Box 2, n.d. 'Observations on the copper trade of England and the dangers of exporting the tools and machines used therein'.

44. *Aris's Birmingham Gazette*, 3 July 1786. *Commons Journals* give only the progressive stages of the passing of the two Tools Acts, without any petition evidence.

45. BCA, MBP, Garbett to Boulton, 19 November 1786; PRO PC 1/123, 14; M. Donaghay, 'The best laid plans; French execution of the Anglo-French Commercial Treaty of 1786', *European History Quarterly*, 14, (1984), 401–22.

46. *Felix Farley's Bristol Journal*, 24 March 1787. I owe this reference to Dr Jeremy Black. For the industrial consultancy of Boulton and Watt in France in 1786, below, p. 501.

47. *Arrêt* of 27 July 1785, given in full in PRO BT 6 112. W. J. Pugh, 'Calonne's "New Deal"', *Journal of Modern History*, 11, (3), September 1939, 297.

48. Lettres Patentes du Roi, registered 10 February 1786. This seems to be a broader revision of an *arrêt* of 13 November 1785 permitting foreign manufacturers to set up in France.

49. In 1776, at the beginning of the break between Britain and her American colonies, there was a memoir to the French government which suggested a campaign to win over English workers to France, including the appointment of an agent in England for that purpose, who was to have the same function as a Prussian agent already there had of learning about leading industries

and seducing their workers. Depression in industries affected by the loss of colonial trade would make such seductions easier. The author of the memoir, passed to Trudaine de Montigny on 26 January 1776, is unknown, nor whether it had any influence, AN F12 676 A.

50. *Manchester Mercury*, 6 March 1781.
51. PRO, Home Office (hereafter HO), 42, vol. 5.
52. PRO HO 42, vol. 1/222, 232, 234.
53. *Aris's Birmingham Gazette*, 18 August 1782.
54. Manchester Central Library, Archives of the Manchester Chamber of Commerce, vol. 1, 1794–96, MS 1/1. Proceedings of the Society of Merchants Trading on the Continent of Europe.
55. *Manchester Mercury*, 19 March 1799.

Notes for Chapter 19

1. PRO, SP 78, State Papers Foreign France, 288.
2. By Josiah Wedgwood FRS, Potter to Her Majesty (Newcastle, Staffs, 1783), Wedgwood Museum. I am most grateful to Miss Gaye Blake Roberts for access to this pamphlet.
3. Above, p. 582, n. 20.
4. Wedgwood Papers, University of Keele. 'Some hints respecting the means of preventing the emigration of our workmen into the service of foreign manufacturers', 24 April 1784.
5. BCA, MBP, Wedgwood Box, Wedgwood to Boulton, 15 March 1783.
6. BCA, B & W, Box 36, bundle 25, Wedgwood, Etruria, to Watt, 30 January 1784. See also JWP, Watt to Wedgwood, 6 February 1784.
7. Wedgwood Papers, Keele University, E18968–26. Draft letter, Wedgwood to Mr Nicholson, 25 October 1785.
8. Of mathematics and astronomy at the University of Kiel, 1770–80, and subsequently at the College of Commerce in Copenhagen.
9. I am most grateful to Professor D. C. Christensen of Roskilde University for correspondence and discussion on Danish industrial espionage in England, and for an early sight of his paper 'Technology transfer or cultural exchange, a history of espionage and Royal Copenhagen Porcelain', *Polhem*, Argang II, (Gothenberg, 1993/94), 310–32.
10. R. Charlesworth, 'Lundberg and Ljungberg, give and take in the ceramic industry of the eighteenth century', in *Opuscula in Honorem C. Hernmarck* (Stockholm, 1967), pp. 39–54. I am most grateful to Mr John Mallet for correspondence on this subject and making this and other sources available to me.
11. Matthew Boulton Papers, Assay Office Letter Boxes, Letters Inwards, Thomas Byerley, 21 August 1789.
12. He had done his espionage first and presented his letter of introduction from Boulton to Wedgwood afterwards!

13. Wedgwood Papers, Keele University, E26–1900, Wedgwood to Sir John Dalrymple, 20 October 1789.

14. Charlesworth, 'Lundberg and Ljungberg', pp. 51–2, states from Danish College of Commerce evidence that there is 'no doubt whatever that Ljungberg was ... an industrial spy in the fullest meaning of the term'.

15. Ibid., p. 46 seq., Christensen, 'Technology transfer', p. 323 seq., and his 'Spying on scientific instruments. The career of Jesper Bidstrup', *Centaurus*, 37, (1994), 230–31, and information from Professor Christensen, who has now discovered Ljungberg's travel diary (Kungl. Myntverkets arkiv, Rigsarkivet, Stockholm, Varia Id, jfr).

16. For Garbett and the Carron Co., see R. H. Campbell, *Carron Company* (1961), especially chs 1 and 5.

17. *Calendar of Home Office Papers*, Geo. III, 1760–65, 1359, Garbett to Lovell Stanhope, 26 June 1764. While he thought the laws against emigrating workmen could be strengthened, at this time he foresaw unnamed 'dangerous contingencies' in doing so.

18. PRO, SP 37, 5, Garbett to Wm. Burke, 4 May 1766.

19. A. Clow and N. Clow, *The Chemical Revolution* (1952), p. 139 seq. The House of Lords gave the additional reason that the substitution of lead for glass was only a slight variation on the older sulphuric acid process, which shows how technologically bizarre the application of patent law could be at this period. Even in 1784, after they had ceased to own it, when the French scientist and inspector Faujas de Saint-Fond tried to visit Prestonpans, he wrote that 'everything is so carefully wrapped in mystery', that the works was surrounded by high walls and continued its no admission policy. B. Faujas de Saint-Fond, *A Journey through England and Scotland to the Hebrides in 1784*, A. Geikie (ed.), 2 vols, (Glasgow, 1907), vol. 1, pp. 151–6.

20. BCA, MBP, Samuel Garbett and Family, Box 1, Samuel Garbett to Boulton, 30 July 1785.

21. Ibid., Garbett to Boulton, 31 August 1786.

22. Ibid., Samuel Garbett Box 2, Tibatts to Garbett, 1 February 1786.

23. R. H. Campbell, *Carron Company*, pp. 148–53.

24. BCA, MBP, Samuel Garbett Box 2, Garbett to Boulton, 28 April 1786.

25. Ibid., Garbett to Boulton, 8 April 1786.

26. Ibid., Samuel Garbett Box 2, 'Observations relative to Mr Gascoigne's letter to Mr Pitt'.

27. E. Robinson, 'The transference of British technology to Russia, 1720–1820: a preliminary enquiry', in B. M. Ratcliffe (ed.), *Britain and her World 1750–1914, Essays in Honour of W. O. Henderson* (Manchester, 1975), p. 7.

28. Ibid., pp. 12–14.

29. Ibid., p. 10. For some additional detail, PRO, Chatham Papers, Correspondence of Pitt the Younger 1783–1806, Garbett to Pitt, 28 April, 11 June, 2 August, 27 September 1786.

30. E. Robinson, 'The international exchange of men and machines, 1750–1800', chapter 6 of A. E. Musson and E. Robinson, *Science and Technology in the Eighteenth Century* (Manchester, 1969), pp. 216–17 and *passim*.

31. W. H. Dickinson, *Matthew Boulton* (Cambridge, 1937), pp. 31–3.
32. *Commons Journals*, 22 April, 1 May 1760.
33. Boulton claimed that an earlier order of 1780 had failed to reach him.
34. Dickinson, *Boulton*, p. 203.
35. BCA, MBP, Letter Book Outwards, K 416, Boulton to Joseph Alcock 'Roanne en Forest', 14 February 1781; K 490, same to same, 7 April and K 506, 21 April 1781.
36. E. Robinson, 'International exchange', p. 222.
37. For de la Houlière see above.
38. BCA, MBP, Letter Box L 1, Marchant de La Houlière to Boulton and Fothergill, London, 31 August 1775.
39. Above, p. 316.
40. Musson and Robinson, *Science and Technology*, p. 217.
41. He had connections with famous scientific clubs of the period, including Benjamin Franklin's Club of Thirteen and was an occasional visitor to the Lunar Society of Birmingham. Musson and Robinson, *Science and Technology*, pp. 126, 144, 220. There is a good life of Raspe by J. Carswell, *The Prospector: Being the Life and Times of Rudolph Erich Raspe (1737–1794)* (1950).
42. Presumably a descendant of Henry Sully's patron, above, p. 26.
43. For this interesting episode and the correspondence discussed here see the valuable letters published in J. Tann, *The Selected Papers of Boulton and Watt*, vol. 1 (London and Cambridge, MA, 1981), pp. 156–65.
44. Musson and Robinson, *Science and Technology*, p. 229.
45. Ibid., p. 216 seq.
46. We will consider the destinations of some of the Birmingham workmen going abroad when examining the efforts of countries other than France to obtain British technology illegally, below, p. 507 seq. See also Musson and Robinson, *Science and Technology*, pp. 223–4.
47. Above.
48. *Calendar of Home Office Papers*, Geo. III, 1760–65, 1818, 3 July 1765. A student and disciple of Linnaeus, Solander came to England in 1760 to propagate his system. He had a post with the British Museum from 1763, and was an active member of the Royal Society from 1764. After extensive travels from 1768 he resumed his work at the British Museum in 1773. He died in London in 1782. It is interesting that though so actively attaching himself to the British scientific establishment, Solander was prepared to help entice Boulton to Sweden.
49. Ibid., 1821, 1765.
50. Ibid., 1919, 19 September 1765.
51. Musson and Robinson, *Science and Technology*, pp. 224–8; Dickinson, *Boulton*, pp. 33–6.
52. The machine had been designed in 1678 by Arnold De Ville. It had fourteen 39-feet water-wheels operating pumps in the Seine and driving three separate sets of flat-rod engines which operated relay pumps at two higher levels. It cost 2.8 million *livres*, delivered 150 hp and needed a supervision and maintenance team of sixty. M. Daumas (ed.), *A History of Technology and Invention*, 2 vols, (New York, 1969), vol. 2, pp. 439–42, 524–7.

53.   Affaires Etrangères, Correspondence Politique, Angleterre, 557, Barthélémy to Rayneval, 14 August 1786; 337, Barthélémy to Monseigneur, 29 August 1786.

54.   Matthew Boulton Papers, Letter box A, 158, Argand to Boulton, 13 September 1786.

55.   Above.

56.   Payen, *Capital et machine à vapeur au XVIIIe siècle* (Paris, 1969), pp. 312–13; Boulton Papers, Box P1, 206, Heads of a Conversation with M. Perier of Paris, 1786: 'we wish to serve the [French] publick to the best of our powers' and they wished to serve the water company 'so far as is consistent with our duty to our Employers [the French state] and to our own characters as honest men. But we find ourselves in a disagreeable predicament, we find our friends of different opinions and of different parties'.

57.   Payen, *Capital et machine à vapeur*, pp. 131–3; for Périer's own abortive scheme for steam-power replacement of the Marly machine, p. 216 seq.; for Boulton on La Charité see J.R. Harris, *Essays in Industry and Technology the Eighteenth Century* (Aldershot, 1992), pp. 154–5.

58.   J. Tann, 'Marketing methods in the international steam engine market: the case of Boulton and Watt', *Journal of Economic History*, 38, (2), June 1978, 382–3.

59.   39 Geo. III c. 96.

60.   Musson and Robinson, *Science and Technology*, p. 229, and E. Robinson, 'The transference of British technology', pp. 4–5.

61.   Information kindly provided by Professor Dan Christensen.

62.   J. R. Harris, 'Sources for the study of industrial espionage by eighteenth century France', in D. C. Christensen (ed.), *European Historiography of Technology* (Odense University Press, Odense, 1993), p. 35; J. Tann, 'Marketing methods', p. 383.

63.   For another merchant making this last point, PRO, BT 6, 112, letter of William Gibbons, 5 December 1786.

64.   Crawshay Letter Books, Glamorgan County Record Office, R. Crawshay to Lord Hawesbury, 10 July 1789.

65.   PRO, BT 6/112, Rd. Crawshay and Josh. Stanley to Lords of Committee on Trade, 16 September 1786.

66.   I am most grateful to Norman Scarfe for making available to me his translation of the journal of the industrial tour of England in 1785 written by François de la Rochefoucauld, and for a very informative correspondence. The journal has now been published. See below, p. 531.

67.   For the Williams–Wilkinson alliance, see J. R. Harris, *The Copper King* (Liverpool and Toronto, 1964), pp. 60 seq., 71–87; for the French report, AN T 591/3 and 4, de Givry papers.

68.   BCA, B & W, Letter Book 8, 418, Watt to John Wilkinson, 6 February 1784; 417, Watt to William Reynolds, 3 February 1784; 419, Watt to Josiah Wedgwood, 6 February 1784.

69.   BCA, B & W, Box 20, 7, John Wilkinson to Watt, Broseley 22 March 1782; W. O. Henderson, *The State and the Industrial Revolution in Prussia 1740–1870* (Liverpool, 1958), pp. 14, 17, 20.

70. Lancashire Record Office, Order of General Quarter Sessions, 11 November 1779.

Notes for Chapter 20

1.   S. Lindqvist, 'Social and Culture Factors in Technology Transfer' in K. Bruland (ed.), *Technology Transfer and Scandinavian Industrialisation* (Oxford, 1991), p. 17. Above, p. 291. I regret that my lack of German means that I have had to neglect material on technical transfer and industrial espionage in the German states.
2.   M. W. Flinn, 'The travel diaries of Swedish engineers of the eighteenth century as sources of technological history', *Transactions of the Newcomen Society*, 31, (1), (1957–58 and 1958–59), 95–106. Flinn relied much on S. Rydberg, *Svenska Studieresor Till England under Frihetstiden* (Uppsala, 1951).
3.   A. Birch, 'Foreign observers of the British iron industry during the eighteenth century', *Journal of Economic History*, 15 (1955), 25.
4.   See above, p. 291.
5.   Birch, 'Foreign observers', 24–9; Flinn, 'Travel diaries', 99–101.
6.   M. W. Flinn, 'Samuel Schröderstierna's "Notes on the English iron industry (1794)"', *Edgar Allen News*, 33, (386), August 1954. Despite the date in brackets in the article's title Schröderstierna was in Britain 1749–50; J. R. Harris, *Essays in Industry and Technology in the Eighteenth Century* (Aldershot, 1992), p. 115 n.3. Professor Dan Christensen and the writer hope to translate and edit the part of the travel journal covering the West Midlands.
7.   Flinn, 'Travel diaries', 103–4; Birch, 'Foreign observers', 29.
8.   Birch, 29–30; Flinn, 103–5.
9.   A. P. Woolrich (ed.), A. den Ouden (trans.), *Ferrner's Journal 1759–1760; an Industrial Spy in Bath and Bristol* (Eindhoven, 1986), pp. 1–3. In this case the sub-title is fully justified.
10. Woolrich, *Ferrner's Journal*, pp. 12–36. Ferrner made some investigation of Bristol window glass and flint glass; ibid., pp. 22–3.
11. Birch, 'Foreign observers', p. 30. M. Fritz, 'British influence on developments in the Swedish foundry industry around the turn of the eighteenth century', in K. Bruland (ed.), *Technology Transfer and Scandinavian Industrialisation* (Oxford, 1991).
12. M. Fritz, 'British influence'.
13. J. R. Harris, *The British Iron Industry 1700–1850* (1988), ch. 3 and pp. 50–53.
14. There may be more archival disposal of records in the French case. Three major reports of the Holkers have now been identified in the Service des Archives économiques et financières, but were not known to me in time to be discussed in the present work. See P. Minard, 'L'inspection des manufactures' (thesis) vol. 1, pp. 23–4.
15. There has to be a tentative element in this judgement, because so many of the Swedish journals and reports remain inaccessible to most English readers.

16. Of course some French industrial officials and investigators, like Hellot, Jars, Faujas de Saint-Fond and Dupont de Nemours acquired connections with the Royal Society or the Society of Arts.

17. Flinn, 'Travel diaries', 102.

18. E. T. Svedenstierna, *Svedenstierna's Tour: Great Britain 1802–3, The Travel Diary of an Industrial Spy* (Newton Abbot, 1973), pp. 8–9.

19. P. Stromstad, 'Artisan travel and technology transfer to Denmark, 1750–1900', in K. Bruland (ed.), *Technology Transfer*, pp. 137–9.

20. Ibid., pp. 139–41.

21. For Nordberg, see T. Parmer, 'How industrial technology first came to Norway', in K. Bruland (ed.), *Technology Transfer*, pp. 42–53.

22. R. P. Amdam, 'Industrial espionage and the transfer of technology to the early Norwegian glass industry', in K. Bruland (ed.), *Technology Transfer*, p. 73 seq.

23. For Waern, see Amdam, 'Industrial espionage', pp. 76–80.

24. I am most grateful to Pyne's descendant, Mr Ole Pein, of Andorra, for a most interesting correspondence and for providing Joseph Pyne's contract.

25. Amdam, 'Industrial espionage', pp. 80–88. I am also grateful to Mr Amdam for helpful conversation and correspondence.

26. D. C. Christensen, 'Spying on scientific instruments. The career of Jesper Bidstrup', *Centaurus*, 37, (1994), 210–44.

27. F. A. Rasmussen, 'The Royal Danish–Norwegian Dockyard. Innovation, espionage and centre of technology', in D. C. Christensen (ed.), *European Historiography of Technology* (Odense, 1993), pp. 41–9, and additional information kindly supplied by him. Of course the remarkable long-term espionage of Ljungberg has to be included in the Danish picture. Professor Christensen has very recently discovered a copy of his Journal in the Swedish Public Records at Stockholm and is currently working on this outstanding source. See above, pp. 484–6.

28. H. Freudenberger, 'Technologie-Transfers von England nach Deutschland und insbes. Österreich im 18. Jahrhundert', *Wolfenbütteler Forschungen*, Band 14 (1991), 105–22. I am grateful for correspondence and the sight of a draft paper on 'Foreign contributions to the development of Habsburg industry'. Dr L. D. Schwarz kindly translated the first item for me.

29. A. G. Cross, *By the Banks of the Thames: Russians in Eighteenth Century Britain* (Newtonville, MA, 1980), pp. 146–56, 157–9.

30. T. S. Ashton, *Iron and Steel in the Industrial Revolution*, 2nd edn (Manchester, 1951), pp. 115–16.

31. Cross, *By the Banks of the Thames*, pp. 175–85.

32. Ibid., pp. 189–93.

33. Ibid., pp. 194–5. For Bentham, *DNB*; E. Robinson, 'The transference of British technology to Russia, 1760–1820: a preliminary enquiry', in B. M. Ratcliff (ed.), *Great Britain and Her World, 1750–1914: Essays in Honour of W. O. Henderson* (Manchester, 1975), pp. 10–12. This essay has been valuable in the present brief account of Russian technological indebtedness to Britain.

34. R. P. Bartlett, 'Charles Gascoigne in Russia. A case study in the diffusion of

British technology 1786–1806', in A. G. Cross (ed.), *Russia and the West in the Eighteenth Century* (Newtonville, MA, 1983), pp. 354–63. The comparative account in this chapter has been confined to the European countries seeking new technology from Britain, and has not attempted to bring America into the comparison. Until the War of Independence the movement of managers and workers was not inhibited, after it the common language, common measures and often tools, the presence of friends and relatives who had previously emigrated, made the process of technological transfer different from that from Britain to Europe, even if the same prohibitory laws now applied.

Notes for Chapter 21

1. National Maritime Museum, Greenwich, MS 85/057; memoir of Lescallier and Forfait to Comte de la Luzerne, Minister for the Navy, 25 January 1790. Margaret Bradley has examined other copies at the Ecole des Ponts et Chaussées and at the French naval archives at Vincennes. See her 'Engineers as military spies? French engineers come to Britain', *Annals of Science*, 49, (1992), 137–61, and her 'Bonaparte's plans to invade England in 1801: the fortunes of Pierre Forfait', *Annals of Science*, 51, (1994), 453–75. For both Forfait and Lescallier there are entries in *Biographie Universelle*, and for Forfait also in Taillemite, *Dictionnaire des Marins Francais*. I am grateful to Dr Bradley for helpful correspondence and discussions.
2. Trans. and ed. A. Geikie, 2 vols (Glasgow, 1907).
3. Ibid., vol. 2, p. 345 seq.
4. Ibid., vol. 1, pp. 96–7.
5. Ibid., vol. 1, p. 133.
6. Ibid., vol. 1, pp. 174–5.
7. Ibid., vol. 1, p. 178 seq.
8. National Maritime Museum, MS 85/07.
9. N. Scarfe, *Innocent Espionage: the La Rochefaucauld Brothers' Tour of England in 1785* (Woodbridge, 1995).
10. N. Scarfe, *A Frenchman's Year in Suffolk, 1784* (Woodbridge, 1988).
11. For the different parts of the narrative deriving from the three see Scarfe, *Innocent Espionage*, pp. 3–8.
12. For the difficulty found in describing and illustrating the stocking frame in the *Encyclopédie*, and the personal interest taken by Diderot, see B. Jacomy, *Une histoire des techniques* (Paris, 1990), pp. 227–37.
13. Scarfe, *Innocent Espionage*, pp. 36–44.
14. Ibid., pp. 51–6, above, p. 183.
15. Ibid., p. 65.
16. Ibid., pp. 69–74.
17. Ibid., p. 83.
18. Ibid., pp. 92–100.
19. Ibid., pp. 100–103.

20. Ibid., pp. 104–6.
21. Ibid., p. 108 seq.
22. Arthur Young, quoted in Scarfe, *Innocent Espionage*, p. 239.
23. Scarfe, *Innocent Espionage*, pp. 255–6.
24. D. C. Coleman, *Industry in Tudor and Stuart England* (1975), pp. 29–32; C. G. A. Clay, *Economic Expansion and Social Change: England 1500–1700*, 2 vols (1984), vol. 2, pp. 16–21, 81–2, 143–52; E. Kerridge, *Textile Manufactures in Early Modern England* (Manchester, 1985), pp. 27, 30–32, 60 seq., ch. 6, ch. 16 esp. 241–3.
25. W. C. Scoville, *The Persecution of the Huguenots and French Economic Development (1680–1720)* (Berkeley, CA, 1960), pp. 120, 125.
26. Ibid., p. 323.
27. Ibid., p. 116.
28. D. C. Coleman, *The British Paper Industry, 1495–1860* (Oxford, 1958), p. 60.
29. Ibid., pp. 68–79; Scoville, *The Persecution*, pp. 327–9.
30. Coleman, *British Paper*, p. 36.
31. D. C. Coleman, *Courtaulds, an Economic and Social History*, 2 vols (Oxford, 1969), vol. 1, pp. 7, 21–2.
32. 'All those secrets, chiefly of the handicraft variety, were closely guarded secrets of French manufacturers: and it would have been more difficult and taken longer for the English to have mastered them without the immigration of skilled artisans' (Scoville, *The Persecution*, p. 325).
33. Coleman, *Courtaulds*, vol. 1, p. 22.
34. Scoville, *The Persecution*, pp. 335–40.
35. Above, p. 343.
36. A. Clow and N. L. Clow, *The Chemical Revolution* (1952), pp. 186, 191–4. A. E. Musson and E. Robinson, *Science and Technology in the Industrial Revolution* (Manchester, 1969), p. 251 seq.
37. Musson and Robinson, *Science and Technology*, pp. 259–60, 284 seq., 314–15, 326.
38. Clow and Clow, *Chemical Revolution*, p. 216 seq.; Musson and Robinson, *Science and Technology*, pp. 344–5.
39. J. G. Smith, *The Origins and Early Development of the Heavy Chemical Industry in France* (Oxford, 1979), p. 209 seq. AN F14 4262.
40. Clow and Clow, *Chemical Revolution*, pp. 100–101, 104. T. C. Barker and J. R. Harris, *A Merseyside Town in the Industrial Revolution: St. Helens 1750–1900*, 3rd impression (London, 1993), pp. 223–39.

Notes for Chapter 22

1. 'Britain's prohibitory laws ... failed originally to stop the flood of technological information spreading abroad, either via men or machines, in this early industrial period. Administering and policing the sort of protection envisaged by the laws required Draconian measures that public opinion

would not tolerate and internal economic and social conditions could not support ... In these circumstances the flood could hardly be dammed', D. J. Jeremy, 'Damming the flood: British government efforts to check the outflow of technicians and machinery, 1780–1843', in D. J. Jeremy (ed.), *Technology Transfer and Business Enterprise* (Aldershot, 1994).

2. AN F12 1342.
3. For the persistence of these fears to the 1820s, see Jeremy, 'Damming the flood', p. 363.
4. AN F12 1340, 1341, 1342.
5. Archives Etrangères, Mémoires et Documents, Angleterre, 65. Third Memoir of Dupont, fol. 88. See also Correspondence Politique, Angleterre, 337.
6. The evidence of the importance of debt in prompting emigration is most complete in the Law scheme of 1718–20, when the means of bringing the workers back home was the discharging of their debts; above, p. 14.
7. T. S. Ashton, *An Eighteenth Century Industrialist: Peter Stubs of Warrington (1756–1806)*, (Manchester, 1939), pp. 10–18, 31–6.
8. W. O. Henderson, *J. C. Fischer and his Diary of Industrial England, 1814–51* (1966), p. 14.
9. Ascribed by P. Boissonade to Trudaine de Montigny. But Trudaine de Montigny was relatively young and inexperienced at this date, while Mignot de Montigny was an Academician appointed as a commissioner to advise the Government on industrial questions. He has been seen as Trudaine's main adviser on the recruitment of Holker in the early 1750s and his installation as an investor in and manager of cotton works at Rouen. P. Boissonade, 'Trois Mémoires relatifs à l'amélioration des manufactures de France sous l'administration des Trudaines (1754)', *Revue d'histoire economique et sociale*, septième année, p. 56; above, pp. 53, 57, 59.
10. AN F12 2204, Le Turc to Citoyen (? 1791).
11. J. A. C. Chaptal, *De L'Industrie Françoise*, 2 vols (Paris, 1819), vol. 2, p. 430.
12. D. Jeremy, 'British textile technology transmission to the United States: the Philadelphia region experience, 1770–1820', *Business History Review*, 47, (1973), 24–52.
13. A. Paulinyi, 'Machine tools in the transfer policy of the Prussian "Gewerbeförderung" (1820s–1840s)', in D. C. Christensen (ed.), *European Historiography of Technology* (Odense University Press, Odense, 1993), p. 20. For an extended discussion of these points, J. R. Harris, 'Skills, coal and British industry in the eighteenth century', in *Essays in Industry and Technology in the Eighteenth Century* (Aldershot, 1992). For the extent that modern technology transfer has depended on non-printed page information, and an interesting example concerning the origins of Sony and Japanese acquisition of American transistor expertise, G. Bassalla, *The Evolution of Technology* (Cambridge, 1988), pp. 83, 86–7. He emphasizes (p. 97) Eugene Ferguson's argument 'that visual, non-verbal thought dominates the creative activity of the technologist'.
14. Linant de Bellefonds, 'Les Techniciens Anglais dans L'Industrie Française au XVIIIᵉ Siècle', thesis (Doctorat en Droit) Paris, 1971, pp. 87–98.

15. M. Audin, 'British hostages in Napoleonic France. The evidence: with particular reference to manufacturers and artisans', M.Soc.Sci. thesis, Birmingham, 1987. Regrettably Mme. Audin's death occurred before she had finished the doctorate which would have enlarged and completed this study.

16. CNAM U1580.

17. CNAM U965.

18. AD Seine Maritime, C1092, n.d. 1787. This report owed much to the observations of the merchants Hurard and Rabasse who had been sent by the Chamber to investigate the situation in England, particularly in textiles. They pointed out that the shears for shearing cloth, made in Birmingham, could no longer be exported under the Tools Acts. Of the greatest importance in early engineering were high quality files in which the French were very deficient. See J. R. Harris, *Essays in Industry and Technology in the Eighteenth Century* (Aldershot, 1992), pp. 92–3, 102–8; J. R. Harris, 'First thoughts on files', *Tools and Trades*, 3, (1985), 27–35; above, pp. 220, 590 n. 18, 229–31.

19. There are two new major inputs to this body of theory. One is an interpretation based on evolutionary theory. Much of the originality here derives from G. Bassalla's *The Evolution of Technology* (Cambridge, 1988). In his view, while the British changes of the late eighteenth and early nineteenth century were 'truly revolutionary' in their economic and social consequences, yet the machines, and the steam-engines that powered them, were the outcome of evolutionary change within technology. A very recent exploration of this approach is J. Mokyr, 'Evolution and technological change: a new metaphor for economic history', in R. Fox (ed.), *Technological Change, Methods and Themes in the History of Technology* (Amsterdam, 1996), p. 63 seq. The implication seems to be that this approach will replace much of the 'new' (now ageing) economic history. The other major input is that which stresses the cultural influence upon the onset of industrialization, by which science became an integral part of western culture. This is the contribution of M. C. Jacob, set out in her *Cultural Meaning of the Scientific Revolution* (New York, 1988). This will be developed in her *Scientific Culture and the Making of the Industrial West* to appear later this year (Oxford, 1996).

20. J. U. Nef, *The Rise of the British Coal Industry*, 2 vols (1932, 2nd impression, Cass, 1966), esp vol. 1, part 2, ch. 2, 'An early industrial revolution' and ch. 3, 'The substitution of coal for wood'; John Hatcher, *The History of the British Coal Industry, Vol. 1: Before 1700: Towards the Age of Coal* (Oxford, 1993) esp. part 1, chs 1–3, and part 4, ch. 12.

21. There was at least a quintupling of the output of coal over the eighteenth century, from approximately 2.6 million tons to 15 million tons. Hatcher, *British Coal*, pp. 68, 556; M. W. Flinn, *The History of the British Coal Industry, Volume 2, 1700–1830: the Industrial Revolution* (Oxford, 1984), p. 26, would give a slightly higher figure for 1700, just under 3 million tons.

22. E. A. Wrigley, *Continuity, Chance and Change: the Character of the Industrial Revolution in England* (Cambridge, 1988), p. 32, and chs 2 ('The advanced agricultural economy') and 3 ('The mineral based economy') *passim*. I find Wrigley's approach both congenial and convincing.

23. N. Rosenberg, 'The direction of technological change: inducement mecha-

nisms and focussing devices', *Economic Development and Cultural Change*, 18, (1), part 1, October 1969, 1–24.
24. Above, pp. 36–8.
25. AN F12 1300, 1313/14, F12 107.
26. AN F12 680.
27. The important *arrêt* of 1723 prevented the creation of new units of furnace industries using wood fuel where there was not a sufficient long-term availability of wood for the general public. If entrepreneurs could show that the works could be supplied with coal permission was normally given. See D. Woronoff, 'La politique des authorisations d'usines et la question du bois', in D. Woronoff (ed.), *Forges et forêts, récherches sur la consommation proto-industrielle de bois* (Paris, 1990), pp. 57–60, which reproduces the *arrêt* of 9 August 1723.
28. E. A. Wrigley, 'The supply of raw materials in the Industrial Revolution', *Economic History Review*, 2nd series, 15, (1962), 1–16.
29. However, Macquer was largely responsible for a successful location of kaolin in France, C. C. Gillispie, *Science and Polity in France at the End of the Old Regime* (Princeton, 1980), pp. 401–6.
30. J. Williams, *Prospectus and Proposals for Publishing an Essay towards a Natural History of the Mineral Kingdom* (1787). I am indebted to Dr Hugh Torrens for this reference to an item in Princeton University Library.
31. *Reports of Minutes of Evidence from the Select Committee on Artisans and Machinery*, first report 23 February 1824, examination of John Martineau 17 February, pp. 5–11.
32. Ibid., evidence of Alexander Galloway, 18 February, pp. 14–25.
33. Ibid., evidence of Bryan Donkin, 20 February, pp. 31–7.
34. Ibid., evidence of Mr Alexander, 2 March, pp. 100–106.
35. P. Mathias, 'Skills and the diffusion of innovations from Britain in the eighteenth century', *Transactions of the Royal Historical Society*, 5th series, 25, (1975), 96. See also L. Perez, 'Invention and the state in eighteenth century France', *Technology and Culture*, 32, (4), (1991), 911. The citations of this author from C. McLeod, *Inventing the Industrial Revolution* (Cambridge, 1988), pp. 210, 219, seem to carry the opposite sense, saying that British 'Inventiveness was ... becoming a source of national pride' in the late eighteenth century, and citing a vehement attack on the canard of there being merely British improvements on French inventions.
36. R. Briggs, 'The Académie Royale des Sciences and the Pursuit of Utility', *Past and Present*, (131), May, 1991.
37. R. Hahn, *The Anatomy of a Scientific Institution: the Paris Academy of Sciences, 1666–1803* (Berkeley, CA, 1971), pp. 185, 194; C. C. Gillispie, *Science and Polity*, pp. 462–78: Dominique de Place, 'Le Bureau de Consultation pour les Arts, Paris, 1791–6', *History and Technology*, 5, (1988), 140 seq.: Gillispie, *Science and Polity*, pp. 463–78.
38. The operations of the officials of the Bureau of Commerce are covered in two elegant and definitive studies by H. T. Parker, *The Bureau of Commerce in 1781 and its Policies with Respect to French Industry* (Durham, NC, 1979), quoted here, p. 190, and *An Administrative Bureau during the Old*

Regime: the Bureau of Commerce and its Relations to French Industry from May 1781 to November 1783 (Newark, DE, 1993). A further volume is in preparation.

List of Archives Consulted

Affaires Etrangères

Archives Départmentales Seine Maritime

Archives Etrangères

Archives Maritime, Lorient

Archives Nationales, Paris

Archives, Conservatoire des Arts et Métiers, Paris

Archives, Saint Gobain

Birmingham City Archives

Birmingham City Library

Birmingham Public Libraries

Ecomusée, Le Creusot

Eleutherian Mills Library, Wilmington, DE, USA

Glamorgan County Record Office

Keele University (Wedgwood Papers)

Manchester Central Library, Archives of the Manchester Chamber of Commerce

Manuscript Division of the Library of Congress, Washington DC, USA

Municipal Library of Lyon

National Maritime Museum, Greenwich

Pilkington Archives, St Helens, Lancashire

Public Record Office, Kew

Service Historique d l'Armée de la Terre, Archives, Vincennes

Service Historique, Port de Lorient

University College of North Wales, Bangor

Select Bibliography

Primary Sources

Aikin, J. (1795), *A Description of the Country from Thirty to Forty Miles round Manchester*.

Annales de l'Industrie, Description des Expositions des produits de l'Industrie Française, vol. 2 (1824), Paris.

Anon. (1780–81), *Lettre d'un Citoyen de Villefranche à M. Roland de la Platière* (n.d. 1780–1781).

Anon. (1784), *An Account of the Manner in which a Standing General Committee was Established at Birmingham*, Birmingham City Library, Local Studies Archives, 240078.

L'Athenée des Arts (1834), *Procès Verbal de la 100ᵉ Séance Publique*.

Ballot, C. (1923), *L'Introduction du Machinisme dans L'Industrie Française*, Lille-Paris.

Boissonade, P. (1914–18), 'Trois Mémoires relatifs à l'amélioration des manufactures de France sous l'administration des Trudaines (1754)', *Revue d'histoire economique et sociale*, septième année.

Bonnasieux, P. and Lelong, E. (1900), *Conseil de Commerce et Bureau de Commerce 1700–1791*, Archives Nationales, Paris.

Bourgin, H. and Bourgin, G. (1920), *L'industrie sidérurgique en France au début de la Révolution*, Paris.

Boussière, G. (1907), 'Une famille anglaise d'ouvriers en soie à Lyon', *Révolution Française*, July.

Boyetet, E. (1789), *Second partie du recueil de divers mémoires relatifs au traité de commerce*, Paris.

Browning, O. (ed.), (1909–10), *Despatches from Paris, Camden Soc. 3rd Series*, **16**, (1), 1784–7 (1909), **19**, (2), 1788–90 (1910).

Chaptal, J. A. C. (1819), *De L'Industrie Françoise* 2 vols, Paris.

Chouiller, E. (1884), *Les Trudaines* (reprinted from *Révue de Champagne et de Brie*, Arcis sur Aube.

Depitre, E. (1914–19), 'Les prêts au commerce et aux manufactures, de 1740 à 1789', *Revue D'Histoire Economique et Sociale*, septième année.

Dietrich, P. F. de (1786), *Description des gîtes de minerai et des bouches à feu de la France, T. 1*, Strasbourg, (reprinted Paris-Geneva, 1986).

Encyclopédie ou dictionnaire raisonné des sciences des arts et des métiers (1765) vol. 17, Neufchatel.

Franklin, B. (1706–90), *The Papers of Benjamin Franklin*, W. B. Willcox (ed.), vols 25 (1986) and 26 (1987); Claude A. Lopez (ed.), vols 27 (1988) and 30 (1990), New Haven.

Gras, L.-J. (1899), *Le Conseil de Commerce de Saint-Etienne*, Saint Etienne.

Gregg, G. G. (n.d.), *The Précis Historique of Charles Albert (a Story of Industrial Espionage in the Eighteenth Century)*, Lancaster Museum, monograph.

Hill, G. B. (ed.), (1900), *The Memoirs of the Life of Edward Gibbon*, London.

Jars, G. (1770), *Manière de préparer le charbon minéral pour le substituer au charbon de bois dans les travaux métallurgiques*, Lyon.

Jars, G. (1774–81), *Voyages métallurgiques*, vol. 1 (Lyon, 1774), vol. 2 (Paris, 1780), vol. 3 (Paris, 1781).

Lang, A. (1897), *Pickle The Spy, or the Incognito of Prince Charles*, London.

Le Play, F. (1843), 'Mémoire sur la fabrication de l'acier en Yorkshire', *Annales des Mimes*, 4th series, 3.

Le Play, F. (1846), *Mémoire ... des fers à acier*, Paris.

Le Turc, J. B. (1781), *Description du camion prysmatique de Mr. De Perronet*, London.

Le Turc, J. B. (1781), *Description des fermes sur lesquelles on ceintre actuellement en France les grandes arches des ponts*, London.

Le Turc, J. B. (1797), *Au Directoire Executif*, Paris.

Muirhead, J. P. (1859), *Life of James Watt*.

Périer, J.-C. (1810), *Sur les machines à vapeur*, Paris.

Perraud, Claud (ed.), (1913–15), *Lettres de Madame Roland*, 2 vols, nouvelle série, 1767–80.

Prosser, E. R. (1881), *Birmingham Inventors and Inventions*, Birmingham, (reprinted Wakefield, 1970).

Rambourg, N. (1823), *De la surabondance et excellence des mines et usines de fer en France*, Paris.

Réaumur, R. A. F. (1722), *L'art de convertir le fer forgé en acier*, Paris.

Roland de la Platière, J.-M. (1780), *L'art du fabricant de velours de coton*, Paris.

Roland de la Platière, J.-M. (1781), *Lettres Imprimés à Lyon, en Octobre*.

Saint-Fond, B. Faujas de (1907), *A Journey through England and Scotland to the Hebrides in 1784*, A. Geikie (ed.), 2 vols, Glasgow.

Sully, H. (1737), *La règle artificielle du temps*, intro. by Julien Le Roy, Paris.

Wedgwood, J. (1783), *An Address to the Workmen in the Pottery, on the Subject of Entering into the Service of Foreign Manufacturers*, Newcastle, Staffs.

Williams, J. (1787), *Prospectus for an Essay towards a National History of the Mineral Kingdom*.

Wood, H. T. (1911), 'Inventions of John Kay', *Journal of the Royal Society of Arts*, 60.

Wright, G. H. (1913), *Chronicles of the Birmingham Chamber of Commerce 1813–1913 and the Birmingham Commercial Society 1783–1812*, Birmingham.

Young, A. (1889), *Travels in France*, M. Betham-Edwards, (ed.).

Secondary Sources

Allen, E. A. (1987), 'Deforestation and fuel crisis in pre-revolutionary Languedoc, 1720–1789', *French Historical Studies*, 13, (4).

Allen, E. A. (1990), 'Business mentality and technology transfer in eighteenth-century France: the Calandre Anglaise at Nîmes, 1752–1792', *History and Technology*, 8.

Allen, J. S. (1969–70), 'The introduction of the Newcomen engine from 1710–1733', *Transactions of the Newcomen Society*, 42.

Amdam, R. P. (1991), 'Industrial espionage and the transfer of technology to the early Norwegian glass industry', in K. Bruland (ed.), *Technology Transfer and Scandinavian Industrialisation*, Oxford.

Ashton, T. S. (1939), *An Eighteenth Century Industrialist: Peter Stubs of Warrington, (1756–1806)*, Manchester.

Ashton, T. S. (1951), *Iron and Steel in the Industrial Revolution*, 2nd edn, Manchester.

Bamford, P. W. (1988), *Privilege and Profit*, Philadelphia.

Barker, T. C. (1960), *Pilkington Brothers and the Glass Industry*.

Barker, T. C. and Harris, J. R. (1954), *A Merseyside Town in the Industrial Revolution: St. Helens 1750–1900* (Liverpool, 1954; Cass, 1959 and 1993).

Barrelet, J. (1950), *La Verrerie en France*, Paris.

Bartlett, R. P. (1983), 'Charles Gascoigne in Russia. A case study in the diffusion of British technology 1786–1806', in A. G. Cross (ed.), *Russia and the West in the Eighteenth Century*, Newtonville, MA.

Bassalla, G. (1988), *The Evolution of Technology*, Cambridge.

Beer, J. J. (1960), 'Eighteenth century theories on the process of dyeing', *Isis*, 51, part 1, (163).

Belhoste, J. F. and Peyre, P. (1982), 'L'une des premières grandes usines hydrauliques: les fonderies de cuivre de Romilly-sur-Andelle', *Actes du IVe Colloque National sur le Patrimoine Industrielle*, Beauvais.

Bergeron, L. (1978), *Banquiers, négociants et manufacturiers parisiens du Directoire à l'Empire*, Paris.

Birch, A. (1955), 'Foreign observers of the British iron industry during the eighteenth century', *Journal of Economic History*, 15.

Birembaut, A. and Thuillier, G. (1966), 'Les cahiers du chimiste Hellot', *Annales*, Mars–Avril.

Bladen, V. W. (1929), 'The Association of Manufacturers of Earthenware (1784–6)', *Economic History*, supplement to the *Economic Journal*, 1.

Bouchary, J. (1946), *L'eau à Paris à la fin du XVIIIe siècle*, Paris.

Bowden, W. (1965), *Industrial Society in England towards the End of the Eighteenth Century*, 2nd edn.

Briggs, R. (1991), 'The Académie Royale des Sciences and the Pursuit of Utility', *Past and Present*, (131), May.

Cahen, L. (1939), 'Une nouvelle interpretation du Traité Franco-Anglais de 1786–1787', *Revue Historique*, 185.

Campbell, R. H. (1961), *Carron Company*.

Carswell, J. (1950), *The Prospector: Being the Life and Times of Rudolf Erich Raspe (1737–1794)*.

Chaloner, W. H. (1949), *Marchant de la Houlière's Report to the French Government on British Methods of Smelting Iron with Coal and Casting Naval Cannon in the Year 1775* five pages, unpaginated. Reprinted from *Edgar Allen News*, December 1948, January 1949, Sheffield.

Chaloner, W. H. (1956), 'Les Frères John et William Wilkinson et leurs rapports avec la métallurgie française', *Actes du Colloque International: Le Fer à travers les ages*, Nancy.

Chaloner, W. H. (1965), 'The textile inventor, John Kay', *Bulletin of the John Rylands Library*, 48.

Chaloner, W. H. (1990), *Industry and Innovation: Selected Essays*, D. A. Farnie and W. O. Henderson (eds).

Chapman, S. D. (ed.), (1967), *Felkin's History of the Machine-Wrought Hosiery and Lace Manufactures*, Newton Abbot.

Chapman, S. D. (1972), 'The genesis of the British hosiery industry 1600–1750', *Textile History*, 3.

Chapman, S. D. and Chassagne, S. (1981), *European Textile Printers of the Eighteenth Century*.

Charlesworth, R. (1967), 'Lundberg and Ljungberg, give and take in the ceramic industry of the eighteenth century', *Opuscula in Honorem C. Hernmark*, Stockholm.

Chassagne, S. (1980), *Oberkampf, un entrepreneur capitaliste au siècle des lumières*, Paris.

Chassagne, S. (1989), 'Une institution originale de la France post-révolutionnaire et impériale: La Société d'encouragement pour l'industrie nationale', *Histoire, Economie et Société*, (2), Paris.

Chassagne, S. (1991), *Le Coton et Ses Patrons, France 1760–1840*, Paris.

Chassagne, S. (1993), 'L'innovation technique dans l'industrie textile pendant la Révolution', *Histoire, Economie et Société*, 1ᵉ trimestre.

Chevalier, J. (1947–49), 'La Mission de Gabriel Jars dans les Mines et les Usines Britanniques en 1764', *Transactions of the Newcomen Society*, 26.

Christensen, D. C. (1993/94), 'Technology transfer or cultural exchange, a history of espionage and Royal Copenhagen Porcelain', *Polhem*, Argang II.

Christensen, D. C. (1994), 'Spying on scientific instruments. The career of Jasper Bidstrup', *Centaurus*, 37.

Clow, A. and Clow, N. (1952), *The Chemical Revolution*.

Cole, A. H. and Watts, G. B. (1952), *The Handicrafts of France as Recorded in the Descriptions des Arts et Métiers, 1761–1788*, Cambridge, MA.

Coleman, D. C. (1958), *The British Paper Industry, 1495–1860*, Oxford.

Coleman, D. C. (1969), *Courtaulds, An Economic and Social History*, 2 vols, Oxford.

Conturie, P. M. J. (1951), *Histoire de la Fonderie Nationale de Ruelle (1750–1940) Première Partie 1750–1855*, Paris.

Cooper, C. (1984), 'The Portsmouth system of manufacture', *Technology and Culture*, 25, (2), April.

Crosland, M. P. (1967), *The Society of Arceuil, A View of French Science at the time of Napoleon I*, London.

Cross, A. G. (1980), *By the Banks of the Thames: Russians in Eighteenth Century Britain*, Newtonville, MA.

Cross, A. G. (1983), *Russia and the West in the Eighteenth Century*, Newtonville, MA.

Crouzet, F. (1967), 'England and France in the eighteenth century: a comparative analysis of two economic growths', in R. M. Hartwell (ed.) *The Causes of the Industrial Revolution in England*.

Crouzet, F. (1985), *De La Supériorité de L'Angleterre sur La France*, Paris.

Crouzet, F. (1990), *Britain Ascendant: Comparative Studies in Franco-British Economic History*, Cambridge.

Dagresco, B. (1993), *English Ceramics in French Archives*, London.

Dane, E. S. (1973), *Peter Stubs and the Lancashire Hand Tool Industry*, Altringham.

Dardel, P. (1942), *Etudes D'Histoire Economique, III, Holker-Guillibaud and Morris (1752–91)*, Rouen.

Daumas, M. (ed.), (1969), *A History of Technology and Invention*, 2 vols, New York.

Davids, K. (1995), 'Openness or secrecy? Industrial espionage in the Dutch Republic', *The Journal of European Economic History*, 24 (2).

Demonfaucon, M.-A. (1974), 'Recherches sur la ville du Creusot et sa population de 1787 à 1836', typescript, Ecomusée, Le Creusot.

Devèze, M. (1966), 'Les forêts françaises à la veille de la Révolution de 1789', *Revue D'Histoire Moderne et Contemporaine*, 13.

Deyon, P. and Guignet, P. (1980), 'The royal manufactures and economic and technological progress in France before the industrial revolution', *Journal of European Economic History*, 9, (3).

Dickinson, H. W. (1937), *Matthew Boulton*, Cambridge.

Dickinson, H. W. (1955), 'The Taylors of Southampton: their ships' blocks, circular saw and ships' pumps', *Transactions of the Newcomen Society*, 29.

Dickinson, H. W. and Jenkins, R. (1927), *James Watt and the Steam Engine*, reprinted 1981, Ashbourne.

Donaghay, M. (1978), 'Calonne and the Anglo-French Commercial Treaty of 1786', *Journal of Modern History*, 50, (3), supplement.

Donaghay, M. (1982), 'Textiles and the Anglo-French Treaty, 1786', *Textile History*, 13, (2).

Donaghay, M. (1984), 'The best laid plans; French execution of the Anglo-French Commercial Treaty of 1786', *European History Quarterly*, 14.

Donaghay, M. (1990), 'The exchange of products of the soil and industrial goods in the Anglo-French Commercial Treaty of 1786', *Journal of European Economic History*, 19, (2).

Donaghay, M. (1995), 'The French debate on the "free trade" treaty of 1786', in I. Zilli (ed.), *Fra Spazio e Temp, Studi in Onore di Luigi de Rosa*, Naples.

Doyon, A. and Liagre, L. (1963), 'L'Hôtel de Mortagne après la mort de Vaucanson', *Histoire des Enterprises*, (11), May.

Dutens, L. (1806), *Mémoires d'un voyageur qui se repose*, London.

Evans, C. (ed.), (1990), *The Letterbook of Richard Crawshay, 1788–97*, Cardiff.

Ferguson, E. S. (1967), 'The steam engine before 1830', in M. Kranzberg and C. Pursell (eds), *Technology in Western Civilisation*, 2 vols, Oxford.

Ferguson, E. S. (1968), *Bibliography of the History of Technology*, Cambridge, MA.

Fitton, R. S. (1989), *The Arkwrights, Spinners of Fortune*, Manchester.

Fitton, R. S. and Wadsworth, A. P. (1958), *The Strutts and the Arkwrights, 1750–1830, a Study of the Early Factory System*, Manchester.

Flinn, M. W. (1954), 'Samuel Schroderstierna's "Notes on the English iron industry (1794)"', *Edgar Allen News*, 33, August 1954.

Flinn, M. W. (1957–58 and 1958–59), 'The travel diaries of Swedish engineers of the eighteenth century as sources of technological history', *Transactions of the Newcomen Society*, 31.

Flinn, M. W. (1962), *Men of Iron, The Crowleys in the Early Iron Industry*, Edinburgh.

Flinn, M. W. (1984), *The History of the British Coal Industry, volume 2; 1700–1830: the Industrial Revolution*, Oxford.

Freudenberger, H. (1981), 'Technologie-Transfers von England nach Deutschland und insbes. Österreich im 18 Jahrhundert', *Wolfenbutteler Forschungen*, Band 14.

Fritz, M. (1991), 'British influence on developments in the Swedish foundry industry around the turn of the eighteenth century' in K. Bruland, *Technology Transfer and Scandinavian Industrialisation*, Oxford.

Gilbert, K. R. (1965), *The Portsmouth Blockmaking Machinery*, HMSO.

Gille, B. (1947), *Les origines de la grande industrie métallurgique en France*, Paris.

Gille, B. (1964), 'La Métallurgie Française d'Ancien Régime', *Revue d'Histoire de la Sidérugie*, 5.

Gille, B. (1965), 'La Psychologie d'un Maître de Forges Français au Debut du XIXe Siècle'. *Revue d'Histoire de la Sidérurgie*, 4.

Gille, B. (ed.), (1978), *Histoire des techniques*, Paris.

Gille, B., Daumas, M. et al. (1951), 'La Machine à Vapeur en France au XVIIIe Siècle', *Techniques et Civilisation*, 2.

Gillispie, C. C. (1980), *Science and Polity in France at the End of the Old Regime*, Princeton.

Glen, R. (1979), 'The Milnes of Stockport and the export of English technology during the early Industrial Revolution', *Cheshire History*, 3.

Glen, R. (1981), 'Industrial wayfarers: Benjamin Franklin and a case of machine smuggling in the 1780s', *Business History*, 23 (3).

Godfrey, E. S. (1975), *The Development of English Glassmaking 1560–1640*, Oxford.

Grosclaude, P. (1961), *Malherbes, témoin et interprète de son temps*, Paris.

Gruder, V. R. (1968), *The Royal Provincial Intendants, a Governing Elite in Eighteenth Century France*, Ithaca, NY.

Hahn, R. (1971), *The Anatomy of a Scientific Institution, the Paris Academy of Sciences, 1666–1803*, Berkeley, CA.

Harris, J. R. (1954), 'The early steam engine on Merseyside', *Transactions of the Historic Society of Lancashire and Cheshire*, 106.

Harris, J. R. (1964), *The Copper King*, Liverpool, Toronto.

Harris, J. R. (1966), 'Copper and shipping in the eighteenth century', *Economic History Review*, 2nd series, **19**.

Harris, J. R. (1967), 'The employment of steam power in the eighteenth century', *History*, **52**.

Harris, J. R. (1972), *Industry and Technology in the Eighteenth Century: England and France*, inaugural lecture, University of Birmingham.

Harris, J. R. (1978–79), 'Recent research on the Newcomen engine and historical studies', *Transactions of the Newcomen Society*, **50**.

Harris, J. R. (1985), 'First thoughts on files', *Journal of the Tools and Trades Society*, **3**.

Harris, J. R. (1988), *The British Iron Industry 1700–1850*.

Harris, J. R. (1992), *Essays in Industry and Technology in the Eighteenth Century: England and France*, Aldershot.

Harris, J. R. (1992), 'Skills, coal and British indusry in the eighteenth century', *Essays in Industry and Technology*, Aldershot.

Harris, J. R. (1993), 'Sources for the study of industrial espionage by eighteenth century France', in D. C. Christensen (ed.), *European Historiography of Technology*, Odense.

Harris, J. R. and Pris, C. (1976), 'The memoirs of Delaunay Deslandes', *Technology and Culture*, **17**, (2).

Harsin, P. (1934), *John Law, Oeuvres Complètes*, T. 1–3, Paris.

Hatcher, J. (1993), *The History of the British Coal Industry, Vol. 1; Before 1700: Towards the Age of Coal*, Oxford.

Henderson, W. O. (1958), *The State and the Industrial Revolution in Prussia 1740–1870*, Liverpool.

Henderson, W. O. (1965), *Britain and Industrial Europe 1750–1870*, 2nd edn, Leicester.

Henderson, W. O. (1966), *J. C. Fischer and his Diary of Industrial England*.

Hilaire-Perez, L. (1995), 'Transferts technologiques et juridiques au siècle des Lumières', *La Revue, Musée des Arts et Métiers*, (12). See also Perez.

Hollister-Short, G. J. (1976–77), 'The introduction of the Newcomen engine into Europe', *Transactions of the Newcomen Society*, **48**.

Hollister-Short, G. J. (1978), 'A new technology and its diffusion: steam engine construction in Europe, 1720–c.1780', Part 1, *Industrial Archaeology*, **13**, (1), Part 2, **13**, (2).

Hyde, H. M. (1948), *John Law: the History of an Honest Adventurer*, London.

Jackson, M. H. and De Beer, C. (1973), *Eighteenth Century Gunfounding*, Newton Abbot.

Jacob, M. C. (1988), *Cultural Meaning of the Scientific Revolution*, New York.

Jacomy, B. (1990), *Une histoire des techniques*, Paris.

Jeremy, D. J. (1973), 'British textile technology transmission to the United States: the Philadelphia region experience, 1770–1820', *Business History Review*, **47** (1).

Jeremy, D. J. (1981), *Transatlantic Industrial Revolution*, Cambridge, MA.

Jeremy, D. J. (1994), 'Damming the flood: British government efforts to check the outflow of technicians and machinery, 1780–1843', in Jeremy, D. J. (ed.), *Technology Transfer and Business Enterprise*, Aldershot.

John, A. H. (1955), 'War and the English economy, 1700–1763', *Economic History Review*, 2nd series, 7, (3).

Kanesfsky, J. and Robey, J. (1980), 'Steam engines in 18th century Britain, a quantitative assessment', *Technology and Culture*, 21, (2), April.

Kerridge, E. (1985), *Textile Manufactures in Early Modern England*, Manchester.

Le Guin, A. (1966), 'Roland de la Platière, a public servant in the eighteenth century', *Transactions of the American Philosophical Society*, New Series, 56, pt 6, Philadelphia.

Léon, P. (1961), *Les techniques métallurgiques Dauphinoises au dix-huitième siècle*, Paris.

Lewis, G. (1993), *The Advent of Modern Capitalism in France 1770–1840: the Contribution of Pierre-François Tubeuf*, Oxford.

Lindqvist, S. (1984), *Technology on Trial, the Introduction of Steam Power Technology into Sweden, 1715–1736*, Uppsala.

Lindqvist, S. (1991), 'Social and culture factors in technology transfer', in Bruland, K. (ed.), *Technology Transfer and Scandinavian Industrialisation*, Oxford.

Lough, J. (1960), *An Introduction to Eighteenth Century France*, London.

Lough, J. (1988), *France on the Eve of the Revolution, British Travellers' Observations 1763–1788*, London.

Luthy, H. (repr. 1969), *La banque protestante en France, de la révocation de l'Edit de Nantes à la fin de l'ancien régime*, Paris.

McCleod, C. (1987), 'Accident or design, George Ravenscroft's patent and the invention of lead crystal glass', *Technology and Culture*, 28, (4).

McLeod, C. (1988), *Inventing the Industrial Revolution: The English Patent System, 1660–1800*, Cambridge.

McLynn, F. J. (1983), *The Jacobite Army in England, 1745. The Final Campaign*, Edinburgh.

McLynn, F. J. (1988), 'Unpopular front; Jews, radicals and Americans in the Jacobite world view', *Royal Stuart Papers XXI*, Huntingdon.

McLynn, F. J. (1991), *Charles Edward Stuart*, Oxford.

Mann, J. de L. (1971), *The Cloth Industry in the West of England*, Oxford.

Mathias, P. (1975), 'Skills and the diffusion of innovations from Britain in the eighteenth century', *Transactions of the Royal Historical Society*, 5th series, 25.

Mercier, A. (1994), *Un conservatoire pour les arts et métiers*, Paris.

Mokyr, J. (1996), 'Evolution and technological change: a new metaphor for economic history', in R. Fox (ed.), *Technological Change, Methods and Themes in the History of Technology*, Amsterdam.

Monod, P. K. (1989), *Jacobitism and the English People 1688–1788*, Cambridge.

Montgomery, F. M. (1977), 'John Holker's mid-eighteenth century livre d'Echantillons', in V. Gervers (ed.), *Studies in Textile History in Memory of Harold B. Burnham*, Toronto.

Morris, R. (1973–80), *The Papers of Robert Morris*, E. J. Ferguson and J. Catanzariti (eds), vol. 1 (1973), vol. 2 (1975), vol. 3 (1977), vol. 4 (1978), vol. 5 (1980), Pittsburg.

Musson, A. E. (1978), *The Growth of British Industry*, New York.

Musson, A. E. and Robinson, E. H. (1959), 'The early growth of steam power', *Economic History Review*, 2nd series, 11.

Musson, A. E. and Robinson, E. (1969), *Science and Technology in the Industrial Revolution*, Manchester.

Nef, J. U. (1932), *The Rise of the British Coal Industry*, 2 vols.

Ozanam, D. (1963), 'La Naisance du Creusot', *Revue d'Histoire de la Sidérurgie*, 4.

Pannell, J. M. (1955), 'The Taylors of Southampton: pioneers in mechanical engineering', *Proceedings of the Institute of Mechanical Engineers*, 165.

Parker, H. T. (1965), 'French administrators and French scientists during the old regime and the early years of the Revolution', in R. Herr and H. T. Parker (eds), *Ideas in History*, Durham, NC.

Parker, H. T. (1979), *The Bureau of Commerce in 1781 and its Policies with Respect to French Industry*, Durham, NC.

Parker, H. T. (1986), 'The transfer of technology between Britain and France in the eighteenth century: administrative activity', *Proceedings of the Consortium on Revolutionary Europe, 1984*.

Parker, H. T. (1993), *An Administrative Bureau during the Old Regime: The Bureau of Commerce and its Relations to French Industry from May 1781 to November 1783*, Newark, DE.

Parmer, T. (1991), 'How industrial technology first came to Norway', in K. Bruland (ed.), *Technology Transfer and Scandinavian Industrialisation*, Oxford.

Payen, J. (1969), *Capital et machine à vapeur au XVIIIe siècle*, Paris.

Perez, L. (1990), 'Invention, politique et société en France dans la deuxième moitié du XVIIIe siècle', *Revue D'Histoire Moderne et Contemporaine*, 27. See also Hilaire-Perez.

Perez, L. (1991), 'Invention and the state in eighteenth century France', *Technology and Culture*, 32, (4). See also Hilaire-Perez.

de Place, D. (1988), 'Le Bureau de Consultation pour les Arts, Paris 1791–6', *History and Technology*, 5.

Pollard, S. (1981), *Peaceful Conquest; the Industrialization of Europe 1760–1870*, Oxford.

Prosser, E. R. (1881), *Birmingham Inventors and Inventions*, Birmingham, (reprinted Wakefield, 1970).

Pugh, W. J. (1939), 'Calonne's "New Deal"', *Journal of Modern History*, 11, (3), September.

Rasmussen, F. A. (1993), 'The Royal Danish–Norwegian Dockyard. Innovation, espionage and centre of technology', in D. C. Christensen (ed.), *European Historiography of Technology*, Odense.

Reddy, W. (1984), *The Rise of Market Culture. The Textile Trade and French Society, 1750–1900*, Cambridge.

Rehder, J. E. (1987), 'The change from charcoal to coke in iron smelting', *Journal of the Historical Metallurgy Society*, 21, (1).

Reilly, R. (1989), *Wedgwood*.

Reilly, R. (1992), *Josiah Wedgwood, 1730–1795*,

Rémond, A. (1946), *John Holker, Manufacturier et Grand Fonctionnaire en France au XVIIIe siècle 1719–1786*, Paris.

Richard, G. (1964), 'Les fonderies de Romilly-sur-Andelle', *Actes du XVIIIe Congrès National des Sociétés Savantes, 1963*, Paris.

Roberts, D. H. (1992), *Eighteenth Century Shipbuilding*, Jean Baudriot Publications, Rotherfield, East Sussex.

Robinson, E. (1975), 'The transference of British technology to Russia, 1720–1820: a preliminary enquiry', in B. Ratcliff (ed.), *Britain and her World 1750–1914, Essays in Honour of W. O. Henderson*, Manchester.

Rolt, L. T. C. (1963), *Thomas Newcomen, the Prehistory of the Steam Engine*, Hartington.

Rolt, L. T. C. and Allen, J. S. (1977), *The Steam Engine of Thomas Newcomen*, Hartington.

Rosenberg, N. (1969), 'The direction of technological change: inducement mechanisms and focussing devices', *Economic Development and Cultural Change*, 18, (1), part 1.

Rosenberg, N. (1976), *Perspectives on Technology*, Cambridge.

Scarfe, N. (1995), *Innocent Espionage, the La Rochefoucauld Brothers' Tour of England in 1785*, Woodbridge.

Scoville, W. C. (1950), *Capitalism and French Glassmaking*, Berkeley.

Seton, B. G. and Arnott, J. G. (1928), *The Prisoners of the '45. Scottish History Society, 3rd Series*, 2 vols,

Silly, J. B. (1969), 'La réprise du Creusot', *Revue d'Histoire des Mines et de la Métallurgie*, 1, (2).

Smeaton, W. A. (1955), 'The early years of the Lycée and the Lycée des Arts', II, 'The Lycée des Arts', *Annals of Science*, 11.

Smith, A. (1978–79), 'The Newcomen engine at Passy, France, in 1725: a transfer of technology which did not take place', *Transactions of the Newcomen Society*, 50.

Smith, A. (1991–92), '"Engines moved by fire and water", the contribution of Fellows of the Royal Society to the development of steam power 1675–1733', *Transactions of the Newcomen Society*, 63.

Smith, A. (1994–95), 'Engines moved by fire and water', *Transactions of the Newcomen Society*, 66.

Smith, J. G. (1979), *The Origins and Early Development of the Heavy Chemical Industry in France*, Oxford.

Stewart, L. (1992), *The Rise of Public Science*, Cambridge.

Stromstad, P. (1991), 'Artisan travel and technology transfer to Denmark, 1750–1900', in K. Bruland (ed.), *Technology Transfer and Scandinavian Industrialisation*, Oxford.

Tann, J. (1978), 'Marketing methods in the international steam engine market: the case of Boulton and Watt', *Journal of Economic History*, 38, (2).

Tann, J. (1981), *The Selected Papers of Boulton and Watt*, London and Cambridge, MA.

Tann, J. and Breckin, M. J. (1978), 'The international diffusion of the Watt engine, 1775–1825', *Economic History Review*, 2nd series, 31, (4).

van Doren, C. (1938), *Benjamin Franklin*, New York.

Vanier, M. G. (1956), 'La Manufacture Royale de Faience Du Faubourg Saint-Sever à Rouen', *Extrait des Actes du 81ᵉ Congrès des Sociétés Savantes, Rouen–Caen 1956*, Paris.

Vayssière, P. (1967), 'Un pionnier de la révolution industrielle en Languedoc au XVIIIᵉ siècle: John Holker', *Annales du Midi*, 79.

Wadsworth, A. P. and Mann, Julia de L. (1931), *The Cotton Trade and Industrial Lancashire*, Manchester.

Woolrich, A. P. (ed.), (1986), den Ouden, A. (trans.) *Ferrner's Journal 1759–1760; an Industrial Spy in Bath and Bristol*, Eindhoven.

Woronoff, D. (1984), *L'industrie sidérurgique en France pendant la Révolution et L'Empire*, Paris.

Woronoff, D. (ed.), (1990), *Forges et forêts, recherches sur la consommation proto-industrielle de bois*, Paris.

Wrigley, E. A. (1962), 'The supply of raw materials in the Industrial Revolution', *Economic History Review*, 2nd series, 15.

Wrigley, E. A. (1988), *Continuity, Chance and Change: the Character of the Industrial Revolution in England*, Cambridge.

Index

643

Molard, Director of the Conservatoire
des Arts et Métiers 145, 392, 401,
402–3
Monge, G., Academician 214, 217,
219, 561
Montereau potteries 61, 530
Montgomery, F. 60
Montigny 108
Morel, M., inspector of textiles 37–8,
50, 60, 544
association with Holker 38, 47–8,
53, 155
Morgan, J.-B. 382, 383
Morris, J. 55, 107
Morris, R. 160–61, 162–3, 164
Moss, P., fustian cutter 43, 45, 46, 54,
107
mule (spinning), introduction to France
377, 380–81, 382, 383
Mulloy, J. 60
Murry, T. 115

Nancy, chemical industry 125
Necker, J., Finance Minister (France)
192, 364, 405, 472, 564
Nef, J. 555
Newcomen engine 21, 37
in Austro-Hungary 290
in Belgium 291, 296, 297, 314, 321
in Britain 228, 232, 245, 292, 321
in France 33, 290–91, 293–4, 296,
298, 299, 300, 306, 307, 309,
310, 314, 319
fuel needs 297
origins 288–9
picture 295
and scientific knowledge 296–7
in Sweden 289, 291–2, 508
Nîmes, silk works 103
Nixon, F. 420
Nock, H., gunmaker 524–5
Nordberg, Danish industrialist 516–18
Norway
glass works 518
industrial espionage 516–21

Oberkampf, C. 420–22
Oberkampf, F. 420
Odhelius, E. 291, 508–9
Ogilvy, Lord 46, 155
O'Kelly, J., Col. 290–91, 292
Oppenheim, M. 341

Orléans, Duke of, French Regent 17,
52, 83, 191, 293, 333, 336, 337,
357, 377, 415, 542
Orsel, A. 192–3, 196–200, 203
Orsel, J. 192–3, 196–200, 203
Oury, D. 343, 353
Ozanam, D. 255

Pagett, J. 16, 20
Papillon, P. 541
Parker, D. 163, 164
Parker, H. 563
*Parliamentary Report on Artisans and
Machinery* 558, 559
Partridge, A. 176–7
Parys Mine Co., Anglesey 265, 271,
272, 273, 275, 276, 344
Passy steam engine 26, 294
Paulinyi, A. 550–51
Payen, J. 313, 314, 318, 320, 321
Payenneville, J. 125
Paynel, L. 58
Pelham, Lord 34
Penn, G. 198
Percival, T., Dr 324, 532
Périer engine, picture 301
Périer, A., engineer 270, 311
Périer, J. C., engineer 26, 131, 250,
270
and spinning machinery 365, 392
and steam engine power 298, 299–
300, 302, 305, 307, 308, 309,
310–11, 312, 313, 316, 317, 318,
320, 321, 406, 495
Sur les machines à vapeur 314
Perret, F. 365
Perronet, J. R. 52, 427–8
Perry, J. 524
Peter the Great 523, 524
Peyre, P. 280
Pickford, P., and the spinning mule
377, 380, 381–2, 383, 413, 414,
415, 417
plate glass, *see* glass making, plate
Polhem, C. 509
Potter, I. 290
pottery manufacture, France 140
Prestonpans works 115, 136, 235,
487, 489, 530, 534
Priestley, J. 530, 533
pulley blocks, naval technology 439–
44, 448, 529

For Product Safety Concerns and Information please contact our
EU representative GPSR@taylorandfrancis.com Taylor & Francis
Verlag GmbH, Kaufingerstraße 24, 80331 München, Germany